Principles of Pharmaceutical Organic Chemistry

Second Edition

Principles of Pharmaceutical Organic Chemistry

Second Edition

Prof. Rama Rao Nadendla
M. Pharm, Ph.D. FIC
Dean, Faculty of Pharmacy,
Acharya Nagarjuna University,
and
Principal,
Chalapathi Institute of Pharmaceutical Sciences,
Chalapathi Nagar, Lam, Guntur-34.

PharmaMed Press
An imprint of Pharma Book Syndicate
A unit of BSP Books Pvt. Ltd.
4-4-309/316, Giriraj Lane,
Sultan Bazar, Hyderabad - 500 095.

Principles of Pharmaceutical Organic Chemistry ***by Rama Rao Nadendla***

Published by

PharmaMed Press

An imprint of Pharma Book Syndicate

A unit of BSP Books Pvt. Ltd.

4-4-309/316, Giriraj Lane, Sultan Bazar, Hyderabad - 500 095.

Phone: 040-23445600, 23445688; Fax: 91+40-23445611

E-mail: info@pharmamedpress.com

ISBN: 978-93-8681-962-8 (Hardbound)

To

Rev Master

Shri Ram Chandra Mission

CONTENTS

?REFACE

'rinciples of Pharmaceutical Organic Chemistry provides a comprehensive coverage of all ıe major concepts in organic pharmaceuticals. This book covers all the changes, ıodifications and revisions made to the syllabi of various Indian universities so as to fulfil ıe needs of undergraduate students of pharmacy and science.

To start with, the book covers fundamentals of organic chemistry and progressively elves into topics that are more complex. Basic concepts of organic chemistry including ıechanisms of chemical reactions are presented in a condensed and easy-to-understand ıanner. A large number of organic pharmaceuticals are added in each chapter and many ommercial syntheses techniques have been incorporated. At the end of each chapter a umber of review questions, including those selected from various university examinations, ave been added. This would ensure a thorough revision of the subject area.

Beginning with a general introduction, the book provides an elaborate coverage of urification, qualitative and quantitative analysis of organic compounds (Chapter 3). rinciples of electron displacement effects and chemistry of reactive intermediates are iscussed in Chapters 4 and 5 respectively. General rules of classification and IUPAC omenclature are thoroughly explained in Chapter 6 while principles of isomerism are covered ı Chapter 7. General methods of preparation, properties, chemical reactions including reaction ıechanisms, chemistry of related drugs or pharmaceuticals of various classes of organic ompounds (alkanes, alkenes, alkynes, dienes, cycloalkanes, alkyl halides, alcohols, ethers, poxides, benzene, aryl halides, and so on) and several other organic compounds and erivatives are comprehensively discussed in Chapters 8 to 26. In addition, a concluding ıapter on Phase-Transfer Catalysis familiarises the reader with the innovative concepts ıvolved in the manufacturing of organic or pharmaceutical compounds.

I sincerely hope that the book will prove useful not only to students and teachers of ıarmacy but also to science students, in general. I shall appreciate any suggestions and ·iticism which would lead to the improvement of the text.

RAMA RAO NADENDLA

\CKNOWLEDGEMENTS

ıave a great pleasure in expressing my sincere thanks to all those teachers and students ıo readily encouraged me while working on the *Principles of Pharmaceutical Organic ıemistry* and sent their constructive comments.

I am greatly indebted to Sri Y. V. Anjaneyulu, President, Chalapati Educational Society, ıntur for his unstinted support and encouragement.

I also record my deep sense of gratitude to my family members who were the real urce of inspiration and without whose cooperation I would not have completed this nture.

I also owe a debt of gratitude to my students, colleagues, friends, professors of various iversities and colleges for encouraging me to author this edition.

I express my indebtedness to the authors of research papers, review articles, monographs d books who helped me to acquire the latest information on the subject.

RAMA RAO NADENDLA

|

TOMIC STRUCTURE

1 FUNDAMENTAL PARTICLES OF ATOM

ie *Atomic Theory of Matter* states that all matter consist of extremely small particles lled atoms. The atom is the fundamental building block of all 'matter'. An individual om is very small. In fact, the smallest atom, hydrogen, has a diameter of 10^{-8} cm. Atoms all elements (except hydrogen) contain three fundamental particles, namely protons, utrons and electrons. In the hydrogen atom, there is only one proton and an electron. otons and neutrons are present in the central core of the atom, called the *nucleus*, while ctrons revolve around the nucleus in fixed paths known as *orbits* or *shells* (Fig. 1.1).

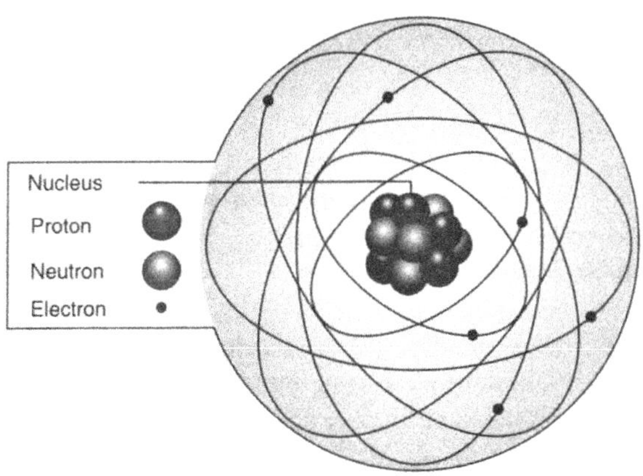

Fig. 1.1 Atomic Structure

(i) *Proton* It is a positively charged particle having a mass of 1.00728 amu on the C^{12} scale.

(ii) *Neutron* It is a neutral particle with a mass equal to 1.00866 amu.

(iii) *Electron* It is a negatively charged particle having negligible mass (1/1836 of the mass of a proton). It has the same magnitude of charge as that of proton but is –ve.

Moseley proposed the concept of atomic number. The total number of positive charges sent inside the nucleus of an atom is called its *atomic number*.

1. Most of the space in the atom is empty.
2. The entire positive charge and mass of the atom is concentrated at its centre knov as nucleus. The size of the nucleus is very small when compared to the size of t atom. The size of the atom is of the order 10^{-8} cm and that of nucleus is of the ord 10^{-12} to 10^{-13} cm.
3. A sufficient number of electrons are revolving around the nucleus at relative larger distances from the nucleus.
4. The number of electrons revolving around the nucleus is equal to the number protons present in the nucleus.
5. Electrons revolve around the nucleus like planets revolve around the sun. Henc Rutherford's model of an atom is also called as planetary model of an atom and tl electrons are called as planetary electrons.
6. The attractive force between electrons and nucleus balances the centrifugal for of the revolving electrons.

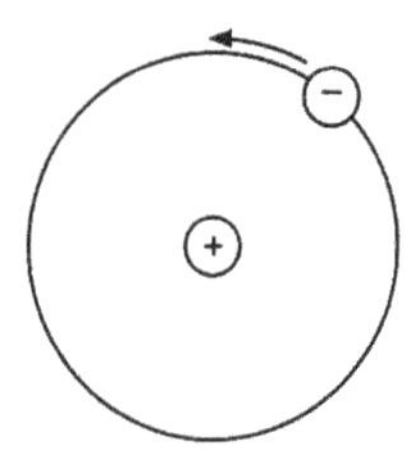

Fig. 1.2 Rutherford's Model

1.2.1 Objections to Rutherford's Model

Whenever an electric charge is subjected to acceleration, it emits radiation and los energy. In other words, a constantly radiating electron will spiral down into nucleus. A a result of this, the orbit will become smaller and the electrons will drop into the nucleu This, however, does not happen.

1.3 BOHR'S MODEL OF THE ATOM

In 1913, Niels Bohr proposed a new model of the atom to rectify the defects (Rutherford's model (Fig. 1.3). Bohr's model of atom was based on Planck's quantu theory and was built on the following postulates:

1. The electrons in an atom revolve round the nucleus in definite amount of energ These orbits are called energy levels. These orbits are numbered as 1, 2, 3 an 4 . . . or named as K, L, M, N . . . starting from the nucleus.
2. So far as an electron revolves in a certain orbit, its energy remains constant an does not radiate energy. These orbits are called stationary orbits or stationar

where m = mass of electron, v = velocity of electron, r = radius of orbit, n =1, 2, 3, 4, . . ., h = Planck's constant.

4. If an electron drops from a higher energy level to a lower energy level, energy is emitted. When an electron jumps from a lower energy level to a higher energy level, energy is absorbed. The absorbed or evolved energy is in the form of quanta, which is equal to the difference in energies of two orbits.

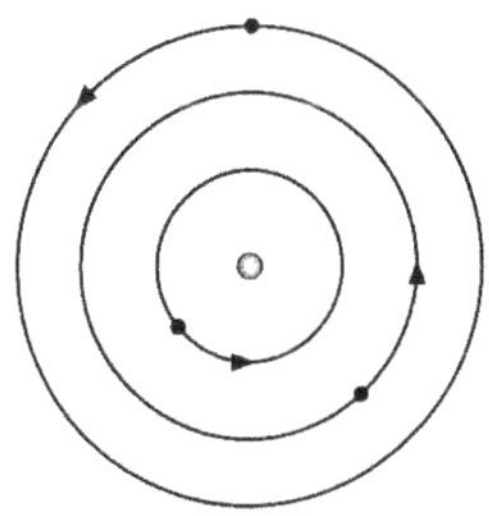

Fig. 1.3 Bohr's Model

$$\Delta E = E_2 - E_1 = h\nu$$

where E_2 = energy of higher orbit, E_1 = energy of lower orbit, h = Planck's constant, ν = frequency.

5. The line spectrum is obtained due to the electronic transition from one stationary orbit to another.

.3.1 Limitations to Bohr's Theory

ohr's theory incorporated the concept of quantisation of energy and predicted the cistence of discrete atomic energy levels. The theory explained large number of features spectroscopic data. It, however, had some limitations:

1. It failed to explain the spectra of atoms or ions having more than one electron.
2. Bohr's theory suggested circular, planar orbits (two-dimensional), but actual atomic model has three-dimensional existence.
3. Shapes of molecules arising out of directional bonding could not be explained.
4. Bohr's theory could not explain the fine structure of lines in the spectra (Division of lines observed under a spectroscope of high resolution).
5. Bohr's theory could not explain Zeeman effect and Stark effect.
6. Bohr's theory considered the corpuscular nature for electron but not the wave nature.
7. Bohr's model could not explain the Heisenberg's uncertainty principle.

4 SOMMERFELD MODEL

magnetic field. Orbits can appear circular or elliptical and can even swing back an forth through the nucleus in a straight line.

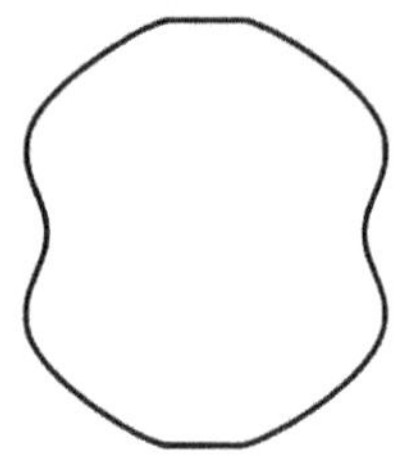

Fig. 1.4 An Elliptical Orbit

2. The electron travelling in an elliptical orbit possesses angular momentum. Thi angular momentum is quantified.

1.5 WAVE NATURE OF THE ELECTRON

The planetary theory of atomic structure forwarded by Rutherford and Bohr considers th electrons as particles moving in orbits around the nucleus. In the 1920s, it was show that moving particles such as electrons behaved in some ways as waves. Followin observations further substantiated this dual nature of electrons:

1. Light also has a dual nature. Some metals such as potassium emit electrons whe irradiated with light of particular wavelength. This phenomenon is called photoelectri effect. It is explained by light travelling as particles called photons. When a photo collides with an electron, it can transfer its energy to the electron. If the energy o the photon is sufficiently large, it can remove the electron from the surface of th metal.
2. However, the phenomena of diffraction and interference of light can only b explained by assuming that light behaves as waves.
3. In 1924, de Broglie postulated that this dual character is applicable to electrons. Th photoelectric effect indicates the particle nature of electrons while electron diffrac tion gives evidence for their wave nature. Diffraction rings were observed photo graphically when a stream of electrons was passed through a thin metal foil Considering wave nature of electrons, the concept of wave mechanics has bee developed which explains the electronic structure of atoms.

1.6 HEISENBERG UNCERTAINTY PRINCIPLE

According to classical mechanics, the position and momentum of a moving electron ca be determined with great accuracy. In 1927, Werner Heisenberg developed a complete

Ieisenberg showed that their product, i.e. product of uncertainty in position and ncertainty in momentum could never be smaller than $h/2\pi$, that is

$$\Delta x \times \Delta p \geq h/2\pi$$

It is impossible to determine accurately both the position and momentum (or velocity) f particle (e.g. electron) simultaneously. It is expressed as

$$\Delta x \cdot p \geq h/2\pi$$

$$\Delta x \cdot m\Delta v \geq h/2\pi$$

/here Δx = uncertainty in position, Δp = uncertainty in momentum, Δv = uncertainty in elocity, m = mass of the particle, h = Planck's constant.

.7 ELECTRONIC CONFIGURATION

'he distribution of electrons among the orbitals of an atom is called the electronic onfiguration. It is obtained by the application of Pauli's exclusion principle, the order of illing the orbitals or relative energies of orbitals. The electronic configuration of atoms f various elements, in their ground state, is governed by the following principles/rules:

. *The Pauli's exclusion principle* The Pauli's exclusion principle was postulated in an attempt to explain some of the properties of electrons in an atom. This principle states that in an atom no two electrons can have identical four quantum numbers. This is an example of a general principle, which applies, not only to electrons but also to other particles (actually, protons and neutrons obey the same principle, while photons do not). By 'state' here we mean a set of properties, such as energy that characterises an electron.

   This principle applies to more complex atoms containing more than one electron. However, in these atoms a complication arises, in that a more rigorous treatment of the problem of an electron orbiting about a proton reveals that, for *each* value of the integer n of the Bohr model, there can be $2n^2$ distinct states that a given electron can occupy.

. *Aufbau's principle* Aufbau's principle states that in the building up of atom, the added electron will occupy an available orbital of lowest energy. According to this principle, the atoms are constructed by adding a proton to the nucleus and an electron to the sub-shell that has the least energy. The sub-shells are filled in the increasing order of energy. The ascending order is

$$1s;\ 2s,\ 2p;\ 3s,\ 3p;\ 4s,\ 3d,\ 4p;\ 5s,\ 4d,\ 5p;\ 6s,\ 4f,\ 5d,\ 6p;\ 7s,\ 5f,\ 6d,\ 7p$$

. *Hund's rule* Electron pairing in any s, p, d or f orbital is not possible until all the available orbitals of the same sub-shell contain one electron each. An electron occupies a vacant orbitals in the same sub-shell and pairing can start when all orbitals are filled up. In other words, electrons fill each and all orbitals in the sub-shell before they pair up with opposite spins

are required. In other words, quantum numbers give the complete identity of an electr
in an atom. They are:

1. Principal quantum number
2. Azhimuthal quantum number
3. Magnetic quantum number
4. Spin quantum number

1. ***Principal Quantum Number*** The principal quantum number was introduced by Nie Bohr and designated by n. It represents the main electronic energy shells from nucleu It can take only integral values like 1, 2, 3, 4, . . ., etc. The corresponding shells are al designated by the English alphabets K, L, M, N, etc.

The principal quantum number gives the size of the orbit. As the value of n increas the size of the electron orbit and its energy increases. The maximum number of electro that can accommodate in a given orbit is known by $2n^2$, where n is the number of t orbit. Thus, the first shell can accommodate $2 \times 1^2 = 2$ electrons, the second shell, 2 $2^2 = 8$, the third shell, $2 \times 3^2 = 18$ and so on.

2. ***Azhimuthal Quantum Number*** Azhimuthal quantum number is also called subsidia or orbital or secondary or angular momentum quantum number which is represented by Sommerfeld introduced this quantum number to represent the number of sub-shells in shell. These sub-levels or orbitals are symbolised by letters s, p, d and f, respectively. T number of sub-shells in any shell can have the values 0 to $(n - 1)$. For example, f principal quantum number $n = 1$, the only possible value for $l = 0$, i.e. there is only o possible orbital (s orbital). For $n = 2$, there are two possible values of l ($l = 0$; $l = 2 - 1 = 1$ Again, $l = 0$ represents s orbital and $l = 1$ indicates a p orbital.

Sub-shell	*Number of Orbitals*
s	1
p	3
d	5
f	7

3. ***Magnetic Quantum Number*** Magnetic quantum number was introduced to explai the number of orbitals in a sub-shell. Magnetic quantum number is denoted by the lett m. It can have all the integral values from – 1 to + 1 through zero. For each value of there will be $(2l + 1)$ values of m.

Sub-shell	*Azhimuthal Quantum Number* (l)	*Magnetic Quantum Number* (m)	*Number of Orbitals* ($2l + 1$) *Values*
s	0	0	1
p	1	– 1, 0, + 1	3
d	2	– 2, – 1, 0, + 1, + 2	5

ɔon the direction of spin. Arrows also represent the direction ↑↓. The two electrons ith the same sign of the spin quantum numbers are said to have parallel spins and at have opposite sign of spin quantum numbers are said to be anti-parallel spin or ıired-up spin.

9 ATOMIC ORBITALS

ıe shape and size of the region in space around the nucleus, where the probability of ıding an electron with certain energy is maximum is called an orbital. There are four pes of orbitals that is *s*, *p*, *d* and *f*. All these four types of orbitals must possess a ıaracteristic shape of their own. According to Schrödinger's wave equation an *s* orbital ıs a spherical shape with the nucleus lying at its centre. *s* orbitals in the quantum levels e spherically symmetrical. The size of *s* orbital increases with *n* (principal quantum number) ılue.

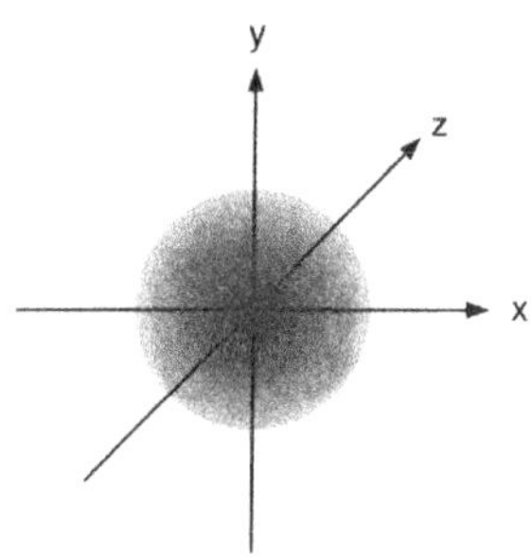

There are three *p* orbitals in each principal quantum level corresponding to $m = -1$, + 1. In p_x orbital, the two lobes are symmetrically oriented along the *x*-axis. In p_y and , the orientation along *y*-axis and *z*-axis, respectively. These three *p* orbitals are of same ergy and are called *degenarate orbitals.*

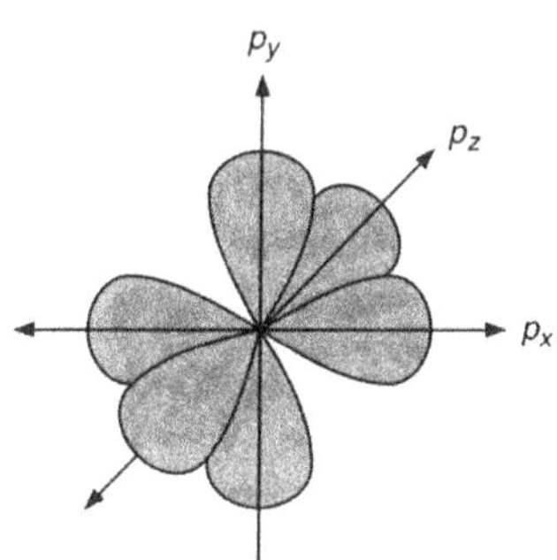

A *p* orbital has a dumb-bell shape with two lobes disposed symmetrically about the ɔleus along a line. This line is referred to as the orbital axis. The two lobes of the orbital ve a position concentric with the atomic nucleus where the probability of finding an

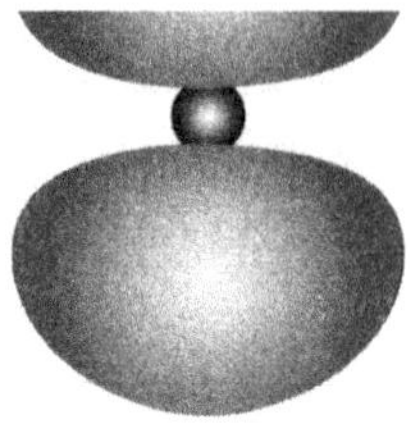

In addition to *s* and *p* orbitals, there are two other sets of orbitals (*d* and *f*) which become available for electrons to inhabit at higher energy levels. At the third level, there is a set of five *d* orbitals (with complicated shapes and names) as well as the 3*s* and 3*p* orbitals ($3p_x$, $3p_y$, $3p_z$). These five orbitals in each level corresponding to $m = -2, -1, 0, +1, +2$. At the third level there are a total of nine orbitals altogether. These are orbitals corresponding to $l = 2$ and are designated as d_{xy}, d_{yz}, d_{zx}, d_{x^2}, d_{y^2}, d_{z^2}.

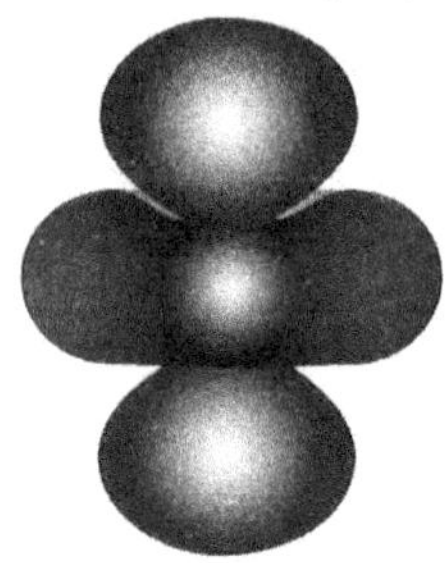

At the fourth level as well the 4*s* and 4*p* and 4*d* orbitals there are an additional seven *f* orbitals, i.e. 16 orbitals in all. *s*, *p*, *d* and *f* orbitals are then available at all higher energy levels as well. The *f* orbitals start from the fourth quantum level, i.e. $n = 4$. The Azhimuthal quantum number is $l = 3$. The magnetic quantum numbers are $m = -3, -2, -1, 0, +1, +2, +3$. These orbitals have complicated shapes.

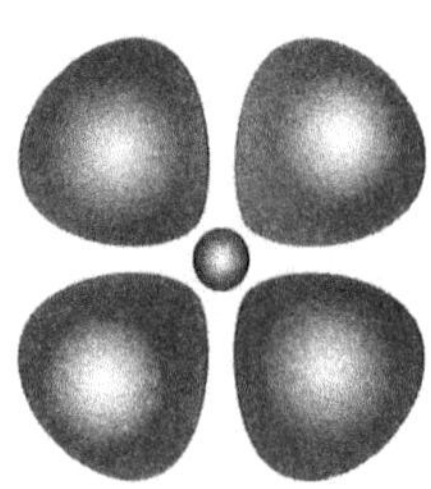

1.9.1 The Order of Filling Orbitals

Electrons fill low energy orbitals (closer to the nucleus) before they fill higher energy ones. Where there is a choice between orbitals of equal energy, they fill the orbitals singly

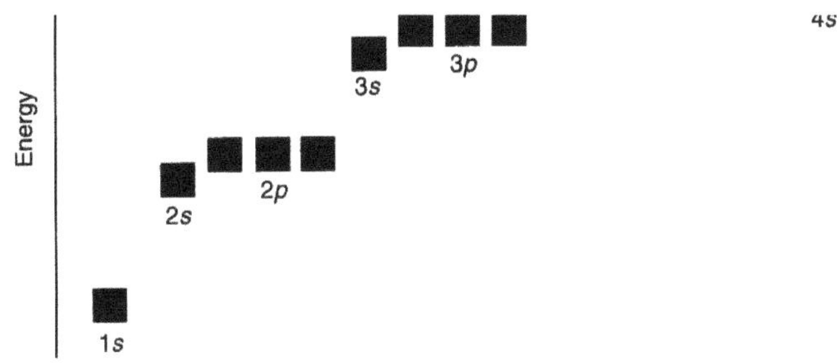

The *s* orbital always has a slightly lower energy than the *p* orbitals at the same energy evel, so the *s* orbital always fills with electrons before the corresponding *p* orbitals. The eal oddity is the position of the 3*d* orbitals. These are at a slightly higher level than the *s* and so it is the 4*s* orbital, which will fill first, followed by all the 3*d* orbitals and then he 4*p* orbitals.

PRACTICE QUESTIONS

1. Explain the fundamental conflict between Bohr's model of hydrogen atom and Heisenberg's uncertainty principle.
2. State and explain Heisenberg's uncertainty principle. Explain why wave nature is observed in small particles only.
3. Describe the wave nature of an electron.
4. What is de Broglie concept.
5. Write notes on:
   (a) *s* orbital
   (b) *p* orbital
   (c) *d* orbital
6. What are the limitations of Bohr's theory?
7. Explain Pauli's exclusion principle and Hund's rule taking oxygen as an example.
8. What is the maximum number of electrons with the principal quantum number 3? How are these distributed in an atom?
9. Explain quantum numbers and wave nature of electrons.
10. Write the importance of quantum numbers.

2

CHEMICAL BONDING AND HYBRIDISATION

When an atom of an element combines chemically with other atoms, which may be of same element or of different element, a compound (molecule) is formed. The term bc is used to describe the linkage between a particular pair of atoms.

2.1 OCTET RULE

G.N. Lewis, in 1916, stated this principle. Atoms form bonds by losing, gaining or shari enough electrons to achieve the outer electronic configuration of noble gases which stable by nature. This stability owes to their electronic configuration; they have f valence shell of electrons (ns^2, np^6). This is known as the octet rule as eight electrc (except a few exceptions like hydrogen) surround each atom.

2.2 CHEMICAL BONDS

Chemical bonds are formed to lower the energy of the system. There are basically t types of chemical bonds, namely, electrovalent and covalent bond. The stable structu can be achieved either by transfer of electrons (electrovalent) or by sharing of electrc (covalent). In both cases the result is a more stable system.

2.2.1 Electrovalent Bond

The bond formed by transfer of electron(s) from one atom to another is called electi valent bond. This is also known as ionic bond. Strongly electropositive elements su as Na, K, Ca, Ba, Sr, Mg, etc., when combined with strongly electronegative elements su as halogen, oxygen and sulphur, form electrovalent bond. An electropositive atom giv up the electron or electrons from the last orbit to form a positive ion called *cation.* electronegative atom takes up electron or electrons forming a negative ion called anic Cations and anions are held together by an electrostatic force. The bond that is form between an anion and a cation is called electrovalent or ionic bond. Compounds involvi electrovalent or ionic bonds are called ionic compounds. Thus, the formation of NaCl frc

The Electrovalent Bond is Strong A considerable amount of energy has to be ıpplied to break greater electrostatic forces of ionic bond because each charged ion is ırrounded by six oppositely charged ions. Hence ionic solids usually have high melting ›ints, for example, sodium chloride melts at 801°C.

Ionic Compounds are Generally Soluble in Polar Solvents (like Water) Upon ssolution, they undergo ionisation. For example, when NaCl is dissolved in water, Na^+ ıd Cl^- ions are formed. Since the solution contains electrically charged particles, it ecomes a good conductor of electricity.

In the Molten State – Good Conductors of Electricity In solid state, however, ions e held to their positions by strong attractive forces and hence are immobile and thus, ıd conductors of electricity.

Bonds in ionic compounds are non-directional.

2.2 Covalent Bond

'hen the electronegativity difference between two combining atoms is small, chemical ›mbination takes place by sharing of electrons to complete the octets in their outermost bits. Each atom contributes electrons and such sharing of electrons is known as ›valent bonding. When one pair of electrons is shared, it is known as a single bond as H_2, Cl_2, CH_4, NH_3, C_2H_6, etc.

$$H\cdot + \cdot H \longrightarrow H:H \quad \text{or} \quad H—H$$

$$H\cdot + \cdot Cl \longrightarrow H:Cl \quad \text{or} \quad H—Cl$$

Each line represents a pair of electrons shared by the two atoms. When two pairs of ectrons are shared, it is known as double bond, as in the case of C_2H_4 and CO_2.

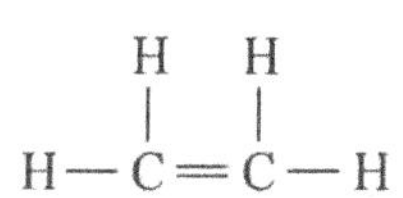

Ethene

$$O{=}C{=}O$$

Carbon dioxide

When three pairs of electrons are shared it is known as triple bond, as in the case of $_2$ and C_2H_2. Triple bond is usually stronger than a double bond, which in turn is stronger an a single bond.

$$H—C{\equiv}C—H$$

Ethyne

$$N{\equiv}N$$

Nitrogen

The covalent compounds have the following characteristics:

Covalent Bond is Weaker in Comparison to Ionic Bond The strength of the valent bond depends on its length. Greater the length, lesser is the strength. For ample, in halogen acids, the bond strength decreases as HF > HCl > HBr > HI

4. ***Isomerism*** These are directional bonds, they may show position isomerism a stereo-isomerism. They are mostly gases or liquids with low boiling points.

5. ***Reactivity*** The chemical reactions between the covalent molecules are generally sl Chemical reactions take place between atoms and hence the covalent bonds between molecules should break up to form atoms.

2.2.3 Coordinate Covalent Bond

When, only one atom contributes both the electrons, to be shared between the two ato then it is known as coordinate–covalent bond. When an atom whose octet is compl has a pair of electrons which it is not sharing with any of the combined atoms, then su a pair of electrons is known as *lone pair* and it can share this pair with any other at which is in need of two electrons. This is coordinate–covalent bond and is represen by → from an atom, which gives lone pair to the atom that receives it. An at contributing lone pair is known as *donor* while the other atom is known as *acceptor*. I example, after the donation of the lone pair by nitrogen to H^+, all the four N—H bo in NH_4^+ are identical.

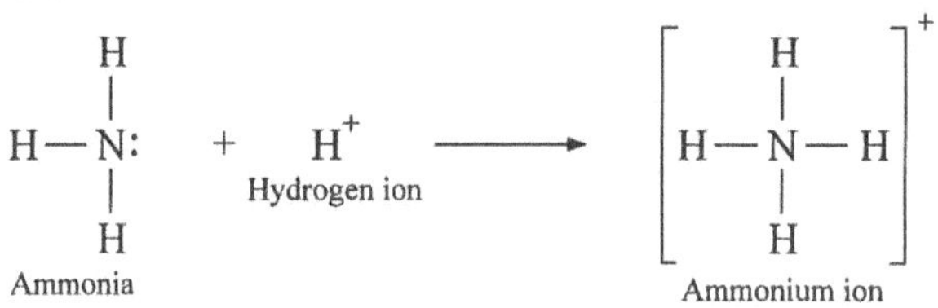

2.3 CHARACTERISTIC FEATURES OF COVALENT BOND

1. ***Bond Length*** Bond length can be defined as the average distance between t centres of nuclei of the two bonded atoms. In a covalent molecule the two bonded ato lie at an optimum distance to each other. The atoms are not stationary but vibrate abo their mean positions with respect to each other. Therefore, it is not reasonable to thi about a single fixed value of the distance between the nuclei. Even though the ato vibrate, the average value of the distance is reasonably constant. The bond lengths a usually expressed in Angstrom units (Å). If the nature of the bond between the two sa atoms changes, the bond length also changes. For example, the table below shows t change in bond length with the bond order.

Molecule	*Bond Length (Å)*	*Molecule*	*Bond Length (Å)*
H—H	0.74	O=O	1.21
F—F	1.42	N≡N	1.09

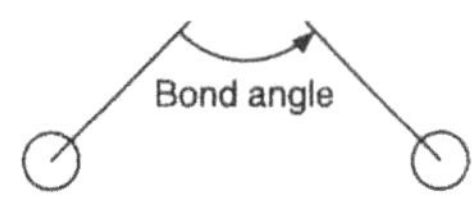

[In hybrid molecules the type of hybridisation of the central atom decides the bond angles.

Hybridisation and Molecular Geometry	*Bond Angle (approximate)*
sp, linear molecule (Ethyne)	180°
sp^2, trigonal (Ethene)	120°
sp^3, tetrahedral (Ethane)	109.5°

ond Dissociation Energy The amount of energy consumed or liberated when a bond roken or formed is known as the bond dissociation energy (D). It is characteristic of articular bond. There are two types of bond dissociations:

Iomolysis In homolytic bond dissociation, the covalent bond dissociates homolytically, one electron goes to each fragment. In this bond dissociation, free radicals are duced. The amount of energy required to dissociate a covalent bond homolytically is ed *homolytic bond dissociation energy.*

$$A:B \longrightarrow A\cdot + \cdot B$$
$$Cl:Cl \longrightarrow Cl\cdot + \cdot Cl$$

Heterolysis In heterolytic bond dissociation the covalent bond dissociates erolytically, i.e. both bonding electrons go to only one of the bonded atoms. Thus erolysis leads to ion formation. The amount of energy required to dissociate a covalent d heterolytically is called heterolytic bond dissociation energy. The heterolytic ociation energy values are higher than homolytic dissociation values because more ı 100 kcal/mole energy is required to separate oppositely charged ions.

$$A:B \longrightarrow A^+ + B^-$$
$$H:Cl \longrightarrow H^+ + Cl^-$$

Molecule	*Bond Dissociation Energy* (kcal/mole) (*Homolytic*)	*Molecule*	*Bond Dissociation Energy* (kcal/mole) (*Heterolytic*)
H—H	104	H—H	204
H—F	136	H—F	236
CH_3—H	104	CH_3—F	206

ond Polarity When a covalent bond is formed between atoms of different elements, bonded pair of electrons is attracted more towards the atom of higher electronega-y. The molecule acquires polarity with a partial negative charge (δ^-) on the more tronegative atom and a partial positive charge (δ^+) on the less electronegative atom. s the ends of the molecules are having different charges, they are also called dipoles.

$\overset{\delta^-}{\text{F}} - \overset{\delta^+}{\text{H}}$

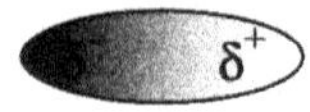

Here the symbols (δ^-) and (δ^+) are read as 'partial minus' (delta minus) and 'partial plu (delta plus). This is the symbolism used to describe a bond dipole, for exampl $H^{\delta+}—F^{\delta-}, H^{\delta+}—Cl^{\delta-}$.

The polarity of molecule (μ) is expressed in terms of its dipole moment. Dipole momei is the product of the magnitude of the charge (δ) on each of the poles and the distanc of separation (d, measured in cm) between the two charges. The dipole moment expressed in Debye units (D). Dipole moment is a vector quantity ($\rightarrow$), which ha magnitude and direction.

$$\mu = \delta \times d$$

Solvent	*Dipole Moment* (μ) *in Debye Units*
CH_3OH	2.87
H_2O	1.84
DMSO	3.96
DMF	3.82
CH_3CN	3.92

A dipole moment of zero means that the 'centre of negative charge' in the molecul corresponds to the 'centre of positive charge'. In case of methane, the 'centre of positiv charge' and the 'centre of negative charge' are focussed on the carbon atom.

2.4 POLAR MOLECULES

(i) The molecules having the property of polarity are known as polar molecules, e.g hydrogen halides (H—F, H—Cl, H—Br and H—I). All the hydrogen halides hav polar bonds – with the hydrogen-end slightly positive and the halogen-end slightl negative.

$$\overset{\delta^-}{\text{F}} - \overset{\delta^+}{\text{H}}$$

$$\overset{\delta^+}{\mathbf{H}} \div \overset{\delta^-}{\mathbf{Br}}$$

(ii) In case of carbonyl group the very electronegative oxygen atom pulls both bondin pairs towards itself – in the sigma bond and the pi bond. That leaves the oxygen fairl negative and the carbon fairly positive.

$$\overset{\delta^+}{\text{C}} = \overset{\delta^-}{\text{O}}$$

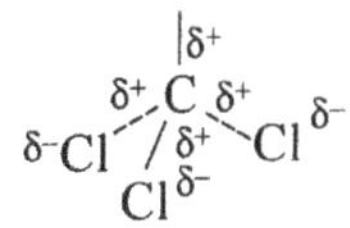

ome other examples of polar molecules are given here.

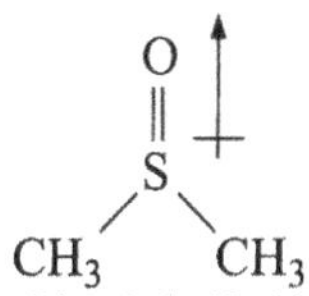

Dimethylsulfoxide

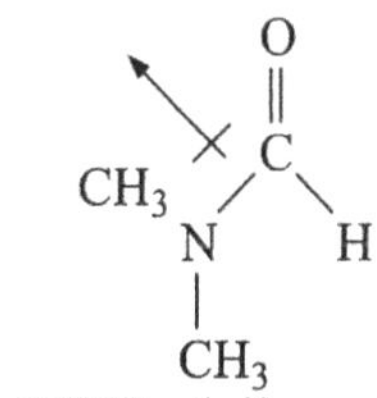

N,N-Dimethylformamide
(DMF)

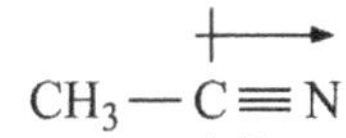

Acetonitrile

5 NON-POLAR BONDS

e covalent bond between two identical atoms is non-polar since the electronegativities the two atoms are identical.

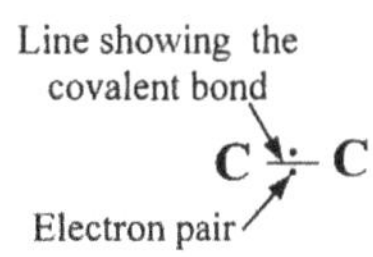

1. The simplest examples are the diatomic molecules such as H_2, N_2, and F_2, the carbon–carbon ($H_3C—CH_3$) is also non-polar.
2. The molecule as a whole, however, is non-polar – in the sense that it doesn't have an end (or a side) which is slightly negative and one which is slightly positive. The entire exterior of the molecule is somewhat negative, but there is no overall separation of charge from top to bottom, or from left to right.

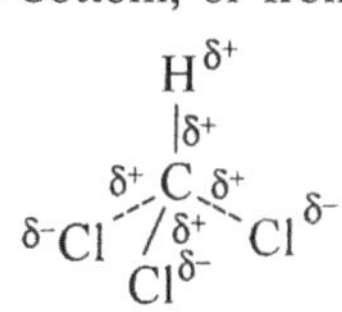

6 APPLICATIONS OF POLARITY

1. Molecular polarity has profound effects on the physical properties of the substance like solubility, boiling point and melting point. Molecular polarity determines the strength and types of intermolecular forces of attraction at work in a sample of the substance. The magnitude of these forces is directly proportional to boiling and melting points. In addition, molecular polarity affects solubility in that polar molecules are best solvated by polar solvent molecules and non-polar molecules are

moment of bond is called bond moment) also explain about shapes of molecules. I a polyatomic molecule, even though each bond has a bond moment the molecule a whole may not possess molecular moment due to cancellation of bond moments th depend on the direction of the bond. The dipole moment of a molecule depends upo the relative orientation of the bond dipoles but not on the polarity of the molecule:

Example

(i) Dipole moment of carbon tetrachloride is zero because of tetrahedral nature of CCl_4. Th bond moment of one C—Cl bond is cancelled by the other C—Cl bond moment.

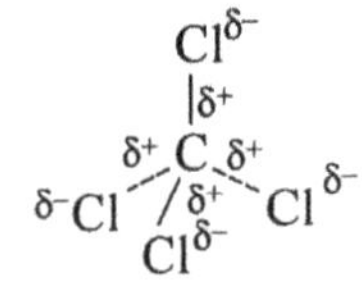

(ii) The dipole moment of carbon dioxide molecule is zero and hence the molecule is linea not bent.

$$\ddot{\underset{..}{O}}=C=\ddot{\underset{..}{O}}$$

(iii) Consider the case of dichlorodifluoromethane (CF_2Cl_2), a component of freon ga This molecule has a dipole moment of 0.51 Debye. While this fact does not prov that dichlorodifluoromethane is tetrahedral, it does distinguish between square plana structures **A** and **B**.

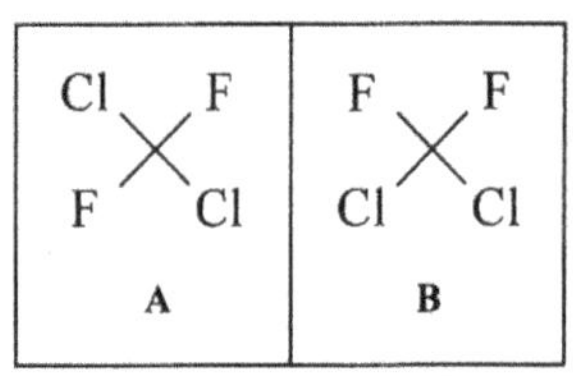

(iv) Polarity of covalent bonds is important to understand chemical reactions:

(a) The polarity of haloalkanes is important to undergo nucleophilic substitutio reactions:

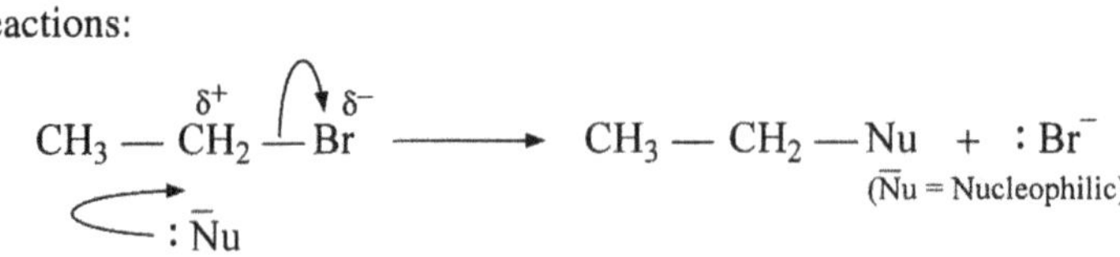

(b) Hydrogen halides add at carbon–carbon double bond due to polarity of hydro gen halides.

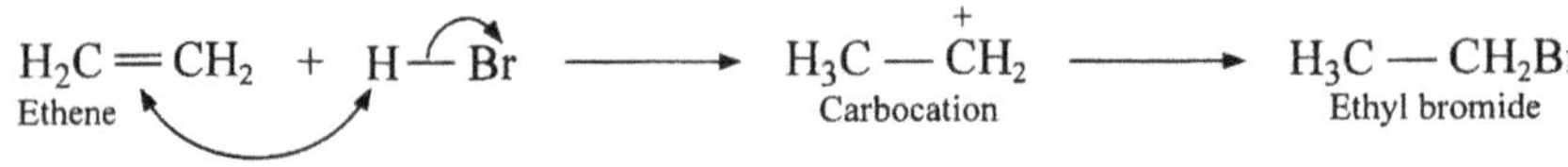

2.7 HYDROGEN BOND

30° from linearity, e.g. hydrogen bonding in NH_3, H_2O and HF.

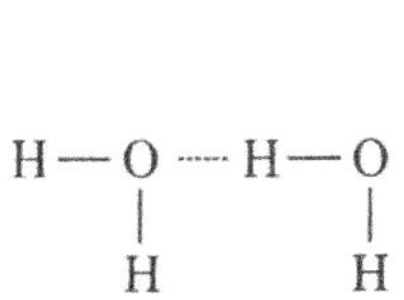

H_2O — H_2O

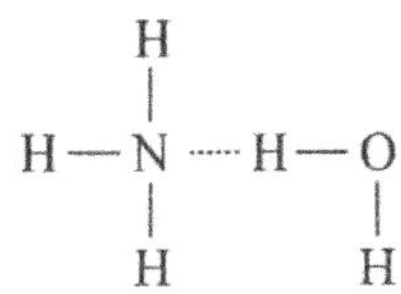

NH_3 — H_2O

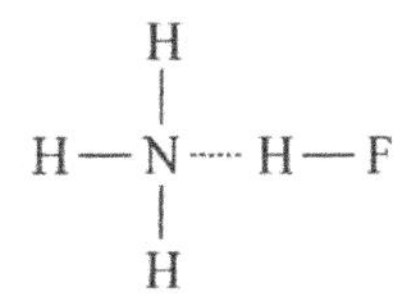

NH_3 — HF

.1 Strength of Hydrogen Bond

: strength of hydrogen bond may vary between 8 and 42 KJ/mol, where the normal d energy is in the order of 200 to 400 KJ/mol. The strength of hydrogen bond is ıker than covalent bond and its strength depends upon the electronegative atom. ger the electronegativity value, greater is the strength of hydrogen bond.

Bond	Bond Strength (KJ/mole)
H······F	42
H······O	30
H······N	12

.2 Types of Hydrogen Bonding

ıerally the hydrogen bonding is classified into two types.

) Intermolecular hydrogen bonding

) Intramolecular hydrogen bonding

Intermolecular hydrogen bonding In this type, hydrogen bonding occurs between or more than two molecules of the same compound and results in the formation of meric aggregate.

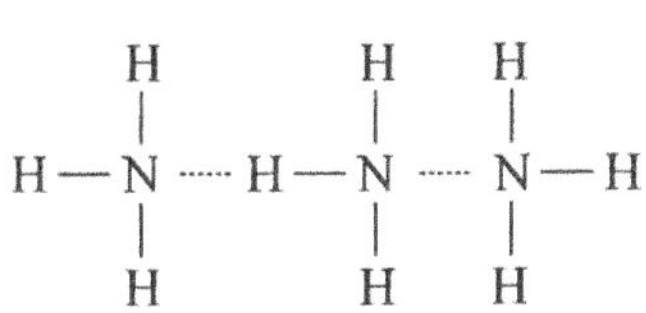

Hydrogen bonding in ammonia

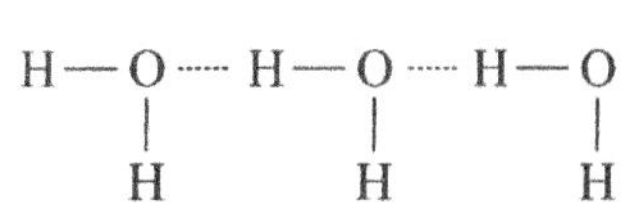

Hydrogen bonding in water

ntermolecular hydrogen bonding increases the boiling point of the compound and its solubility in water. The increase in boiling point is due to association of several ecules of the compound. As a result the effective molecular weight of the compound

Ethanol (C_2H_6O)	46	78°C
Dimethyl ether (C_2H_6O)	46	−25°C.
Diethyl ether ($C_4H_{10}O$)	74	61°C
1-Butanol ($C_4H_{10}O$)	74	118°C

(ii) *Intramolecular hydrogen bonding* In this type, hydrogen bonding occurs in atoms of the same molecule. This type of hydrogen bonding is commonly knowr chelation and frequently occurs in organic compounds. Sometimes intramolecular hy(gen bonding develops a six- or five-membered ring.

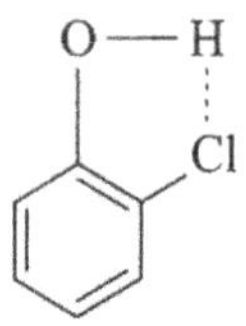

Hydrogen bonding in *o*-chlorophenol

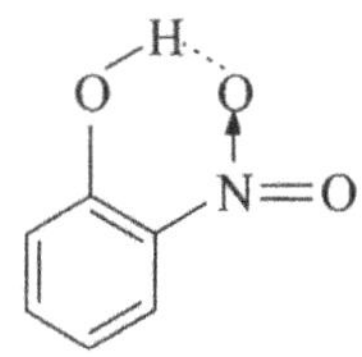

Hydrogen bonding in *o*-nitro phenol

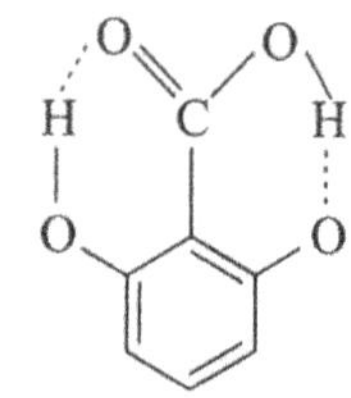

Hydrogen bonding in 2, 6-dihydroxybenzoic aci(

Intramolecular hydrogen bonding decreases the boiling point of the compound ; also its solubility in water. This is because of the fact that the chelation between ortho-substituted groups restricts the possibility of intermolecular hydrogen bond with water and thus prevents association of the molecules, which would have raised melting point and boiling point. Chelation is not possible in the corresponding meta ; para isomers because the two groups are far away from each other. Hence in such ca: intermolecular hydrogen bonding takes place, which in turn increases the boiling po Thus we can explain the lower melting point and boiling point of the ortho isomers hydroxy, nitro and carbonyl compounds than the corresponding meta and para isom(

o-Nitrophenol

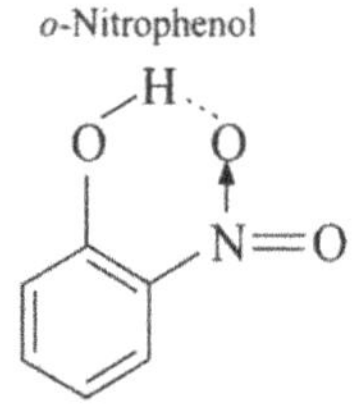

Hydrogen bonding in *o*-nitrophenol
Boiling point = 215° C

p-Nitrophenol

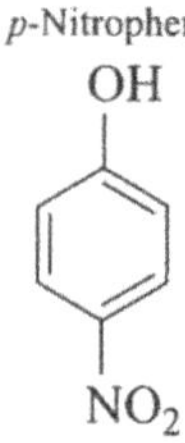

Boiling point = 279° C

m-Nitrophenol

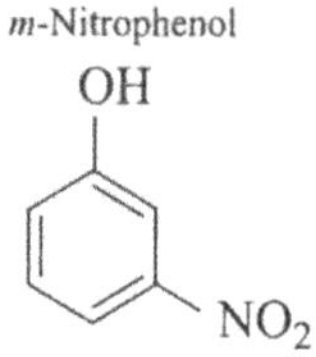

Boiling point = 279° C

2.7.3 Effects of Hydrogen Bonding

Almost all physical properties are affected by hydrogen bonding. Here only those propert

ıding decreases the boiling point of the compound. This is because the chelation ween the groups of same molecule restricts the possibility of intermolecular hydrogen ıding and thus prevents association of the molecules, which would have raised the lting point and boiling point.

Vater Solubility Solubility of a substance increases tremendously when hydrogen ıding is possible between the solvent and the solute, for example, methanol and anol are highly soluble in water due to hydrogen bonding between molecules.

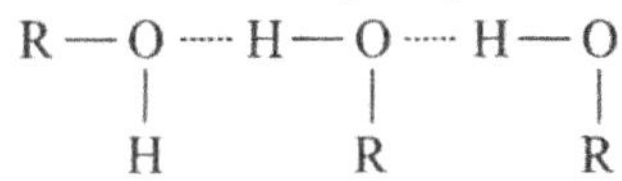

The high solubility of polyhydric phenols and sugars may be attributed to the fact that se compounds make available greater number of hydroxyl (—OH) groups for hydrogen ıding.

Strength of Acids Any structural feature that contributes for the greater stability of ɔn in comparison to free acid will shift the ionisation equilibrium to the right. Thus if anion of acid were stabilised due to intramolecular hydrogen bonding, there would narked increase in the strength of acid, for instance, the ionisation constant of salicylic l is higher than the other two isomers.

Spectroscopic Properties The hydrogen bonding shifts the position of bands in ared and NMR spectra of organic compounds. Infrared spectrum of ethyl alcohol in our phase shows absorption band at 3700 cm^{-1} due to free hydroxyl group. In solution band is completely replaced by a broad band around 3500 cm^{-1} which is characteristic ıydrogen bonded hydroxyl groups.

On Surface Tension and Viscosity The compounds which possess hydrogen bonding found to have higher surface tension and viscosity. Glycerol, glycol, sulphuric acid, ar syrup, phosphoric acid, etc., are viscous liquids due to extensive hydrogen bonding veen their molecules. Due to more number of hydroxyl (OH) groups, the extent of hydrobonding is more in glycerol. So, it is more viscous than glycol.

Biological Products The three-dimensional structures of proteins and nucleic acids is to hydrogen bonding. In α-helices, hydrogen bonds extend from the hydrogen atoms olar N—H units in peptide group to oxygen atoms of polar carbonyl (C=O) units.

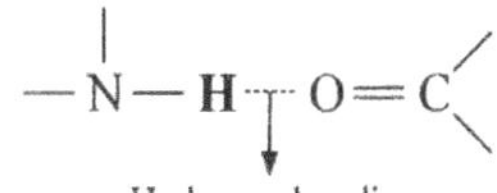

Hydrogen bonding

Hydrogen bonds are extremely important in the chemistry of the genetic code. As we study later, the double strands of DNA are held together by hydrogen bonds. The

INTERMOLECULAR FORCES

Attractive forces between molecules are called intermolecular forces. They are m weaker and responsible for the bulk properties of matter like melting point, boiling po etc. The following are different types of intermolecular forces: (1) Ion–dipole forces, dipole–dipole forces, (3) dipole–induced dipole forces, and (4) dispersion forces. Dipc dipole, dipole–induced dipole and dispersion forces are commonly referred to as *van Waals forces*.

1. ***Ion–Dipole Forces*** These forces occur between an ion (either a cation or an ani and a polar molecule, e.g. in an aqueous solution of NaCl, the Na^+ and Cl^- ions surrounded by water molecules.

2. ***Dipole–Dipole Forces*** These forces act between polar molecules – the molecules t possess dipole moments. Molecules that have permanent dipoles will have higher boil points rather than molecules, which only have temporary fluctuating dipoles. For examp the boiling points of ethane (CH_3CH_3) and fluoromethane (CH_3F) are

Ethane

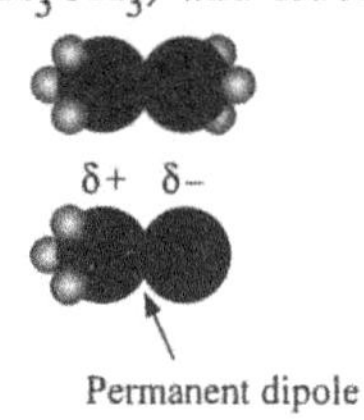

Boiling point = 184.5 K

Fluoromethane

Boiling point = 194.7 K

The higher boiling point of fluoromethane is due to the large permanent dipole on molecule because of the high electronegativity of fluorine.

3. ***Dipole–Induced Dipole Forces*** The attractive interaction between a polar molec and the induced dipole (The dipole in an atom or molecule is said to be induced dip because the separation of positive and negative charges in the atom or a non-po molecule is due to the proximity of an anion or a polar molecule) is called dipole–induc dipole interaction, e.g. forces between water and CCl_4 molecules.

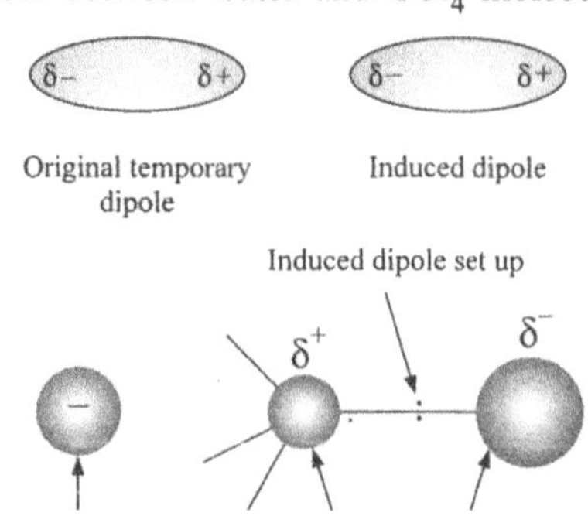

n molar mass, for example, forces present between the molecules of CCl_4.
As the right-hand side molecule approaches, its electrons will tend to be attracted by slightly positive end of the left-hand side molecule.

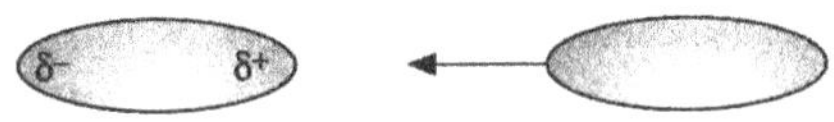

There is no reason why this has to be restricted to two molecules. As long as the lecules are close together this synchronised movement of the electrons can occur over ;e numbers of molecules.

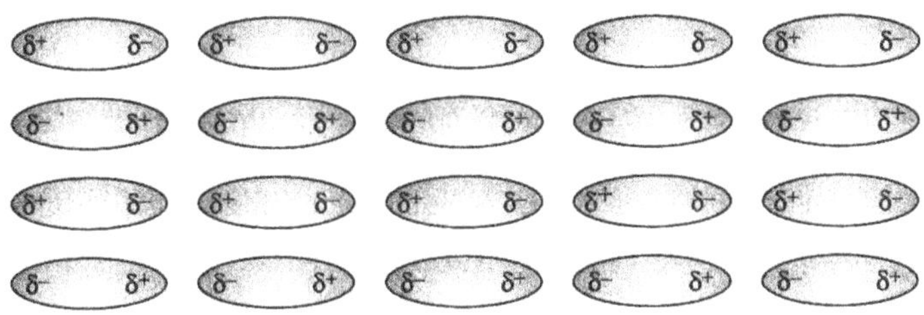

Surprisingly, dipole–dipole attractions are fairly minor compared with dispersion forces, their effect can only really be seen if you compare two molecules with the same nber of electrons and the same size.

MOLECULAR ORBITAL THEORY

:mists view molecules as combinations of atoms. They consider molecular orbitals as nbinations of atomic orbitals. To explain the nature of covalent bond, Mulliken, Huckel Hund developed molecular orbital theory. According to this theory, the orbitals of atoms combine to form a reactant orbital known as molecular orbital. Molecular orbital O) is an orbital of an entire molecule rather than an orbital of a single atom. All the :trons pertaining to both the atoms are considered to be moving along the entire lecule under the influence of all the nuclei. The electrons in the molecular orbitals can described by the four quantum numbers, i.e. principal quantum number (n), azhimuthal ntum number (l), angular momentum (quantified by wave function = λ) and spin ntum number (s). A fundamental rule of molecular orbital theory is that the number nolecular orbitals must be equal to the number of atomic orbitals. For two hydrogen ns, there are two atomic orbitals, which means that there must be two molecular itals for dihydrogen. The second molecular orbital is described by the equation $= 1s_A - 1s_B$. There is no valence bond equivalent of ψ^*.
The wavefunction describing a molecular orbital is obtained by two methods: linear combination of atomic orbitals (LCAO) and (b) united atom method.

.1 LCAO Approximation

atomic orbitals overlap. There is increased electron density between the nuclei beca each of the electrons in this region is electrostatically attracted to both nuclei. This is sim to two light waves or two sound waves that reinforce or enhance each other. The bond orbitals are designated as σ (sigma), π (pi), δ (delta), etc.

The second-half of the molecular orbitals are associated with higher energies than atomic orbitals which are termed as anti-bonding molecular orbitals (designated by : as σ*, π*). The anti-bonding orbitals are formed when two out-of-phase atomic orbi overlap. The electrons placed in such anti-bonding orbitals decrease the stability of sı bond. This is similar to the darkness that occurs when two light waves cancel each otl

1. ***Hydrogen Molecule*** (H_2) In the formation of the hydrogen molecule H_2, the t 1*s*-electrons – one from each of the atoms concerned with opposite spin passes int σ1*s*-molecular orbital. This is a bonding orbital and constitutes the single covalent bo in the hydrogen molecule. The σ^*1s-anti-bonding molecular orbital is unoccupied.

There are several features of Fig. 2.1:

- The electron distribution about the separated hydrogen atoms is spherica symmetrical. In contrast, the electron distribution in the MO ψ is not. Rather, electron density is concentrated in the inter-nuclear region where both electr can experience the Coulombic attraction of both nuclei. (This is the result constructive interference.)

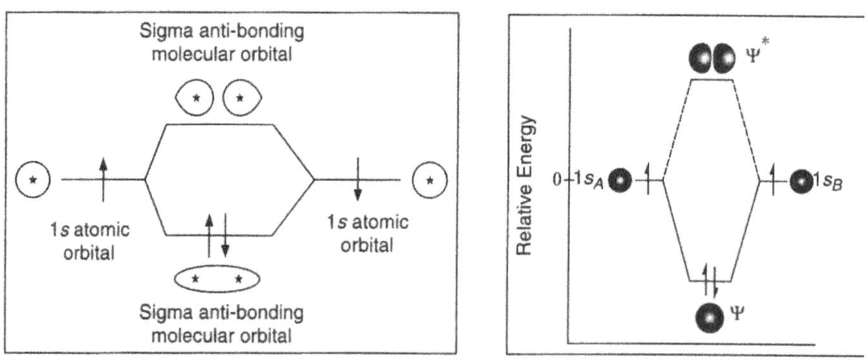

Fig. 2.1 An Orbital Picture of the Formation of Dihydrogen

- In the ground state there are no electrons in ψ^*. However, if an electron is *exci* from ψ to ψ^*, the probability of the resulting electron density being in the int nuclear region of ψ^* is very low. (This is the result of destructive interferenc
- The inter-nuclear distance in ψ is less than the sum of the atomic radii of the tv hydrogen atoms. The inter-nuclear distance in ψ^* is greater than the sum of t atomic radii of the two hydrogen atoms.

The MOs ψ and ψ^* are called the Highest Occupied Molecular Orbital (HOMO) a

Oxygen Molecule

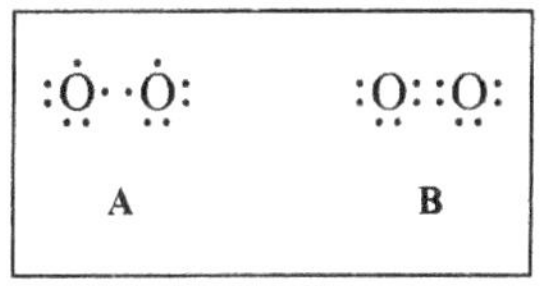

Two Lewis structures for O_2

Figure 2.2 shows the MO diagram for dioxygen. Only the valence shell atomic orbitals e shown.

The important feature of the figure is that there are two HOMOs that have the same iergy. Each one contains a single electron. According to Hund's rule the energy of the stem will be lower if the spins of these two electrons are unpaired than if they are paired. other words, the most stable form of dioxygen should be paramagnetic, not diamagnetic.

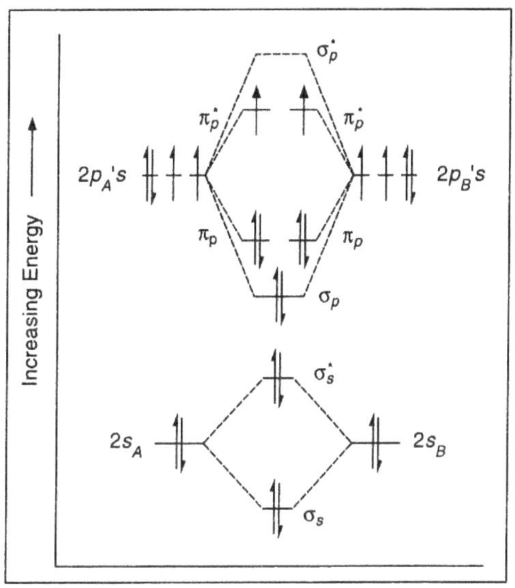

Fig. 2.2 Molecular Orbital Diagram for Dioxygen

10 HYBRIDISATION

ybridisation may be defined as the phenomenon of 'mixing up' of orbitals of an atom nearly equal energy, giving rise to entirely new orbitals equal to the number of mixing bitals and having same energy contents and identical shapes.

10.1 Rules of Hybridisation

or hybridisation to occur thc atom has to satisfy the following conditions:

1. Orbitals on a single atom only would undergo hybridisation.

character of the hybrid orbitals.
5. It is the orbitals that undergo hybridisation and not the electrons.
6. The hybridising orbitals may or may not contain electrons.
7. The angle between any two hybrid orbitals is the same.
8. While occupying the hybrid orbitals electrons follow Hund's rule of maximu multiplicity and Pauli's exclusion principle.

Throughout the course of organic chemistry, carbon exhibits only three types c hybridisation. They are (a) sp^3 hybridisation, (b) sp^2 hybridisation, and (c) sp hybridisatio

2.10.2 sp^3 Hybridisation (Tetrahedral Hybridisation)

In this type of hybridisation, one 2*s* orbital and three 2*p* orbitals merge together to for four identical orbitals known as sp^3 hybrid orbitals. These hybrid orbitals are directed i space towards the four corners of a regular tetrahedron with a bond angle of 109° 28′ wit one another. Each sp^3 hybrid orbital has ¼ *s* and ¾ *p* character. This type of hybridisatio is observed in carbon–carbon single bond compounds like methane, ethane, etc.

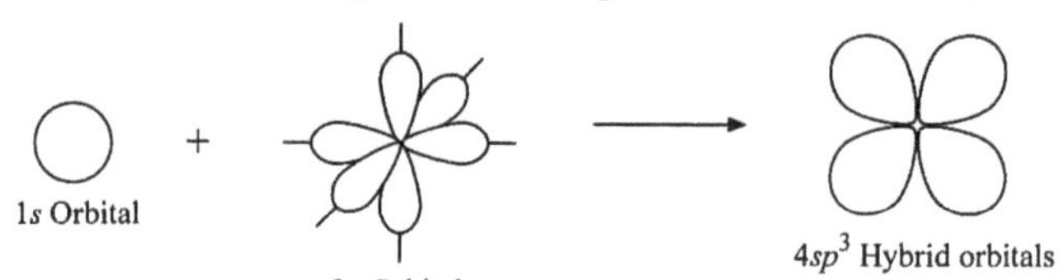

1. ***Methane Molecule*** The four sp^3 hybrid orbitals of the central carbon atom overla the 1*s* orbitals of the four hydrogen atoms, which are situated at the corners of tetrahedron. Each carbon–hydrogen bond has a length of 1.10 Å and each H—C—H angle has a measure of 109° 28′. The following is the molecular model of methane molecule

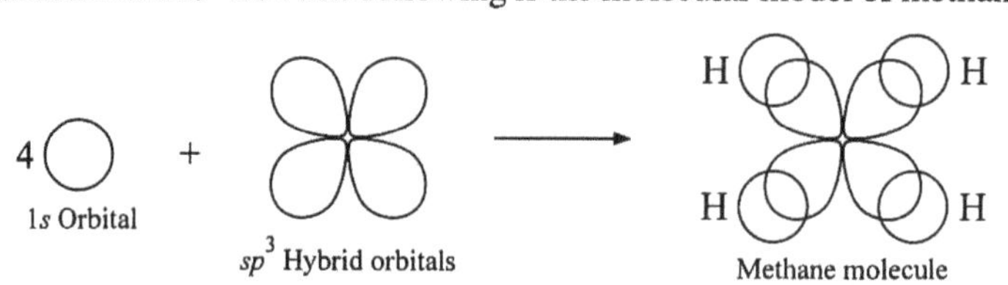

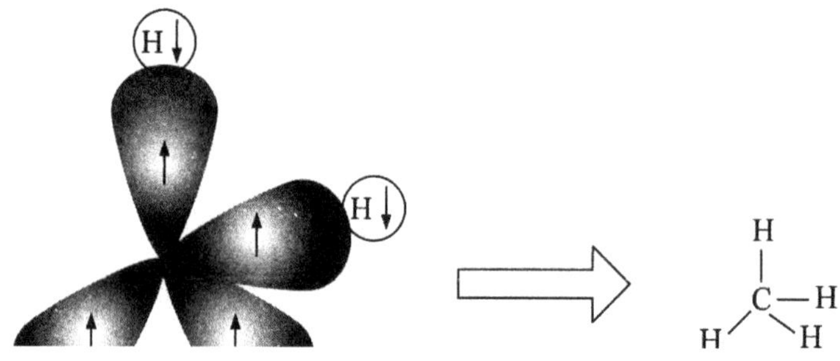

ach carbon overlap with 1s orbitals of three hydrogens forming (sp^3–s) three σ bonds.
ethane molecule exhibits different conformations due to free rotation of methyl ıps about the C—C sigma bond.

0.3 sp^2 Hybridisation (Trigonal Hybridisation)

his type of hybridisation, one 2s orbital and two 2p orbitals coalesce together to form e identical orbitals known as sp^2 hybrid orbitals, leaving one 2p orbital unhybridised. se three sp^2 hybrid orbitals are directed towards the three corners of a triangle with nd angle of 120° with one another. Each sp^2 hybrid orbital has one-third s and two-d p character. This type of hybridisation is observed in carbon–carbon double bond ıpounds like ethene, propene, etc.

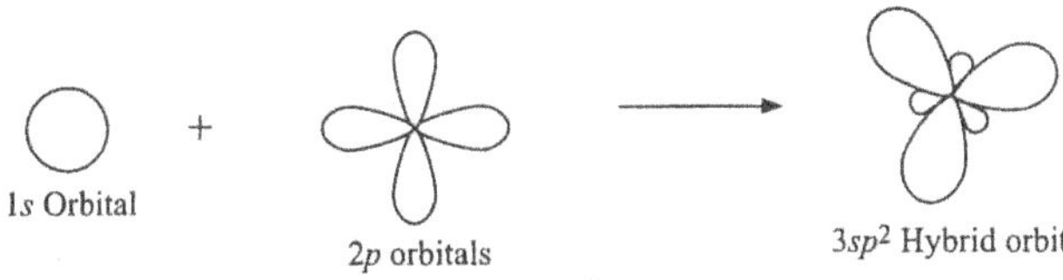

n ethene the two carbon atoms are of sp^2 hybridised state. The two carbon atoms ed themselves by the overlap of one sp^2 hybrid orbital from each carbon. Each carbon n forms two C—H bonds by the overlap of sp^2 hybrid orbital of carbon atom with 1s tal of hydrogen. All these bonds are sigma bonds (σ) with bond angles of 120°. The aining unpaired electron at each carbon atom in $2p_z$ orbital, which is perpendicular to plane of sigma bonds. These p_z orbitals overlap in lateral way and form π bond. Thus carbon–carbon double bond in alkene is made of one σ bond and one π bond. The carbon atoms in ethene are held more tightly than in ethane, with the result the C bond distance in ethene is less than C—C bond distance in ethane. The alkenes more reactive due to availability of π electrons and the free rotation of carbon atoms so restricted. Hence, alkenes exhibits geometrical isomerism.

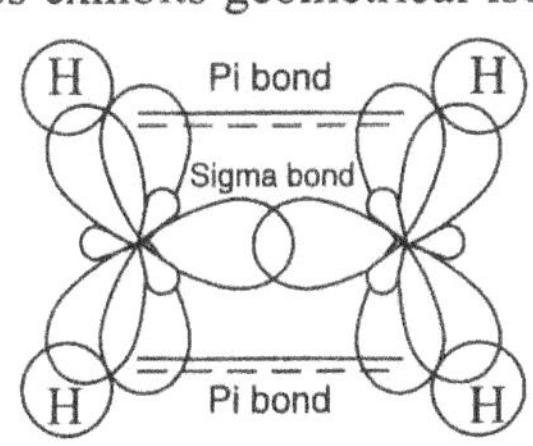

Ethene molecule

0.4 sp Hybridisation (Linear Hybridisation)

ıis type of hybridisation, one 2s orbital and one 2p orbitals coalesce together to form

1s Orbitals

In the formation of ethyne (acetylene), one of the *sp* hybrid orbitals of one carbon a overlaps with the similar orbital of the second carbon atom to give a σ bond. The sec *sp* orbital of each carbon atom overlaps with 1*s* orbital of hydrogen atom to form ano σ bond. The remaining two perpendicular unhybridised *p* orbitals of one carbon a overlap sideways with 2*p* orbitals of the second carbon atom to form two π bonds. ' electron cloud of one π bond is considered to lie above and below the line joining two nuclei. Thus, acetylene molecule contains one σ bond and two π bonds between two carbons and each carbon is linked to one H-atom with a σ bond. Because of smaller effective size of *sp* orbitals and two π bonds, the carbon–carbon triple bond ler is only 1.20 Å. Similarly, due to the smaller size of *sp* orbitals the C—H distanc acetylene is also shorter than in ethane and ethene. Unlike alkenes, alkynes do not exh geometrical isomerism because of the linear shape of molecule.

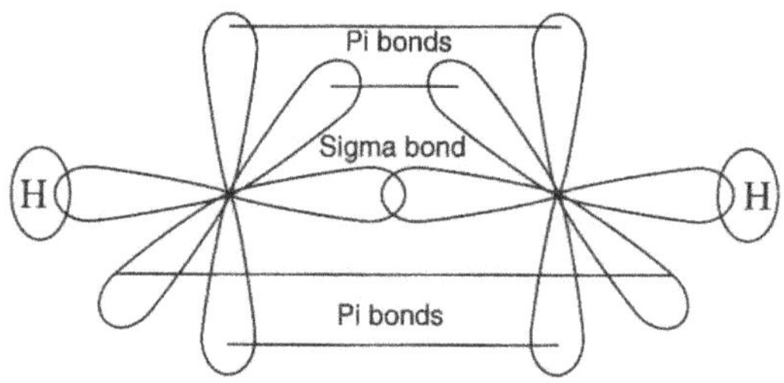

Acetylene molecule

PRACTICE QUESTIONS

1. What do you mean by chemical bond? How many types of chemical bonds are there? Exp different chemical bonds with examples.
2. Give a brief account on the differences between covalent and ionic bonds.
3. Enumerate different properties of covalent compounds.
4. Discuss various characteristic features of covalent bond.
5. Differentiate bond energy from bond dissociation energy.
6. Define bonding molecular orbital, anti-bonding molecular orbital, sigma molecular orbital pi molecular orbital? Discuss the formation of O_2 molecule.
7. Boiling point of ortho-nitrophenol is lesser than that of para-nitrophenol or meta-nitrophe Why?
8. Though the hydrogen bonds are stronger in HF than in H_2O, the former has relatively boiling point. Why?
9. Explain, why:
   (a) Ionic compounds melt at higher temperatures than covalent compounds?
   (b) Sodium chloride is soluble in water?

Write notes on:

(a) Bond polarity
(b) Bond dissociation energy
(c) Dipole moment
(d) Polar and non-polar molecules

Enumerate various applications of hydrogen bond.

3

PURIFICATION AND CHARACTERISATIO OF ORGANIC COMPOUNDS

3.1 INTRODUCTION

The structural formula of an organic compound isolated from a natural source or prepare the laboratory can be determined by following a systematic procedure. The different st employed in the study of organic compounds are: (a) purification, (b) qualitative analysis, quantitative analysis, (d) molecular mass determination, (e) calculation of the empirical molecular formulae, and (f) determination of structure by one or more of several meth including chemical synthesis. In this chapter, we shall deal with some of the meth commonly employed for the purification and characterisation of organic compounds.

3.2 PURIFICATION

Before investigating the structure and properties of an organic compound, it is essen to obtain it in the pure form. Many substances obtained from natural sources or fr chemical reactions may contain some undesirable components. These components called *impurities* and the process of removal of impurities from the concerned compou is called *purification*. Methods of separating organic compounds from one another purifying them depend on the differences in their physical properties. The comn techniques used are (a) crystallisation, (b) sublimation, (c) distillation, (d) differen extraction, and (e) chromatography.

3.2.1 Crystallisation

This process is very useful for the solid compounds with low percentage of impuriti The basis of crystallisation is that the solubility of organic compounds usually increa considerably with increase in temperature. Briefly, the method consists of dissolving solid in a solvent in which it is sparingly soluble at room temperature but apprecial soluble at higher temperatures. This is achieved by heating. Once the bulk of the so has dissolved, any insoluble impurities present are removed by filtration. On cooling, pure solid crystallises out. Frequently, to enhance the recovery of the solid, the soluti is either concentrated by partial evaporation of the solvent or diluted with a solvent

sible, because both naphthalene and benzoic acid are quite soluble in benzene.
n case the difference in solubility of two substances in the solvent is not discernable, tional crystallisation, involving a series of repeated crystallisations is carried out.

.2 Sublimation

s is a method of limited application and is used to purify those solids, which sublime lily and contain non-volatile impurities. If the vapour pressure of the impurities in a d is significantly lower than that of a solid sample, then sublimation can be used as ırification method. On heating the mixture, the volatile substance is converted into our, leaving behind the other components. On cooling, the vapour of the volatile stance is changed into solid. This process of conversion of a solid directly into our is called *sublimation*.

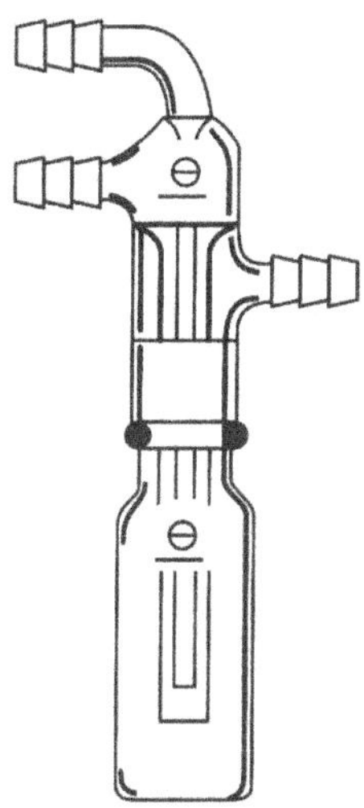

Fig. 3.1 Apparatus for Sublimation

$$\text{Solid} \xrightarrow{\text{Heat}} \text{Vapour} \xrightarrow{\text{Cool}} \text{Solid}$$

ertain substances like naphthalene, benzoic acid and camphor on heating are verted to vapours without passing into liquid state. Naphthalene is commercially fied by sublimation (Fig. 3.1).

3 Distillation

is an important method for purifying liquids and is based on differences in boiling ts. Simple distillation involves the conversion of a liquid into vapour by heating and condensation of the vapour to liquid into another flask. For example, distillation can

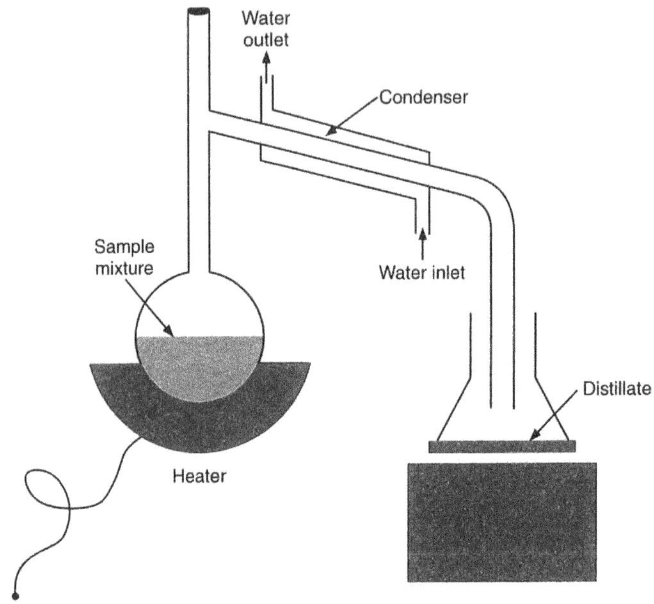

Fig. 3.2 Distillation Apparatus

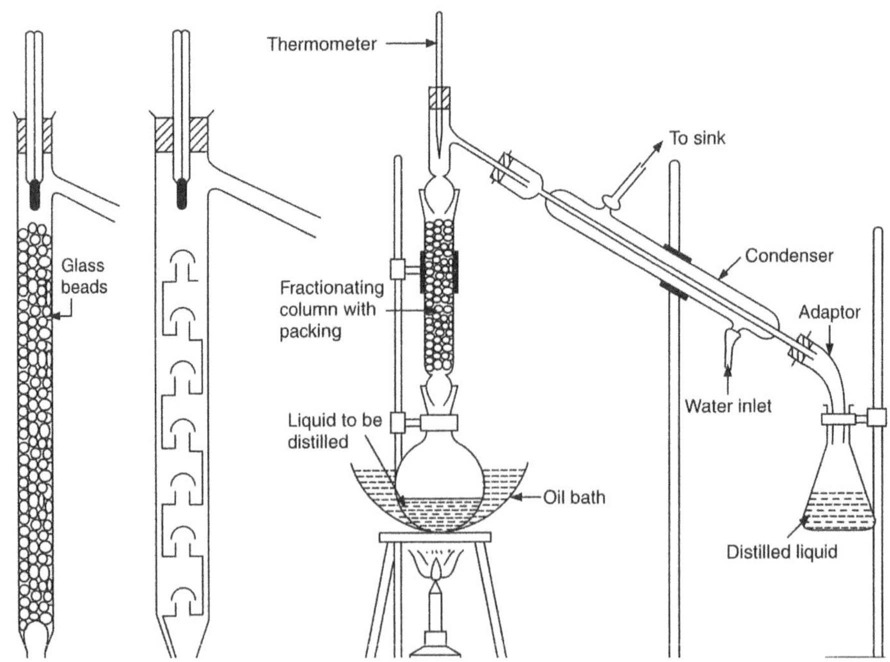

creases the cooling surface and the vapours go up from the distillation flask through
: column. The liquids with high boiling are condensed in the lower portions, the more latile components will volatise and condense in the upper, cooler portion of the column.

Liquids with high boiling point as well as liquids, which decompose at, or below their rmal boiling points are generally distilled at lower temperatures under reduced pressure. th an ordinary vaccum pump, a pressure of 10–20 mm Hg can be obtained and under se conditions boiling points are reduced by about 100 degrees. Lower pressures 1 mm Hg) may be obtained with better vacuum pumps.

It is often convenient to separate organic compounds from non-volatile organic or rganic impurities by distillation with steam. This is applicable to only those compounds, ich are, steam volatile and are sparingly soluble in water [e.g. aniline ($C_6H_5NH_2$)]. am distillation can be carried out by passing steam through a heated flask containing liquid to be distilled (Fig. 3.4). The mixture of steam and the volatile organic npounds (that distils out) is later condensed and the components separated from each er. We know that a liquid boils when its vapour pressure becomes equal to the nospheric pressure. In steam distillation, water and organic substance vapourise ether and their vapour pressures together equal the atmospheric pressure.

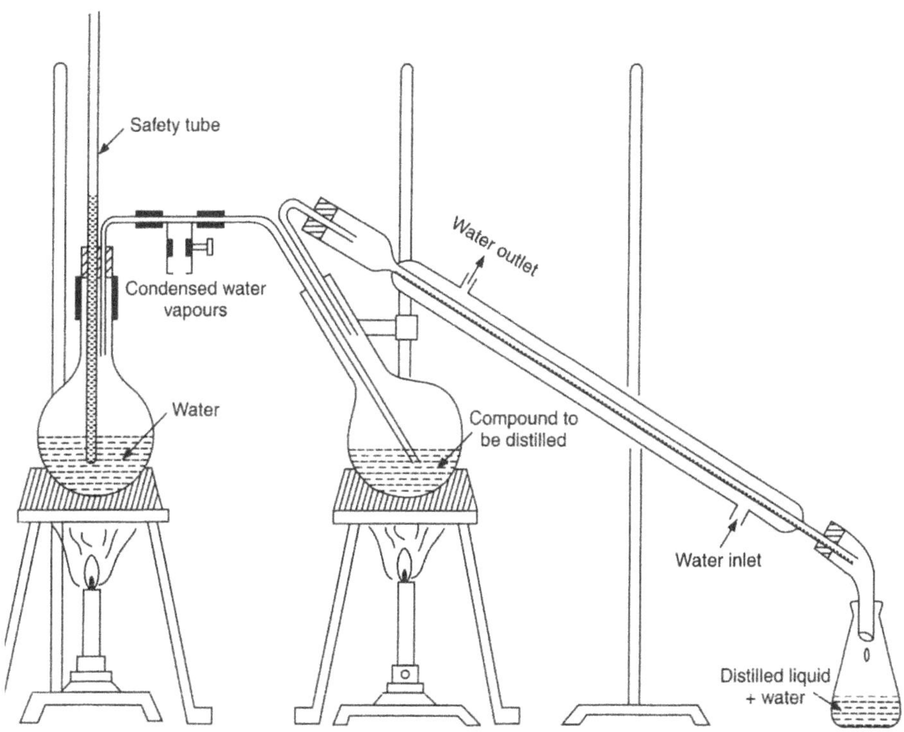

at lower temperatures.

The proportion of the organic substance that distils over with steam is related to vapour pressures as well as molecular masses by the following equation:

$$\frac{W_1}{W_2} = \frac{P_1 M_1}{P_2 M_2}$$

where W is the mass, P is the vapour pressure and M is the molecular mass with subscripts 1 and 2 standing for water and the organic substance, respectively.

3.2.4 Differential Extraction

When an organic compound is present in aqueous solution, it can be recovered shaking it with a suitable organic solvent (the compound should be more soluble in organic solvent than in water). The organic solvent should be immiscible with water that the organic and water layers can be easily separated. The solvent on evaporat leaves behind the recovered substance. This method is normally applicable on n volatile organic compounds. For example, benzoic acid can be extracted from aque solution using benzene (see Fig. 3.5).

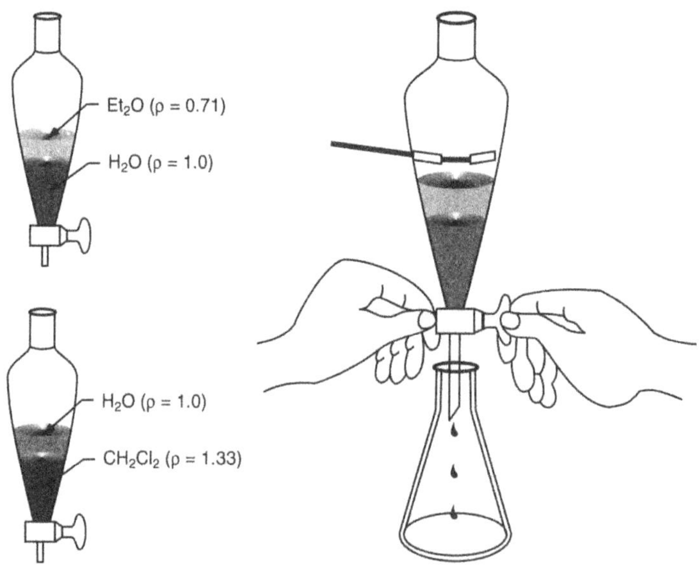

Fig. 3.5 Extraction Process using Separating Funnel

3.2.5 Chromatography

Chromatography is a separation method that relies on differences in partitioning ehaviour between a flowing mobile phase and a stationary phase to separate the omponents in a mixture. The working principle is based on the differences in the extent of ıteraction (adsorption) of various substances with a stationary phase and a mobile phase.

ypes of Chromatographic Techniques There are various types of chromatographic echniques which differ from one another on the basis of difference between the moving hase and the stationary phase.

) *Column chromatography* The simplest chromatographic method is column hromatography. A suitable adsorbent, like alumina (Al_2O_3), is packed in a column and ıis constitutes the stationary phase. The mixture to be separated is taken in suitable olvent and the solution poured on the top of the column of the adsorbent. The omponents are then eluted out by a suitable solvent (which acts as a mobile phase). The veakly adsorbed component will be eluted more rapidly than a more strongly adsorbed omponent. Such a progressive separation of a mixture is diagrammatically shown in ig. 3.6. We may see separate bands in columns formed by different compounds in the ıixture, if they are coloured.

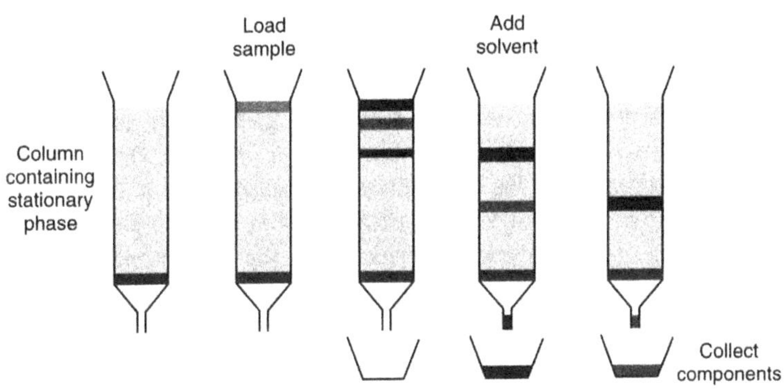

Fig. 3.6 Column Chromatography

ii) *Thin-layer chromatography (TLC)* Thin-layer chromatography (TLC) is a hromatographic technique that is useful for separating organic compounds. Because of s simplicity and rapidity, TLC technique is often used to monitor the progress of organic eactions and to check the purity of products.

Aethod Thin-layer chromatography consists of a stationary phase immobilised on a lass or plastic plate and an organic solvent. The sample, either liquid or solid dissolved ı a volatile solvent, is deposited as a spot on the stationary phase. The constituents of sample can be identified by simultaneously running standards with the unknown. The ottom edge of the plate is placed in a solvent reservoir, and the solvent moves up the

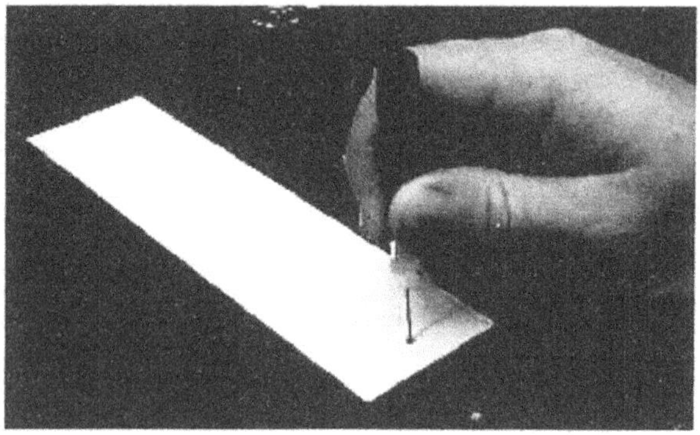

Spotting a TLC plate with sample

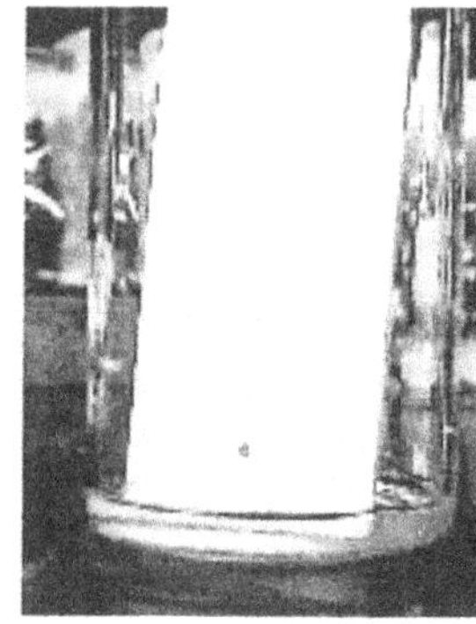

Running the TLC plate in solv

Fig. 3.7 Thin-layer Chromatography (TLC)

(iii) *Gas chromatography (GC)* Gas chromatography is a chromatographic technique t can be used to separate volatile organic compounds. A gas chromatograph consists c flowing mobile phase, an injection port, a separation column containing the stationary ph and a detector. The organic compounds are separated due to differences in their partition behaviour between the mobile gas phase and the stationary phase in the column.

Instrumentation Mobile phases are generally inert gases such as helium, argon, nitrogen. The *injection port* consists of a rubber septum through which a syringe nee is inserted to inject the sample. The injection port is maintained at a higher temperat than the boiling point of the least volatile component in the sample mixture. Since partitioning behaviour is dependent on temperature, the separation column is usua contained in a thermostat-controlled oven. Separating components with a wide range boiling points is accomplished by starting at a low oven temperature and increasing temperature over time to elute the high-boiling point components. Most columns cont a liquid stationary phase on a solid support. Separation of low-molecular weight ga is accomplished with solid adsorbents. Separate documents describe some specific (Columns and GC Detectors. Figure 3.8 gives a schematic representation of a g chromatograph.

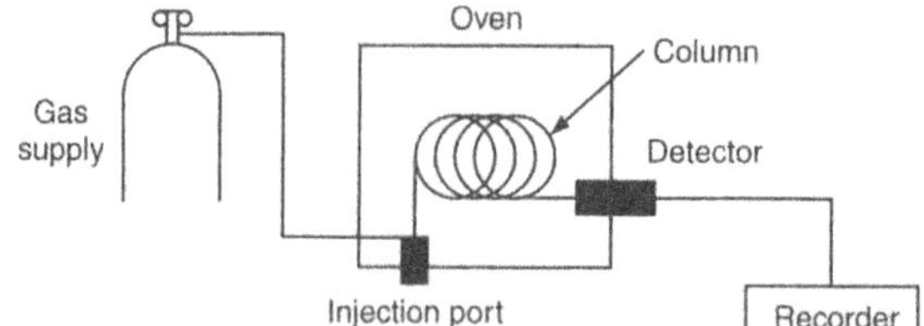

Fig. 3.8 Schematic representation of a Gas Chromatograph

ixture pass through the column at different rates due to differences in their partitioning :haviour between the mobile liquid phase and the stationary phase.

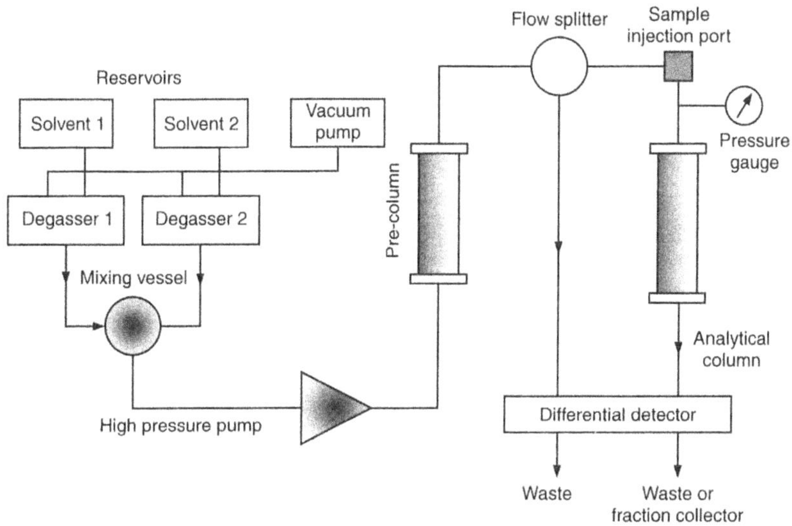

Fig. 3.9 Schematic representation of an HPLC Instrument

urce: © 1995 CHP.

strumentation Solvents must be degassed to eliminate formation of bubbles. The .mps provide a steady high pressure with no pulsating, and can be programmed to vary ɜ composition of the solvent during the course of the separation (see Fig. 3.9). The [uid sample is introduced into a sample loop of an injector with a syringe. When the ɔp is filled, the injector can be used to inject the sample into the stream by placing the mple loop in line with the mobile phase tubing. The presence of analytes in the column fluent is recorded by detecting a change in refractive index, UV-VIS absorption at a set ıvelength, fluorescence after excitation with a suitable wavelength or electrochemical ;ponse. Mass spectrometers can also be interfaced with liquid chromatography to ɔvide structural information and help to identify the separated analytes.

3 QUALITATIVE ANALYSIS OF ORGANIC COMPOUNDS

ıalysis of an organic compound first involves the detection of elements. The elements mmonly present in organic compounds are carbon, hydrogen, oxygen, nitrogen, logens, sulphur and phosphorus. Carbon and hydrogen are normally detected by ongly heating a mixture of the organic compound and cupric oxide.

Nitrogen, sulphur and halogens in the organic compounds are detected by Lassaigne's

$$\longrightarrow NaCN + Na_2S + NaX \text{ (X = Cl, Br or I)}$$

If both, nitrogen and sulphur, are present in the organic compound, they may g sodium thiocyanate (NaSCN), which in the presence of excess sodium, forms sodi cyanide and sodium sulphide.

$$Na + C + N + S \longrightarrow NaSCN$$

$$NaSCN + 2Na \longrightarrow NaCN + Na_2S$$

A systematic analysis of the products obtained from the sodium fusion test enab us to identify the elements present in the organic compound of interest.

A small piece of sodium is heated in a small, dry fusion tube till the sodium melts. T fusion tube is removed from the flame, the organic compound (about 50–60 mg) is add and the tube heated strongly for 2-3 minutes. After cooling, the tube is carefully brol in a mortar containing water, when the sodium salts formed in the above reactions (NaCN, Na_2S, NaX or NaSCN) dissolve. Excess of sodium reacts with water to give sodi hydroxide. This alkaline solution is called Lassaigne solution. The solution is first filte to remove insoluble materials and the clear filtrate is used for further testing.

1. ***Tests for Nitrogen*** The filtrate from the sodium fusion test is heated to boiling w ferrous sulphate crystals and then acidified with dilute sulphuric acid. If nitrogen present, a blue precipitate is formed.

The reaction involved in this test are as follows. Sodium cyanide on reaction w ferrous sulphate gives sodium ferrocyanide. On heating, some of the ferrous salt oxidised to the ferric salt and this reacts with sodium ferrocyanide.

$$6NaCN + FeSO_4 \longrightarrow \underset{\text{Sodium ferrocyanide}}{Na_4Fe(CN)_6} + Na_2SO_4$$

$$3Na_4Fe(CN)_6 + 2Fe_2(SO_4)_3 \longrightarrow \underset{\text{Prussian blue}}{Fe_4[Fe(CN)_6]} + 6Na_2SO_4$$

2. ***Test for Sulphur*** (i) Lassaigne's solution is first acidified with acetic acid and le acetate solution is added to it. A black precipitate of lead sulphide indicates the preser of sulphur.

$$(CH_3COO)_2Pb + Na_2S \longrightarrow \underset{\text{Black ppt}}{PbS} + 2CH_3COONa$$

(ii) Lassaigne's solution is treated with sodium nitroprusside solution. A violet colo indicates the presence of sulphur. This colour slowly fades on standing.

$$Na_2S + Na_2Fe(CN)_5NO \longrightarrow \underset{\text{Violet}}{Na_4[Fe(CN)_5NOS]}$$

If sulphur is present along with nitrogen and sodium thiocyanate is formed duri fusion due to insufficient sodium, then a blood red colouration appears on heating w ferrous sulphate, which is invariably contaminated with ferric sulphate

white precipitate soluble in ammonia shows chlorine, a yellowish precipitate, sparingly luble in ammonia indicates bromine and a yellow precipitate insoluble in ammonia ows the presence of iodine.

$$NaX + AgNO_3 \longrightarrow AgX + NaNO_3$$

Test for Phosphorus Phosphorus is detected by fusing the organic compound with dium peroxide followed by extraction with water. This aqueous solution is boiled with ncentrated nitric acid followed by the addition of ammonium molybdate solution. A llow solution or precipitate indicates the presence of phosphorus. The yellow precipitate of ammonium phosphomolybdate $[(NH_4)_3PO_4.12MoO_3]$.

4 QUANTITATIVE ANALYSIS

ıce we have qualitatively determined the presence of various elements in an organic mpound, we shall have to quantitatively determine the proportions (or percentages) of se elements in the compound. We shall now discuss the principles involved in antitative determinations (estimations) of elements in organic compounds.

4.1 Carbon and Hydrogen Estimation

known mass of the organic compound is heated in a current of dry oxygen (free from bon dioxide) in the presence of cupric oxide, till all the carbon is oxidised to carbon ıxide and all the hydrogen is oxidised to water.

$$\text{Organic compound} + O_2 \xrightarrow[\text{Heat}]{\text{Excess CuO}} x\,CO_2 + \frac{y}{2}H_2O$$

Water and carbon dioxide thus produced are absorbed in U-tubes; the one containing ıydrous calcium chloride or anhydrous magnesium perchlorate is for absorbing water d the other, having a strong solution of potassium hydroxide or ascarite (NaOH-CaO), or absorbing carbon dioxide. The containers (with the absorbents) are weighed before combustion is performed. The increase in the mass after the experiment would give amount of water and carbon dioxide produced.

Let the mass of the organic compound taken be W g, increase in the calcium chloride tube (i.e. mass of water formed) be W_1 g, and increase in mass of potash U-tube be g (i.e. mass of CO_2 formed).

$$\text{Percentage of carbon} = \frac{12}{44} \times \frac{W_2}{W} \times 100$$

18 g of $H_2O \equiv 2$ g of hydrogen.

i.e. 18 g (Mol. wt. of H_2O) of H_2O constitutes 2 g of hydrogen.

Kjeldahl's method.

1. ***Dumas' Method*** A known mass of the organic compound is heated with cupric o› in an atmosphere of carbon dioxide. The carbon and hydrogen are oxidised to car dioxide and water, respectively while nitrogen is set free. If any oxide of nitroge produced during this process, it is reduced to free nitrogen by passing over a he copper gauze. This gaseous mixture is collected over an aqueous solution of potass hydroxide. All gases except nitrogen are absorbed in the solution. The volume of the collected is measured and this is equivalent to the nitrogen set free from the compo

Let the mass of the organic compound be Wg.

Volume of nitrogen collected = V_1 cm^3

Atmospheric pressure = P_1 mm Hg (after subtracting aqueous tension)

Room temperature = T_1 K

$$\text{Volume of nitrogen at STP} = \frac{P_1V_1 \times 273}{760 \times T_1} = A \text{ cm}^3$$

$$\text{Mass of } A \text{ cm}^3 \text{ of nitrogen at STP} = \frac{28 \times A}{22400} \text{ g}$$

$$\text{Percentage of nitrogen} = \frac{28 \times A \times 100}{22400 \times W}$$

2. ***Kjeldahl's Method*** The method was developed by the Danish chemist Jol Kjeldahl (1849–1900). Many nitrogen-containing organic compounds when heated stron with concentrated sulphuric acid are converted quantitatively into ammonium sulph

The solution is heated with excess of sodium hydroxide. The ammonia gas t liberated is absorbed in a known volume (taken excess) of a standard solution of an a The amount of acid neutralised can be determined by titrating the solution agains standard alkali solution and this would correspond to the amount of ammonia produc

$$\left\{\begin{matrix}\text{Organic compound}\\ \text{with nitrogen}\end{matrix}\right\} + H_2SO_4 \longrightarrow (NH_4)_2SO_4 \xrightarrow{2NaOH} Na_2SO_4 + 2NH_3 + 2H$$

$$2NH_3 + H_2SO_4 \longrightarrow (NH_4)_2SO_4$$

Let the mass of the organic compound taken be W g.

Volume of acid of normality N_1 neutralised by ammonia = V_1 cm^3

But 1000 cm^3 of normal ammonia ≡ 17 g of ammonia

≡ 14 g of nitrogen

V_1 cm^3 of N_1 of acid ≡ V_1 cm^3 of N_1 ammonia

$\frac{14}{} \times V_1 \times N_1$ g of nitrogen ≡ $\frac{14V_1N_1}{}$ g of nitrogen

ours) in the presence of silver nitrate in a special sealed tube known as Carius tube. The eating is done in a furnace, carbon and hydrogen are oxidised to carbon dioxide and ater while halogen forms a precipitate of silver halide (AgX). After filtration and ashing, the precipitate is dried and weighed.

Let the mass of the compound be W g.

Let the mass of the AgX formed be W_1 g.

Molecular mass of AgX ≡ Atomic mass of X

$$\therefore \quad \text{Mass of halogen in } W_1 \text{ g of AgX} = \frac{\text{Atomic mass of X} \times W_1}{\text{Molecular mass of AgX}} \text{ g}$$

$$\therefore \quad \text{Percentage of halogen} = \frac{\text{Atomic mass of X} \times W_1}{\text{Molecular mass of AgX}} \times \frac{100}{W}$$

.4.4 Other Elements

Estimation of Sulphur A known mass of organic compound is strongly heated in a ealed tube (Carius tube) with fuming nitric acid. Sulphur present in an organic compound oxidised (by fuming nitric acid) to sulphuric acid which is then quantitatively precipitated s barium sulphate by the addition of excess barium chloride. The precipitate is filtered, ashed, dried and weighed.

Let the mass of the organic compound be W g.

Let the mass of the precipitate be W_1 g.

233 g of $BaSO_4$ ≡ 32 g of sulphur

$$\therefore \quad \text{Percentage of sulphur} \equiv \frac{32}{233} \times \frac{W_1}{W} \times 100$$

Estimation of Phosphorus A known mass of the organic substance is heated with uming nitric acid. The phosphorus present is oxidised to phosphoric acid. The phosphoric cid thus obtained is treated with magnesia mixture (a solution containing magnesium hloride, ammonium chloride and ammonia) to give a precipitate $MgNH_4PO_4$ which on gnition is converted into $Mg_2P_2O_7$.

Let the mass of the organic compound be W g.

Mass of the $Mg_2P_2O_7$ obtained on ignition = W_1 g

222 g of $Mg_2P_2O_7$ ≡ 62 g of phosphorus

$$\text{Percentage of phosphorus} = \frac{62}{222} \times \frac{W_1}{W} \times 100$$

Estimation of Oxygen The percentage of oxygen in an organic compound is normally

3.5 DETERMINATION OF MOLECULAR MASS

Molecular mass of organic compounds is determined by a number of methods. Thi information becomes essential to fix the molecular formulae of compounds. We shall no discuss the principles of some of these methods.

3.5.1 Victor Meyer's Method

This is a convenient method for the determination of molecular masses of volatil substances. A known mass of a substance is converted into vapour. The vapour is mad to displace an equal volume of air, which can be collected over water.

Let the mass of the organic compound be W g

Volume of air displaced = V_1 cm^3

Pressure of the air = P mm Hg

Room temperature = T_1 K

Volume, V_2 of air displaced at STP,

$$\frac{P \times V_1 \times 273}{T_1 \times 760} = \text{volume of vapour at STP}$$

Thus, V_2 cm^3 of the vapour of the substance at STP weighs = W g

Therefore, 22400 cm^3 of vapour of the substance at STP should weigh

$$= \frac{W \times 22400}{V_2} g$$

$$\text{Molecular mass of the substance} = \frac{W \times 22400}{V_2}$$

3.6 CALCULATION OF EMPIRICAL AND MOLECULAR FORMULAE

The empirical formula of a compound is defined as the simplest formula that shows the ratio of the atoms of various elements in a molecule. This is normally calculated from the percentage composition of the elements in the molecule according to the following rules

1. The percentages of all the elements are divided by their respective atomic masses
2. The numbers thus obtained are divided by the lowest of the above numbers.
3. The quotients are normally whole numbers. If they are not whole numbers, they are converted to whole numbers by multiplication with a suitable common factor

Let us take an example where we need to calculate the empirical formula of an organic compound which has 61.00% of carbon and 11.88% of hydrogen. Now the sum of the

Carbon	61.00	$\frac{\;}{12} = 5.08$	$\frac{\;}{1.70} = 2.99$	3
Hydrogen	11.88	$\frac{11.88}{1} = 11.88$	$\frac{11.88}{1.70} = 6.9$	7
Oxygen	27.12	$\frac{27.12}{6.0} = 1.70$	$\frac{1.70}{1.70} = 1$	1

On the basis of simple whole number ratio the empirical formula is, therefore, C_3H_7O.

The molecular formula of a compound gives the actual number of atoms of each ment present in the molecule. The molecular formula may be the same as the empirical mula or a simple multiple of it.

Molecular formula = Empirical formula × n

$$\therefore \quad n = \frac{\text{Molecular formula}}{\text{Empirical formula}}$$

In the problem on empirical formula worked out earlier, if the molecular mass of the npound is 118, the value of n will be 2. This is because the empirical formula (C_3H_7O) ss is 59 and n = 118/59 = 2. The molecular formula is, therefore, $C_6H_{14}O_2$.

MODERN METHODS OF STRUCTURE ELUCIDATION

e rapid development of scientific instrumentation has progressed to a point that the nplete structure of a compound can be obtained in a matter of days. Molecular weights l molecular formulae are readily determined from mass spectrometry. The types of ctional groups present in a molecule are found from electronic, infrared and nuclear gnetic resonance spectroscopies. Finally, the complete three-dimensional structure of molecule, including bond lengths and bond angles is determined from x-ray diffraction. contrast to the classical methods discussed earlier these methods need very small ounts of the sample. All these methods have made the structure determination of a npound a much simpler task than it was a few decades ago. A detailed discussion of scope and application of these methods is beyond the scope of this book.

PHYSICAL PROPERTIES OF CHEMICAL COMPOUNDS

/sical properties are those properties that can be observed or measured without nging the identity of the material. These properties are important in order to provide omplete description of the material and to provide a means for the identification of the terial. Physical properties may be classified as extensive or intensive. Extensive 'sical properties are those which depend upon the amount of matter present such as ss, length and volume. Intensive physical properties are independent of the amount matter present. Density, melting point, boiling point, ductility, malleability, colour, stalline shape, and refractive index are examples of intensive physical properties.

liquid displaced is equal to the volume of the solid. If it is too difficult to measure mass and/or volume, the density of the solid could be determined indirectly. A solid wl is less dense than the liquid into which it is placed will float in the liquid. A solid wl is denser than the liquid into which it is placed will sink in the liquid. When the s and liquid have the same density, the solid will be suspended in the liquid. Since the s and liquid have the same density, the mass of a known volume of liquid can be measu and, thus, the density of the solid determined.

3.8.2 Boiling Point

The boiling point of a substance is the temperature at which the vapour pressure of liquid is equal to the atmospheric pressure. At this temperature the liquid changes t gas. Pure compounds have a definite boiling point. Impurities in the liquid elevate boiling point. The purity of a liquid can be estimated by comparing its boiling point v the boiling point of a pure sample of the substance. The boiling point is characteri of a substance and may be used to identify the substance. In addition, mixtures of liqu can usually be separated by distillation based upon their individual boiling points.

Procedures for Determination of Boiling Point There are several methods usec determine the boiling point. The choice of method depends on the amount of mate available. In order of decreasing amounts of sample required, we have:

(i) distillation
(ii) mini-scale
(iii) micro-scale

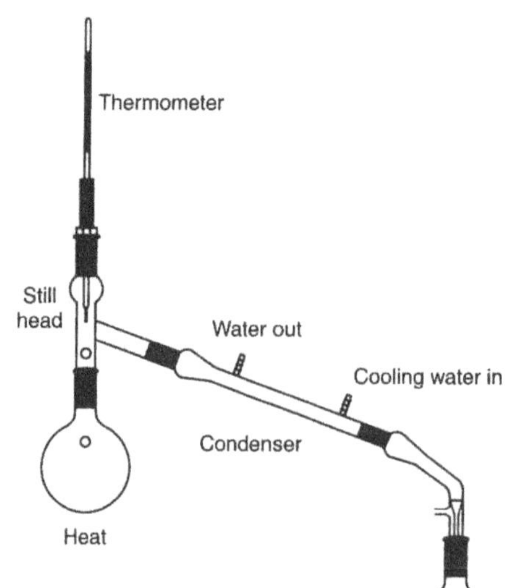

hich the distillation of the sample occurs. The distillation takes a reasonable amount of ne so that temperature reading can be done easily (Fig. 3.10).

i) *Mini-scale boiling point determination* This method is reasonably accurate : 0.5° C) and requires a reasonably small amount of sample (approx. 2 ml). The procedure nsists of bringing a small amount of sample in a mini test tube to a boil. Since the mperature of the vapour will not get appreciably higher than the boiling point as long it is in the tube with more liquid, the boiling point can be read as the highest mperature achieved as the vapour condenses on the thermometer bulb. The process much the same.

- Put a boiling stone in the mini test tube
- Add about 2 ml of liquid
- Clamp in stand in the fume hood
- Insert thermometer into test tube with bottom of mercury bulb about $^1/_2$ to 1 inch above the liquid
- Carefully heat until the temperature remains constant
- Read temperature

i) *Micro-scale boiling point determination* This method is more accurate than dis-lation or mini-scale (± 0.2° C) and requires a small amount of sample (approx. 0.2 ml). The ocedure consists of determining the temperature at which the external pressure on the iling liquid is large enough to overcome the vapour pressure in a capillary tube inserted osed-side up in the liquid. When this happens, the vapour will condense and liquid will rise to the capillary (Fig. 3.11). Usually a melting-point apparatus is used to heat the sample.

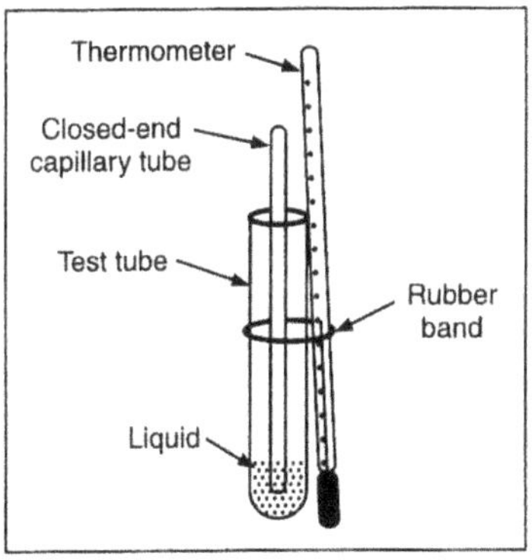

Fig. 3.11 Test Tube Assembly

- Using a micro pipette, fill about a half inch of a melting point tube with sample, insert a Bell capillary tube with open-end down.
- Push the Bell capillary down into the liquid with a section of a long capillary tube. The long capillary tube resting on top will keep the Bell capillary submersed. Make

the nucleation point for formation of vapour is at the capillary rim; the inside nearly filled with pure sample vapour by now).

- Turn off the heater.
- Carefully note the temperature at which the liquid *starts to rise into the invert Bell capillary* (as soon as the temperature drops below the boiling point unc these conditions, the vapour condenses to liquid and liquid fills the capillary).
- Record the temperature.

3.8.3 Melting Point

The melting point of a substance is the temperature at which the solid melts to becor a liquid. Pure compounds have a definite melting point. Impurities in the solid lower melting point. The purity of a solid can be estimated by comparing its melting point wi the melting point of a pure sample of the substance. The melting point is characteris of a substance and may be used to help identify the substance.

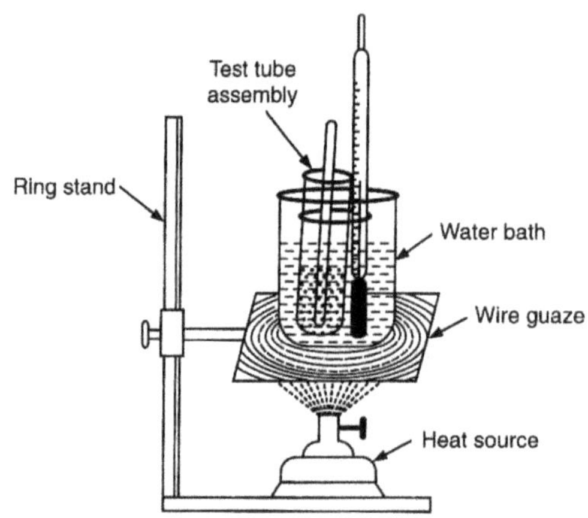

Fig. 3.12 Heating Assembly

The melting point, as a parameter, is used in research, development and quality contrc for purity determination or for the identification of different samples. The classical visu observation of a sample in a capillary tube is automated by recording the change of tl light transmittance during the melting process. The melting point or the melting range reported. The experimental method to determine melting point involves heating of a sma amount of the sample substance in a capillary tube attached to a thermometer, which immersed in a suitable bath of liquid. The bath is heated slowly. The temperature at whic the compound commences to liquify and at which it is completely liquid is recorded a the melting range (Fig. 3.12).

Nowadays a number of commercially useful apparatus are available. They require n

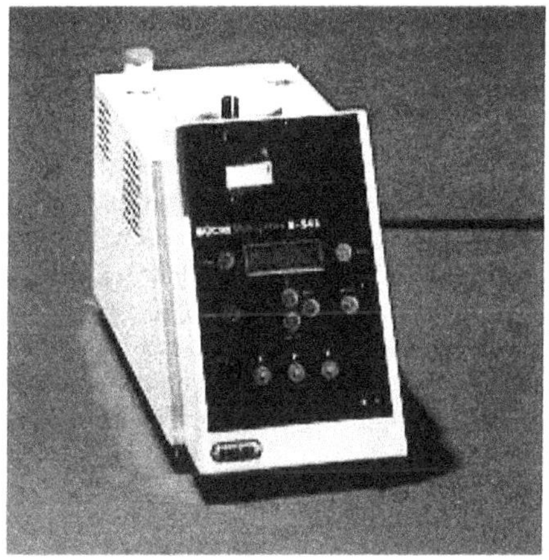

Fig. 3.13 Electrically Heated Melting Point Apparatus

PRACTICE QUESTIONS

1. Explain with an example the following terms:
   (i) Crystallisation (ii) Sublimation (iii) Simple distillation (iv) Fractional distillation (v) Distillation under reduced pressure (vi) Steam distillation (vii) Extraction with a solvent (viii) Chromatography.
2. (i) Will you get any precipitate if you add silver nitrate solution to chloromethane? If not, why?
   (ii) Write the chemical equations involved in the detection of nitrogen, halogens, sulphur and phosphorus, present in an organic compound.
3. 0.45 g of an organic compound gave on combustion 0.792 g of CO_2 and 0.324 g of water. 0.24 g of the same substance was Kjeldahlised and the ammonia formed was absorbed in 50.0 cm^3 of $(NH_4)_2SO_4$. The excess acid required 77.0 cm^3 of N/10 NaOH for complete neutralisation. Calculate the empirical formula of the compound.
4. 0.45 g of an organic compound containing only carbon, hydrogen and nitrogen on combustion gave 1.1 mg of carbon dioxide and 0.3 mg of water. What is empirical formula of the compound?
5. What is the empirical formula of the compounds whose analysis percentages are given below:
   (i) C = 41.35, H= 6.89, N = 24.12
   (ii) C = 60, H = 13.3
   (iii) C = 65.73, H = 15.06, N = 19.21
   (iv) C = 50.4, H = 9.25
   (v) C = 10, H = 0.84, Cl = 89.2
   (vi) C = 71.4, H = 3.78, N = 7.57, S = 17.3

of the compound gave 5.00 mg of silver chloride in Carius estimation. Find the molecı formula of the compound.

8. 0.246 g of an organic compound containing 58.33% of carbon and 4.06% of hydrogen g 22.4 cm^3 of nitrogen at STP. What is the empirical formula of the compound?
9. 0.246 g of an organic compound gave 0.198 g of carbon dioxide and 0.1014 g of water complete combustion. 0.37 g of the compound gave 0.638 g of silver bromide. Wha the molecular formula of the compound if its vapour density is 54.4?
10. 0.1 g of an organic monobasic acid gave 0.2545 g of CO_2 and 0.4428 g H_2O on combusti 0.122 g of the acid required for neutralisation 10 cm^3 of a N/10 alkali. Determine molecular formula of the acid.
11. An acid of molecular mass 104 contains 34.6% carbon and 3.85% of hydrogen. 3.812 of the acid required 7.33 cm^3 of 0.01 N NaOH for neutralisation. Suggest a structure the acid.
12. Write notes on: (a) Melting Point (b) Boiling point (c) HPLC (d) Thin-layer chromatograı (e) Fractional distillation.
13. What is boiling point? How do you determine the boiling point of a sample?

ł

LECTRON DISPLACEMENT EFFECTS

e changes or effects involved in the displacement of electrons in the substrate molecule referred as electron displacement effects. There are four types of displacement effects quently observed in organic molecules: (1) Inductive effect, (2) Electromeric effect, Resonance or Mesomeric effect and (4) Hyperconjugative effect.

I INDUCTIVE EFFECT

ıen an atom or group of atoms is substituted for another atom or group of atoms in nolecule the distribution of electron density changes. The effect of the new atom or ›up of atoms on this electron density distribution is termed the 'inductive effect' of the m or group. If the new atom or group of atoms (the substituent) is more electronegative n the one that it replaced, then electrons will be withdrawn from other parts of the lecule toward the new substituent. On the other hand, if the new substituent is less ctronegative than the group that it replaced then the electron density will increase in rest of the molecule. To illustrate inductive effect let us consider the following example.

$$\underset{4}{C} \longrightarrow \underset{3}{C} \longrightarrow \underset{2}{C} \longrightarrow \underset{1}{\overset{\delta^+}{C}} \longrightarrow \underset{4}{\overset{\delta^-}{Cl}}$$

In this example the bond, C_1—Cl, is a polar covalent bond. Due to greater ctronegativity of chlorine, the electron pair shared between C_1 and Cl is displaced ›ards chlorine atom. As a result chlorine acquires a small negative charge (δ^-) while becomes slightly positively charged (δ^+). The partially positively charged C_1 withdraws ctrons from C_1—C_2 bond, the positive charge on C_1 is partially neutralised while a small ;itive charge develops on C_2. The C_2 in turn may have effect on C_3 and C_3 in turn on of course in a decreasing manner. However, it should be noted that the effect on the ıstituent atoms of the chain is not the same. It decreases as we move away from the m involved in the initial polar bond and is negligible from fourth atom upward.

The process of electron shift along the length of atoms due to the presence of a polar ·alent bond in a molecule is known as *inductive effect*. The inductive effect is a *permanent* *ct* in the ground state of the molecule and operates through the single bond.

.1 Types of Inductive Effect

2. ***Electron-releasing Inductive Effect*** *(+ I effect)* Atoms or groups that have le electron attracting capacity than hydrogen and lose electrons towards a carbon are to have + I effect, for example, $(CH_3)_3C^+$, $(CH_3)_2HC^+$, $^+C_2H_5$, $^+CH_3$ (+ I effect decrea order).

4.1.2 Applications of Inductive Effect

1. ***Strength of Acids*** Changes in substituents can have a profound effect on acidity basicity of molecules, and the relative strengths of structurally related acids and b can be predicted on the basis of inductive effects of substituents.

(a) A more electronegative substituent X will increase the acidity of an oxy (or hydr acid by greater withdrawal of electron density from the oxygen–hydrogen bond. ' weakens the O—H bond and increases the positive charge on hydrogen. A similar ef is present for the conjugate base XO^-; here the presence of a more electronega substituent stabilises the anion by withdrawing charge from the oxygen and effecti delocalising the charge over more of the molecule. The pK_a values for the X(O)—(simple acids are:

Simple Acids	pK_a
Cl—OH	7.5
Br—OH	8.7
I—OH	10.7
HO—OH	11.8
H—OH	15.7
CH—OH	16.63

(b) The difference of strengths of aliphatic acids may be explained on the basis of induc effect, e.g. formic acid is strongly acidic than acetic acid.

H— COOH
Formic acid

CH_3—COOH
Acetic acid

(c) + I effect increases in the order H, CH_3, C_2H_5. H has little or no + I effect on the car of COOH of formic acid hence HCOOH loses H^+ easily. Methyl (CH_3) group has more effect than H hence COOH of CH_3COOH gives H^+ slowly. So HCOOH is strongly ac than H_3C—COOH.

2. ***Strength of Bases*** The basic strengths of different bases can be explained on basis of inductive effect, e.g. methyl amine is strongly basic than ammonia due to effect of CH_3 group on nitrogen; makes it richer in electrons and can more readily do the lone pair of electrons than ammonia.

3. ***Bond Lengths*** Increase in inductive effect decreases the bond length, e.g.

ıductive effect also plays a very important role in organic chemistry in understanding ıe cause of reactivity of many compounds.

.2 ELECTROMERIC EFFECT

.2.1 Introduction

. molecular polarisability effect occurring by an intramolecular electron displacement ,ometimes called the 'conjugative mechanism' and, previously, the 'tautomeric mechanism') ıaracterised by the substitution of one electron pair for another within the same atomic :tet of electrons. It can be indicated by curved arrows symbolising the displacement of .ectron pairs, as in:

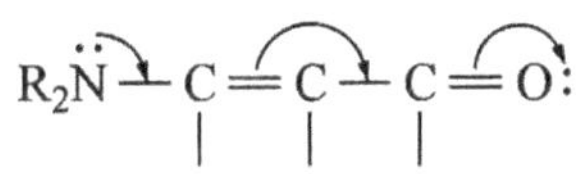

Electromeric effect represents the hypothetical electron shift:

$$R_2N-C=C-C=O \dashrightarrow R_2N^+=C-C=C-O^-$$

The effect involves instantaneous and complete transfer of a shared pair of electrons f the multiple bonds to one of the linked atoms, depending upon the requirements of ıe attacking reagent. This effect involves π-electrons.

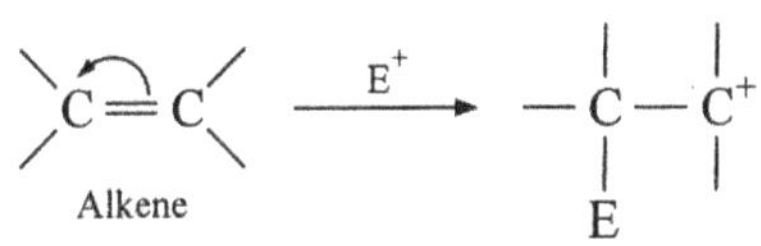

Electromeric effect is a temporary effect and comes into play when an attacking reagent :mands it. On removal of the reagent, the original electronic position is restored. This 'fect is indicated by 'E' and represented by a curved arrow showing the direction of ıifting of electron pair. When both inductive and electromeric effects operate at the same me the latter predominates. The effect may be either + E or – E accordingly, as the π ectrons are either transferred to the atom to which the attacking reagent is added or to .e other atom of the double bond.

.2.2 Applications of Electromeric Effect

+ *E Effect* Though ethylene is not ionic in character, when the attacking bromine .olecule approaches, bromine molecule is polarised under the influence of electrons and ectromeric shift of electrons to one of the carbons takes place.

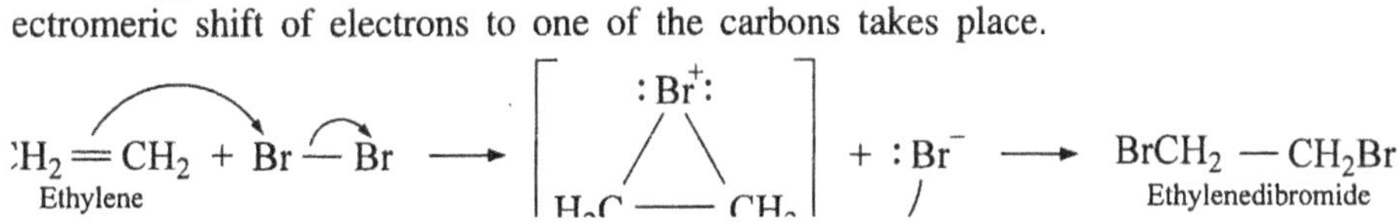

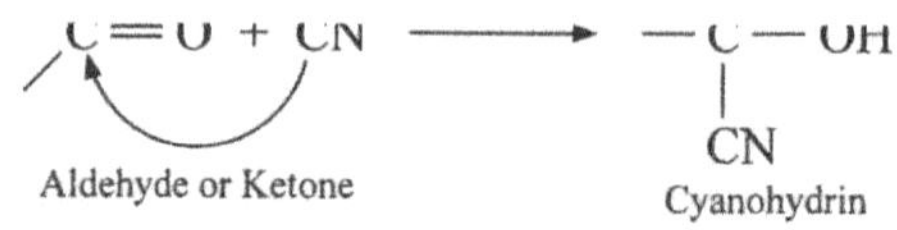

4.3 RESONANCE

4.3.1 Introduction

There are, however, molecules whose electronic distribution is inadequately represer by a single Lewis formula. In these cases, two or more Lewis formulae may be necess to satisfactorily represent the molecule. Resonance is a phenomenon involved when m than one Lewis formula is needed to adequately describe the electronic distribution molecule. This theory states that whenever a molecule or an ion can be represented two or more Lewis structures (contributing or canonical or resonance structures) differ only in the position of electrons (each of which explain most but not all the obser properties, i.e. chemical or physical properties), the actual structure of molecule or ioi resonance hybrid) will be somewhere in between the various possible contribut structures. The resonance structures (*contributing or canonical*) are not structures the actual molecule or ion; they exist only in theory. As such they can never be isola The actual structure is called *resonance hybrid* which is generally represented by putt double-headed arrows (↔) among the contributing structures. The resonance hybri an entirely new and individual structure and it neither oscillates between the vari contributing structures nor is in equilibrium with the contributing structures.

Resonance is an important feature of many organic molecules. It can have a profo influence on their structure, chemical reactions and physical properties.

For example, consider the sulphur dioxide (SO_2) molecule. Structural studies show t both S—O bonds in SO_2 are of equal length and strength. This electronic distributioi not explained by either single Lewis structure, but is explained when both Lewis formu are taken into consideration.

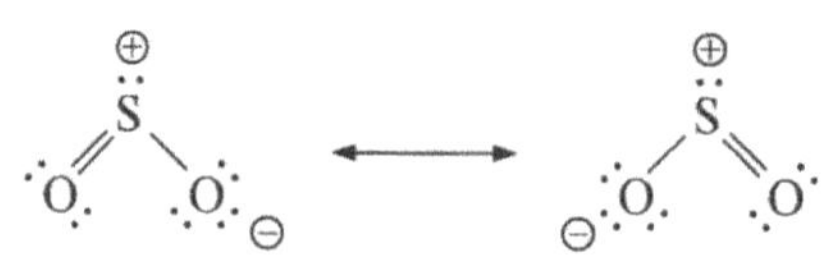

Resonance contributors of sulphur dioxide

Both Lewis structures are called resonance structures or resonance contributors. T actual molecule is not an equilibrium mixture of the imaginary resonance structures, rather a single unchanging composite structure called the resonance hybrid. Resonar hybrids are often represented by the 'partial-bond' or combined notation. The resonar

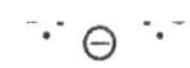

Resonance hybrid of sulphur dioxide

Fundamentally, the phenomenon of resonance is involved because of the inability of ngle Lewis structure to show *electron delocalisation* over the molecule. In fact, resonance often called delocalisation. For instance, in SO_2, the pi electron pair is delocalised or read over both S—O bonds and not localised in a single S—O bond. Thus, the existence f electron delocalisation in a molecule means that more than a single resonance structure ust be drawn to fully describe the electronic structure of the molecule. Further, since ectronic delocalisation is stabilising, the existence of resonance implies molecular abilisation. Generally, the more are the resonance contributors, the more stable is the olecule.

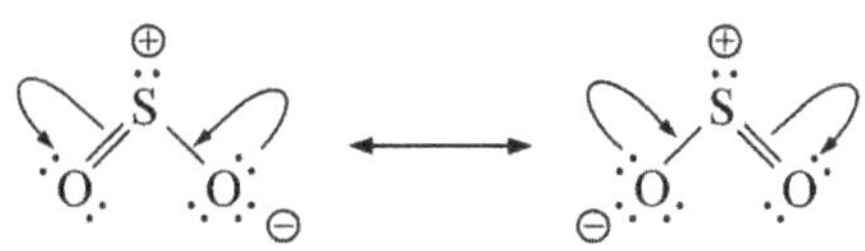

Resonance contributors of sulphur dioxide

Resonance structures differ only in the location of their π electrons; the atomic nuclei not move and the bond angles do not change. All resonance structures must contain ual numbers of electron pairs and/or unpaired electrons. Electronic movement denoted curved arrows can convert one resonance structue to another. For instance, the two sonance structures for SO_2 are interconverted by the electron movements shown.

Resonance in Benzene

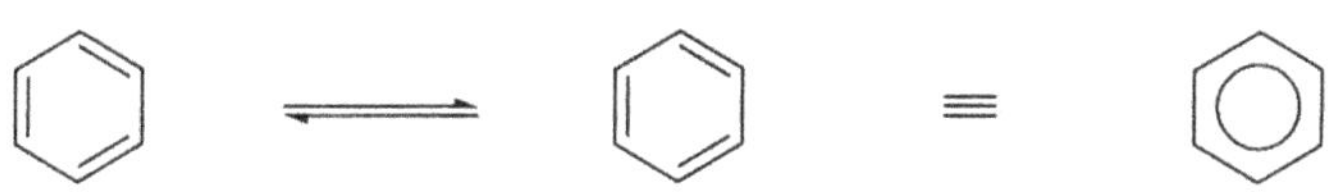

Contributors for benzene

Resonance hybrid of benzene

3.2 Conditions for Resonance or Rules for Writing Resonance Structures

ccording to the resonance or mesomerism theory, the various contributing structures ust satisfy the following conditions:

- Resonance structures exist only on paper; they have no real existence of their own.
- The various contributing structures should differ from each other only in the positions of electrons whereas the relative arrangement of atoms must be the same.

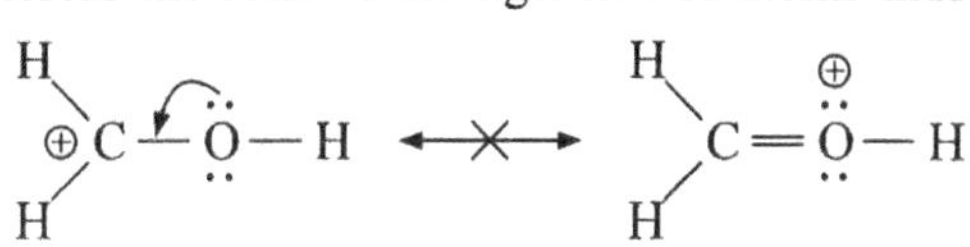

A B

- All resonance structures must have the same number of unpaired electrons.

C D

Resonance structure **C** is acceptable. Structure **D** is not acceptable because the carb(has ten valance electrons.

- The *more stable a structure is the greater is its contribution to the hybrid.* Structur(that are not equivalent *do not make equal contributions.*
- *The energy* of actual molecule is lower than the energy that might be estimated for ar contributing structure. *Nuclei do not change positions in space between resonan(structures*. Resonance structures differ only in the arrangement of valence electron

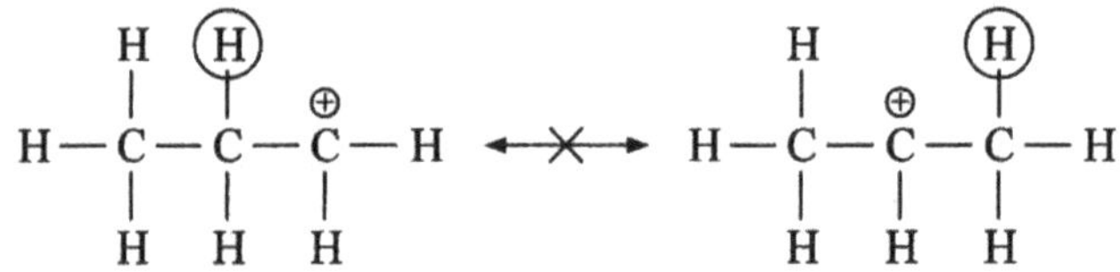

E **F**

- Both structures, **E** and **F**, are acceptable Lewis structures, but they are not relat(by resonance because the circled hydrogen atom has changed position in spac(
- Resonance structures are *interconvertible* by one or a series of electron shifts.

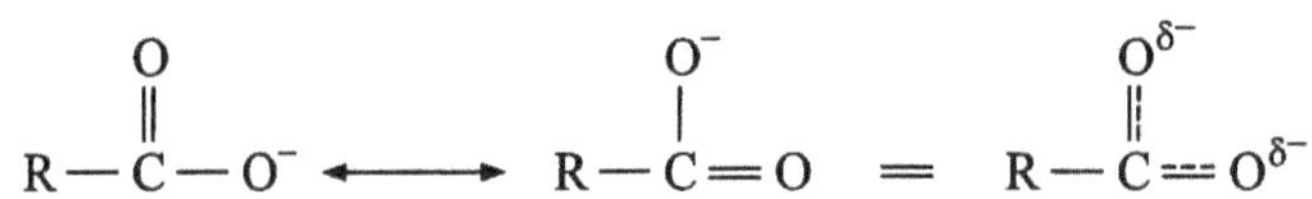

Contributors of carboxylate ion Resonance hybrid of carboxylate ion

4.3.3 Determination of Relative Stability of Resonance Structures

The following rules will help us making decisions about the relative stabilities of resonanc structures.

Resonance structures may or may not contribute equally to the resonance hybri Resonance structures contribute in proportion to their stability; that is, the more stabl the resonance structure, the greater its contribution to the hybrid. Thus, it is importa to evaluate the relative energies, and hence relative importance, of various resonanc contributors. In this regard, there are several situations to consider. These are detaile below with examples.

1. Equivalent resonance contributors have equal energies and, therefore, make an equ contribution to the hybrid. The larger the number of equivalent resonance structure the more stable the molecule. For instance, consider the allyl carbocation, stabilise by the existence of equivalent resonance structures.

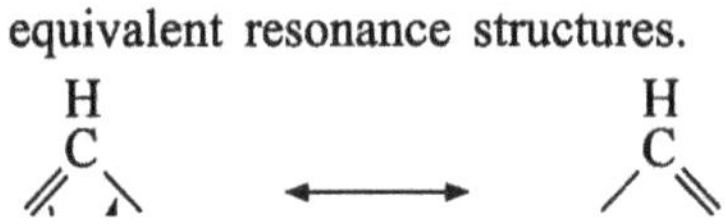

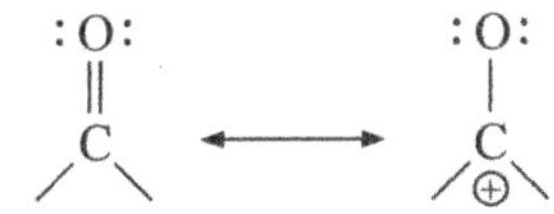

Major contributor Minor contributor

3. Contributors with formal negative charges on more electronegative atoms or formal positive charge on less electronegative atoms contain less energy than those with formal negative charges of less electronegative atoms or formal positive charges on more electronegative atoms. Both structures generally make a contribution to the hybrid, although unequal.

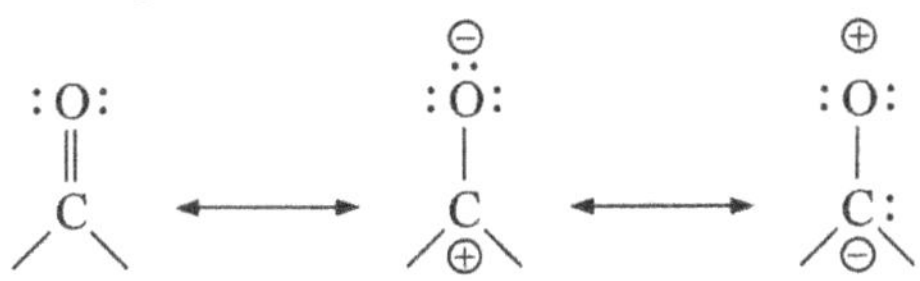

Major contributor Minor contributor Very minor contributor

4. Contributors with more bonds are more important than those with fewer bonds.

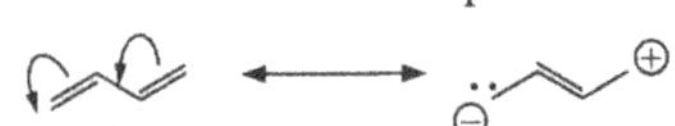

Major Minor

5. Contributors with a complete octet have a lower energy than those with an incomplete octet.

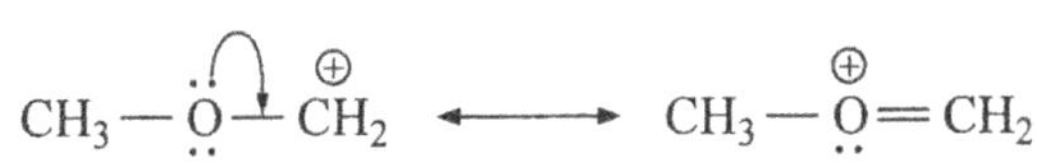

Major Minor

5. All atoms taking part in the resonance structure must lie in the same plane to maximise orbital overlap.

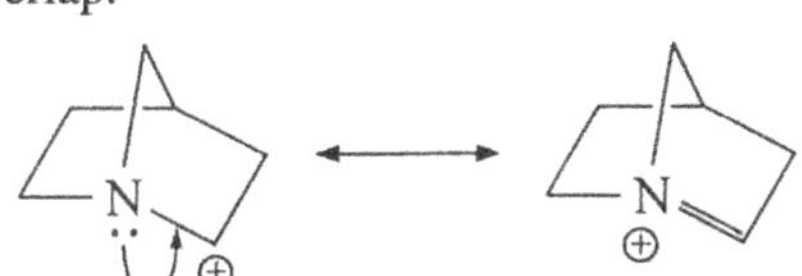

Major Minor

.4 Properties of Resonance Hybrid

Stability A *resonance hybrid* always has *lesser energy* and is more stable than any he contributing structures. The difference in energy of the resonance hybrid and most ıle contributing structure is called *resonance energy or delocalisation energy*. The re the resonance energy of a molecule, the more the stability.

or mesomeric effect. It involves overlap of its p or π orbitals with the p or π orbitals the rest of the molecular entity. Delocalisation is thereby introduced or extended, a electronic charge may flow to or from the substituent. The effect is symbolised by M Strictly speaking, the mesomeric effect operates in the ground electronic state of t molecule. When the molecule undergoes electronic excitation or its energy is increas on the way to the transition state of a chemical reaction, the mesomeric effect may enhanced by the electromeric effect. The mesomeric effect refers to the polarity produc in a molecule as a result of interaction between two π bonds or a π bond and a lone pa of electrons. This effect is also transmitted along a chain, like inductive effect.

Atoms which lose electrons towards a carbon atom are said to have (+) mesomer effect (+ M), e.g. Cl, Br, I, NH_2, OH, etc. Those atoms that draw electrons away from carbon atom are said to have a (–) mesomeric effect (– M), e.g. NO_2, CN, C=O, etc. is permanent and does not depend upon the presence of a reagent.

4.3.6 Applications

Resonance effect is of great importance in conjugated compounds. In such systems, th π electrons get delocalised as a consequence of mesomeric effect, giving a number resonance structures of the molecule.

For example, in a carbonyl group, the π electrons of C—O double bond get displace toward the oxygen atom. Thus gives the following structures:

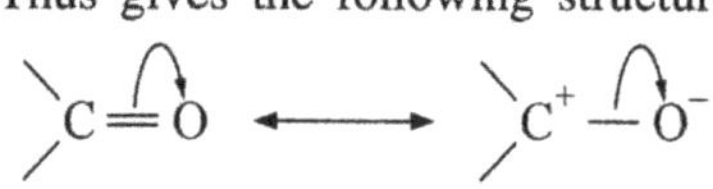

The stability of conjugated dienes could be explained basing on resonance phenomeno

$$CH_2=CH-CH=CH_2 \longleftrightarrow \bar{C}H_2-CH=CH-\overset{+}{C}H_2 \longleftrightarrow \overset{+}{C}H_2-CH=CH-\bar{C}H$$

Resonance contributing structures of a conjugated diene

$$|||$$

$$CH_2 \overset{\cdots}{=} CH \overset{\cdots}{=} CH \overset{\cdots}{=} CH_2$$

Resonance hybrid

4.4 HYPERCONJUGATIVE EFFECT

4.4.1 Introduction

Hyperconjugation is the stabilising interaction that results from the interaction of th electrons in a σ-bond (usually **C—H** or **C—C**) with an adjacent empty (or partially fille p orbital or an π orbital to give an extended molecular orbital that increases the stabilit of the system. Based on the valence bond model of bonding, hyperconjugation can b described as 'double bond–no-bond resonance phenomena'.

Hyperconjugation is a special type of resonance and was put forward by Baker an

Hyperconjugation phenomenon helps explaining the stability [illegible] carbocations, many addition, elimination and substitution reactions.

Example

Ethyl radical is explained by the following structures:

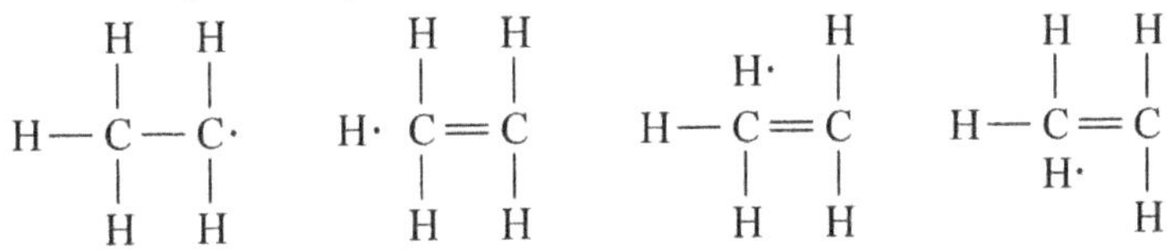

I II III IV

In Structures II, III and IV there is a double bond that joins two carbons and a hydrogen ›m holds the odd electron. Structures II to IV are called no-bond resonance structures. means that carbon–carbon bond has some double bond character and the odd electron partly accommodated by hydrogen atoms. A contribution from these unstable structures not important. However, due to existence of these hyperconjugative structures ethyl lical is more stable to methyl radical by 6 kcal /mole (104–95). In Structures II, III and there is no definite bond between one of the carbon atom and one of the hydrogen ›ms hence, hyperconjugation is also known as no-bond resonance. The stabilisation carbocations arises because the orbital interaction leads to the electrons being in a ver energy orbital (Fig. 4.1).

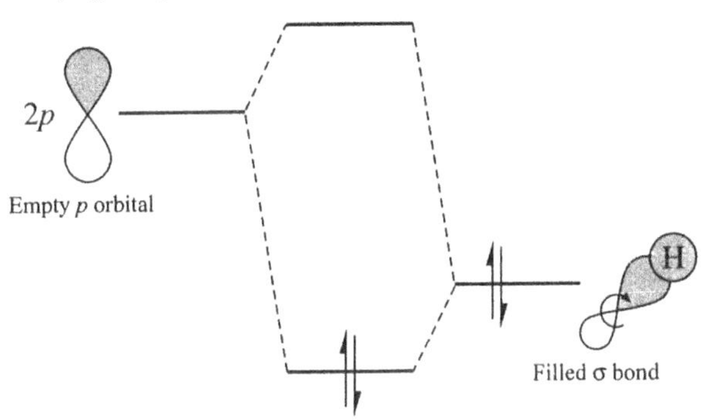

Fig. 4.1 Hyperconjugative Effect of Empty *p* Orbital with Hydrogen

The **C—C** σ-bond is free to rotate, and as it does so, each of the **C—H** σ-bonds in n undergoes the stabilising interaction. So the ethyl cation has 3 **C—H** σ-bonds that n be involved in hyperconjugation. The more hyperconjuagtion there is, the greater is e stabilisation of the system. For example, the *t*-butyl cation has 9 **C—H** σ-bonds that n be involved in hyperconjugation. Hence, $(CH_3)_3C^+$ is more stable than $CH_3CH_2^+$. ie effect is not limited to **C—H** σ-bonds, appropriate **C—C** σ-bonds can also be involved hyperconjugation.

The interaction between filled p orbitals and adjacent antibonding σ * orbitals is

4.5 THEORIES OF REACTION RATES

To understand how a chemical reaction takes place, the two theories were propo collision theory and transition state theory.

4.5.1 Collision Theory

According to collision theory, a chemical reaction occurs only when the molecule: reactants come nearer and collide with each other. During the collisions, the exis bonds will be disturbed or broken and new bonds will be formed between the molecu (Breaking up of the old bonds and formation of new bonds is a chemical reaction.) all collisions do not result in the formation of products.

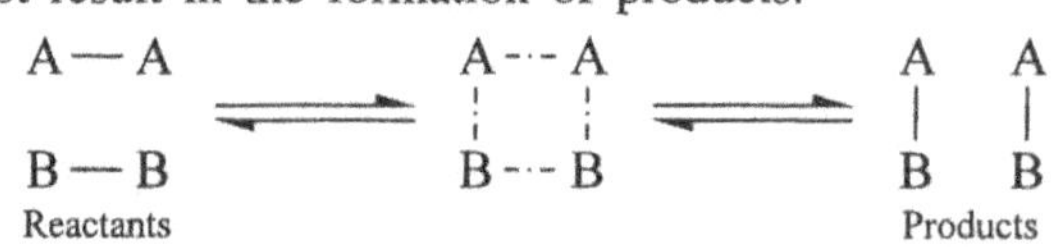

For collisions to be effective, there must be considerable force in the collisions. ' slower moving molecules do not have enough kinetic energy to react when they col and they bounce off one another and retain their identity. Only the molecules movin high speed have enough energy for collisions to result in a reaction. A reaction coordi diagram can explain the energy changes that take place during the course of a react

4.5.2 Reaction Coordinate Diagram

In a reaction coordinate diagram, the energy of the species involved in the reactio plotted against the progress of the reaction. The reaction coordinate diagram is represen in Fig. 4.2.

In order to be effective in bringing about the reaction, the collisions must fulfil following conditions:

1. ***The Colliding Particles must have Threshold Energy*** The molecules that do possess threshold energy can not give the products because the collisions are not effecti The minimum amount of additional energy required by the reactants to attain the thresh energy to give products is known as energy of activation (E_a). In other words, the activat energy of a reaction is the amount of energy needed to initiate the reaction. It represe the minimum energy needed to form an activated complex during a collision between reactants. In slow reactions, the fraction of molecules in the system moving fast eno to form an activated complex when a collision occurs is low, as a result most collisi do not produce a reaction. However, in a fast reaction this fraction is high and, theref

proper orientation to form an activated complex.

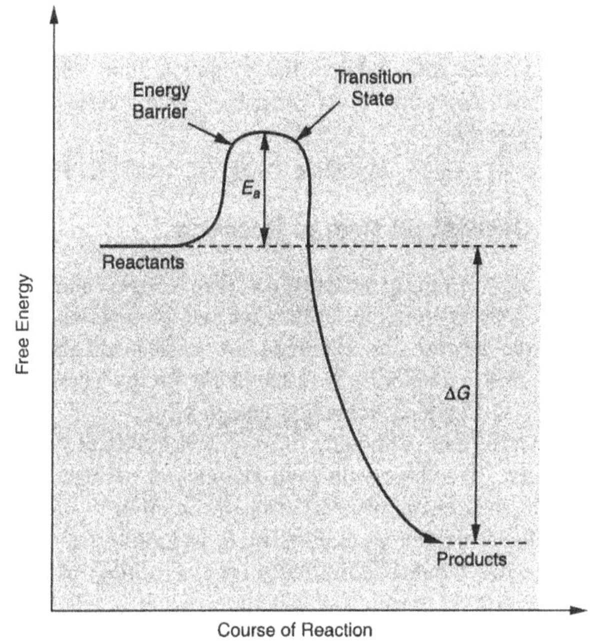

Fig. 4.2 Energy Diagram and Activation Energy Barrier

Activation energy = Threshold energy – Energy possessed by the reactant molecules

t is important to distinguish between the free energy of activation ($\Delta G^{\cdot}$), and the erimental energy of activation, E_a. The free energy of activation has both, an enthalpy nponent and an entropy component. The experimental energy of activation has only enthalpy component. The energy of activation is an approximate energy barrier to a ction. The true energy barrier to a reaction is given by free energy of activation, since ne reactions are driven by a change in enthalpy, some by a change in entropy, but most a change in both enthalpy and entropy.

he Colliding Particles must be Properly Oriented with respect to each other at the e of Collision If the orientations of the colliding molecules are proper, the products formed. If the orientation is not proper, the products do not form. The energy required poorly oriented molecules is more than the energy required for properly oriented ecules.

3 Transition State Theory

occurs at a potential energy maximum, which corresponds to the top of energy barr
and has an arrangement of atoms with partly broken bonds and partially formed r
bonds (see Fig. 4.2). Factors that stabilise the transition state relative to the reactа
facilitate the reaction and vice versa. On the other hand, if E_a were low the transition s
would be reached quite early.

$$\text{Reactants} \rightleftharpoons \text{Activated complex} \longrightarrow \text{Products}$$

4.5.4 Influence of Catalyst on Rate of Reaction

The activation energy (E_a) for an uncatalysed reaction is higher than that for a cataly reaction. The activation energy directly affects the rate of reaction, and the presence a catalyst speeds up the reaction by changing the mechanism and thus lowering activation energy. Figure 4.3, depicting two activation energy profile, clearly shows importance of enzymes in lowering activation energy (E_a).

This energy of activation can be thought of as a barrier or wall that must be overco for the reaction to occur. Reactions with high energies of activation (high wall/barri require the input of larger amounts of energy for the reaction to occur. The smaller activation energy, the lesser the energy needed for a reaction to occur. (Think of jump over a fence. A high fence would require more energy to jump over than a low fenc By lowering the barrier of a reaction (decreasing the amount of energy needed to get o the wall), enzymes work to increase the rate of a reaction.

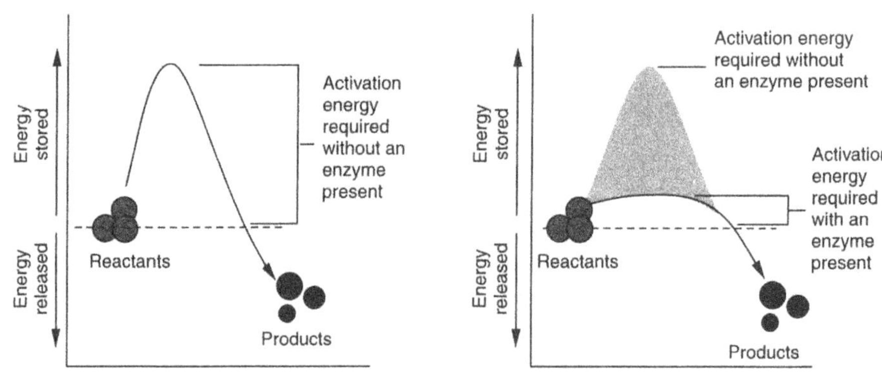

Fig. 4.3 A Schematic showing Effect of a Catalyst on Rate of Reaction

1. What are electron displacement effects? Enumerate various electron displacement effects.
2. Write the differences between:
   (a) Inductive effect and electromeric effect
   (b) Mesomerism and mesomeric effect
   (c) Resonance and hyperconjugation
3. What is hyperconjugation? Explain with examples.
4. Explain electromeric effect with examples.
5. Explain the terms resonance, resonance contributors, resonance hybrid critically with examples.
6. Arrange the following acids in the order of increasing strength:
   (a) CH_3COOH (b) Cl_3CCOOH (c) $Cl_2CHCOOH$ (d) $ClCH_2COOH$

5

REACTIVE INTERMEDIATES

5.1 INTRODUCTION

In a laboratory synthesis, a product may be prepared, isolated and purified, then us as the starting material for a subsequent step in the total sequence. Such products often termed as synthetic intermediates. In most of the organic reactions, the reacta first change into intermediate substances, which ultimately give the product. Su intermediates are known as reactive intermediates. The reactive intermediates are qu unstable and their half-lives range from a fraction of a second to several minut Although all the intermediates cannot be isolated, yet their existence is proved spectroscopic studies. The most important of reactive intermediates are: (1) Free radic (2) Carbocations, (3) Carbanions, (4) Carbenes, and (5) Nitrenes.

5.2 FREE RADICALS

An atom or a group of atoms, which contains one or more odd or unpaired electron, called a free radical. It is denoted by putting a dot (·) against the symbol of atom or gro of atoms, for example, Cl·, H_3C·, etc.

5.2.1 Formation

Free radicals are formed by the homolytic bond dissociation of a covalent bond. Th are produced by the following methods:

1. ***Thermal Decomposition*** Free radicals are produced by thermal decomposition compounds containing weak bonds, for example

$$\underset{\text{Tetraethyl lead}}{(C_2H_5)_4\,Pb} \xrightarrow{600^\circ C} \underset{\text{Ethyl free radical}}{4H_5C_2^{\cdot}}$$

2. ***Photochemical Decomposition*** When molecules absorb visible or UV light, they g sufficient energy, which can break the chemical bonds homolytically to form free radic for example

.2.2 Properties

1. Free radicals are formed by homolytic fission.
2. They are neither positively charged nor negatively charged. Hence they are electrically neutral.
3. They are short-lived species.
4. They are paramagnetic due to the presence of an unpaired electron.
5. They are highly reactive to pair up the odd electron.
6. They are less stable.
7. They do not undergo rearrangements.

.2.3 Reactions

ree radicals undergo the following chemical reactions:

Substitution Reactions Free radicals undergo substitution reactions, in which a free ıdical substitutes for another free radical, for example

$$CH_4 + Cl\cdot \longrightarrow H_3CCl + H\cdot$$

Combination One free radical combines with another free radical to get octet ɔnfiguration, for example

$$H_3C\cdot + \cdot CH_3 \longrightarrow CH_3 - CH_3$$

Addition Free radical may be added to the unsaturated carbon atoms. For instance, ıe presence of peroxides, which yield free radicals readily, initiates addition of HBr to kenes, for example

$$HBr + H_2C = CH_2 \longrightarrow H_3C - CH_2Br$$

Disproportionation In this reaction, one free radical abstracts a hydrogen atom from ıother free radical, for example

$$\cdot C_2H_5 + \cdot C_2H_5 \longrightarrow C_2H_6 + C_2H_4$$

Decomposition A free radical may decompose to give a neutral molecule and another ee radical, for example

$$C_2H_5COO\cdot \longrightarrow \cdot C_2H_5 + CO_2$$

.2.4 Alkyl Free Radicals

he free radicals in which free radical character (possessing of odd or unpaired electron) associated with carbon atom, for example

$$H_3C\cdot,\quad H_5C_2\cdot$$

Methyl free radical Primary free radical Secondary free radical |

CH_3

Tertiary free radical

2. ***Structure of Alkyl Free Radical*** The geometry of the free radicals has not bee established clearly, but it is believed that the carbon free radicals are either pyramidal ‹ planar. The carbon atom having odd electron is sp^2 hybridised. The three coplanar hybr: orbitals are involved in the formation of three bonds with three alkyl groups or hydroge atoms. The unhybridised p_z orbital lies in a plane at a right angle to the plane of hybri orbital that carries the odd electron.

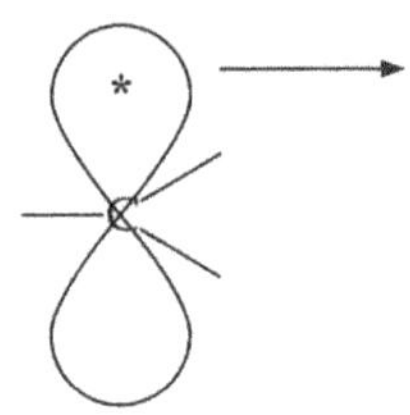

p_z Orbital associated with odd electron

3. ***Stability of Alkyl Free Radicals*** The relative stability of alkyl free radicals : determined from homolytic bond dissociation energy values.

$$CH_3-H \longrightarrow \underset{\text{Methyl free radical}}{H_3C\cdot} + H\cdot \qquad \Delta H = 104 \text{ kcal/mole}$$

$$CH_3CH_2-H \longrightarrow \underset{\text{Primary free radical}}{CH_3H_2C\cdot} + H\cdot \qquad \Delta H = 98 \text{ kcal/mole}$$

$$CH_3\overset{\displaystyle CH_3 \atop |}{C}H-H \longrightarrow \underset{\text{Secondary free radical}}{CH_3H\overset{\displaystyle CH_3 \atop |}{C}\cdot} + H\cdot \qquad \Delta H = 95 \text{ kcal/mole}$$

$$H_3C-\overset{\displaystyle CH_3 \atop |}{\underset{\displaystyle | \atop CH_3}{C}}-H \longrightarrow \underset{\text{Tertiary free radical}}{H_3C-\overset{\displaystyle CH_3 \atop |}{\underset{\displaystyle | \atop CH_3}{C}}\cdot} + H\cdot \qquad \Delta H = 91 \text{ kcal/mole}$$

The amount of energy needed to form various classes of radicals decreases in the orde methyl free radical > primary free radical > secondary free radical > tertiary free radica This implies, more energy is needed to make a primary free radical than a secondary one

If lesser energy is needed to form one radical than another, it implies that relative t the alkane from which it is formed this radical contains *lesser energy* than the other, i.e it is more stable. So the order of stability of free radicals is 3° > 2° > 1° > methyl fre

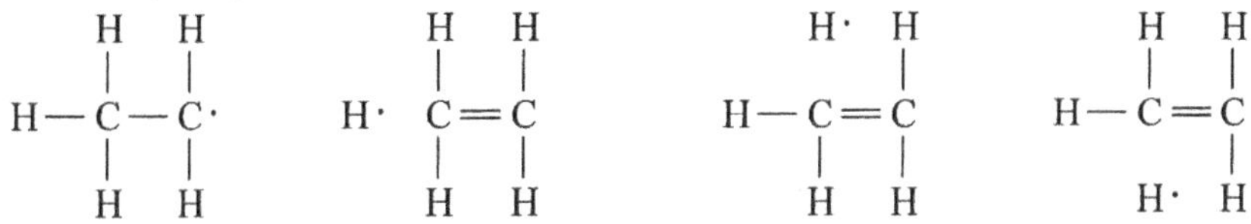

I II III IV

The larger the number of contributing structures *more extensive the delocalisation* of e odd electron and hence greater the stabilisation of the radical.

3 CARBOCATIONS

arbocation is a group of atoms that contains a carbon atom bearing only six electrons, r example, H_3C^+, $H_5C_2^+$, etc.

3.1 Classification

arbocations are classified into four groups on the basis of nature of carbon bearing posi- ve charge. These are methyl cation, primary cation, secondary cation and tertiary cation.

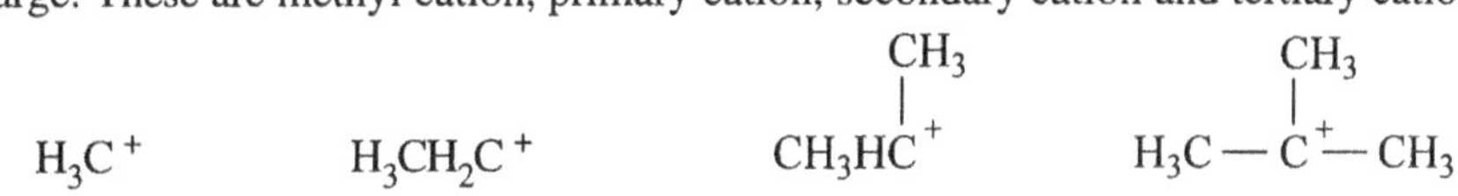

Methyl carbocation | Ethyl carbocation (Primary carbocation) | Isopropyl carbocation (Secondary carbocation) | Tertiary butyl carbocation (Tertiary carbocation)

3.2 Formation

arbocations are produced by heterolytic cleavage of a covalent bond. These are oduced by the following methods:

(i) *Heterolysis of a polar covalent bond*

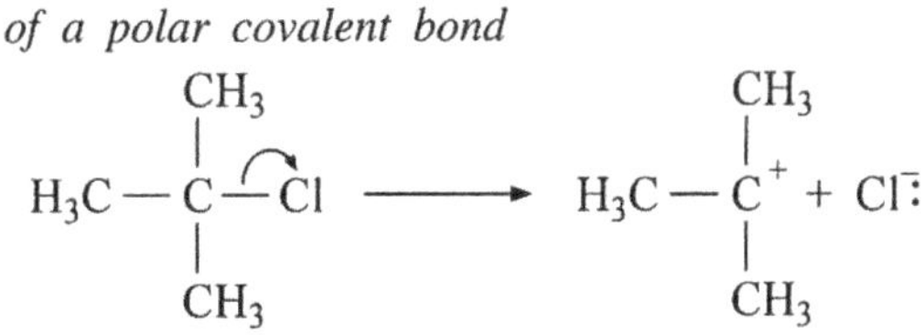

Tertiary butyl chloride — Tertiary butyl carbocation

(ii) *Protonation*

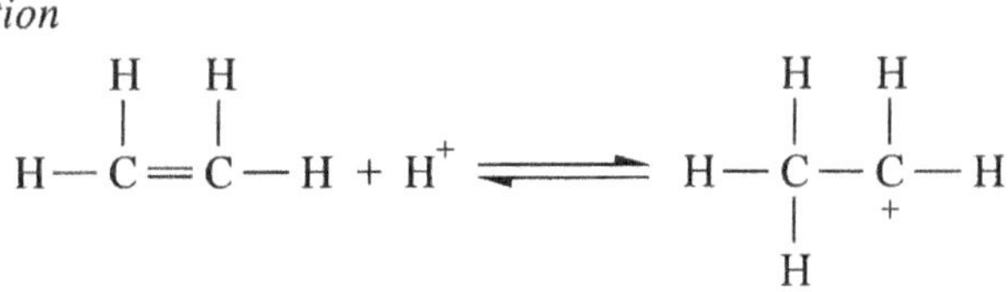

2. They are short-lived.
3. They are highly reactive and get octet configuration for stability.
4. They are positively (+ve) charged.
5. They are less stable.
6. They undergo rearrangements.

5.3.4 Structure

The positively charged carbon of the carbocation is in sp^2 state of hybridisation. Tł three sp^2 hybrid orbitals lie in the same plane and are involved in the formation of thre sigma covalent bonds with other atoms or groups. The unhybridised p_z orbital remair vacant. Thus, the carbocation has a flat structure. The bond angle around the positivel charged carbon is nearly 120°.

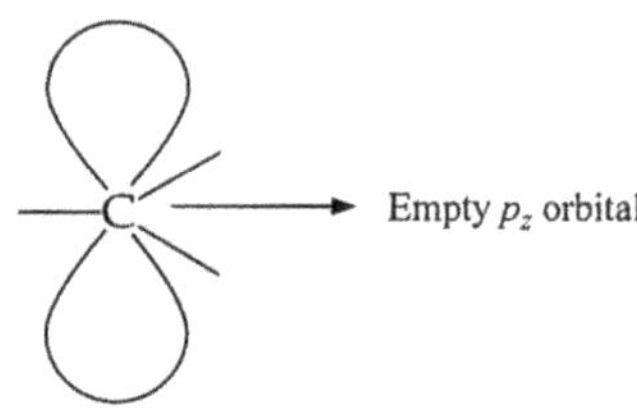

5.3.5 Stability

The relative stability carbocations on the basis of heterolytic dissociation energy value is 3° > 2° > 1° > methyl. Inductive effect and hyperconjugation can explain this order c stability. The carbocation is a positively charged species. The stability of a charge system is increased by dispersal of the charge. An electron-releasing substituent (alky groups) reduce the positive charge at the electron-deficient carbon, thus stabilise carbocation. The more the number of alkyl groups, the greater the dispersal of positiv charge and, therefore, more the stability of carbocation. For instance, 3° carbocation i having three alkyl groups attached to the +ve carbon is more stable than a secondar carbocation with two alkyl groups.

Greater electron flow   Less electron flow

The relative stability of these carbocations may be explained partly on the basis o hyperconjugation. There are only four hyperconjugative forms from a 1° carbocation while the 3° butyl carbocation can exist in 10 canonical forms. Since the greater th number of canonical forms the greater is the stability, 3° butyl carbocations would be mor stable than primary.

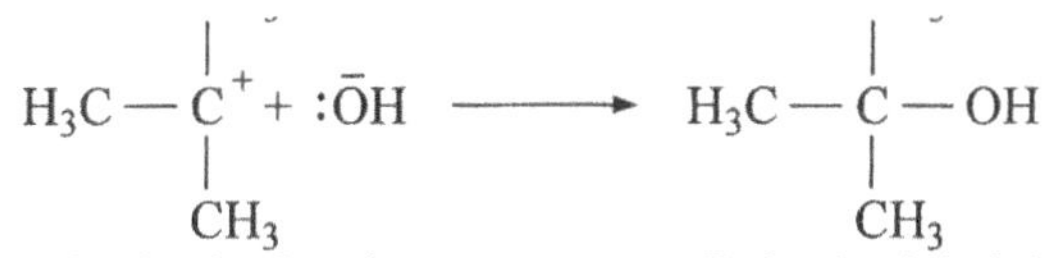

Tertiary butyl carbocation Tertiary butyl alcohol

Elimination of a Proton A carbocation may expel a proton to form an alkene.

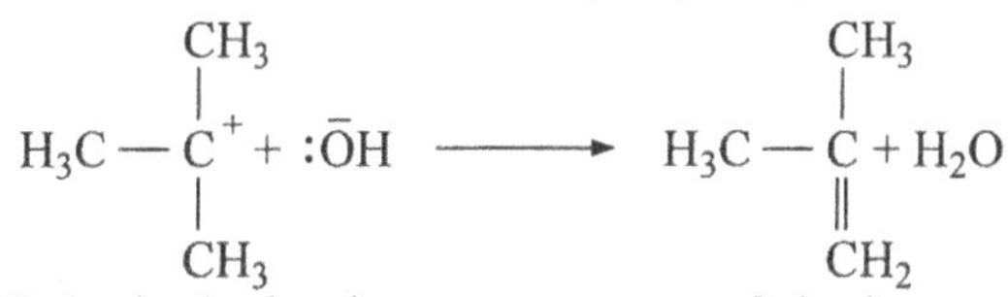

Tertiary butyl carbocation Isobutylene

Rearrangement If the structure permits a carbocation may undergo rearrangement to rm a more stable carbocation either by hydride shift (a migration of hydrogen with a ir of electrons) or by alkyl shift (migration of an alkyl group with a pair of electrons).

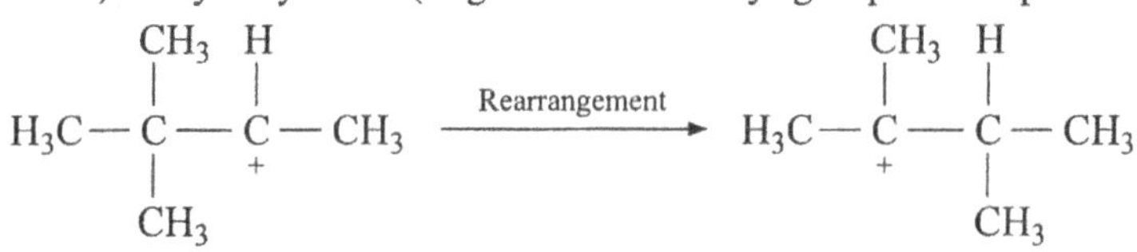

Secondary carbocation Tertiary carbocation

4 CARBENES

irbenes are highly reactive neutral chemical species in which the carbon atom is having electrons in the valence shell out of which two are unshared, e.g. H_2C:, Cl_2C:, etc.

4.1 Types

irbenes may exist in two distinct states:

Singlet Carbenes In these carbenes the unshared electrons are paired. Both electrons in same orbital, hence singlet carbenes does not have magnetic moment.

Triplet Carbenes Carbenes in which the unshared electrons are not paired. A triplet rbene has a permanent magnetic moment.

4.2 Generation

irbenes are produced during the following organic reactions:

Thermal or Photochemical Decomposition Diazomethane decomposes to yield me-ylene.

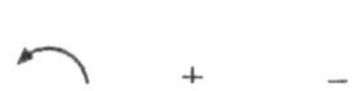

followed by the loss of a nucleophile from the same carbon leads to form carbene

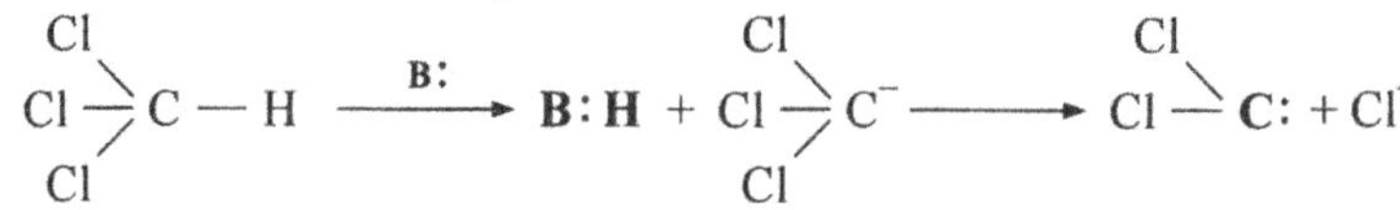

5.4.3 Structure

In singlet carbenes, the central carbon is in a state of sp^2 hybridisation. Of the three hybrid orbitals, two are used in forming two single bonds with the monovalent atom groups attached to carbon. The third sp^2 orbital contains the unshared pair of electi while the unhybridised p orbital is empty.

In triplet carbenes, the central carbon is in a state of sp hybridisation. The twc hybrid orbitals are used in forming two single bonds with the two monovalent atom groups attached to carbon. The two unhybridised p orbitals contain one unshá electron each.

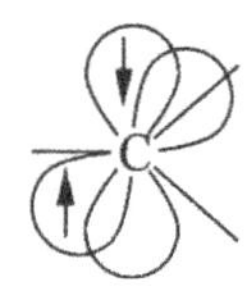

Triplet carbene

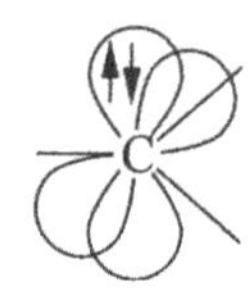

Singlet carbene

5.4.4 Properties

1. Carbenes are neutral chemical species.
2. They are highly reactive electrophilic entities.
3. Triplet carbenes are paramagnetic.

5.4.5 Reactions

Carbenes shows the following reactions.

1. ***Insertion into Single Bonds*** Carbenes undergo insertion reactions at C—H bonc hydrocarbons, e.g. CH_2 reacts with propane to give normal butane and isobutane.

$$\underset{\text{Propane}}{CH_3-CH_2-CH_3} \xrightarrow{H_2C:} \underset{n\text{-Butane}}{CH_3-CH_2-CH_2-CH_3} + \underset{\text{Isobutane}}{CH_3-\overset{CH_3}{\overset{|}{CH}}-CH_3}$$

2. ***Addition to Multiple Bonds*** Carbenes add to olefines to give cyclopropane derivati

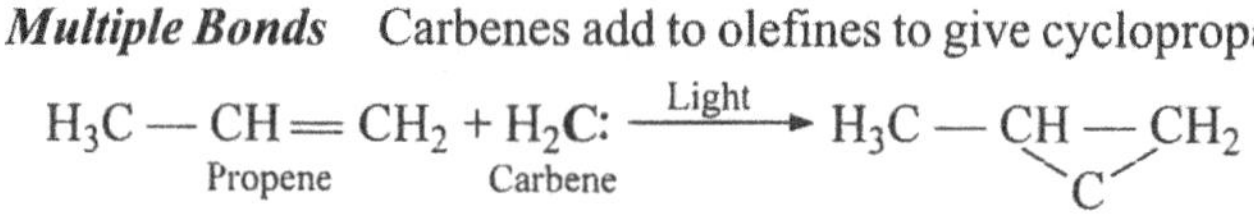

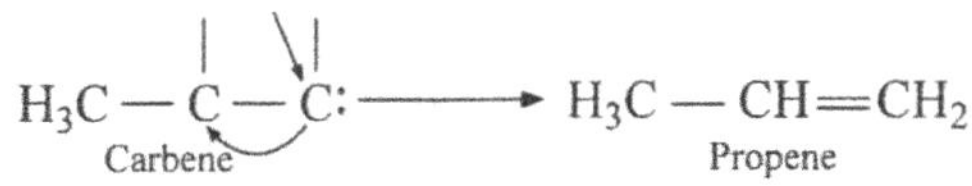

NITRENES

renes are highly reactive intermediates resembling carbenes. They have a monovalent ogen atom with a sextet of electrons. They are also called azenes and may be resented by R—N:

.1 Generation

: nitrenes are produced by the following processes:

'hermal and Photochemical Decomposition A wide variety of azides on decomposi- ı yield nitrenes.

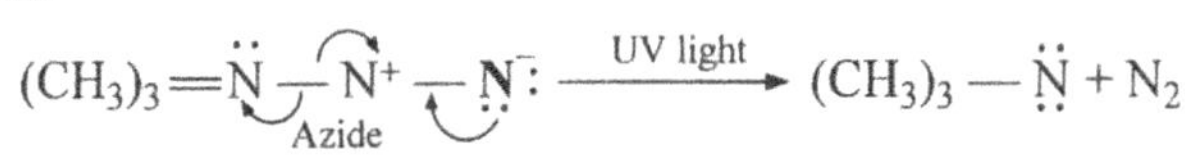

)xidation of Primary Amino Groups The removal of two hydrogen atoms (H^- and from an amino group forms a nitrene, e.g. lead tetraacetate on oxidation of the owing hydrazine derivative forms an amino nitrene.

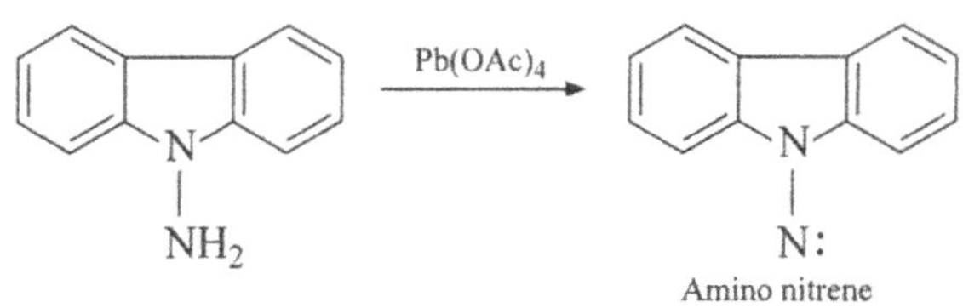

2 Reactions

enes undergo the following reactions:

\ddition Reactions The addition of nitrenes have been very little investigated, since most easily formed nitrenes undergo rearrangement and not addition. However, ition reactions occur when nitrene is formed from a precursor other than an azide. The ition is stereospecific with a singlet nitrene but non-specific with a triplet nitrene.

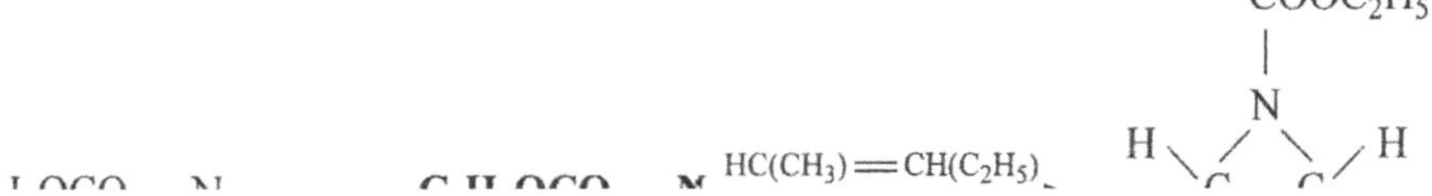

3. The Hofmann, Curtius, Lossen, Schmidt group of molecular rearrangements are reactions which proceed through the intermediate formation of nitrenes.

5.6 CARBANIONS

Carbanions are negatively charged species in which the carbon atom possess unshared pair of electrons and thus behave as bases, e.g. methyl carbanion (H_3(primary alkyl carbanion (RH_2C^-), etc.

5.6.1 Types of Alkyl Carbanions

There are different types of alkyl carbanions depending up on the number of alkyl gro attached to negatively charged carbon atom. These are

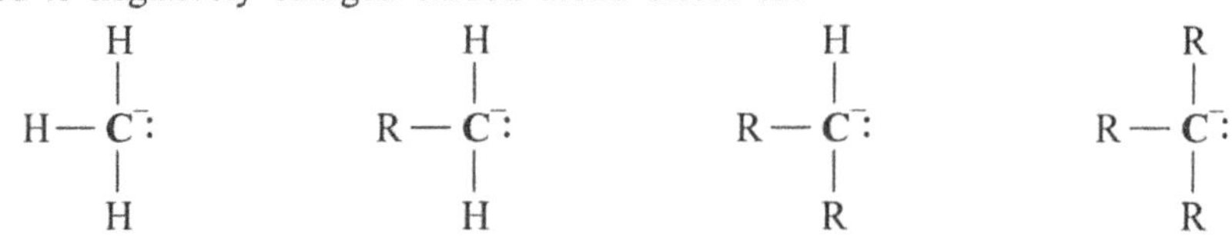

Methyl carbanion | Primary alkyl carbanion | Secondary alkyl carbanion | Tertiary alkyl carbanion

5.6.2 Structure

The central carbon (negatively charged) of carbanion is sp^3 hybridised. The four hybrid orbitals are directed to four corners of a tetrahedron. One of the hybrid orbit possesses an unshared pair of electrons.

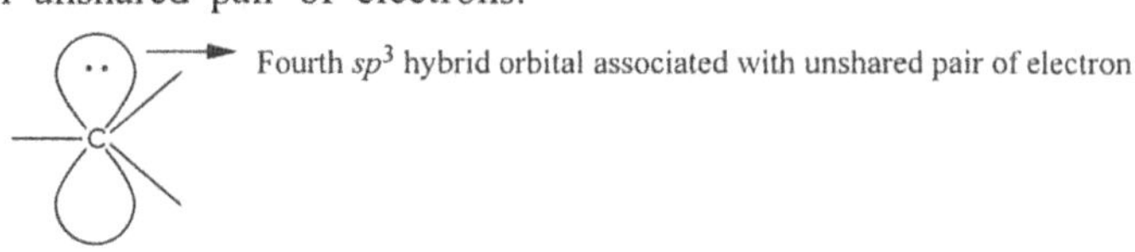

5.6.3 Formation

Carbanions are formed by heterolytic bond dissociation during the following reactio

- Heterolysis of organometallic compounds yield carbanions.

$$H_3C - Li \longrightarrow H_3C^{\bar{:}} + Li^+$$

- By heating alkynes having terminal hydrogen atoms with a base like amide io

$$CH \equiv CH + NaNH_2 \longrightarrow NH_3 + CH \equiv C{:}Na$$

rimary alkyl carbanions > Secondary alkyl carbanions > Tertiary alkyl carbanions. This er of stability is explained by considering inductive effect. When we move from methyl banion to tertiary alkyl carbanion the number of alkyl groups (electron releasing) is reased hence the stability is decreased.

.5 Properties

1. Carbanions are produced by heterolysis of a covalent bond.
2. They are short-lived.
3. They are highly reactive to give the unshared pair of electrons.
4. They are relatively charged.
5. They are less stable.

.6 Reactions

banions undergo the following reactions:

ddition Reactions The following addition reactions proceeds through the interme-e formation of carbanions:

Aldol condensation Two molecules of an aldehyde or a ketone having α-hydrogen ns undergo self-condensation in presence of dilute base or dilute acid at room perature to form product called aldol (β-hydroxy aldehyde or ketone). This reaction hrough intermediate carbanion mechanism and is represented below:

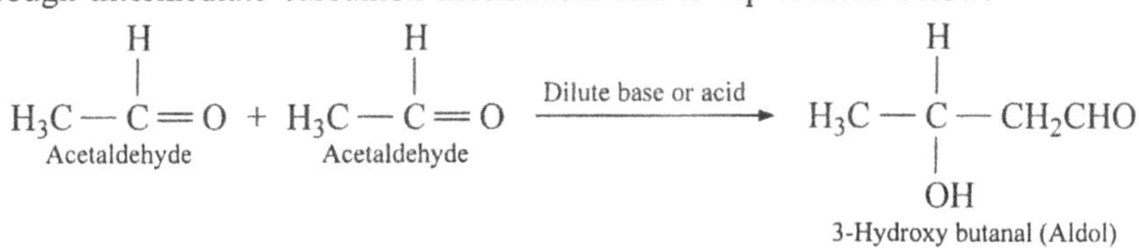

Perkin condensation Aromatic aldehydes on reaction with acid anhydrides in sence of base yields α,β-unsaturated acid. The reaction is known as Perkin reaction ch proceeds via carbanion mechanism.

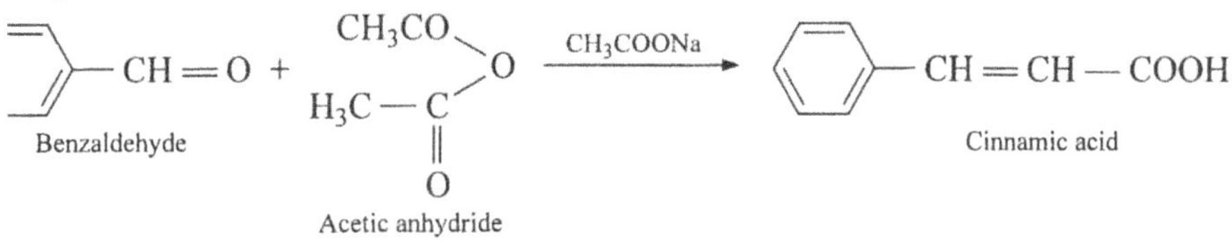

Benzoin condensation Aromatic aldehydes containing no α-hydrogen atoms un-go self-condensation in presence of KCN to form benzoins (ArCHOHCOAr). This tion also proceeds through carbanion intermediate.

condensations and proceeds through *carbanion mechanism.*

$$\underset{\text{Ethyl acetate}}{2CH_3COOC_2H_5} \xrightarrow{C_2H_5ONa} C_2H_5OH + \underset{\text{Sodioacetoacetic ester}}{CH_3CO\bar{C}HCOOC_2H_5} \xrightarrow{HCl} \underset{\text{Ethyl acetoacetate}}{CH_3COCH_2COOC}$$

2. ***Displacement Reactions*** Carbanions do undergo the following displacement reactic
(i) *Reimer–Tiemann reaction* Phenol, on treatment with a NaOH and $CHCl_3$, an aldeh group (—CHO) is introduced to the ortho position of —OH group on to the aromatic ri This reaction is known as Reimer–Tiemann reaction. In this reaction, the base conv chloroform to carbanion (trichloro carbanion) which decomposes to a carbene.

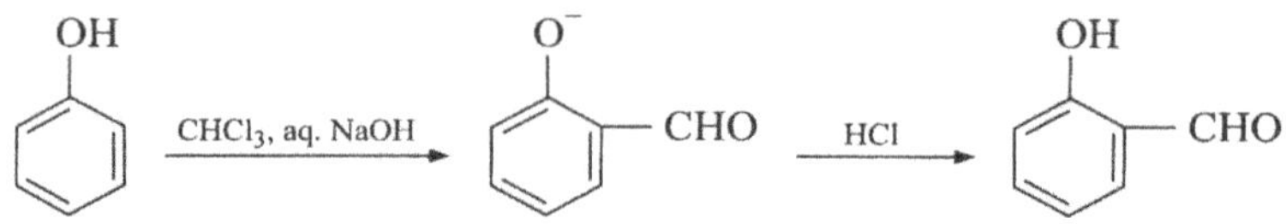

Phenol Salicylaldehyde

(ii) *Special types of reactions (Haloform reaction)* The haloform reaction proce through the intermediate formation of carbanion.

$$\underset{\text{Methyl ketone}}{R-\overset{\overset{\displaystyle O}{\|}}{C}-CH_3} + 3I_2 + 4NaOH \longrightarrow \underset{\text{Sodium carboxylate}}{RCOONa} + 3NaI + H_2O + \underset{\text{Iodoform}}{CHI_3}$$

5.7 ORGANIC REAGENTS

There are three types of reagents taking part in organic reactions. These are:

5.7.1 Electrophilic Reagents

An electrophilic reagent or an electrophile (i.e. electron-loving particle) is a reag containing an atom, which is deficient in electrons. Because of the presence electron-deficient atom, electrophile tries to seek electrons from other sources, th behaves as a Lewis acid. The electrophilic reagents are of two types:

1. ***Positive Electrophiles*** They are deficient in two electrons and carry a positive char e.g. carbocations, bromonium ion, nitronium ion.

2. ***Neutral Electrophiles*** These are electrophilic reagents in which the electron defici atom does not carry any charge, e.g. $AlCl_3$, BF_3, $FeCl_3$.

5.7.2 Nucleophilic Reagents

carry negative charge, e.g. carbanions, Cl^-, Br^-, CN^-, ^-OH, ^-OR.

leutral Nucleophiles These nucleophilic reagents have atoms with lone pairs of :trons but do not carry any charge, e.g. water (H_2O), ammonia (NH_3), Alcohol -O—H).

.3 Free Radicals

Section 5.2 for free radicals.

ACIDS AND BASES

early chemists classified inorganic compounds into three main groups: acids, bases salts. Towards the end of seventeenth century, Robert Boyle studied and described properties of acids.

.1 Properties of Acids

. Acids are sour to taste.
:. These turn blue litmus red.
'. These are good conductors of electricity.
-. These precipitate sulphur from alkaline solutions of sulphur.
. These dissolve active metals like zinc and liberate hydrogen.
. These lose the acid character when they react with alkalies to give salt and water.

2 Properties of Bases

elle studied and described the following properties of bases:

. Bases are bitter to taste.
. Their solutions in water are often soapy to touch.
. They have detergent property.
. They can dissolve oils and sulphur.
. They turn red litmus blue.
. They react with acids to form salts.

3 Modern Concepts of Acids and Bases

owing are the three important theories of acids and bases.

. Arrhenius theory of acids and bases

compound that contains hydroxyl group and gives hydroxide ions in aqueous solution

$$H{-}Cl \xrightleftharpoons{\text{Water}} H^+ + Cl^-$$

$$CH_3COOH \xrightleftharpoons{\text{Water}} H^+ + CH_3COO^-$$

$$NaOH \xrightleftharpoons{\text{Water}} Na^+ + OH^-$$

Limitations

(i) Arrhenius theory of acids and bases is limited to aqueous solutions only. Sc substances, such as CO_2, SO_2, SO_3, etc., behave as acids even though they not contain hydrogen ions (H^+).

(ii) Some substances exhibit the properties of a base, though they do not cont hydroxide ions, e.g. liquid ammonia.

(iii) The reaction between HCl (gas) and NH_3 (gas) to give NH_4Cl is a neutralisat reaction, though H^+ and OH^- ions are not involved.

(iv) Solutions of acids in water contain hydronium ions (H_3O^+) only and not hydro; ions (H^+).

$$H_2O + H_2O \longleftrightarrow H_3O^+(aq) + OH^-(aq)$$

2. ***Bronsted–Lowry Theory*** To overcome the limitations of Arrhenius concept, J Bronsted and T.M. Lowry in 1923 proposed, independently and almost simultaneou a general definition of acids and bases. According to them, 'an acid is a substance t exhibits a tendency to lose one or more protons and a base is a substance that exhil a tendency to gain protons.' In other words, an acid is 'proton-donor' and a base 'proton-acceptor'. When an acid loses a proton, the remaining part of it will have tendency to regain the proton. So the remaining part behaves as a base.

Thus, A^- is called the conjugate base of acid HA. The acid and the base differ he by a proton. They are known as acid–base conjugate pair. According to this theory strong acid is one, which has a greater tendency to donate a proton. If the tendency less, the acid is weak.

$$\underset{\text{Acid}}{H{-}A} \xrightleftharpoons{\text{Water}} \underset{\text{Proton}}{H^+} + \underset{\text{Base}}{A^-}$$

$$H{-}Cl \xrightleftharpoons{\text{Water}} H^+ + Cl^-$$

Limitations This theory serves very well in explaining the behaviour of acids and ba: in protonic solvents. But it fails in the case of some reactions, which do not invol proton transfer. For example, CaO, BaO does not involve any transfer of proton.

$$CO_2 + CaO \longrightarrow CaCO_3$$

3. ***Lewis Theory*** In 1923, G.N. Lewis proposed a new concept of acids and ba:

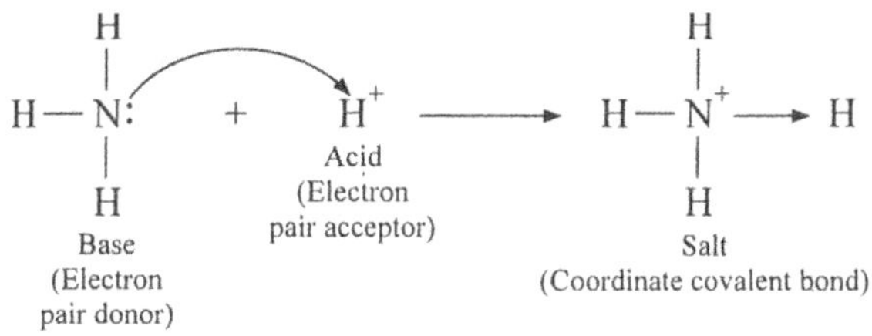

itations Lewis theory has the following limitations:

(i) Lewis theory failed to explain the strength of acids and bases.
ii) Acids such as HCl, H_2SO_4 do not form coordinate covalent bonds with bases, which is essential for this theory.
ii) In certain cases the formation of coordinate bond is very slow.
v) Catalytic activity of proton $[H^+]$ is the property of an acid.

4 Strength of Acids and Bases

strength of an acid depends on its ability to transfer its proton (H^+) to a base to form onjugate base. A monoprotic acid (HA) transfers a proton to water to form hydrorium and a conjugate base.

$$HA + H_2O \rightleftharpoons H_3O^{\oplus} + A^{\ominus}$$

n dilute solutions, the molar concentration of water can be taken as fairly constant. lying law of mass action to the above ionic equilibrium,

$$K_a = \frac{[H_3O^{\oplus}][A^{\ominus}]}{[HA]}$$

imilarly, the dissociation constant of a base (K_b) to measure the strength of the base.

$$\text{Dissociation of constant of base } (K_b) = \frac{[BH^+][OH^-]}{[B]}$$

'he strength of an acid and base is usually expressed in terms of K_a and K_b values. larger the value of K_a or K_b stronger will be the base. However, the strength of the s may also be expressed in terms of pK_a value to provide a continuous scale for acids bases. The low pK_a value represents strong acid whereas high pK_a value represents ıg base. For example,

ormic acid (pK_a = 3.72) is strongly acidic than acetic acid (pK_a = 4.75).

Water (pK_a = 14.0) is strongly basic than ethanol (pK_a = 10.0).

5 Factors influencing Dissociation Constants

Acidity of Halogenated Acetic Acids

Acid	*pH of 0.1-M Solution*
CH_3CO_2H	2.91
$ClCH_2CO_2H$	2.00
Cl_2CHCO_2H	1.39
Cl_3CCO_2H	1.23
F_3CCO_2H	1.21

Methyl group of acetic acid has greater electron-releasing inductive effective effect) than hydrogen atom of formic acid and, consequently, acetic acid is a weaker a than formic acid. In the case of halogen substituted acetic acids, the halogen atoms electron-withdrawing inductive effect (– I effect). Therefore, they are stronger than for and acetic acids. Similarly, the electron-releasing inductive effect (+ I effect) of a groups make the nitrogen atom of amines to donate the lone pair easily, making them m basic than ammonia.

2. ***Influence of Resonance Effect*** Resonance effect influences the dissociation of acid or a base, making the compound a stronger or weaker acid or base. For example, resonance-stabilised structures of carboxylate ion are more stable than those of phenox ion and, hence, carboxylic acids are more acidic than phenols.

3. ***Influence of Hybridisation*** The attachment of a multiple bond to an atom increa its effective electronegativity. For example, the protons of ethyne are more acidic t ethene and ethane. The carbon–hydrogen bond of ethyne, ethene and ethane hybridisat of carbon changes from *sp* to sp^3, the *s*-character of hybrid orbitals decreases from 5(25% and hence the electronegativity is decreased (tendency of the atom to keep bonding electron pair closer to it).

4. ***Steric Factors*** On the basis of electron-releasing inductive effect (+ I effect) of th alkyl groups on nitrogen, tertiary amines may be expected to be more basic than prima secondary amines. Practically, tertiary amines are less basic because of steric hindra or crowding created by three alkyl groups.

5.9 CHEMICAL REACTIONS: AN OVERVIEW

5.9.1 Introduction

One of the greatest challenges that organic chemistry presents to students is seemingly overwhelming number of reactions and reagents that must be learned. Wh it is true that organic chemists have developed thousands of reactions, it is also true t all of those reactions, every one can be classified into one of three categories, sub

at organic chemists use. The vocabulary includes the following definitions:

(i) *Reactant* The organic molecule that is transformed from starting material to product in a chemical reaction.

(ii) *Reagent* The compound that effects the transformation of the reactant to the product.

(iii) *Catalyst* The compound or combination of compounds that is used to accelerate the rate of the reaction.

(iv) *Solvent* The medium in which the reactant, reagent, and catalyst are dissolved.

9.3 Substitution Reactions

ll substitution reactions result in the replacement of one atom or group by another. gure 5.1 presents 4 specific examples of different types of substitution reactions.

While the reactions shown in Fig. 5.1 undergo substitution reactions under a wide nge of reaction conditions. In each case an atom or group attached to a carbon atom replaced by another atom or group. Scheme 1 presents a general representation of all bstitution reactions.

$$\boxed{C-G + X/Y \longrightarrow C-Y + G-X}$$

Scheme 1 General Scheme for Substitution Reactions

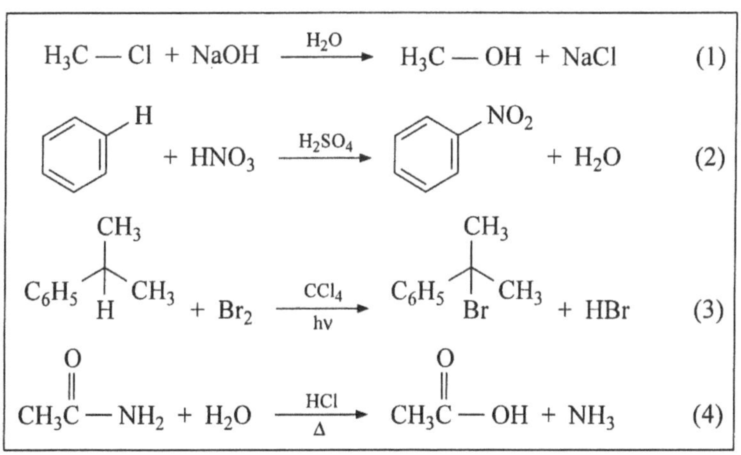

Fig. 5.1 Substitution Reactions

9.4 Elimination Reactions

mination reactions are processes in which two atoms or groups are removed from

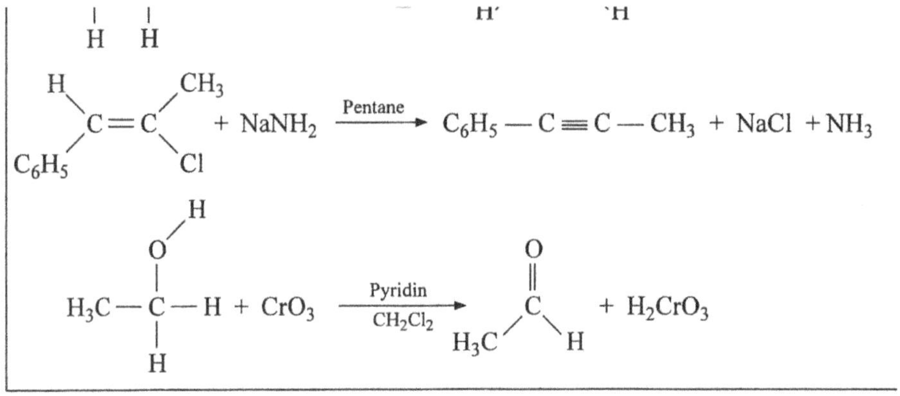

Fig. 5.2 Elimination Reactions

Scheme 2 depicts the minimal features of the various types of elimination reactic

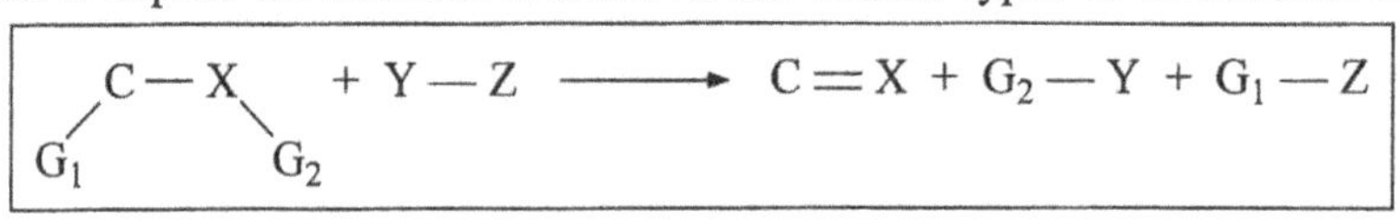

Scheme 2 General Scheme for Elimination Reactions

Two features of Scheme 2 are worth mentioning here. First, since the atoms or groups t are eliminated are attached to adjacent atoms, this type of reaction is often referred to a 1,2-elimination. Second, Reaction 7 (Fig. 5.2) makes apparent that X may represent atc other than C.

5.9.5 Addition Reactions

Addition reactions are the reverse of elimination reactions. Three examples are giver

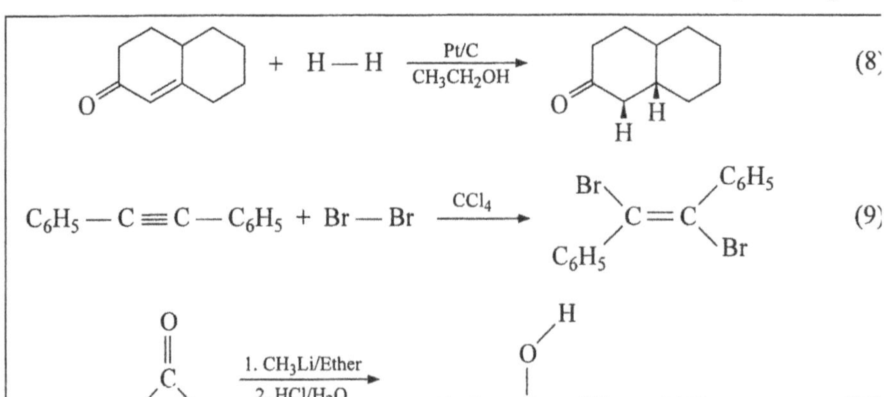

Scheme 3 illustrates the essential features of Reactions 8 to 10.

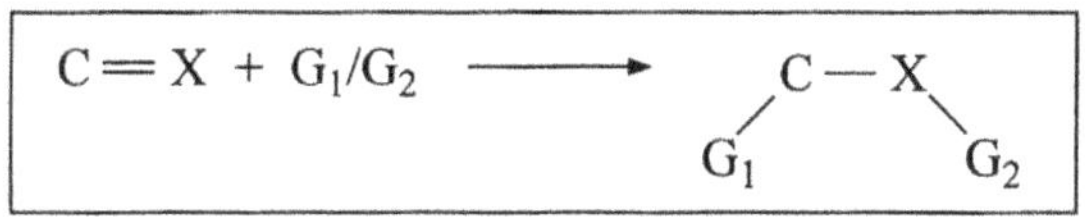

Scheme 3 General Scheme for Addition Reactions

The implication of the notation G_1/G_2 is that the two atoms or groups that add to the ultiple bond may be the elements of a single molecule as they are in Reactions 8 and or they may come from different molecules as they do in Reaction 10. An organic emist would say that Reaction 10 described the addition of the 'elements of' methane the C—O double bond of acetaldehyde, the elements of methane being CH_3 and H.

.10 SOLVENTS

10.1 Introduction

solvent is a liquid that can dissolve another material. In industry, the term solvent is nerally applied to the kind of substances known as 'organic solvents' that are widely ed to dissolve organic chemicals. Organic solvents are often used as cleaners or greasers, and as ingredients in paints, inks, glues and varnishes. The vast majority of emical reactions are performed in solutions. The solvent fulfils several functions during chemical reaction. It solvates the reactants and reagents so that they dissolve. This cilitates collisions between the reactant(s) and reagents that must occur in order to ansform the reactant(s) to product(s). The solvent also provides a means of temperature ntrol; either to increase the energy of the colliding particles so that they will react more ickly, or to absorb heat that is generated during an exothermic reaction. Generally, a od solvent should meet the following criteria:

(i) *Inertness* It should be inert to the reaction conditions.
(ii) *Solubility* It should dissolve the reactants and reagents.
(iii) *Boiling point* It should have an appropriate boiling point.
(iv) *Separability* It should be easily removed at the end of the reaction.
(v) *Dipole moment* The solubility of a drug is due in large measure to the polarity of the solvent, that is, to its dipole moment.
(vi) *Dielectric constant* Gorman and Hall obtained a linear relationship between log mole fraction of solute (methyl salicylate) versus the dielectric constant of isopropanol–water mixture.
(vii) *Miscibility with water* It should be miscible with water.

The solvents have been broadly classified into three categories according to their larity.

The polarity of the polar protic solvents stems from the bond dipole of the O—H boı The large difference in electronegativities of the oxygen and the hydrogen ato combined with the small size of the hydrogen atom, warrant separating molecules with (group from those polar compounds that do not have an OH group, e.g. water (HOI methanol (CH_3OH), and acetic acid (CH_3CO_2H).

5.10.3 Dipolar Aprotic Solvents

Solvents that have polar bonds but do not have hydrogen bond directly to oxygen nitrogen are called *polar aprotic*. They are not capable of acting as hydrogen-bo donors. Solvents that have hydrogen bond directly to N or O tend to solvate nucleophi through a process resembling hydrogen bonding. The heavily solvated nucleophile is le reactive in an S_N2 reaction since it is stabilised and must also drag a cage of solve molecules into any reaction site.

Solvents in this class all contain a bond that has a large bond dipole. Typically, tl bond is a multiple bond between carbon and either oxygen or nitrogen. Most dipo aprotic solvents contain a C=O double bond. Examples are acetone [$(CH_3)_2C{=}O$] a ethyl acetate ($CH_3CO_2CH_2CH_3$).

5.10.4 Non-Polar Solvents

Non-polar solvents are compounds that have low dielecrtic constants and are not miscit in water. Examples include benzene (C_6H_6), carbon tetrachloride (CCl_4), and diethyl eth ($CH_3CH_2OCH_2CH_3$).

Table 5.1 presents a list of solvents that are commonly used in chemical reactions. T boiling point, dipole moment, and dielectric constant of each solvent is included. All the solvents are clear, colourless liquids.

It should be apparent from the table that there are no sharp boundaries between pol and non-polar solvents, at least if you use dielectric constants or dipole moments as measure. There is, however, a correlation between chemical structure and dielectı constant that provides a useful way to think about polarity.

			Moment	*Constant*
Water	$H—OH$	100	1.85	80
Methanol	$CH_3—OH$	68	1.70	33
Ethanol	$CH_3CH_2—OH$	78	1.69	24.3
1-Propanol	$CH_3CH_2CH_2—OH$	97	1.68	20.1
1-Butanol	$CH_3CH_2CH_2CH_2—OH$	118	1.66	17.8
Formic acid	$H—C(=O)—OH$	100	1.41	58
Acetic acid	$H_3C—C(=O)—OH$	118	1.74	6.15
Formamide	$H—C(=O)—NH_2$	210	3.73	109
Acetone	$H_3C—C(=O)—CH_3$	56	2.88	20.7
Methylethyl ketone	$CH_3—C(=O)—C_2H_5$	80	2.78	18.5
Ethyl acetate	$H_3C—C(=O)—OCH_2CH_3$	78	1.78	6.02
Acetonitrile	$H_3C—C\equiv N$	81	3.92	36.6
N,N-Dimethylformamide	$H—C(=O)—N(CH_3)_2$	153	3.82	38.3
Diemthyl sulphoxide (DMSO)	$H_3C—S(=O)—CH_3$	189	3.96	47.2
Hexane	$CH_3(CH_2)_4CH_3$	69	–	2.02
Benzene	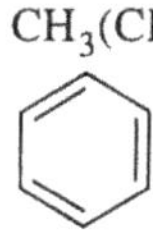	80	0	2.28
Diethyl ether	$CH_3CH_2OCH_2CH_3$	35	1.15	4.34
Tetrahydrofuran (THF)	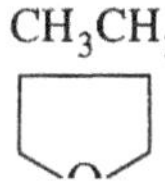	66	1.63	7.52

intermediates?

2. What are alkyl free radicals? Explain about their formation, relative stabilities and proper
3. Write notes on:
   (a) Carbanion
   (b) Nitrenes
   (c) Carbenes
   (d) Carbocations
4. Arrange the following acids in the order of increasing strength.
   (a) CH_3COOH
   (b) $Cl_2CHCOOH$
   (c) Cl_3CCOOH
   (d) $ClCH_2COOH$
5. Explain, why
   (a) Primary free radical is less stable than secondary or tertiary free radical?
   (b) Tertiary carbocation is more stable than secondary or primary carbocation?
   (c) Tertiary carbanion is less stable than secondary or primary carbanion?
6. Write notes on:
   (a) Polar protic solvents
   (b) Dipolar aprotic solvents
   (c) Lewis acids
   (d) Non-polar solvents
7. Discuss with examples about various types of chemical reactions do you encounter in orga compounds.

LASSIFICATION AND NOMENCLATURE F ORGANIC COMPOUNDS

CLASSIFICATION OF ORGANIC COMPOUNDS

: of the striking features of organic chemistry is the vast number of organic com-nds known to exist. Over ten million organic compounds are already known and every r thousands of new compounds are discovered. To facilitate the study of very large iber of these compounds, they have been divided into different classes depending n the nature of carbon skeleton present in their molecules.

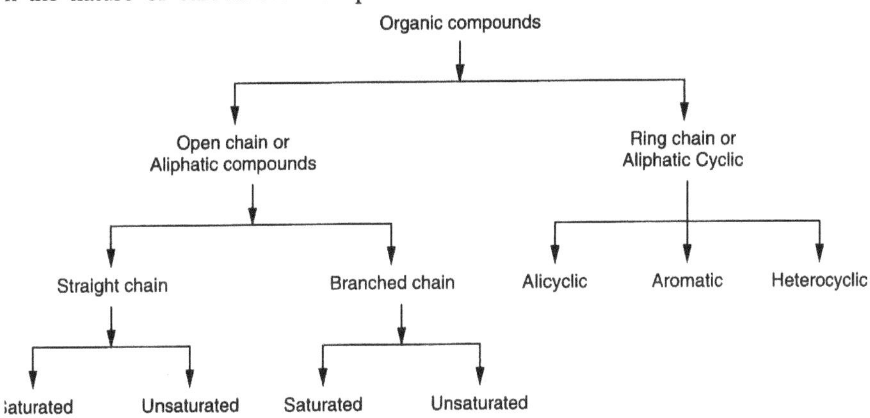

FUNCTIONAL GROUP

atom or group of atoms, which is responsible for the characteristic property of a

Table 6.1

Name of Compound	*Functional Group*	*Name of Compound*	*Functional Group*
Alkene	$>C=C<$	Ketone	—CO—
Alkyne	$-C\equiv C-$	Carboxylic acid	—COOH
Halide	X(F, Cl, Br or I)	Amine	$-NH_2$

summarises the broader categories of compounds and their respective functional grou

6.3 HOMOLOGOUS SERIES

A homologous series may be defined as a series of compounds in which the vario members have similar structural features and similar chemical properties, and the succe sive members differ in their molecular formulae by CH_2. The members of such series a known as *homologous* of each other.

6.4 NOMENCLATURE OF ORGANIC COMPOUNDS

The nomenclature to organic compounds is an important aspect of organic chemistry. Th following are various methods:

6.4.1 Earlier Methods of Naming Organic Compounds

1. Prior to the end of the ninteenth century, organic compounds were named after tho parent compounds from which these were synthesised. Usually they were named r flecting the source of the compound. These are now called common or trivial nam and some are still in use today. For example, the simplest alcohol has a common trivial name of 'wood alcohol'. This compound was given this name because the chi source of this alcohol was the destructive distillation of wood chips. Destructiv distillation is distilling in the absence of air. Wood chips can be distilled in this mann and will yield a very complex mixture. Analysis of this mixture will result in a large pa of this alcohol. Another alcohol, the second member of the alcohol family is calle 'grain alcohol'. This trivial name came from the fact that one of the principal sourc of this alcohol is the fermentation of grains and fruits.
2. Later in the century, a second nomenclature system developed, called the derive system. In the derived system, the major hydrocarbon portion of the molecule w named as an alkyl group followed by the family name. The same simplest member the alcohol family would be called 'methyl alcohol' because the formula CH_3OH show a methyl group attached to the functional group for the alcohol family. The secon member's name in the derived system would be 'ethyl alcohol' because the formula this alcohol $CH_3—CH_2—OH$ shows the ethyl group attached to an OH group.

In systematic nomenclature system for organic compounds (IUPAC) it became ver clear early into the twentieth century that the use of common names and derived name was not going to work very efficiently for the organic compounds that were being rapidl synthesised with greater complexity. The International Union of Pure and Applied Chem ists (IUPAC) developed a systematic approach to organic nomenclature. The organisatio meets periodically beginning in 1921 in Geneva, Switzerland in order to form committee

\ unique feature of this system is that it permits the writing of only one name for a :n structure. At the same time, a given name of a compound can clearly direct in ing of only one molecular structure. The system of nomenclature is designed to reflect, ' closely, the name of the compound with the structure, because the structure is very ortant in establishing the physical and chemical behaviour of organic molecules. A set ules was set up for each family of compounds and these rules were to be consistent veen the families. Usually the rules involve a general core of rules that apply to every ily. Then there are specific rules that apply to just one family that establish:

. The *identity of branching groups*
. The *location of these branched groups*
. The *identity of the functional group* that differentiates the families from one another
. The *location of the functional group*
. The *identity of the family name*

'he IUPAC name of a compound can be split up into following parts:

Word Root The word root is the basic carbon skeleton. It depends upon the number of carbon atoms present in the parent chain, which contains functional group. The following are IUPAC word roots:

Carbon Chain Length	*Word Root*	*Carbon Chain Length*	*Word Root*
C1	Meth-	C6	Hex-
C2	Eth-	C7	Hept-
C3	Prop-	C8	Oct-
C4	But-	C9	Non-
C5	Pent-	C10	Dec-

Prefixes Prefixes preceed the word root. There are three types of prefixes.

(i) *Primary prefix* Primary prefix (cyclo) is added before the word root to indicate carbocyclic compound.

(ii) *Secondary prefixes* These are added before the word root in an alphabetical order to indicate side chains or substituents.

Side Chain or Substituent	*Secondary Prefix*	*Side Chain or Substituent*	*Secondary Prefix*
—F	Fluoro	$—NO_2$	Nitro
—Cl	Chloro	—NO	Nitroso
—Br	Bromo	—R	Alkyl
—I	Iodo	—OR	Alkoxy

(iii) *Numerical prefixes* They are added before the designations of side chains or

Nature of Carbon Chain	*Suffix*
Saturated	-ane
Unsaturated (C═C double bond)	-ene
Unsaturated (C≡C triple bond)	-yne

(ii) *Secondary suffix* It is written after the word root to indicate the partic functional group present in the carbon chain. The secondary suffixes for s functional groups are given here:

Functional Group	*Secondary Suffix*	*Functional Group*	*Secondary Suffix*
—OH	-ol	—$CONH_2$	-amide
—CO—	-one	—COOR	-oate
—CHO	-al	—CN	-cyano
—COOH	-oic acid	—NH_2	-amine

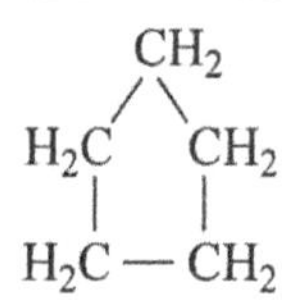

Cyclo — pent — ane

Cyclo → Primary prefix; pent → Word root; ane → Primary suffix

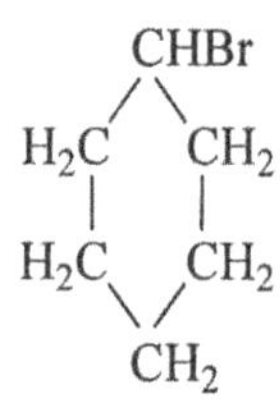

Bromo — cyclo — hex — ane

cyclo → Primary prefix; hex → Word root; ane → Primary suffix

4. The longest continuous chain of carbon atoms in the molecule is first selected. chain does not necessarily have to be straight. The carbon atoms of the main chai parent chain are numbered by numerals (1, 2, 3,...) from one end to the other (ei from left to right or from right to left) to get lowest possible numbers to substituent side chains.

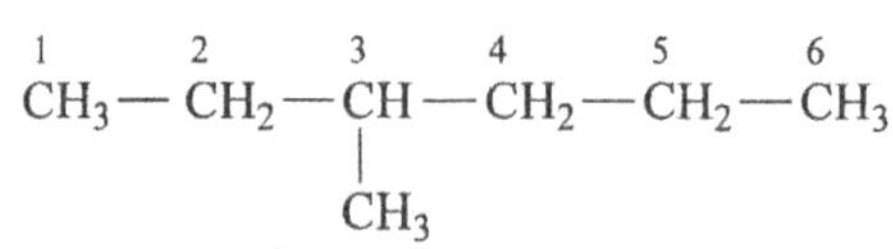

3-Methyl hexane but not, 4-Methyl hexane

5. Writing the lower number of two carbon atoms involved in the bond indic multiple bonds (double bond or triple bond) present in the chain between car atoms.

functional group. (In such cases the sum of the numbers of carbon atoms carryir the different groups may or may not be minimum possible.)

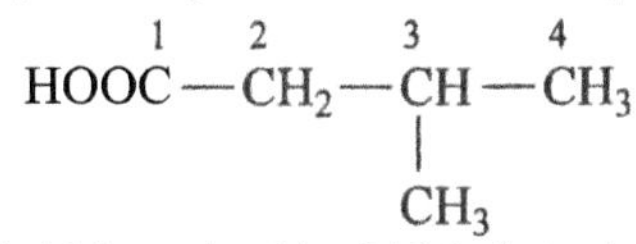

3-Methyl-1-butanoic acid or 3-Methylbutan-1-oic acid

. When a chain terminating group (such as —CHO, —COOH, —COOR, —CONH —CN, etc.) is present as functional group, it must be assigned the number 1.

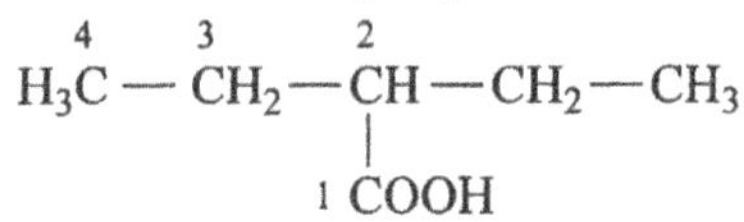

2-Ethyl-1-butanoic acid or 2-Ethylbutan-1-oic acid

. If two different alkyl groups are at equal distance in relation to the ends of th parent chain numbering is generally done from that end of the chain, which i nearest to the smaller group. But in case of other groups, the numbering is don from that end which gives lower number to the group coming first in alphabetic order as shown below:

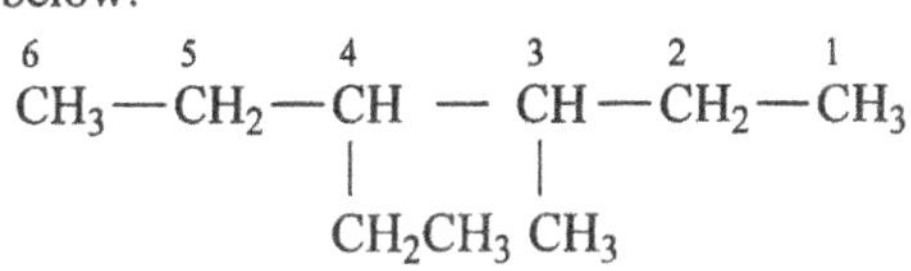

4-Ethyl-3-methylhexane

. The name of the compound is written as one word. Numbers are separated fror the designations of prefixes or suffixes by hyphens and numbers are separated fror each other by commas.

. In case of compounds containing two or more functional groups including C=C C≡C, the principal group forms the suffix of the compound and the other group are considered as substituents and are designated by prefixes. The principal func tional group is chosen in the following order of preference.
Acids > Acid derivatives except nitriles > Aldehydes > Nitriles > Ketones > Alcohol > Amines > Ethers > Carbon-carbon double or triple bond. In such cases, the longes chain is selected to include the principal functional group and the maximum numbe of other functional groups.

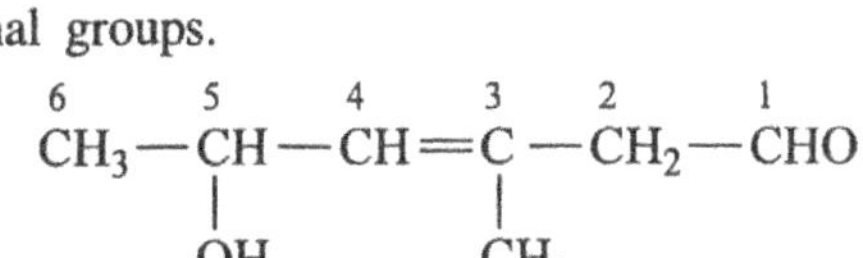

3-Methyl-5-hydroxy-3-hexenal

4-Hydroxy-3-(2-hydroxyethyl)-pentanoic acid

6.5 RULES TO WRITE THE STRUCTURE OF A COMPOUND

(a) Note the word root and write down a linked straight chain or ring in case the w root carries the prefix cyclo of that many carbon atoms and number it from any e
(b) Note the primary suffixes, which indicate the number, kind and positions of carb carbon, multiple bonds in the parent chain and fill the double or triple bonds in parent chain at the proper places.
(c) Attach the substituent and functional groups indicated by prefixes and suffixes the specified carbon atoms.
(d) Attach suitable number of hydrogen atoms to satisfy the tetra-covalency of e carbon atom. For instance

   (i) As the word root is pent, write down a linked straight chain of 5 carbon ato and number it from any end.

$$\overset{5}{C}-\overset{4}{C}-\overset{3}{C}-\overset{2}{C}-\overset{1}{C}$$

   (ii) The word root carries the primary suffix -en, it indicates the presence of a dou bond. The position of this double bond is between carbon numbers 3 and 4 indicated by number 3 before the word root.

$$\overset{5}{C}-\overset{4}{C}=\overset{3}{C}-\overset{2}{C}-\overset{1}{C}$$

   (iii) Attach a methyl group at number 2 and hydroxy group at number 4 and ha a carboxyl group at carbon number 1 as suggested by the name.

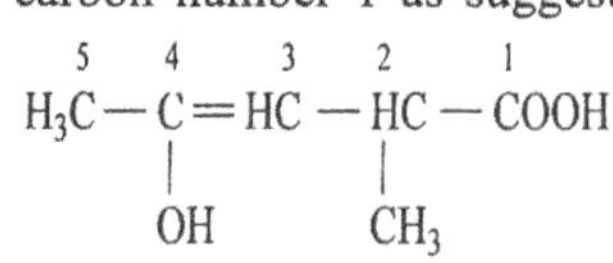

   (iv) Attach the required number of hydrogen atoms to various carbon atoms to the final structure.

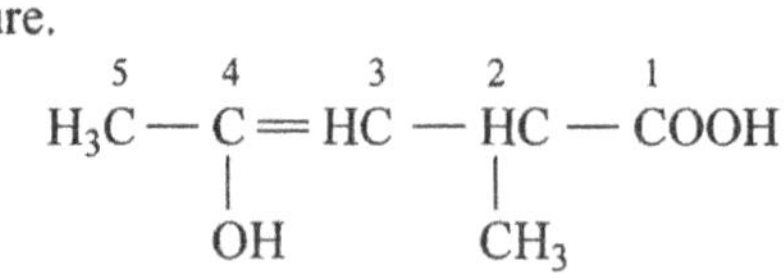

4-Hydroxy-2-methyl-3-penten-1-oic acid

PRACTICE QUESTIONS

1. Write IUPAC names for the following:

H

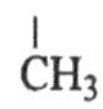

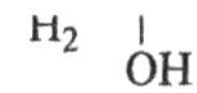

(e) 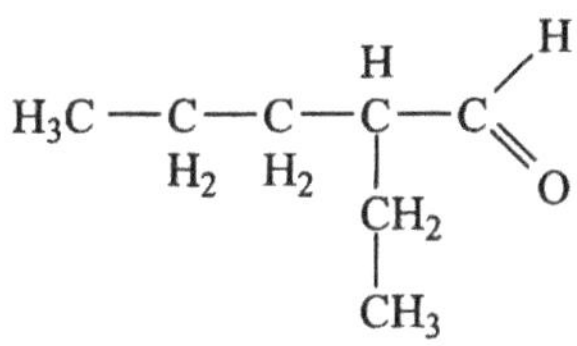

(f) 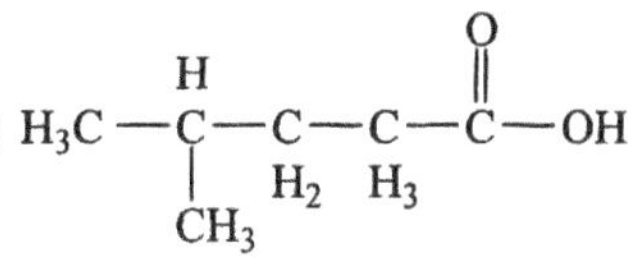

(g) 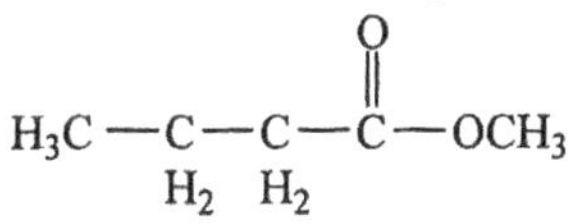

(h) 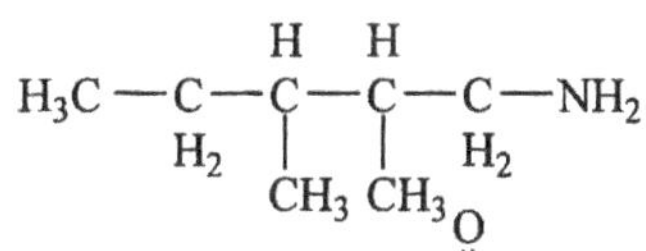

(i) 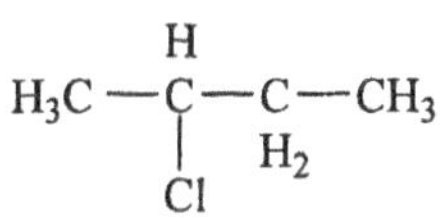

(j) 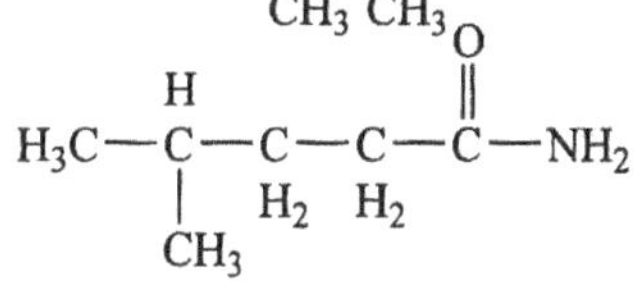

(k) 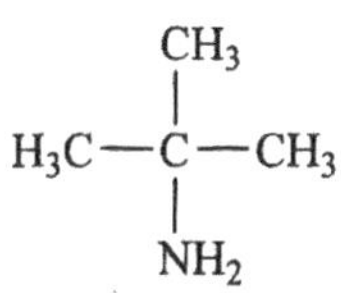

(l) 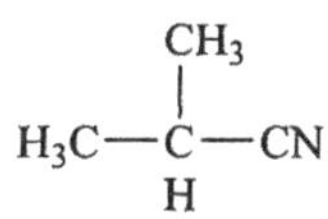

2. State the IUPAC rules for naming a monofunctional organic compound.
3. Write the structural formula of the following compounds:
   (a) 1-Bromo-3-methylhexane
   (b) 3-Chloro-2,4-dimethylpentane
   (c) 3-Methylbutenal
   (d) Ethylpropanoate
   (e) Cyclohexane
   (f) 2-Methylbutanenitrile
   (g) 3-Methyl-2-hexanone
4. Define a functional group. Write the functional group present in the following compounds: Lactic acid, methyl salicylate, dimercaprol, Vanillin, ethyl oleate, chloramine-T, hydroquinone, chlorbutol, sodium lauryl sulphate, and diethyl malonate.

7

PRINCIPLES OF ISOMERISM

There are a number of organic compounds which have the same molecular formula different physical and chemical properties. They are known as isomers (Greek: *iso* = eq *meros* = parts) and the phenomenon is known as isomerism. There are two main t of isomerism. They are

- Structural isomerism
- Space or stereoisomerism

7.1 STRUCTURAL ISOMERISM

When the isomerism occurs because of the difference in the arrangement of atoms wi the molecule (without any reference to space) it is termed as structural isomerism. Struct isomerism can be further divided into following five types.

7.1.1 Chain Isomerism

This type of isomerism arises because of the difference in the nature of the carbon ch i.e. straight or branched chain. For example,

$$CH_3 - CH_2 - CH_2 - CH_3$$

n-Butane

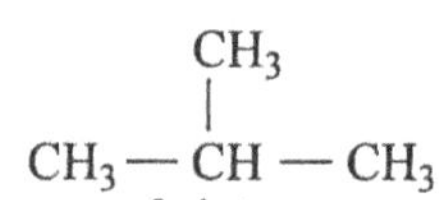

Isobutane

$$CH_3 - CH_2 - CH_2 - CH_2 - CH_3$$

n-Pentane

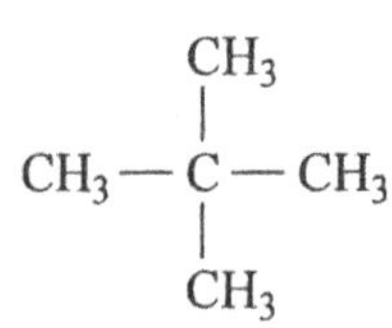

Neopentane

7.1.2 Position Isomerism

n-Propanol Isopropanol

1-Chloropropane and 2-chloropropane are position isomers.

$$CH_3-CH_2-CH_2-Cl$$

1-Chloropropane

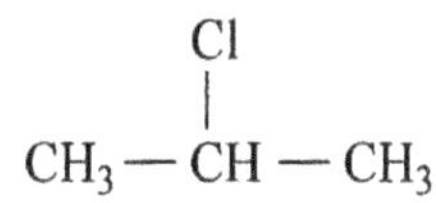

2-Chloropropane

1.3 Functional Isomerism

iis type of isomerism is because of the difference in the nature of functional group. For stance, ethyl alcohol and dimethyl ether, both, have the same molecular formula, C_2H_6O, t they contain different functional groups.

$$CH_3-CH_2-OH \qquad CH_3-O-CH_3$$

Ethyl alcohol Dimethyl ether

$$CH_3-CH_2-CHO \qquad CH_3-CO-CH_3$$

Propionaldehyde Acetone

1.4 Metamerism

occurs because of difference in the nature of alkyl groups attached to the same functional oup. Compounds of the same homologous series show this type of isomerism, e.g. ethyl ether and methylpropyl ether represents a pair of metamers.

$$CH_3-CH_2-O-CH_2-CH_3 \qquad CH_3-O-CH_2-CH_2-CH_3$$

Diethyl ether Methylpropyl ether

1.5 Tautomerism

is may be regarded as a special case of functional group isomerism. It arises due to the gration of a proton, e.g. acetone exhibits tautomerism between the following two forms.

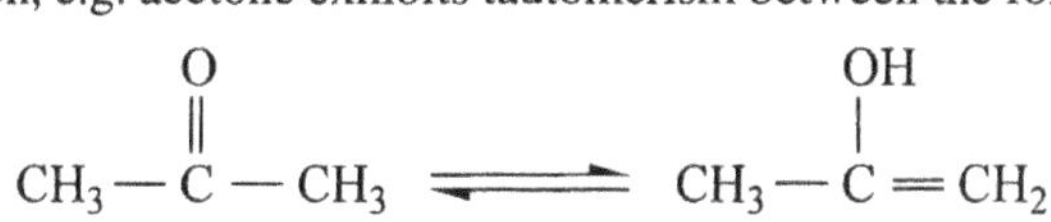

(Keto form) (Enol form)

2 STEREOISOMERISM

hen the isomers have the same structural formulae but differ in relative arrangement of ms or groups in space within the molecule, they are known as stereoisomers and the enomenon as stereoisomerism. Stereoisomers have atoms that differ only by their

substance, could be rotated clockwise or counterclockwise depending on optical axi: the substance. Stereoisomerism can be further classified into three types: (a) geometr isomerism, (b) optical isomerism, and (c) conformational isomerism.

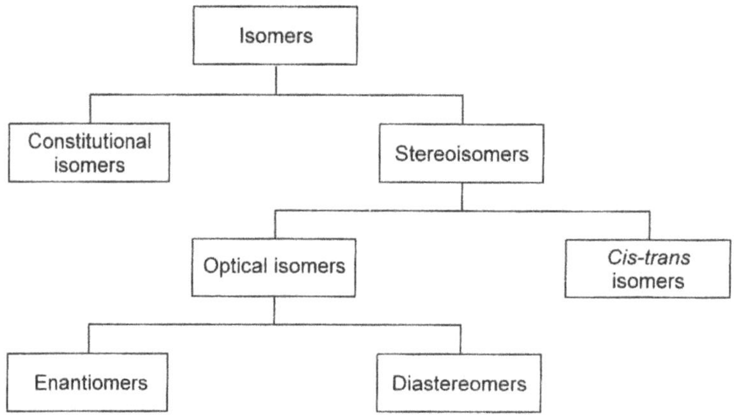

7.3 GEOMETRICAL ISOMERISM

7.3.1 Principles of Geometrical Isomerism

Geometrical isomerism is a form of stereoisomerism and describes the orientation functional groups at the ends of a *molecule* which has a double bond. The isomers wh are having the same structural formulae but differ in spatial arrangement of the grou or atoms around the double bond are termed as geometrical isomers. Geometrical isomeri is exhibited by carbon–carbon double bond molecules, carbon–nitrogen double bc compounds (oximes), cyclic aliphatic hydrocarbons and nitrogen–nitrogen double bc molecules. The double bond present in these cases *restricts free rotation*. The t geometric isomers are not superimposable.

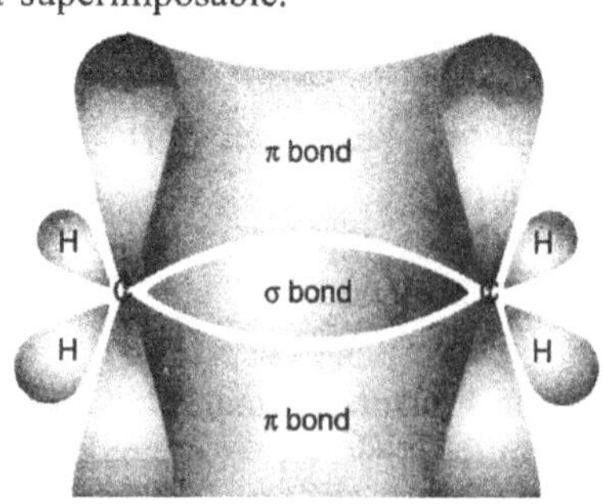

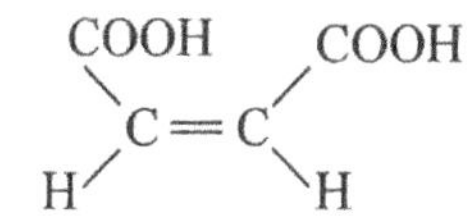

Maleic acid (*cis* isomer)

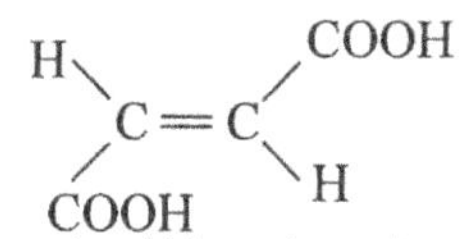

Fumaric acid (*trans* isomer)

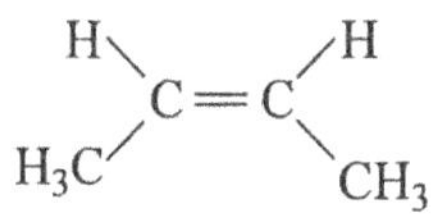

cis-2-Butene

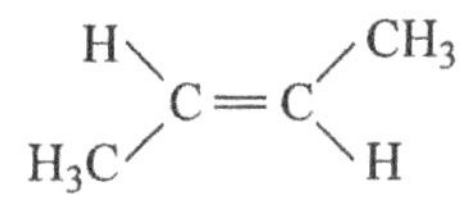

trans-2-Butene

The *necessary and sufficient condition for geometrical isomerism* in an alkene C = CCD is that A ≠ B and C ≠ D. The groups A, B, C and D can be arranged in e different ways as:

Type I

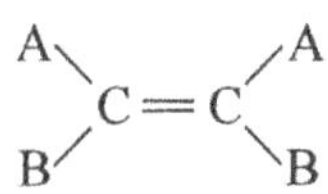

cis

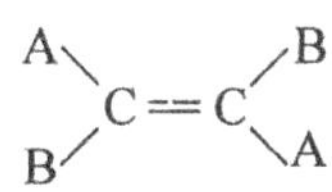

trans

Type II

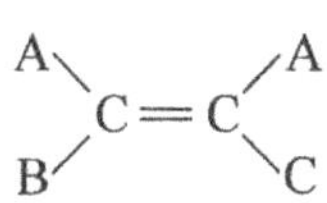

cis

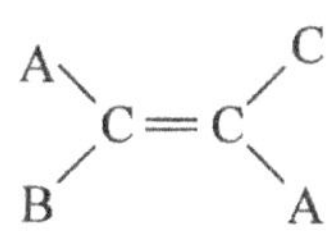

trans

Type III

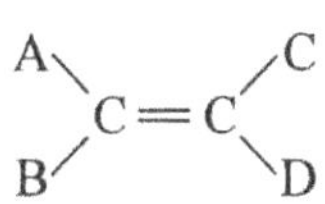

cis

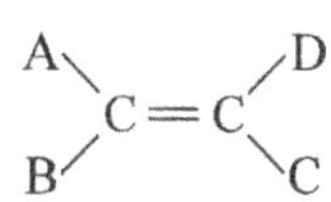

trans

n Types I and II, *cis* and *trans* can be used to distinguish these (because at least one ıp is common to both the carbon atoms), whereas in Type III four different substituents present hence E and Z system is used.

Cyclic compounds also exhibit this form of isomerism because the bonds cannot rotate to the ring structure. e.g. 1,2-dichlorocyclohexane:

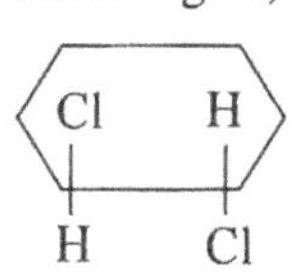

trans-1,2-Dichlorocyclohexane

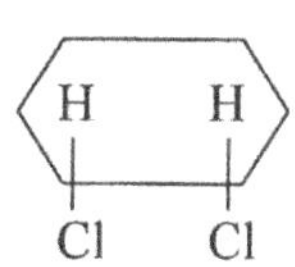

cis-1,2-Dichlorocyclohexane

2 E–Z Nomenclature

bonded to one of the sp^2 orbitals of carbons and then the relative priorities of the two gro bonded to the other sp^2 hybridised carbon. Priorities of the groups depend upon ato number, the atom of higher atomic number gets higher priority. If the high-priority gro are on the same side of the double bond the isomer is said to have Z configuration (Z for *Zusammen* which means together). If the high-priority groups are on opposite side: the double bond the isomer has the E configuration (E is for *Entgegen* means opposi

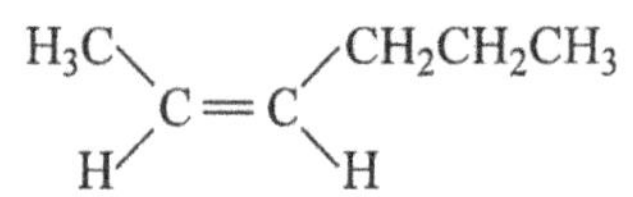

cis-2-Hexene or Z isomer

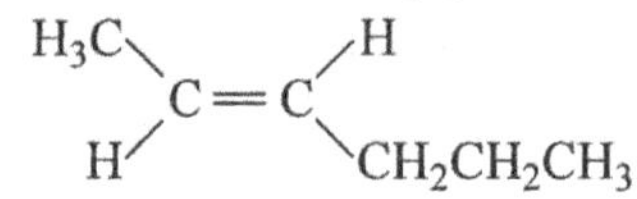

trans-2-Hexene or E isomer

The two groups attached to each carbon of the double bond are assigned priorit if the two with the highest priority are on the same side of the double bond, the molec would be designated as the Z form. If not, it is the E form.

(Z)-1-Bromo-2-chloro-2-fluoro-1-iodoethene	(E)-1-Bromo-2-chloro-2-fluoro-1-iodoethene
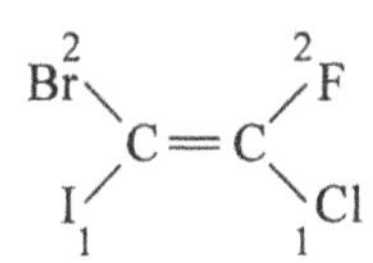	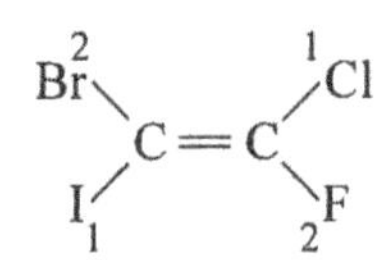

(The Z stands for the German zusammen, which means together, while the E stai for the German Entgegen, which means opposite.)

7.3.3 Determination of Configuration of Geometrical Isomer

The following methods are used to determine the configuration of geometrical isome

1. ***Physical Methods*** The *physical properties* of geometrical isomers are usually quite differ The configuration of *cis-* and *trans-* isomers is determined by the following physical metho

Some physical properties of *cis*-butenedioic (maleic) acid and *trans*-butenedioic (fumai acid are shown here:

(i) *Dipole moment* In general, the *cis*-isomer possesses higher dipole moment as compa to *trans*-isomer, e.g. *cis*-1,2-dichloroethene has a dipole moment of 1.89 D, wher *trans*-isomer of 0.01 D.

(ii) *Melting point* In general, *trans* molecules can pack more closely than *cis* in the sc state and this results in the *trans* form having the highest melting point. For instance, mal acid (a *cis*-isomer) melts at 130.5° C whereas fumaric acid (a *trans*-isomer) melts at 287°

(iii) *Boiling point* The *cis*-isomers generally have higher boiling points than t corresponding *trans*-isomers

i) Spectroscopic methods Spectroscopic methods (UV, infrared, NMR, XRD, electron
ffraction) are used to determine configuration.

Physical Property	*cis-Butenedioic Acid*	*trans-Butenedioic Acid*
Melting point (°C)	130–131	286
Density (g/cm^3)	1.590	1.635
Solubility in water at 25° C (g per 100 ml water)	Very soluble	Soluble

Chemical Methods

Cyclisation method Geometrical isomers are normally *chemically similar* because ey have the same functional groups in the same environment. There are a few exceptions this rule, e.g. the butenedioic acids. The *cis*-isomer loses water to form a cyclic anhydride ıen heated to 120°C but the *trans* form must be heated to 250° C before this happens this temperature the double bond breaks down and the molecule can rotate to the *cis*-nfiguration and lose water).

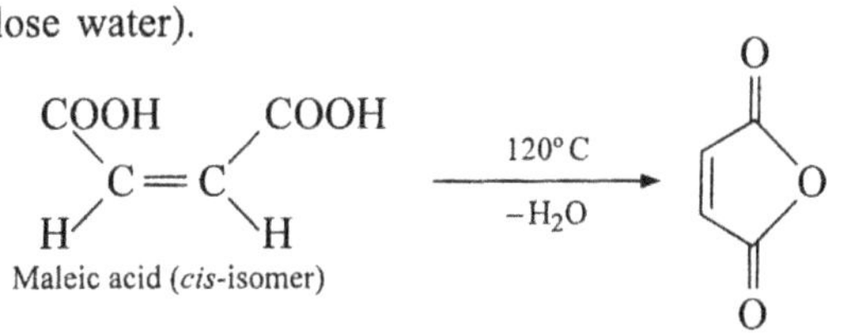

Maleic acid (*cis*-isomer)

Maleic anhydride

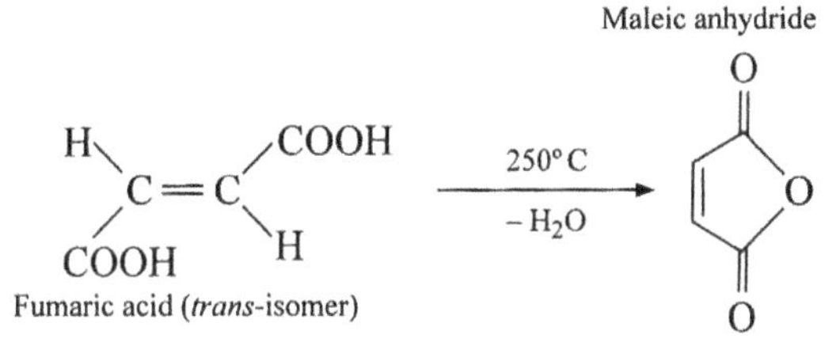

Fumaric acid (*trans*-isomer)

Maleic anhydride

This method has been based on the observation that because of the proximity of the ›ups the *cis*-isomers readily undergo elimination reaction to give a cyclic compound ereas the *trans*-isomer requires more drastic conditions for cyclisation, e.g.

A simple example involves the geometrical isomers of butenedioic acid (Fig. 7.1).

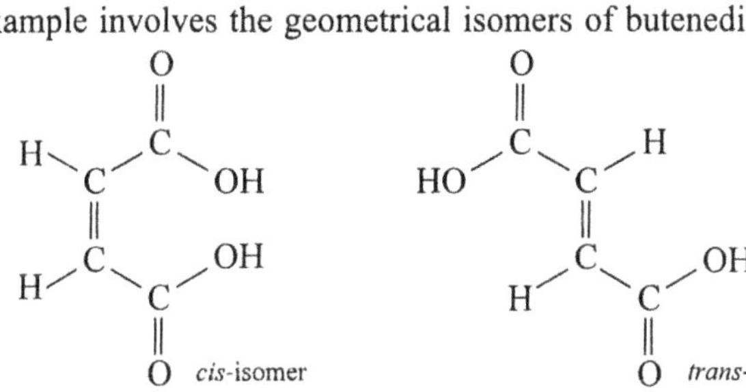

cis-isomer *trans*-isomer

MP = 142° C MP = 300° C

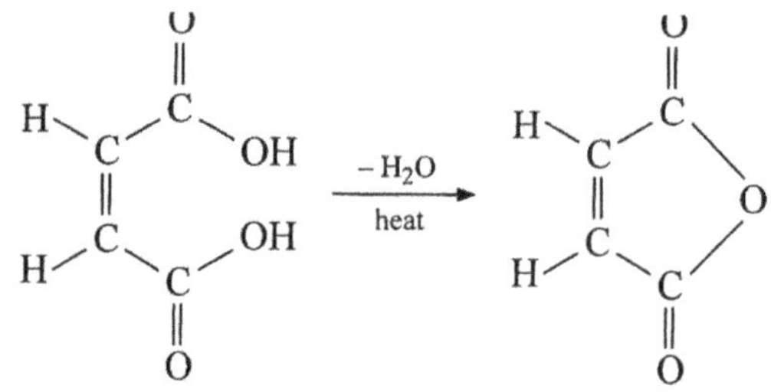

Fig. 7.2 Dehydration of *cis*-Butenedioic Acid

(ii) *Rearrangement reaction* By identifying the product of a rearrangement reaction th configuration of these isomers can be ascertained, e.g. the configuration of oximes is be: determined by Beckmann rearrangement reaction. According to Beckmann rearrangemen oximes rearrange to substituted amides under the influence of mineral or Lewis acid ($SOCl_2$, H_3PO_4, P_2O_5, PCl_5, H_2SO_4, HCl, CH_3COCl, C_6H_5COCl, etc.). The rearrangement i stereospecific and the group that migrates normally is the one that is anti to the hydroxy group of oxime. The function of acidic reagent is to convert the hydroxyl group to a bette leaving group.

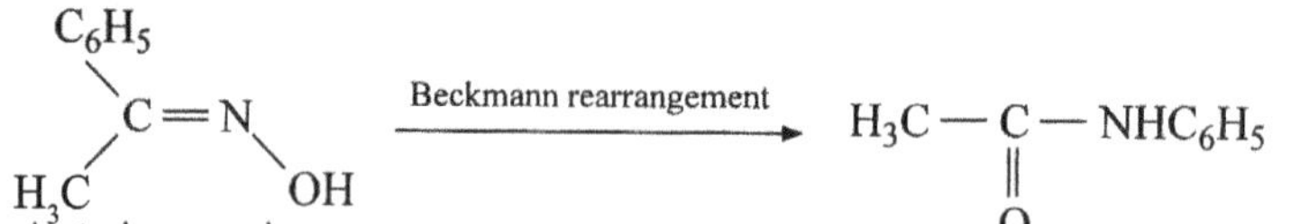

Acetophenone oxime

Acetanilide

Mechanism The mechanism involves the following steps:

- The mechanism of Beckmann rearrangement begins by the conversion of hydroxy group of oxime into a good leaving group under the influence of an acid.

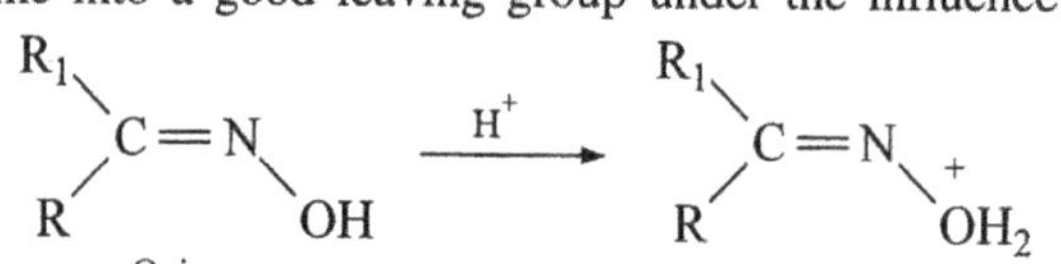

Oxime

- Migration of alkyl or aryl groups (that is anti to the hydroxyl group of oxime) witl bonding electrons to electron-deficient nitrogen and forms nitrilium ion.

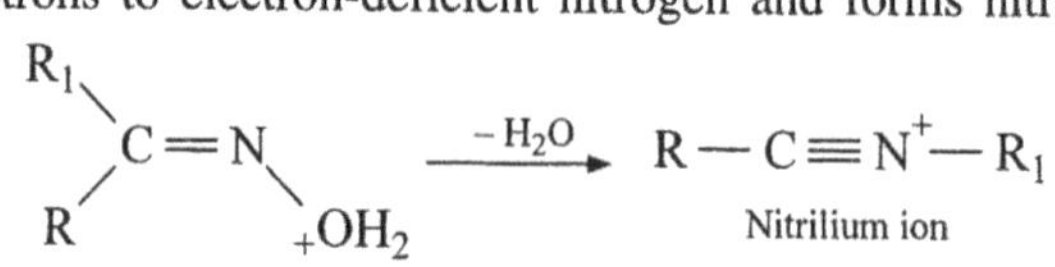

- Attack of weak electrophile (like water) on highly active nitrilium ion, followed by deprotonation and tautomerisation gives amide.

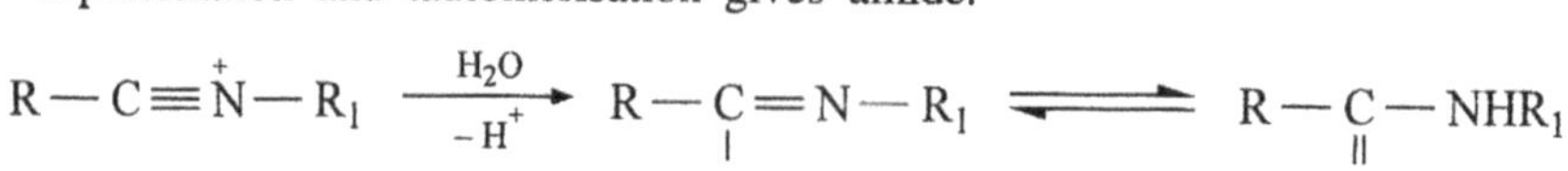

/ substance that rotates the plane of polarised light is optically active, and the phenomenon ted to it is called optical isomerism. The substance can rotate the plane of polarised light er in a clockwise direction or anticlockwise direction. The former is called dextrorotatory, le the later is laevorotatory and is denoted by *d* (or '+') and *l* (or '–') respectively, e.g. lactic acid or dextrorotatory lactic acid rotates plane-polarised light to right. (–) 2-methyl, utanol or laevorotatory form rotates plane-polarised light to left.

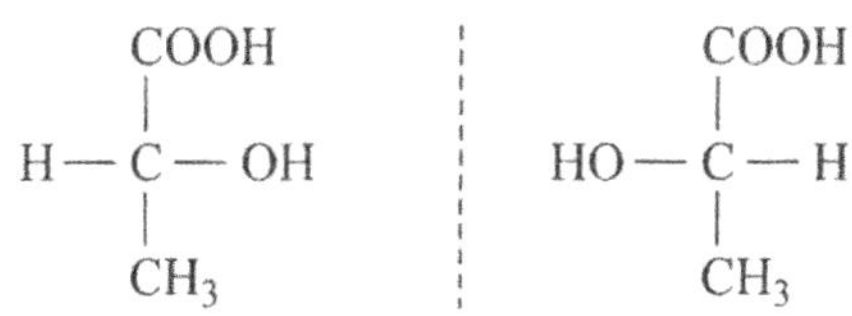

Enantiomers of lactic acid (Optically active)

.2 Chirality and Chiral Molecules

necessary and sufficient condition for the optically active compound is *chirality*. A ›on atom to which four different groups are attached is a *chiral carbon* (Greek = chiral ins *handedness*). Our hands are mirror images of each other, which are not identical. ley were, then we would not need a right-hand and left-hand glove. We can prove by trying to lay one hand on top of the other palms up. When we attempt to do this, observe that the thumbs and fingers do not lie on top of one another. We say that ' are non-superimposible upon one another. Since they are not the same and yet are or

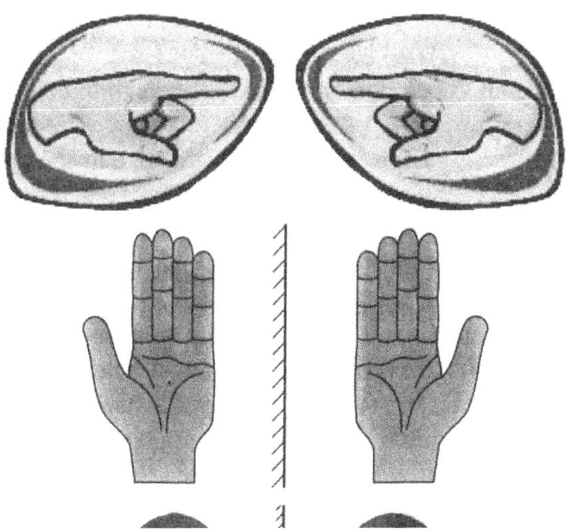

hand. The mirror image of a left hand is a right hand, and these two objects are superimposable. Examples include hands, screws, propellers, and keys.

Molecules like objects are capable of exhibiting chirality. These chiral molecules h: certain characteristics which are different from other molecules that do not exhibit chiral Chiral molecules have the following characteristics:

1. Chiral molecules will have their mirror images non-superimposible as we saw w all chiral objects above.
2. Chiral molecules must have no internal plane of symmetry. Molecule's that do h: an internal plane of symmetry will be able to be split in half and each half will a mirror image of the other. An example of this is 2-propanol (Fig. 7.3). If we constr a plane that cuts the molecule in half that would run through the hydrogen at of the middle carbon and the hydroxyl group, the two halves would be mirror ima of one another (See Fig. 7.3). Such a molecule would be achiral, i.e. not capable exhibiting chirality.

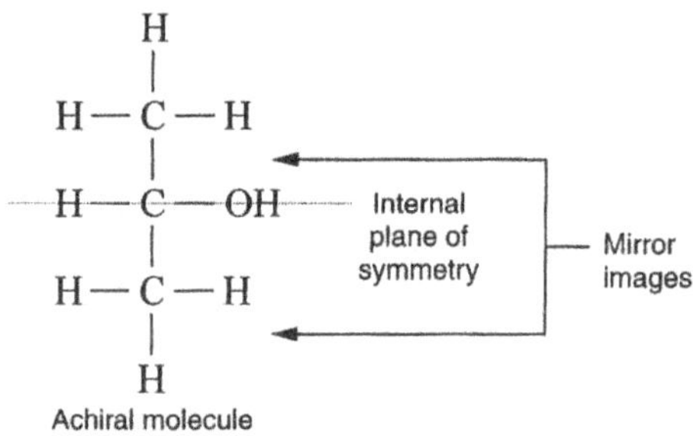

Fig. 7.3 Achirality and Internal Plane of Symmetry in 2-Propanol

On the other hand, 2-butanol does not have an internal plane of symme (See Fig. 7.4). Constructing a plane that runs through the molecule at any part the molecule will not result in the two halves being mirror images of one anoth Such a molecule, for example, 2-butanol is said to be chiral. If we construct the mir image of 2-butanol, and then try to superimpose it on each other it cannot be do: They are non-super imposable mirror images and constitute an enantiomeric p:

3. Chiral molecules will have one stereocentre (or chiral) carbon. A stereocentre carb has four non-equivalent groups bonded to it. As seen in case of 2-propa (See Fig. 7.3) there are no stereocentres in the molecule. Each carbon has less th four non-equivalent groups bonded to it. Each of the two end carbons have th hydrogens which are equivalent (the same). The middle carbon has two hydroge besides the two methyl groups bonded to it. Since 2-propanol has no stereocen carbon, it is not expected to exhibit chirality. It is, therefore, achiral.

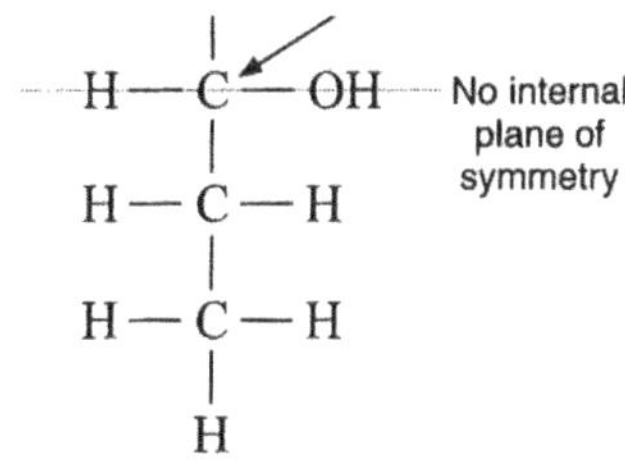

Chiral Molecule

Fig. 7.4 Chirality, Internal Planes, and Stereocentres

On the other hand, 2-butanol (See Fig. 7.4) does have a stereocentre carbon which is e C2 carbon (carbon number 2). The number 2 carbon will have a hydrogen, a hydroxyl, methyl, and an ethyl group bonded to it. Such a molecule would be chiral – possessing) internal plane of symmetry and non-molecules (which contain chiral carbon) are non- ıperimposable on their mirror images and are called chiral molecules. A stereogenic :ntre is also known as a chiral centre. It is characterised by an atom which has different 'oups bound to it in such a manner that its mirror image is non-superimposable. The 'esence of a single stereogenic centre in a molecule results in a chiral molecule.

Molecules can, however, possess more than one stereogenic centre. Such molecules ay or may not be chiral.

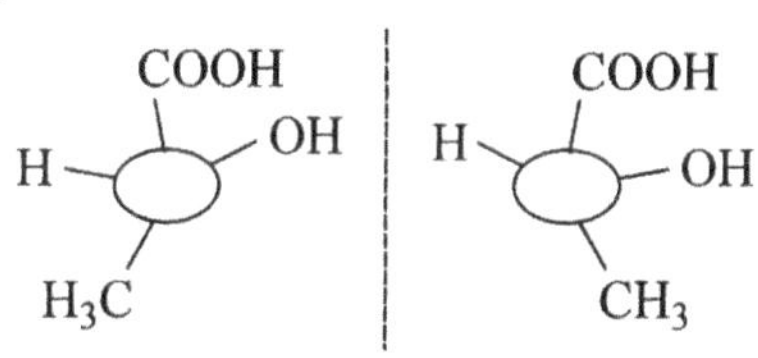

Non-superimposable mirror images of lactic acid

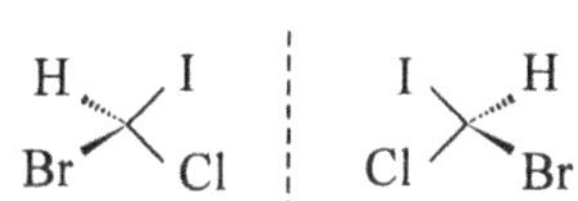

4.3 Achirality and Achiral Molecules

:hiral molecule does not possess a plane of symmetry or centre of symmetry or an ternating axis of symmetry. An *Achiral* object is superimposable on its mirror image. (amples include ball, buckets, nails, and T-shirts (no pockets). Achiral objects possess ther a plane, centre, or alternating axis of symmetry.

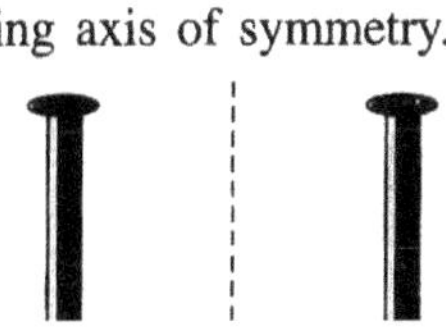

common of these atoms, with which an organic chemist should be familiar, are Si, N a P. They may be tetrahedral molecules (where the four different groups or atoms) or trigo pyramidal molecules (where a lone pair is included as one of the four different grou

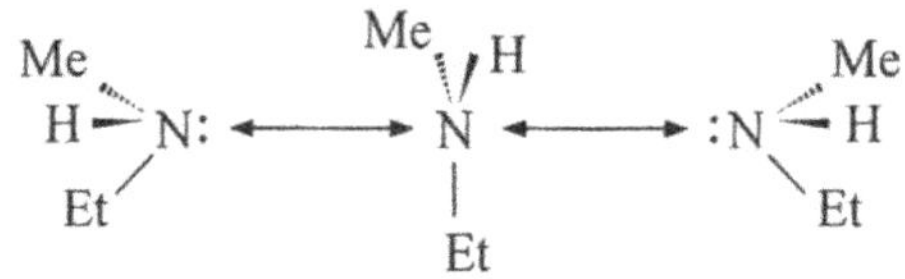

Stereogenic centres containing nitrogen

In this case, even though a stereogenic centre is present in each molecule, a sam is optically inactive as the optical activity of the two extremes of inversion averages c

7.4.5 Plane-Polarised Light

Ordinary light consists of waves vibrating in all possible planes perpendicular to its pa Ordinary day light is turned into plane-polarised light by passing it through a lens ma of polaroid or calcite. A light beam filtered in this manner is said to be a plane-polaris light beam. Plane-polarised light is light whose vibrations take place in only one directi

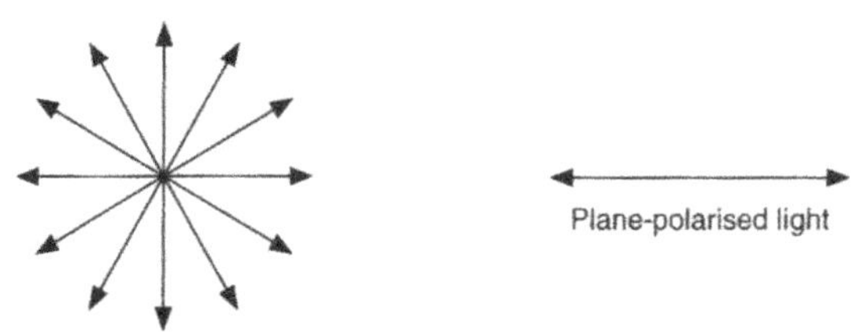

7.4.6 Polarimeter

The instrument used to measure light rotation is called a polarimeter. It consists of monochromatic light source usually a Sodium D-Lamp that is capable of emmitting a pu single wavelength of light which is bi-planar (Fig. 7.5). A polariser filters out one pla of this bi-planar light and allows only one plane to pass through the polariser. This plar polarised light beam is then split into two beams and one beam is routed around t sample while the other split beam is passed through the sample. If the beam passi through the sample, shows any rotation, then the intensity of the light passing throu the sample will be different than the beam that was passed around the sample. This w appear to an observer, looking through an eyepiece, as two semi-circular spots of ligh one brighter than the other. By rotating a calibrated analyser in such a way that the tv half circles of light become of the same intensity the boundary will disappear in t

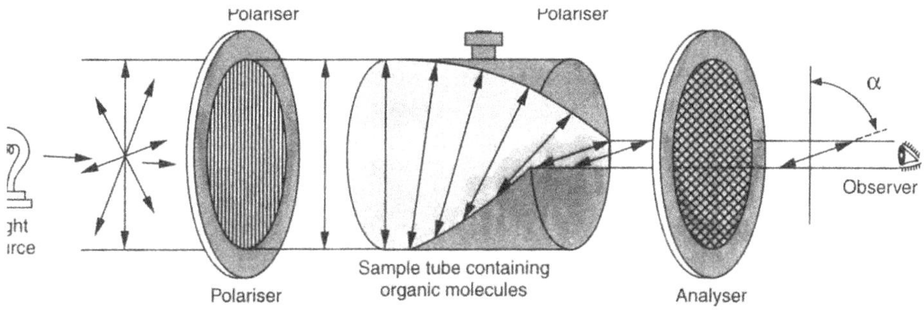

Fig. 7.5 Schematic Representation of a Polarimeter Plane-Polarised Light passes through an Analyser

ł.7 Specific Rotation

e optical activity of a compound is reported in terms of specific rotation, which is ıstant and characteristic for a particular compound. Specific rotation, [α], is the number degrees of rotation observed if a one-decimetre tube is used, and the compound being ımined is present to the extent of one g/cc. This is calculated from the following formula:

$$\text{Specific rotation} = [\alpha]_D^T = \frac{\alpha}{l \times c}$$

ere

α = observed rotation angle

l = length of sample tube in decimetres

c = concentration of substance in solvent

Specific rotation is a physical property like boiling point, melting point, solubility, ısity, etc., of a sample. Specific rotation depends on the nature of the substance, velength of the light used, concentration of the solution, thickness of the layer, nature the solvent and temperature at which the experiment is conducted.

.8 Enantiomers

ʾrinciples of Enantiomerism The isomers whose structures are non-superimposable ror images of each other and which rotate the plane of polarised light but in opposite ections are known as enantiomers or enantiomorphs. Enantiomers cause the plane of arised light to rotate in opposite directions, but to the same extent (clockwise = +ve, ınterclockwise = –ve). The phenomenon of existence of enantiomers is called ntiomerism. Enantiomers have the same chemical and physical properties (melting points, ling points, heat of combustion, etc.), except for their interaction with plane polarised

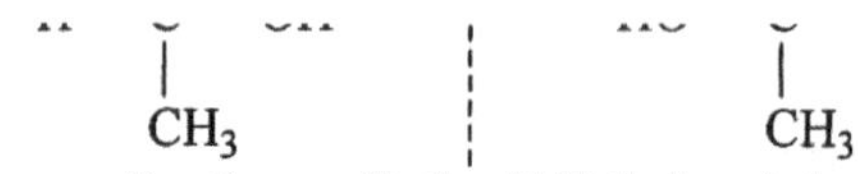

Enantiomers of lactic acid (Optically active)

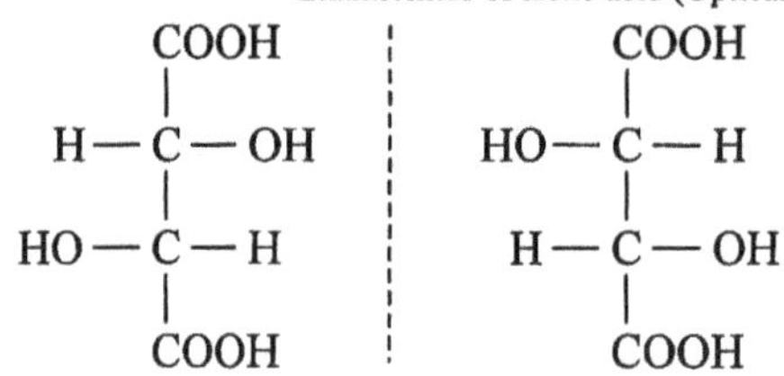

Enantiomers of tartaric acid (Optically active)

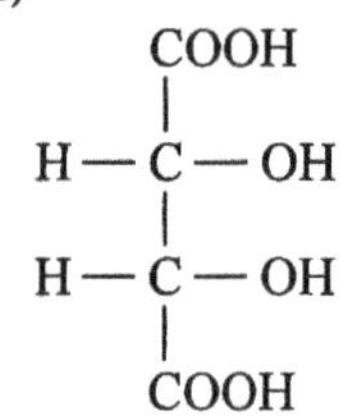

Meso-tartaric acid

2. ***Characteristic Features of Enantiomers***

(i) Enantiomers have identical physical properties (melting point, boiling poin density, solubility, and refractive index) but there is a difference in direction c rotation of plane-polarised light, as described here in case of lactic acid.

Property	*(+)-Lactic Acid*	*(–)-Lactic Acid*
Specific rotation	+ 2.24°	– 2.24°
Melting point	26° C	26° C

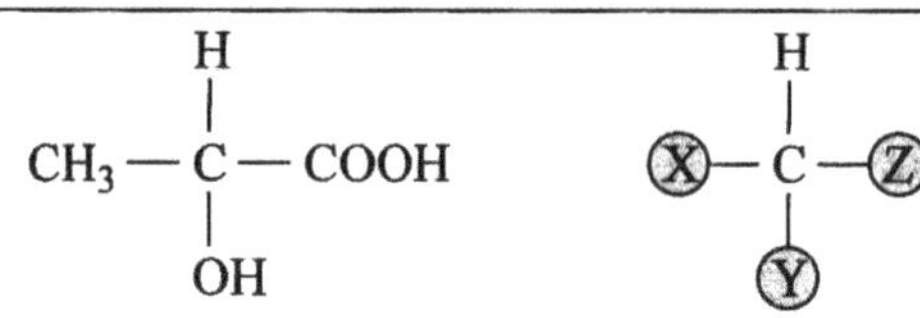

Lactic acid: Molecule of general formula CHXYZ

Mirror

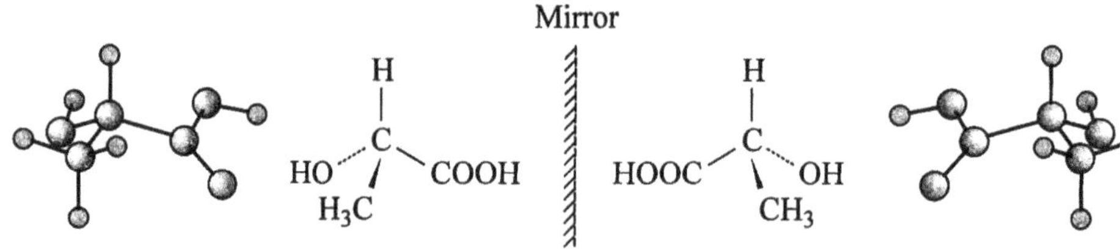

(+)-Lactic acid $[\alpha]_D = +3.82°$

(–)-Lactic acid $[\alpha]_D = -3.82°$

Lactic acid: Molecule of general formula CHXYZ

(ii) They have identical chemical properties except in chemical reactions with othe optically active compounds.

(iii) Enantiomers have identical physical properties, and consequently cannot b directly separated by conventional methods such as distillation, crystallisation sizing, or chromatography on conventional stationary phases.

(iv) They have different biological properties, i.e. (+) dextrose plays an importan role in animal metabolism, whereas (–) dextrose is not metabolised.

ach other are termed as diastereomers. Diastereomers can have quite different physical
chemical properties from one another. For example, the following structures of 2,3-
hlorobutane are diastereoisomers of each other.

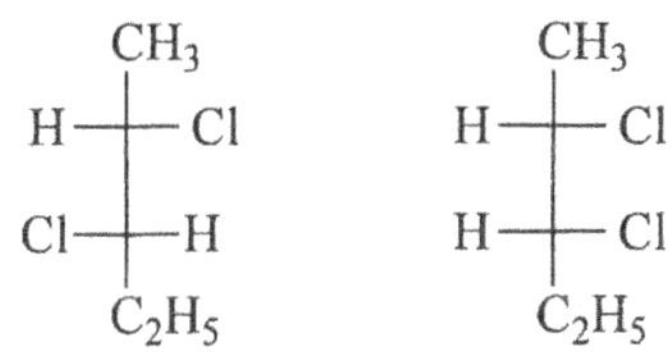

Characteristics

(i) Diastereomers are the members of the same family hence their chemical properties are similar but not identical due to the differences in their E_{act} values and transition states.

(ii) They exhibit different physical properties like melting point, boiling point, solubility, density, refractive index, etc.

(iii) Diastereomers exhibit different specific rotation but they may have same or opposite sign of rotation.

.10 Meso Compound

ners of *achiral molecules*, that possess two or more stereogenic centres, are known
neso isomers (stereoisomers that are superimposable). A meso compound is one whose
ecules are superimposable on their mirror images even though they contain chiral
tres. A meso compound is optically inactive for the same reason as any other compound
ose molecules are achiral: the rotation caused by any one molecule is cancelled by an
al and opposite rotation caused by another molecule that is the mirror image of the
, e.g. meso-2,3-dichlorobutane. This molecule has a plane of symmetry and cannot be
al. Further, one-half of the molecule is the mirror image of the other.

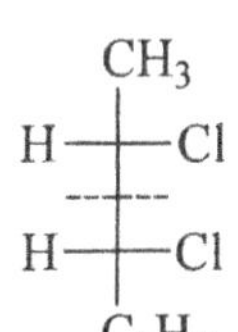

Meso-2,3-dichlorobutane

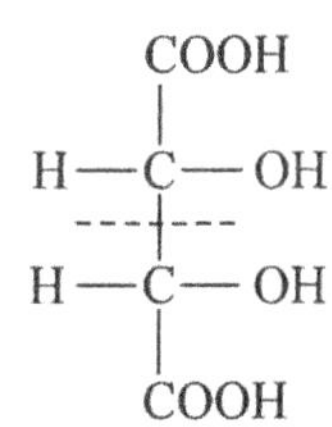

Meso-tartaric acid

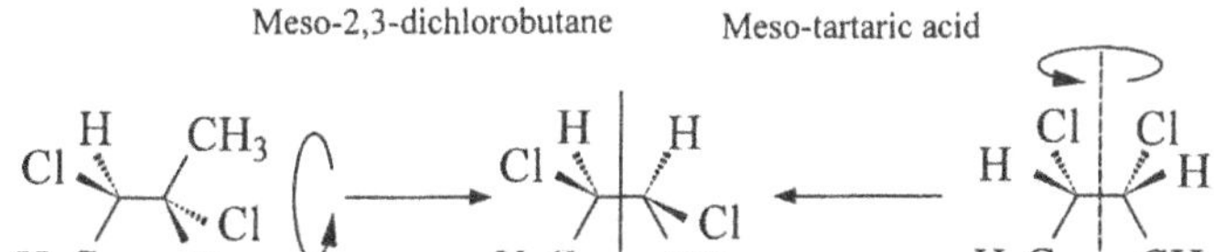

7.4.11 Fischer Projections and the DL-Nomenclature System

Fischer invented this system in 1891. It works by having horizontal lines represent bonds coming out of the plane of the page and vertical lines representing bonds go into the plane of the page. Fischer Projections provide a way to deal with the thr dimensional properties of molecules using a two-dimensional representation.

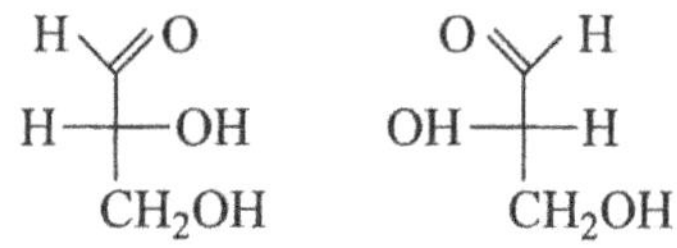

D-Glyceraldehyde L-Glyceraldehyde

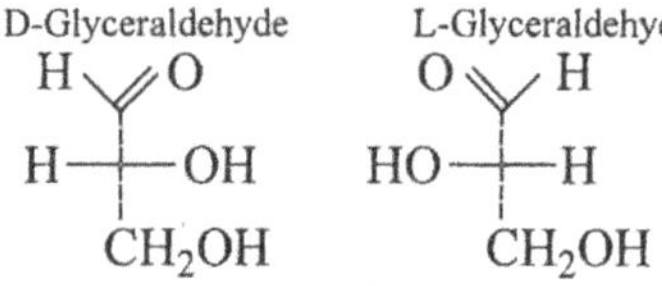

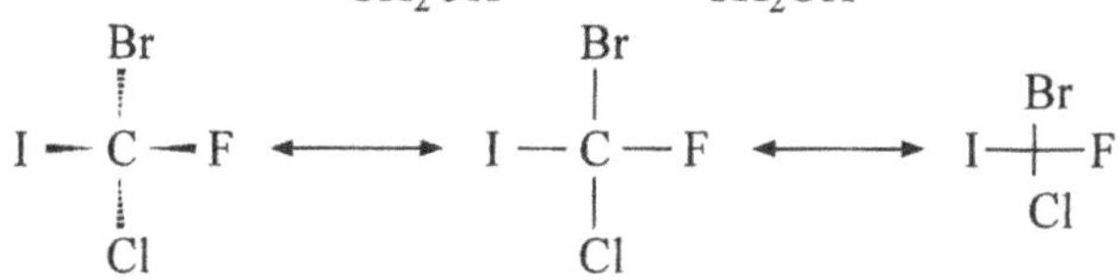

Still Fischer Projections are used for sugars, but generally discouraged.

7.4.12 Elements of Symmetry

The optically inactive molecules have one or more elements of symmetry. These molecu are also known as achiral molecules. These are three main elements of symmetry.

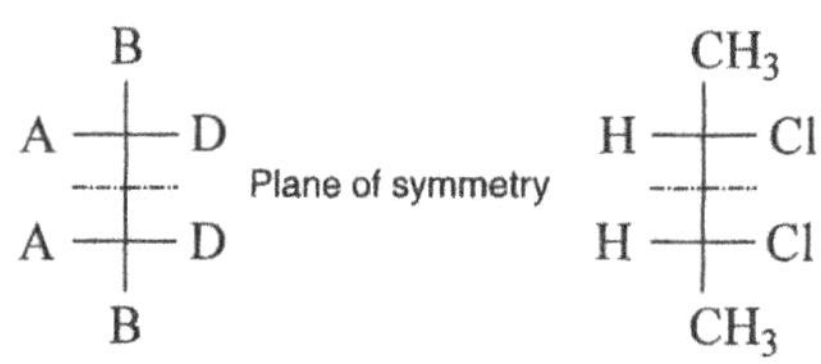

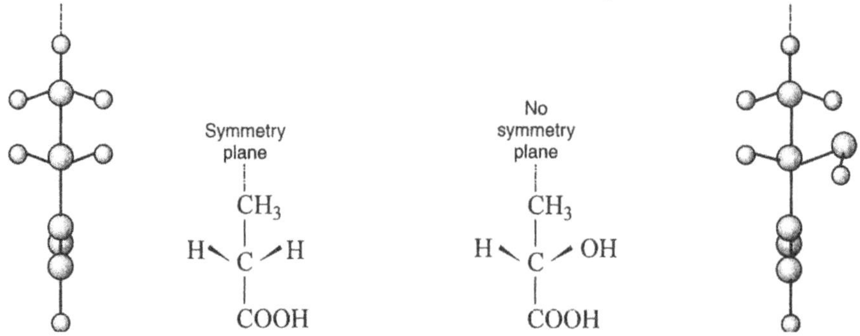

nmetry are achiral (see Fig. 7.6).

Centre of Symmetry Centre of symmetry is a point in the centre of a molecule from ıich any line drawn through the molecule finds similar environment in opposite directions.

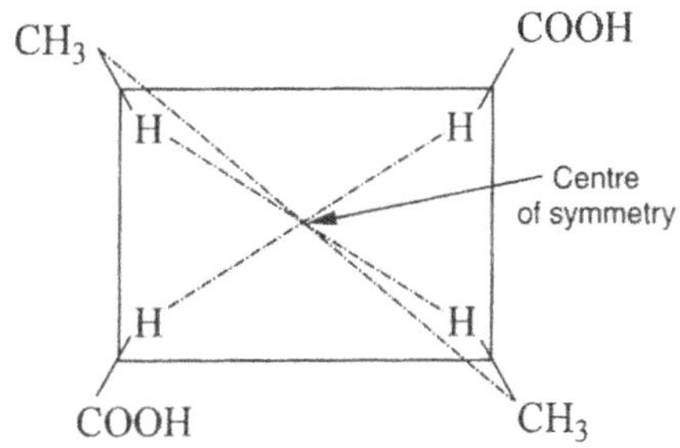

Alternating Axis of Symmetry Alternating axis of symmetry is a line, which passes ough the molecule so that a rotation of 360° about this axis leads to a three-dimensional ıcture, which is similar to the original one. All molecules possess a onefold axis of nmetry ($n = 1$) since rotation of 360° about an axis leads to the identical structure. The ernating axis of symmetry is also known as rotation–reflection axis of symmetry. For ımple, 1,2,3,4-tetramethylcyclobutane is optically active because it possess four–fold ernating axis of symmetry.

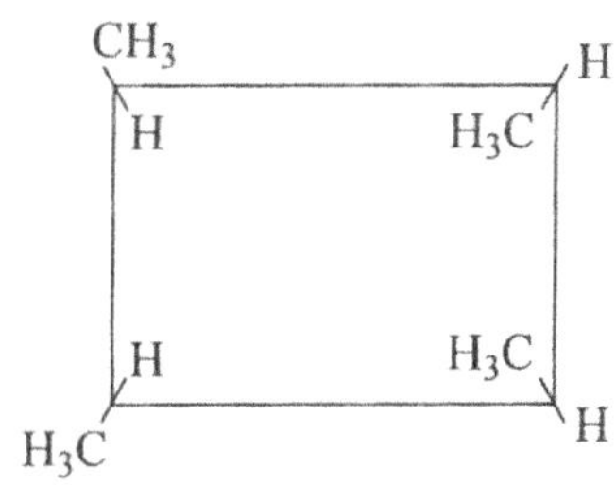

.13 Racemic Mixture

ıixture having equal amounts of enantiomers is called as racemic modification. A racemic ture is optically inactive due to external compensation of rotation caused by both ntiomers. This is generally represented by the prefix dl (or) (±), for example, (±) lactic l and (±) tartaric acid.

The process of conversion of an enantiomer (dextro or laevo form) into a racemic ture (optically inactive) is called *racemisation.* For instance, when d-tartaric acid is ted at 165°–170° C, dl-tartaric acid is formed.

.14 Resolution of Racemic Modification

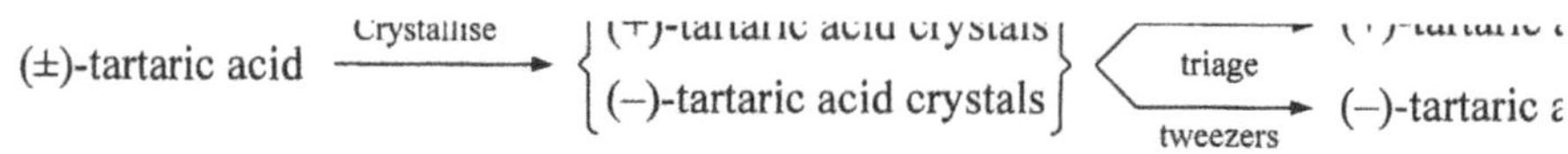

2. ***Biochemical Method*** In biochemical method, a dilute solution of racemic mix is mixed with certain microorganisms (bacteria or mould) and these microorgan consume one enantiomer without affecting the other, e.g. (+) ammonium tartra rapidly destroyed than (–) form.

3. ***Chemical Method*** This method involves conversion of enantiomers of race modification into diastereomers by reaction with an optically active substance. The obta diastereomers exhibit different physical properties (solubility) hence can be separate fractional crystallisation, e.g. (±) alanine is separated by using (–) brucine.

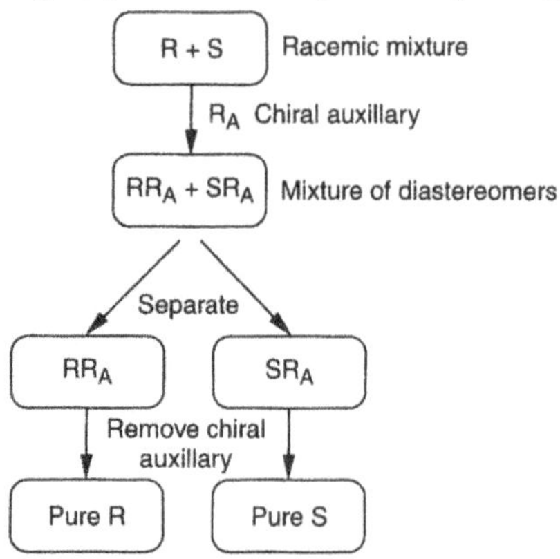

4. ***Chromatographic Method*** In this process, the racemate gets adsorbed by s optically active adsorbents, e.g. wool and casein is able to adsorb selectively (+)-manc acid from an aqueous solution of (±)-mandelic acid.

5. ***Kinetic Resolution*** Racemic mixture reacts with a pure chiral catalyst or enzyme. enantiomer of the racemic mixture reacts faster than the other.

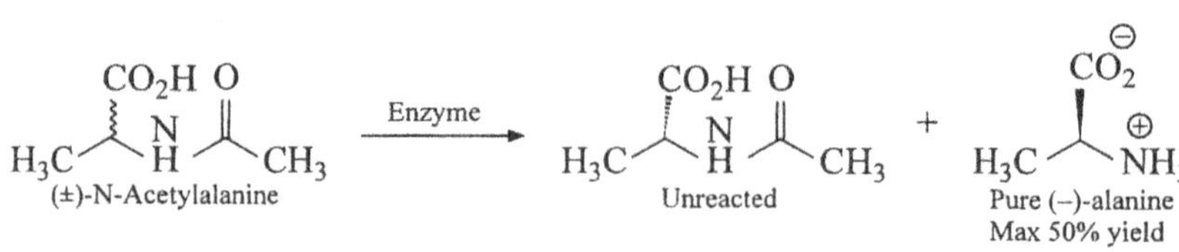

7.4.15 Configuration

The arrangement of atoms that characterises a particular stereoisomer is called

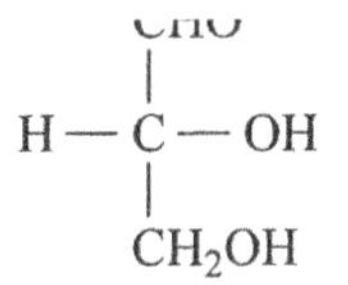

D or (+)-Glyceraldehyde

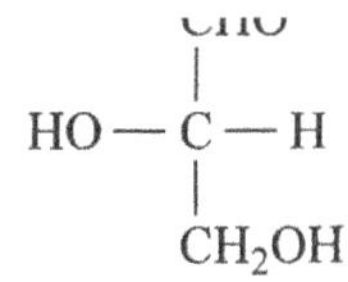

L or (–)-Glyceraldehyde

f the configuration at the asymmetric carbon atom of a compound can be related to +)-glyceraldehyde, it belongs to D-series and if it can be related to L(–)-glyceraldehyde compound belongs to L-series, e.g. natural alanine relates to L-lactic acid which relates (–)-glyceraldehyde, hence belongs to L-series.

bsolute Configuration (R and S System) The most generally useful method gested by Cahn, Ingold and Prelog is the use of the prefixes R and S. The following s are used to assign absolute configuration:

(i) To assign the R or S configuration to a Fischer Projection, you must arrange the projection so that the lowest priority group is either on the top or the bottom of the diagram by using allowable manipulations.

ii) Then assign priorities to the groups as usual followed by moving from the highest priority group to the next highest and the next. If that movement is clockwise, then it is the R isomer. If the movement is counterclockwise, then it is the S isomer.

mple The projection must first be manipulated to place the lowest priority group (F) he top, or bottom position.
n moving from the highest to lower priority groups (1, 2, 3), the movement is nterclockwise and this must therefore be an S isomer.

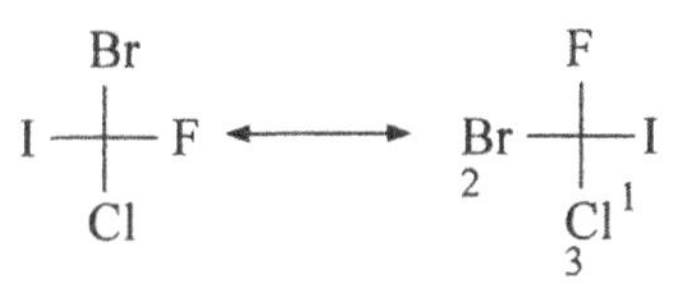

1 We assign a sequence of priority to the four atoms or groups of atoms that is the four ligands attached to the chiral centre. Priority depends simply on atomic number – the atom of higher atomic number gets higher priority. In the case of bromochloroiodomethane the priority depends on atomic number thus the order of priority is I > Br > Cl > H.

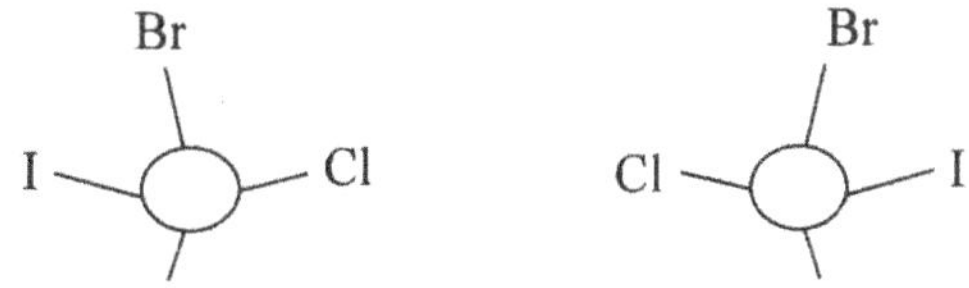

if, in proceeding from the ligand of highest priority to the ligand of seco priority and thence to the third, our eye travels in a clockwise direction, t configuration is specified R (Latin: *rectus* = right): if it travels counterclockwi the configuration is specified S (Latin: *Sinister* = left). Thus, configurations structures (i) and (ii) are viewed like this:

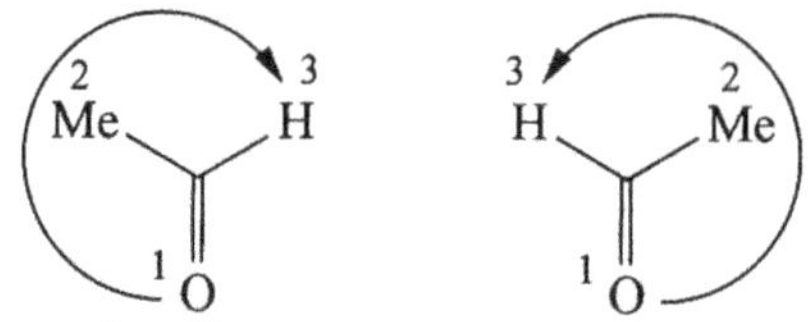

Rectus face Sinister face

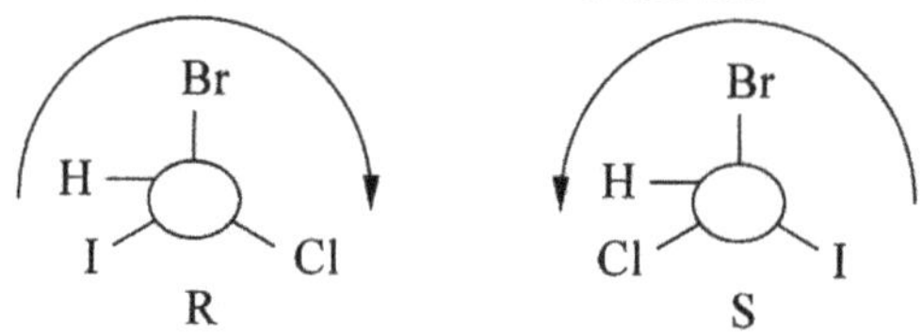

Bromochloroiodomethane

An enzyme can recognise these two diffferent faces which can be referred to as tl *rectus* face or the *sinister* face or *re/si* faces.

Sequence Rule 1 If all the four atoms attached to the chiral centre are differer priority depends on atomic number, with the atom of higher atomic number gets high priority. If two atoms are isotopes of the same element, the atom of higher mass numb has the higher priority, e.g. in chloroiodomethanesulphonic acid, the sequence is I, C S, H while in a deuterioethyl bromide it is Br, C, D, H.

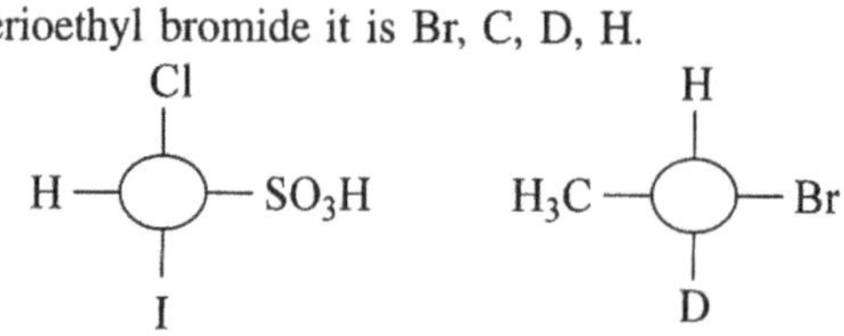

Chloroiodomethanesulphonic acid Deuterioethyl bromide

Sequence Rule 2 If the relative priority of two groups cannot be decided by Rule 1 the priority shall be determined by a similar comparison of the next atoms in the group (and so on, if necessary, working outward from the chiral centre). This is to say, if tw atoms attached to each of these first atoms.

Sequence Rule 3 Where there is double or triple bond, both atoms are considere to be duplicated or triplicated, e.g. in glyceraldehyde, the priority order is

$$—OH, —CHO, —CH_2OH, —H.$$

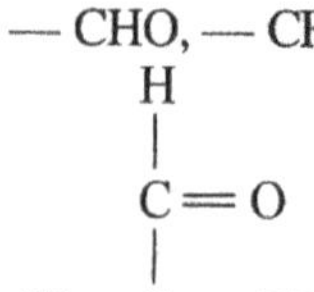

ve substances.

$$M \xrightarrow{R_A} M-R_A \xrightarrow{\text{Reaction}} \underset{\text{(Minor)}}{R-R_A} + \underset{\text{(Major)}}{S-R_A} \xrightarrow{\text{Separate}} S-R_A \xrightarrow{\text{Remove}} \text{Pure S}$$

'or example, optically active lactic acid is prepared from pyruvic acid by converting rst into L-menthylpyruvate.

$$\underset{\text{Pyruvic acid}}{CH_3-CO-COOH} + \underset{\text{L-Menthyl}}{C_{10}H_{19}OH} \longrightarrow \underset{\text{L-Menthylpyruvate}}{CH_3COCOOC_{10}H_{19}}$$

Reduction

$$\longrightarrow \text{L-Menthyl-}d\text{-lactate} + \underset{\text{L-Menthyl-}l\text{-lactate}}{CH_3CH(OH)COOC_{10}H_{19}}$$

Hydrolysis

$$\longrightarrow \underset{\text{L-Lactic acid}}{CH_3CH(OH)COOH} + \underset{\text{L-Menthol}}{C_{10}H_{19}OH} + d\text{-Lactic acid}$$

16 Optical Inversion (Walden Inversion)

conversion of dextro form into laevo form or vice versa by certain chemical sformations without recourse to resolution was discovered by Walden, in 1993, hence ıame Walden inversion. There is an inversion of configuration of the atoms or groups ınd the asymmetric carbon atom.

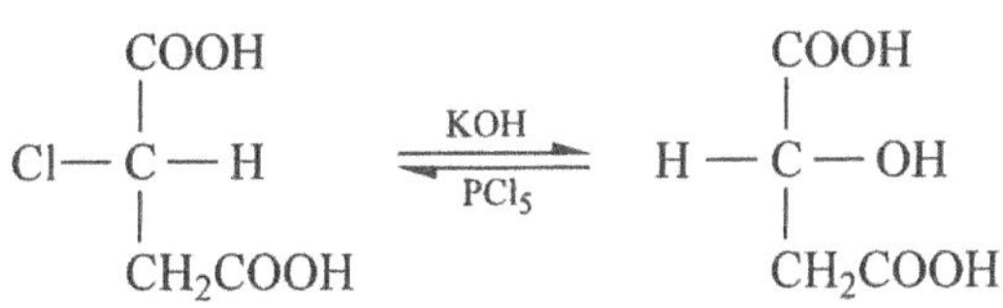

l-Chlorosuccinic acid   *d*-Malic acid

17 Importance of Optical Isomerism

cal isomerism is immensely important in biological systems. In most biological systems one optical isomer of each organic compound is usually present. For example, when amino acid alanine is synthesised in the laboratory, a mixture of the two possible ıers (a racemic mixture) is produced (Fig. 7.7). When alanine is isolated from living , only one of the two forms is seen.

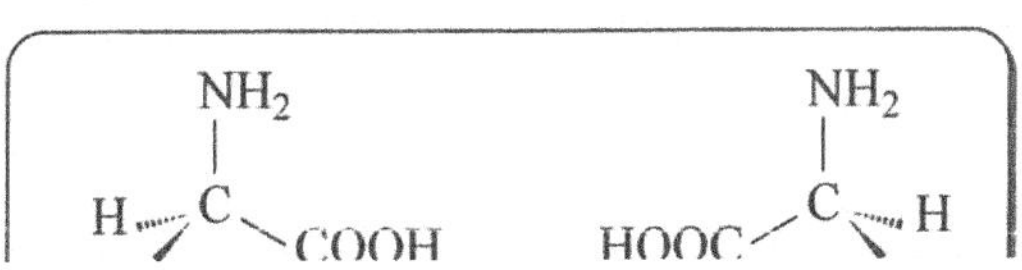

(Fig. 7.8) occurs naturally in organisms such as humans. Since amino acids are the monome in proteins, such as enzymes, therefore, enzymes themselves will be chiral. The active si of an enzyme will only be able to operate on one type of optical isomer. An interestii example of this is the action of penicillin, which functions by preventing the formati of peptide links involving the enantiomer of alanine present in the cell walls of bacteri This enantiomer is not found in humans. Penicillin can, therefore, attack and kill bacter but not harm the human host, as this enantiomer is not present in human cells.

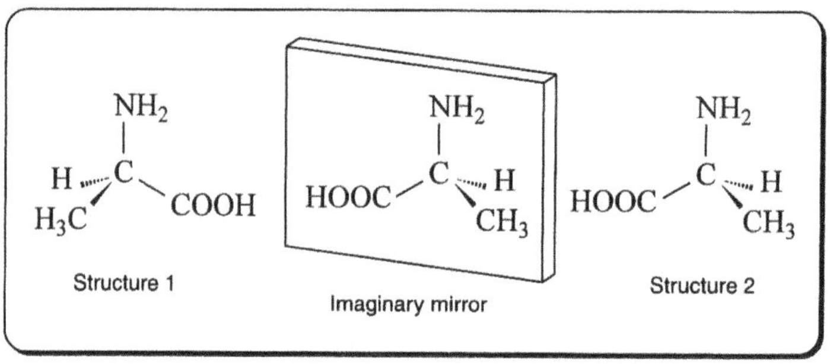

Fig. 7.8 Optical Isomers of alanine

Many medicines are produced as a mixture of enantiomers, only one of which pharmacologically active, as it can prove expensive to separate the isomers. One of tl enantiomers of salbutamol used in the treatment of asthma, is 68 times more effective tha the other. Great caution has to be taken when using drugs with enantiomeric forms as th might be risky, specifically in the case of thalidomide (Fig. 7.9). To quote an example, mixture of the isomers was used to treat nausea during pregnancy, and one enantiome which was thought to be inactive, turned out to cause damage to the unborn child. Mar handicapped babies were born before the drug was recognised as being responsibl Screening of pharmaceuticals has to be very thorough. Regulations were tightene significantly after the thalidomide tragedy to ensure that both enantiomeric forms of chir drugs are tested.

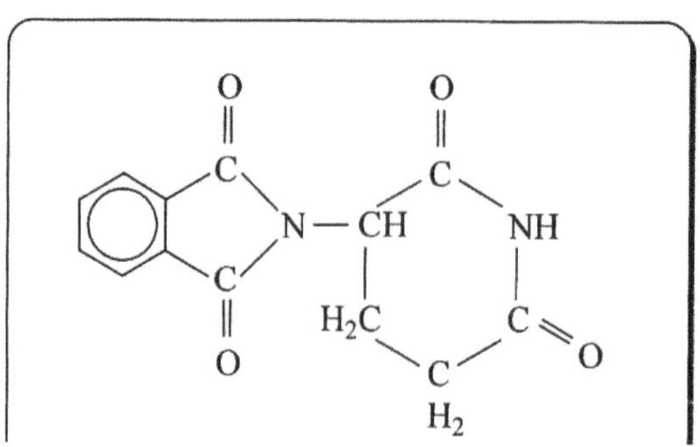

ıe molecules, which differ from one another only by rotation about single bonds, are ıown as conformational isomers or rotational isomers or conformers or rotomers. ɔnformers are not isomers but they are equivalent structures that arise as a result of the tation of carbon atoms about a sigma bond. Usually at normal room temperatures, the fferent conformers are not distinguishable because the energy required to convert one ınformer into another (due to rotation about a sigma bond) is small enough to allow pid conversion and unhindered rotation. Instruments are incapable of detecting the istence of different conformers because of the very high speed of rotation at room nperature where there is enough energy to convert through the conformers, as rotation curs about the sigma bond. However, if one lowers the temperature of the environment, is slows the molecular motion and eventually the rotational speed is slowed to the point ıere instruments are capable of recording differences between conformers. Indeed, the wering of amount of kinetic energy available to cause rotation about the sigma bond ll eventually be restricted enough so that rotation is stopped, and the molecule settles r the most stable conformer. This study of the energy relations between conformers is lled *Conformational Analysis.*

5.2 Modes of Representations

ıe following modes are used to represent the conformations:

- *Dotted line-wedge structure* The dotted lines in the structure, which represents the bonds, are on the plane of paper. The wedges indicate that the bonds are projecting out of the paper.
- *Sawhorse structure* In this type, the bond between the two carbon atoms is drawn diagonally backwards.
- *Newman structure* In this representation, the molecule is viewed from front to back. The two carbon atoms overlap each other, which are represented as superimposed circles. In case of front carbon, the bonds terminate at the centre, whereas in the case of back carbon atom the bonds terminate at the periphery of the circle.

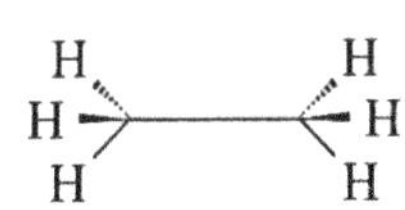

Dotted line-wedge structure

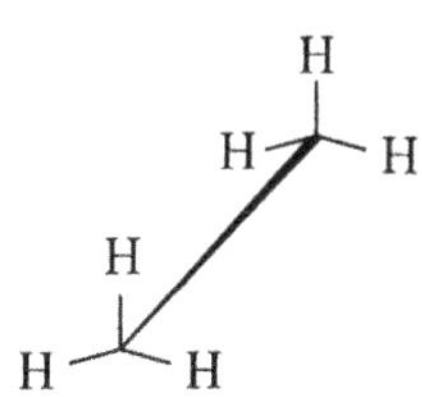

Sawhorse structure

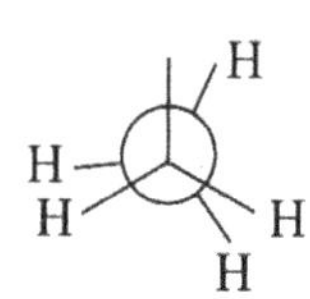

Newman projection structure

into one another by rotation about single bonds are known as conformations.

In case of ethane molecule, one methyl group is imagined to be stationary and tl other methyl group rotates about the C—C sigma bond to give infinite number of structure The angle through which the methyl group is rotated is known as the angle of torsio The following are various conformations of ethane:

- *Eclipsed conformation* In the eclipsed conformation, the hydrogens on the forwa carbon are directly in front of those on the back carbon.
- *Staggered conformation* In this type, the hydrogens on the forward carbon a set between each of the hydrogen on the back carbon.
- *Skew conformation* This conformation is intermediate between eclipsed ar staggered conformation.

The staggered conformer is the most stable by 2.8 kcal/mole because the hydroge in the staggered conformer are farthest away from one another and, therefore, do n physically hinder each other as much. This hindrance, because atoms are too close each other, is called van der Waals Strain (Steric Strain). This steric strain is minimise in the staggered conformer. Furthermore, the sigma bonding pairs holding the hydroge atoms to the carbons are as far away from each other as possible. Since electrons rep each other and this repulsion causes instability, the bonding electron pairs in the staggere conformer are as far away as possible and, therefore, their repulsion is minimised thereb maximising the stability of the molecule. This repulsion of sigma bonding pairs on adjace carbons is called *torsional strain*. In the eclipsed conformer, the amount of steric strai and the tortional strain is much increased thus making the molecule less stable.

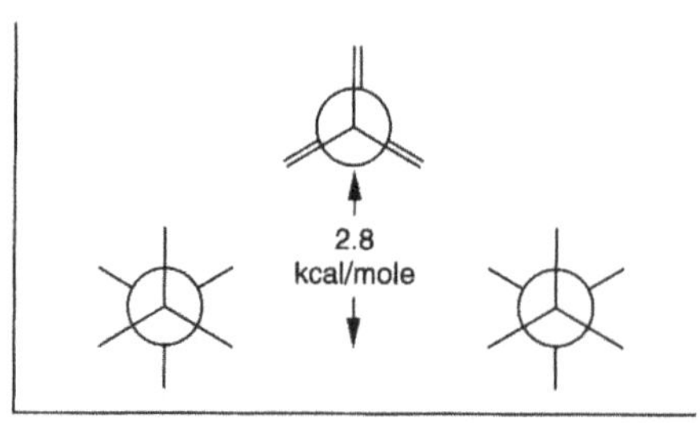

Fig. 7.10 Conformational Analysis of Ethane

7.5.4 The Conformations of Butane

The free rotation of the C2 and C3 carbons of butane give rise to several conformers th differ in their energy states. The most stable of the six conformers of butane is the anti conformer (see Fig. 7.11a) where the two end CH_3 groups (the C1 and C4 carbons o butane) are as far away from each other as possible. This minimises any van der Waal

creases the van der Waals strain since the hydrogen atom and the methyl groups are very ose. In addition, the torsional strain would be increased, and this conformer is 3.8 kcal/ ole more in energy than the anti-conformer and is less stable than the anti (see Fig. 7.12b).

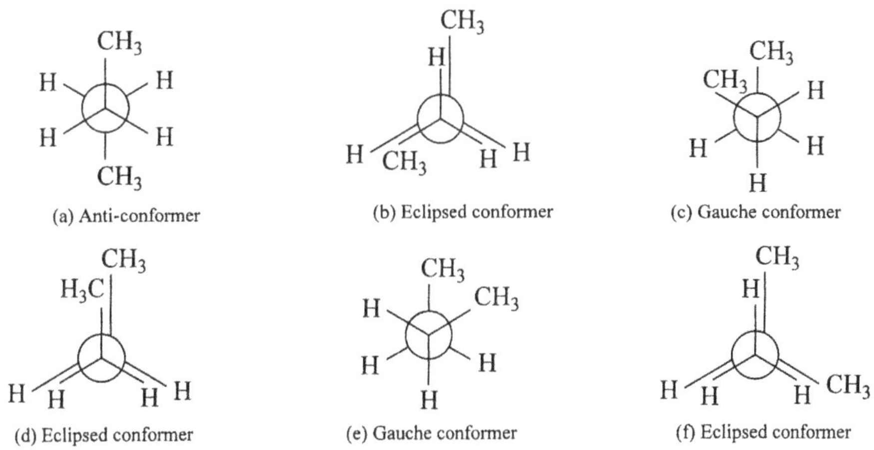

Fig. 7.11(a–f) Conformers of Butane

Another 60-degree rotation about the C2 and C3 sigma bond will place the methyl oups, representing the C1 and C4 carbons, as close to each other as possible. This lipsed conformer [see Fig. 7.11(d)] has maximum van der Waals strain since the bulky ethyl groups are rubbing up against each other and strongly repelling each other. In ldition, the bonding pairs on the C2 and C3 carbons are eclipsing one another, thus aximising the torsional strain. This eclipsed conformer is the highest in energy – being 5 kcal/mole more in energy than the anti-conformer and is, therefore, the least stable of e six conformers (see Fig. 7.12d).

Another 60-degree rotation (the fourth such rotation since the anti-conformer) will lead another gauche conformer where the methyl groups (C1 and C4 carbons) are about as r away from each other as in the first gauche conformer (see Fig. 7.11e). This gauche nformer is equivalent to the first gauche conformer in the amount of van der Waals ain and torsional strain it possesses, so it has the same energy state (0.9 kcal/mole more an the anti) (see Fig. 7.12e).

A fifth 60-degree rotation will give us a third eclipsed conformer (see Fig. 7.11f) which terms of van der Waals strain and torsional strain is equivalent to the first eclipsed form e saw in Fig. 7.12c and is 3.8 kcal/mole above in energy state compared to the anti- nformer (see Fig. 7.12f).

A sixth 60-degree rotation will bring us back to the anti-conformer. At room temperature,

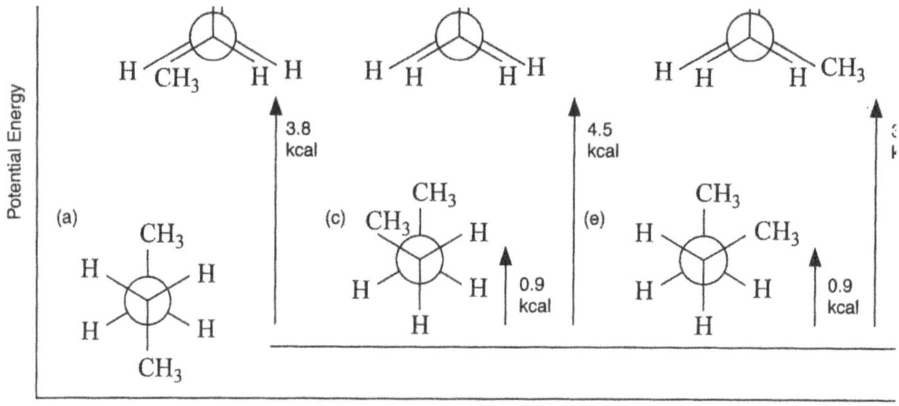

Fig. 7.12 Energy States of Butane Conformers

This rotation at room temperature is so rapid that we are not able to detect the individ conformers. It is similar to what happens when one tries to capture a very rapid ev on film. If the shutter speed of the camera is much slower than the rapidly occurring eve then the event will be blurred at best, and a distinct picture of it will be impossible. C has to either speed up the shutter speed or slow down the event. With sigma bc rotation, we can slow down the event (rotational speed) by lowering the temperature the environment to well below 0° C. This slows down molecular motion since the kine energy is reduced. The rotational speed is reduced because there is no longer as mu kinetic energy to draw upon to get through the energy barriers that must be travers during the rotation (see Fig. 7.12). At one point, there is not enough energy available overcome these energy barriers, and thus the molecule settles for the most stable (low energy) anti-conformer. This would also be true if we were to lower the temperature ethane (see Section 7.5.3).

7.5.5 Cyclohexane Conformations

Cyclohexane seems to be the most stable of the cycloalkanes. Even though cycloalkan have restricted rotation about the sigma bonds between the ring carbons, there is so limited rotation which is enough cyclohexane to have conformers. Of the several conform of cyclohexane, the most stable is the chair conformer. This conformer's stability can attributed to the minimal van der Waals strain of the hydrogens of the C1 and C4 carbo in the ring. In the chair conformer, these positions are the head rest and the foot r (see Fig. 7.13a). In addition to the minimal steric strain at these positions, there is a minimal torsional strain between adjacent carbons because the hydrogens on these carbo in the ring, are staggered. The chair conformer of cyclohexane will undergo a 'ring fl

bons in what is called the twist boat. This is 5.5 kcal/mol more than the chair
e Fig. 7.13c). The twist boat converts into the boat conformer where the C1 and C4 bons form the bow and stern of a boat. The other four carbons are planar. The boat ıformer is less stable than the chair by 7.1 kcal/mol because of the increased steric ıin of the hydrogens on the C1 and C4 carbons (see Fig. 7.13d). The boat twists in effort to bring the C1 carbon down below the plane, which forms an equivalent twist ıt conformer – 5.5 kcal/mol more energetic (less stable) than the chair conformer e Fig. 7.13e). The C1 carbon then becomes planar to the C2, C3, C5 and C6 carbons form a half-chair conformer, which is equivalent to the above half-chair which is 10.8 ıl/mol more energetic than the chair conformer (see Fig. 7.13f). The C1 carbon then ves down below the plane to assume the flipped chair conformer becoming the foot t (see Fig. 7.13g).

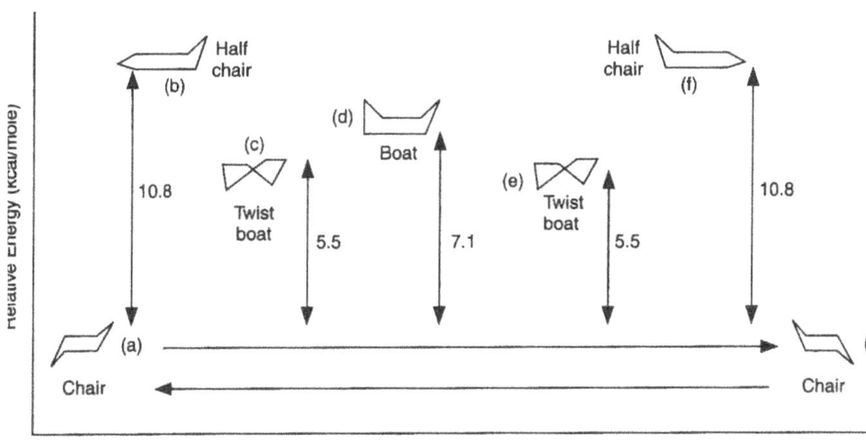

Fig. 7.13 Conformers and Conformational Analysis of Cyclohexane

At room temperature, there is more than enough energy available for the ring flip to ːrcome the energy transitions shown in Fig. 7.13 with over one million such conversions ing place, but because of the more stable state of the chair conformer, it is estimated t 99% of the molecules are in that conformation at any given time.

Axial and Equatorial Hydrogens of Cyclohexane Not all of the hydrogens attached he ring carbons in cyclohexane are equivalent. We can prove this by replacing all, but ;, of the 12 hydrogens with deuterium leaving one position as regular hydrogen. Because ring flip occurs so rapidly at room temperature, there will be only one *nuclear magnetic onance* signal for the one hydrogen. Deuterium atoms do not have a spin state that ıld generate an NMR signal. However, when we slow down the molecular motion by ering the temperature of the sample to an extremely low level, the ring flip occurs much

sigma bonds are perpendicular to their axis (see Fig. 7.14a). The equatorial bonds approximately horizontal to the molecule. During the ring flip process, the axial hydrog become equatorial and the equatorial hydrogens become axial (see Fig. 7.14b).

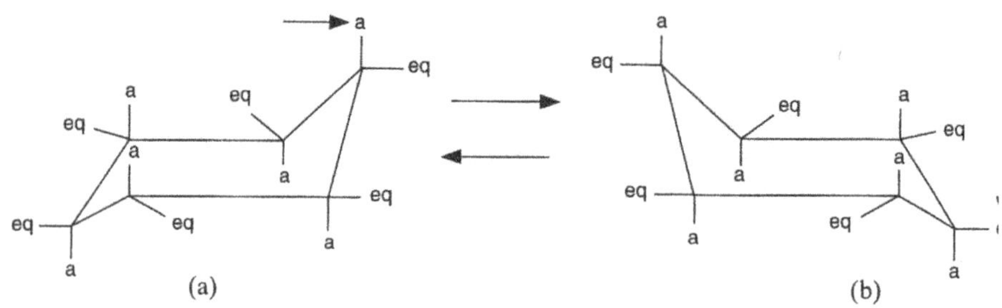

Fig. 7.14 Ring Flip of Cyclohexane

PRACTICE QUESTIONS

1. (a) Explain geometrical isomerism with examples. What type of compounds exhibits i phenomenon?
   (b) Discuss the different methods of determination of configuration of geometrical isom
   (c) Explain conformational analysis.
2. Explain the following terms with examples:
   (i) Enantiomorphs
   (ii) Centre of symmetry
   (iii) Partial asymmetric synthesis
   (iv) A plane of symmetry
   (v) A centre of symmetry
   (vi) Alternating axis of symmetry
   (vii) Molecular symmetry
   (viii) Walden inversion
   (ix) Resolution of racemic modifications
   (x) Asymmetric synthesis
3. Define the following terms giving suitable examples:
   (i) Stereoisomerism
   (ii) Conformation
   (iii) Mesoform
4. (a) What are different methods involved in determination of configuration of geometrical isome Illustrate with suitable examples.
   (b) Explain briefly the modern theory of double bonds.
   (c) What are the evidences in favour of tetrahedral nature of carbon atoms?
5. (a) Draw the Fischer projection formulae for the following:

(ii) Specific rotation
(iii) Enantiomers
(iv) Superimposable
(v) Diasteromers
(vi) Meso compound
(vii) Configuration
(viii) Optical activity
(ix) Conformational isomers
(x) Configurational isomers
(xi) Explain sequence rules

(a) State the necessary and sufficient condition for a compound to show
(i) Geometrical isomerism
(ii) Optical isomerism
Illustrate your answer with two examples of each giving reason for the phenomena.
(b) What is Walden inversion? Explain with examples. What are the factors that affect Walden inversion.

(a) What are the different elements of symmetry? Explain with examples.
(b) Discuss asymmetric synthesis with examples.
(c) Suggest important methods for the resolution of recemic mixture.
(d) What do you understand by conformational analysis? Discuss with examples.

(a) What do you understand by Z and E conformation and mesostructure?
(b) What is meant by resolution of racemic mixture? Discuss three important methods of resolution.
(c) Write stereochemical structures of:
(i) R. Chlorobromoiodomethane
(ii) Z. 2-Heptene
(iii) S. Butanol
(d) Draw stereochemical formula of all possible stereoisomers of 2,3 dichlorobutane and show their inter relationship. Specify configuration (R or S) at each carbon in any two structures.

Write notes on:
(i) Resolution of racemic mixture
(ii) Walden inversion

(a) What is meant by absolute configuration? Explain with suitable examples.
(b) Discuss the types of isomers that can be distinguished due to rotation across a single and across a double bond between unsymmetrically substituted carbons. Illustrate with suitable examples and diagrams.

(a) What do you understand by the following terms?
(i) Stereoisomers
(ii) Optical isomers
(iii) Diastereomers
(iv) Plane of symmetry

(i) Chiral centre
(ii) E and Z notation
(iii) Polarised light
(iv) Racemic and meso forms

(d) What is confirmation? Which of the confirmations of cyclohexane is more stable and w

16. (a) Which of the following are optically active?
(b) Specify the configuration of the following as (R) or (S):

$$\text{(i)}\ \begin{array}{c} CH_3 \\ | \\ H-C-OH \\ | \\ COOH \end{array} \qquad \text{(ii)}\ \begin{array}{c} COOH \\ | \\ H_2N-C-H \\ | \\ CH_2OH \end{array} \qquad \text{(iii)}\ \begin{array}{c} CH_2OH \\ | \\ H-C-CH_3 \\ | \\ C_2H_5 \end{array}$$

(c) Define enantiomerism and diastereomerism. Explain these terms with suitable examp
(d) Which of the following are chiral and why?
(i) Spool of thread
(ii) A pair of scissors
(iii) Tennis ball
(iv) Your nose

17. Write a note on the following:
(a) Restricted rotation about single bond in cyclohexane
(b) Geometrical isomerism due to C=N
(c) Resolution of recemic mixtures

18. (a) What are the necessary and sufficient requirements for a diphenyl derivate to be optic. active?
(b) Explain Walden inversion and enumerate the factors influencing it.
(c) Write a note on geometrical isomerism of oximes and methods used for determining tl configuration.

19. Differentiate between the following:
(a) Asymetric and disymetric molecules
(b) Configuration and conformation
(c) Absolute and partial asymmetric synthesis
(d) Enantiomers and diastereoisomers

20. Explain the following:
(a) Lactic acid exhibits optical isomerism where as propionic acid does not.
(b) What is required for a compound to show optical activity?
(c) Distinguish between the following terms giving examples:
(i) Absolute and relative configuration
(ii) Meso compound and racemic mixture
(iii) Absolute and relative configuration

3

;HEMISTRY OF ALKANES

kanes are the saturated aliphatic hydrocarbons, having the general formula C_nH_{2n+2} here n = 1, 2, 3, 4, . . ., and so on). The carbon atoms in these molecules are bonded each other by single covalent bonds.

I NOMENCLATURE OF ALKANES

Common System

(i) In this system, the first four members of the series are called by their trivial or common names: methane (CH_4); ethane (C_2H_6), propane (C_3H_8) and butane (C_4H_{10}). Rest of the members are named by prefixing Greek numerals *pent* (5), *hex* (6), *hept* (7), *Oct* (8) and so on, respectively, indicating the number of carbon atoms in the molecule.

(ii) The alkanes, having a straight or normal chain, are called normal alkanes by prefixing *n*- to the name of the alkane.

$CH_3CH_2CH_2CH_3$ — *n*-Butane

$CH_3CH_2CH_2CH_2CH_3$ — *n*-Pentane

(iii) The alkanes, in which the carbon chain is branched, are called branched-chain alkanes. Alkanes, which possess a one-carbon branch on the second carbon of the basic normal chain, are referred to as *iso* alkanes.

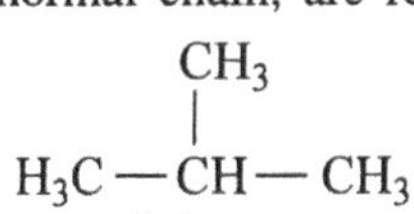
Isobutane

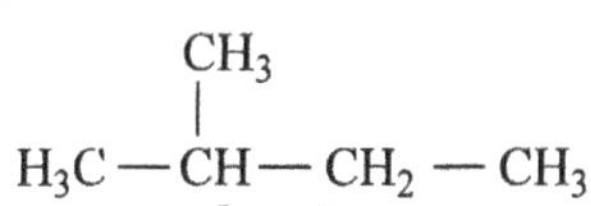
Isopentane

(iv) From pentane onwards, when the normal carbon chain present in the molecule has two one-carbon branches, on the second carbon, the alkane is referred to as *neo* alkane.

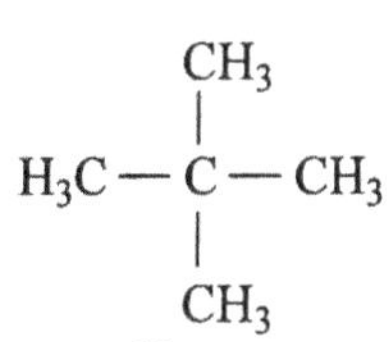

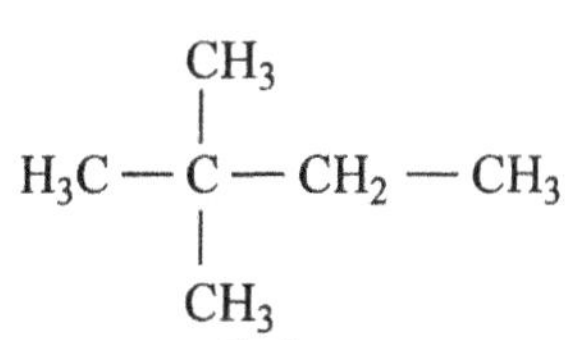

2	Ethane	C_2H_6	CH_3CH_3
3	Propane	C_3H_8	$CH_3CH_2CH_3$
4	Butane	C_4H_{10}	$CH_3CH_2CH_2CH_3$
5	Pentane	C_5H_{12}	$CH_3CH_2CH_2CH_2CH_3$
6	Hexane	C_6H_{14}	$CH_3CH_2CH_2CH_2CH_2CH_3$
7	Heptane	C_7H_{16}	$CH_3CH_2CH_2CH_2CH_2CH_2CH_3$
8	Octane	C_8H_{18}	$CH_3CH_2CH_2CH_2CH_2CH_2CH_2CH_3$
10	Decane	$C_{10}H_{22}$	$CH_3CH_2CH_2CH_2CH_2CH_2CH_2CH_2CH_2CH$

(i) Determine the longest continuous chain of carbons. The longest continuous ch does not necessarily have to be straight.

(ii) Identify the various branching groups attached to this continuous chain of carb by name.

(iii) Number the carbons in the chain so that the groups would be attached to carbons with the lowest designated number. This means that you have to dec whether to begin numbering on the right-end or left-end of the chain.
For example, if you number one way so that three branched groups are attacl on number designated carbons 3, 5, 6 in a six-carbon continuous chain and tl number the six carbons in the opposite direction so that these same brancl groups are attached to carbons designated as 1, 2, 4, then the proper number would be the second way where the designated numbers would be 1, 2, 4. suitable way to decide is to add up the designated numbers in the sequence. ٦ lowest sum would be the direction you would number of the carbons in continuous chain.

(iv) Name the branched groups in an alphabetical order attaching (hyphenating) carbon number it is attached to along the continuous chain of carbons to the fr of the branch name.

(v) If more than one of the same kind of branched group is attached to the cha identify the designated number of carbon each group is attached to, as a ser of numbers separated by commas between each number then a hyphen and fina use a Greek prefix attached to the branch name.

8.2 ALKYL GROUPS

A group of atoms derived from alkanes (R—H) by the removal of hydrogen atom a called alkyl groups. The name of an alkyl group is obtained by replacing the -ane of t corresponding name of alkane by the suffix -yl.

Alkane	*Alkyl Group*	*Name of the Alkyl Group*

ture of many hydrocarbons and most of them belong to alkane series. Petroleum refining he process of separating the various compounds present in crude petroleum. The iciple used is that the longer the carbon chains the higher the temperature at which compounds will boil. The crude petroleum is heated and changed into a gas. The es are passed through a distillation column, which becomes cooler as the height eases. When a compound in the gaseous state cools below its boiling point, it denses into a liquid. The liquids may be drawn off the distilling column at various ghts (Fig. 8.1).

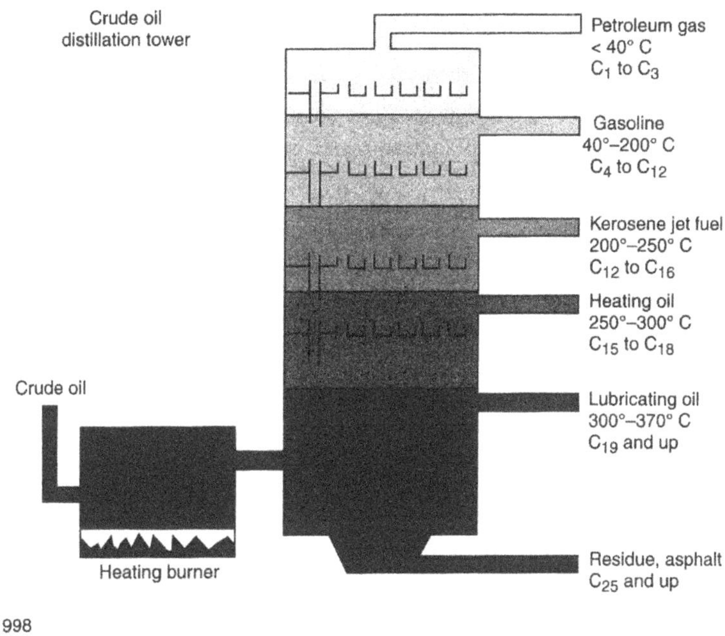

Fig. 8.1 Fractional Distillation of Crude Oil

'he individual alkanes are obtained from petroleum by refining in a refinery. Natural obtained from petroleum fields contains about 80% methane, 10% ethane and the aining 10% mixture of higher members.

GENERAL METHODS OF PREPARATION

Iydrogenation of Unsaturated Hydrocarbons Alkenes or alkynes on treating with ecular hydrogen gas in presence of catalyst like Ni, Pt, Pd (heterogeneous ogenation) or Wilkinson's catalyst (homogeneous hydrogenation) give alkanes. This

Ethyne Ethane

2. ***Reduction of Alkyl Halides*** Alkyl halides on reduction with nascent hydrogen f(alkanes. The nascent hydrogen required for reduction may be obtained by using Z HCl, Zn + CH_3COOH, $LiAlH_4$, H_2 + Ni or Pt reagents. However, primary and second alkyl halides are readily reduced to alkanes with lithium aluminium hydride.

$$\underset{\text{Alkyl halide}}{R - X} + H_2 \longrightarrow \underset{\text{Alkane}}{R - H} + HX$$

$$\underset{\text{Methyl iodide}}{CH_3I} + H_2 \longrightarrow \underset{\text{Methane}}{CH_4} + HI$$

$$\underset{\text{Ethyl bromide}}{CH_3CH_2Br} + H_2 \longrightarrow \underset{\text{Ethane}}{CH_3CH_3} + HI$$

3. ***Wurtz Reaction*** Higher alkanes are obtained by the condensation of two molecu of an alkyl halide (RX) with sodium metal in presence of alcohol-free dry ether.

$$\underset{\text{Alkyl halide}}{R\,X} + 2Na + \underset{\text{Alkyl halide}}{X\,R} \longrightarrow \underset{\text{Alkane}}{R - R} + 2NaX$$

$$\underset{\text{Methyl iodide}}{CH_3\,I} + 2Na + \underset{\text{Methyl iodide}}{I\,CH_3} \longrightarrow \underset{\text{Ethane}}{H_3C - CH_3} + 2NaI$$

$$\underset{\text{Ethyl iodide}}{CH_3CH_2\,I} + 2Na + \underset{\text{Ethyl iodide}}{I\,H_2CCH_3} \longrightarrow \underset{n\text{-Butane}}{CH_3CH_2CH_2CH_3} + 2NaI$$

Wurtz reaction may follow either of the following two mechanisms.

(i) Intermediate formation of organo sodium.

$$\underset{\text{Alkyl halide}}{RX} + 2Na \longrightarrow \underset{\text{Alkyl sodium}}{R - Na} + NaX$$

$$\underset{\text{Alkyl halide}}{RX} + \underset{\text{Alkyl sodium}}{R - Na} \longrightarrow \underset{\text{Alkane}}{R - R} + NaX$$

(ii) Intermediate formation of free radicals.

$$\underset{\text{Alkyl halide}}{RX} + Na \longrightarrow \underset{\text{Alkyl free radical}}{R\cdot} + NaX$$

$$\underset{\text{Alkyl free radicals}}{R\cdot + R\cdot} \longrightarrow \underset{\text{Alkane}}{R - R}$$

The main feature of Wurtz reaction is that it leads to the formation of a carbon–carb bond. Thus higher alkanes are synthesised by this method. It is suitable only for preparati of symmetrical alkanes.

Limitations This method of preparation is unsuitable for unsymmetrical alkanes becau a mixture of all possible alkanes is formed. It is not used for the preparation of metha

ι carbanion. The partially bonded carbanion is a Lewis base. It reacts with strong acids ;ive an alkane. Any compound possessing of acidic hydrogen (water, alcohols, terminal ynes, phenols and carboxylic acids) will bring about this reaction.

$$\underset{\text{Alkyl magnesium halide}}{R-MgX} + H-OH \longrightarrow \underset{\text{Alkane}}{R-H} + Mg(X)OH$$

$$\underset{\text{Methyl magnesium halide}}{CH_3MgI} + HOH \longrightarrow \underset{\text{Methane}}{CH_4} + Mg(I)OH$$

:orey–House Synthesis This is a highly versatile method in synthesising alkanes. In method, an alkyl halide is first converted into lithium dialkyl cuprate (LiR_2Cu) in anhydrous :r. This on treatment with the same or different alkyl halide an alkane is formed.

$$R-X \xrightarrow{2Li} R-Li + LiX$$

$$2R-Li + CuI \xrightarrow[\text{Ether}]{0^\circ C} R_2CuLi + LiI$$

ylation with R_2CuLi

$$R-X + R_2CuLi \xrightarrow[\text{Ether}]{0^\circ C} R-R + R-Cu + LiX$$

X = Cl, Br, I

mples

$$(CH_3)_2CuLi + CH_3(CH_2)_4-I \longrightarrow CH_3-(CH_2)_4-CH_3$$

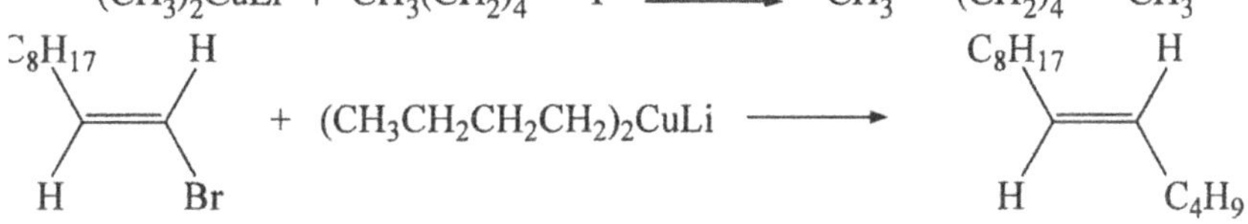

Corey–House reaction

Decarboxylation of Carboxylic Acid When the sodium salt of a carboxylic acid is ed strongly with sodalime (NaOH + CaO), an alkane is formed. The alkane, so obtained, ains one carbon less than the original acid. This reaction is known as decarboxylation.

$$\underset{\text{Sodium carboxylate}}{RCOONa} + \underset{\text{Sodalime}}{NaOH/CaO} \longrightarrow \underset{\text{Alkane}}{RH} + Na_2CO_3$$

$$\underset{\text{Sodium acetate}}{CH_3COONa} + NaOH/CaO \longrightarrow \underset{\text{Methane}}{CH_4} + Na_2CO_3$$

:olbe's Synthesis When a concentrated solution of sodium or potassium salt of a

At Anode

$$\underset{\text{Carboylate ion}}{RCOO^-} \longrightarrow \underset{\text{Carboxylate radical}}{RCOO\cdot} + e^-$$

$$\underset{\text{Carboxylate radical}}{RCOO\cdot} \longrightarrow \underset{\text{Alkyl free radical}}{R\cdot + CO_2}$$

$$\underset{\text{Alkyl free radicals}}{R\cdot + R\cdot} \longrightarrow \underset{\text{Alkane}}{R - R}$$

At Cathode

$$2H_2O + 2e^- \longrightarrow H_2 + 2OH^-$$

$$Na^+ + OH^- \longrightarrow NaOH$$

Importance The Kolbe's electrolytic method is widely employed to prepare lipids.

8. ***From Carbonyl Compounds*** Aldehydes and ketones can be reduced to hydrocarbc with zinc amalgam (Zn/Hg) in presence of HCl (Clemmensen reduction) or hydrazi ($NH_2 - NH_2$) in presence of sodium ethoxide (Wolf–Kishner reduction).

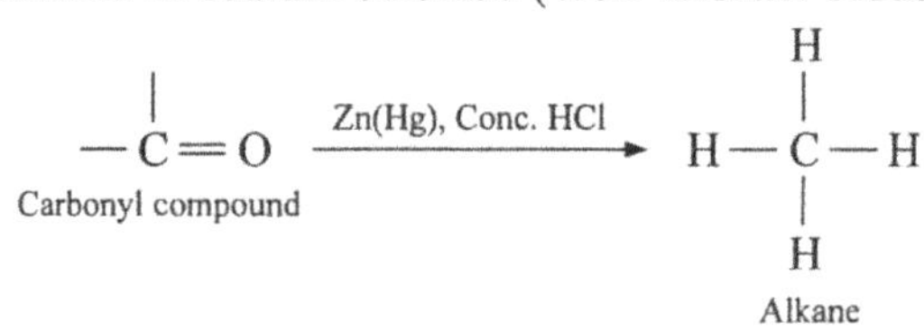

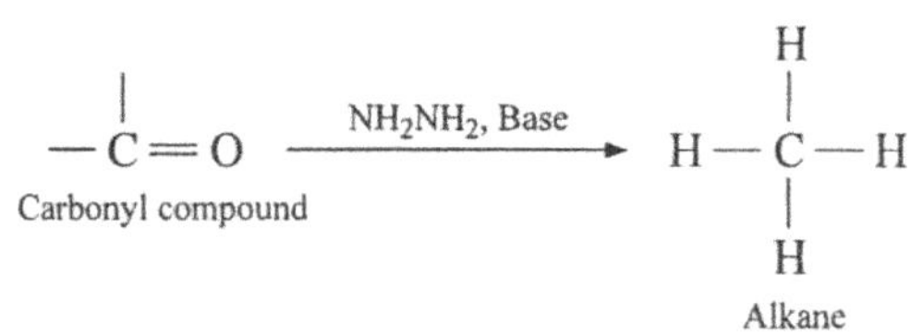

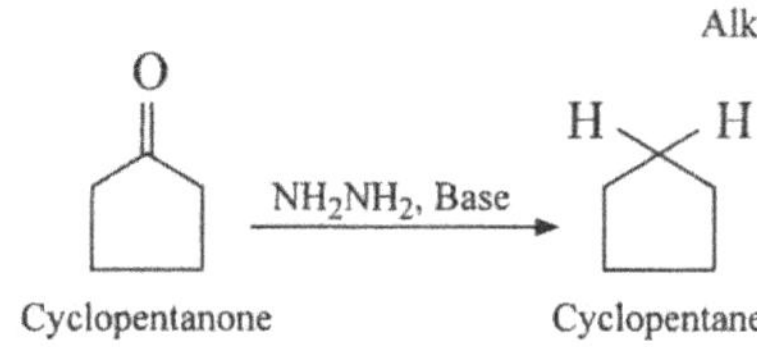

8.5 PHYSICAL PROPERTIES

1. The first four members of alkanes are gases, next 12 are liquids and higher membe are colourless solids.
2. Alkanes are insoluble in water because the polar water molecules are not attract to the non-polar alkane molecules. However, alkanes are soluble in non-polar solver such as carbon tetrachloride (CCl_4).

thereby the boiling point decreases. A comparative view is given here.

Alkane	*Boiling Point* (°C)
n-Butane	– 0.5
Iso-Butane	– 10.2

(i) The symmetrical neopentane molecules escape from the liquid the way marbles might pop out of a box when it is shaken vigorously. The pentane and isopentane molecules tend to get tangled, like coat hangers, and must be heated to higher temperatures before they can boil. Unsymmetrical molecules, therefore, tend to be liquids over a larger range of temperatures than molecules that are symmetrical.

(ii) Pentane and isopentane molecules have zigzag structures, which differ only in terms of whether the chain of C—C bonds is linear or branched. These less symmetrical molecules are harder to pack to form a solid, so these compounds must be cooled to much lower temperatures before they become solids. Pentane freezes at – 130° C. Isopentane must be cooled to almost – 160° C before it forms a solid.

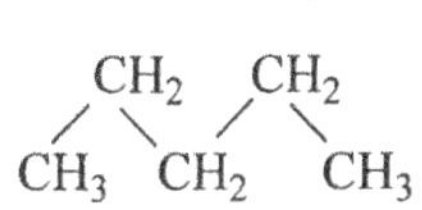

Pentane

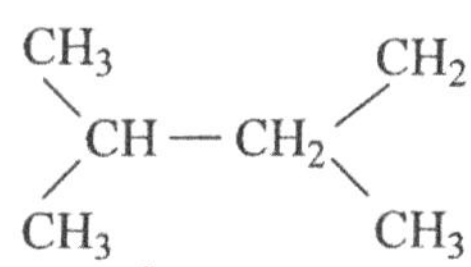

Isopentane

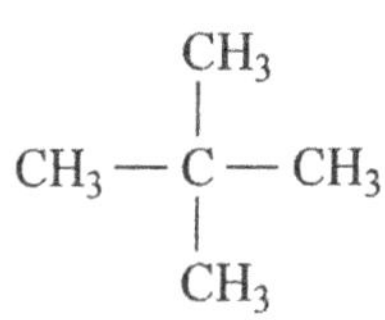

Neopentane

Alkane	*Freezing Point*	*Boiling Point*
Pentane	– 130	36.1
Isopentane	– 159.9	27.8
Neopentane	– 16.5	9.5

Alkane, with even number of carbon atoms, has higher melting point than the one, having one carbon atom less or the next higher alkane with odd number of carbon atoms. This is probably due to the fact that alkanes, with even number of carbon atoms, fold so as to permit greater intermolecular attraction, which in turn results in higher melting points.

IUPAC Name	*Molecular Formula*	*Structural Formula*	*Boiling Point* (°C)	*Melting Point* (°C)	*Density* (g/ml, 20°C)
Methane	CH_4	CH_4	– 161.5	– 182.5	
Ethane	C_2H_6	CH_3CH_3	– 88.6	– 183.3	
Propane	C_3H_8	$CH_3CH_2CH_3$	– 42.1	– 189.7	
Butane	C_4H_{10}	$CH_3(CH_2)_2CH_3$	– 0.5	– 138.4	
Pentane	C_5H_{12}	$CH_3(CH_2)_3CH_3$	36.1	– 129.7	0.626
Hexane	C_6H_{14}	$CH_3(CH_2)_4CH_3$	68.7	– 95.3	0.659

thus are fairly stable. The bonded electrons in C—H bond are equally shared betwee them and the bond is almost non-polar. The C—C bond is completely non-polar, therefor polar reagents find no reaction sites on alkane molecules.

Alkanes are stable to acids (H_2SO_4, HNO_3), alkalies (NaOH) and oxidising agen ($KMnO_4$, $K_2Cr_2O_7$, etc.) at room temperature. This low reactivity of alkanes toward reagen accounts for the fact that alkanes were originally called paraffins. However, at hig temperatures or in the presence of UV light alkanes undergo *free-radical substitutic reactions* through the formation of free radicals.

8.6.1 Free-Radical Substitution Reactions

The most important and characteristic reaction of saturated hydrocarbons is free-radic substitution. In free-radical substitution reactions of alkanes, another atom or group replace a hydrogen atom. Some important free-radical substitution reactions of alkanes ar represented below:

1. ***Halogenation*** Alkanes react with halogens in which a hydrogen atom of alkane i replaced by a halogen atom. This is an example of free-radical substitution reaction. Th order of reactivity of halogens is $F_2 > Cl_2 > Br_2 > I_2$.

$$\underset{\text{Alkane}}{RH} \xrightarrow{X_2,\ \text{UV light}/350^\circ\text{–}450^\circ C} \underset{\text{Alkyl halide}}{R—X}$$

(i) *Fluorination* Fluorination of alkanes is an agressive/vigorous reaction and results i a mixture of carbon, fluoroalkanes and HF. It can, however, be controlled by dilutin fluorine with an inert gas.

(ii) *Chlorination and Bromination* Alkanes react with chlorine or bromine to form alky chlorides or alkyl bromides. These reactions take place only at high temperatures (350°- 500° C) or in presence of UV light.

(iii) *Iodination* Iodine reacts with alkanes reversibly. The HI formed in the reaction reduce the iodoalkane back to alkane. Hence, alkanes can be iodinated in presence of oxidisin agents such as iodic acid (HIO_3), periodic acid (HIO_4) or nitric acid (HNO_3) which oxidis hydroiodic acid (HI) back to iodine or which will destroy HI.

$$CH_4 + I_2 \rightleftharpoons CH_3I + HI$$

Halogenation is used to prepare many solvents like chloroform (general anaesthetic) dichloromethane (paint stripper), 1,2-dichloroethane (dry cleaning fluid), etc.

Mechanism The halogenation of alkanes is a free-radical chain reaction, which involve a series of steps. Each step generates a free radical that brings the next step till the chai of these steps finally terminates. Halogenation involves the following steps:

(a) *Chain-initiating step* In the chain initiating step, the free radicals are produce by homolytic bond dissociation of halogen molecule by consuming heat or ligh

$$X\cdot + RH \longrightarrow HX + R\cdot$$

Halogen (Free radical) — Alkane — Alkyl (Free radical)

- In the second propagating step, alkyl free radical abstracts a halogen atom from halogen molecule to form alkyl halide and another halogen radical, which can abstract a hydrogen atom from another alkane molecule.

$$R\cdot + X—X \longrightarrow RX + X\cdot$$

Alkyl (Free radical) — Alkyl halide — Halogen (Free radical)

Thus these two steps are repeated several times.

c) *Chain-terminating steps* The above chain reaction terminates, when any two free radicals combine.

$$X\cdot + \cdot X \longrightarrow X—X$$

$$R\cdot + \cdot X \longrightarrow R—X$$

$$R\cdot + \cdot R \longrightarrow R—R$$

tive Reactivities of Halogens in Halogenation of Alkanes Halogenation of alkanes lves three steps (chain-initiating steps, chain-propagating steps and chain-termination ;). Of these the first chain-propagating step, i.e. abstraction of hydrogen atom by gen free radical is considered to determine the relative reactivities of halogens because step is most difficult one. To know the relative reactivities of halogens the E_a values lese steps derived from homolytic bond dissociation energies are given here:

s

	X	= F	Cl	Br	I
$X—X \rightarrow 2X^\bullet$	E_a (in kcal-mol^{-1})	= + 38	+ 58	+ 46	+ 36
$X\cdot + CH_4 \rightarrow HX + \cdot CH_3$	E_a (in kcal-mol^{-1})	= – 32	+ 4	+ 18	+ 34
$^\bullet CH_3 + X_2 \rightarrow CH_3X + X\cdot$	E_a (in kcal-mol^{-1})	= – 70	– 02	– 24	– 20

(i) The *first* step involves homolytic dissociation of halogen molecules. In first step, the E_a values with all halogens are positive and the reaction is, therefore, endothermic.

(ii) In *second* step (involves the abstraction of hydrogen of methane by a halogen atom) the E_a values show that, the reaction with fluorine atom is highly exothermic, while with iodine atom is highly endothermic. This step is most difficult one, *a low E_a in the second step means the reaction takes place rapidly* and *a high E_a means that reaction will take place slowly*. In addition, low E_a values of a reaction shall have more number of *effective collisions*. The effective collisions

the reaction is exothermic in all the four cases. For all these reactions, E quite small, hence all reactions take place at the same rate. Hence in determin the relative reactivities of halogens this step need not be considered. Theref the order of reactivities of halogens with alkanes towards free radical substitut was found to be fluorine > chlorine > bromine > iodine.

1. ***Relative Reactivities of Alkanes in Halogenation*** Different alkanes exhibit diffe degrees of reactivity while reacting with a particular halogen. The different reactivitie alkanes are due to the presence of different classes of hydrogen atoms (methyl, prim secondary, tertiary). Of the three steps of halogenation, abstraction of hydrogen at (first chain-propagating step) controls overall rate of reaction. The ease of abstraction different hydrogens should be in the order: tertiary > secondary > primary > methyl. relative ease of abstraction of hydrogen atoms may be explained by considering relative stabilities of alkyl free radicals formed. For example, propane is more reactive w chlorine than ethane because secondary alkyl free radical formed from propane is m stable than 1° free radical formed from ethane.

2. ***Nitration*** When a mixture of an alkane and nitric acid vapours is heated at 400°–500° one hydrogen atom of the alkane is replaced by a nitro group. The product is called ni alkane. This process is called vapour-phase nitration.

$$R-\boxed{H + HO}-NO_2 \longrightarrow R-NO_2 + H_2O$$

$$CH_3-\boxed{H + HO}-NO_2 \longrightarrow CH_3-NO_2 + H_2O$$

Mechanism Nitration of alkanes proceeds through free-radical mechanism.

$$HO-NO_2 \xrightarrow{X_2,\ \text{UV light}/400°\text{–}500°C} HO\cdot + O_2N\cdot$$

$$R-H + HO\cdot \longrightarrow R\cdot + H_2O$$

$$R\cdot + O_2N\cdot \longrightarrow R-NO_2$$

3. ***Sulphonation*** This reaction involves the replacement of a hydrogen atom of an alk by a sulphonic acid ($-SO_3H$) group. Only higher alkanes undergo sulphonation reaction with fuming H_2SO_4 at 400° C.

$$\underset{\text{Alkane}}{R-H} + HO-SO_3H \longrightarrow \underset{\text{Alkyl sulphonic acid}}{R-SO_3H} + H_2O$$

Mechanism Sulphonation also involves free-radical mechanism.

$$HO-SO_3H \longrightarrow HO\cdot + HO_3S\cdot$$

$$R-H + HO\cdot \longrightarrow R\cdot + H_2O$$

$$R\cdot + HO_3S\cdot \longrightarrow R-SO_3H$$

8.6.2 Pyrolysis or Cracking

$$CH_3CH_2CH_3 \longrightarrow \underset{\text{Ethene}}{H_2C = CH_2} + CH_4$$

$$CH_3CH_2CH_3 \xrightarrow{600^\circ C} CH_3CH = CH_2 + H_2$$

A mixture of saturated and unsaturated hydrocarbons are produced in cracking process. gaseous hydrogen is also present during the cracking, only saturated hydrocarbons are oduced. The hydrocarbon mixtures produced by these cracking processes have a high oportion of branched chain isomers. These branched isomers improve the quality of fuel.

$$C_{16}H_{34} + H_2 \xrightarrow[\text{Heat}]{\text{Catalyst}} 2C_8H_{18}$$

6.3 Combustion

'hen alkane is burnt in excess of air or oxygen, alkanes undergo complete oxidation to oduce carbon dioxide, water and large quantities of heat.

$$C_nH_{2n+2} + O_2 \text{ (Excess)} \longrightarrow nCO_2 + (n + 1)\ H_2O + \text{Heat}$$

6.4 Aromatisation

ιis process involves the conversion of aliphatic hydrocarbons into aromatic hydrocarbons the presence of suitable catalyst. The reaction involves dehydrogenation, cyclisation ıd even isomerisation.

$$\underset{n\text{-Hexane}}{CH_3CH_2CH_2CH_2CH_2CH_3} \longrightarrow$$

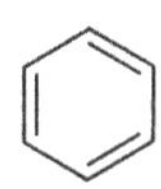

Benzene

7 PHARMACEUTICAL COMPOUNDS

Hard Paraffin It is a mixture of solid hydrocarbons obtained from petroleum or shale l. Hard paraffin is a colourless or translucent mass. It is practically insoluble in water, :ohol and is soluble in solvent ether. Hard paraffin is used as a pharmaceutical aid tiffening agent) in the preparation of semi-solid dosage forms.

Soft Paraffin Soft paraffin is a semi-solid translucent mixture of hydrocarbons produced ɔm petroleum. The soft paraffin may be colourless or yellow in colour. It is insoluble water, in alcohol and soluble in solvent ether. Soft paraffin is used in the preparation ointment bases.

Liquid Paraffin (Mineral oil) Liquid paraffin is a mixture of liquid hydrocarbons ıtained from petroleum. It is a transparent, colourless, oily liquid. Liquid paraffin is soluble in water, alcohol and soluble in solvent ether. Liquid paraffin is used as ıarmaceutical aid in the preparation of ointments, emulsions and creams. It is also used

PRACTICE QUESTIONS

1. Explain the mechanism of halogenation of alkanes. What evidence can you offer in sup of this mechanism?
2. Answer the following giving justification of your answers:
   (a) Traces of 2,3-dimethythexane have been observed in the free-radical chlorination of prop
   (b) All the four carbon–hydrogen bonds in methane are identical.
   (c) Chlorination of methane requires UV light or high temperatures.
   (d) Ethane does not react with halogens in dark.
   (e) Chlorination is faster than bromination.
   (f) Iodination of methane is difficult.
   (g) Bioling points of branched alkanes are lesser than normal alkanes.
3. Write and explain the mechanism of free-radical substitution reaction between methane chlorine.
4. How will you distinguish between the following pairs of compounds in the laboratory?
   (a) Propylene and propane
   (b) Butene and butane
5. Complete the following reduction schemes stating the products and any essential conditic

$$CH_4 + Cl\cdot \longrightarrow$$

6. Write the structures and IUPAC names of various isomers of pentane.
7. Explain the type of hybridisation and bonding in methane?
8. Write notes on: (a) paraffins, (b) icthammol, (c) pyrolysis.
9. How do you convert:
   (a) Methane to ethane
   (b) Ethane to methane
   (c) Ethene to ethane
   (d) N-Butane from ethane
   (e) 2,3-Dimethylbutane from isopropyl bromide
10. What are active hydrogens?
11. What happens when:
    (a) Ethyl magnesium bromide is reacted with acidified water.
    (b) 2-Chlorobutane is reacted with sodium metal.
    (c) Acetic acid is heated with sodalime.
    (d) N-Propylbromide is treated with lithium aluminium hydride.
12. Write notes on:
    (a) Wurtz reaction
    (b) Corey–House synthesis
    (c) Sabatier–Senderen's reaction

HEMISTRY OF ALKENES

INTRODUCTION

enes are unsaturated hydrocarbons with general formula C_nH_{2n}, where n is the number :arbon atoms. The members of this class of compounds have two hydrogen atoms less ı the corresponding saturated hydrocarbons (alkanes). In general, alkenes are referred ›lefins because lower members of this series react with chlorine to form oily products. enes contain at least one carbon–carbon double bond. The carbon–carbon double d in alkenes is known as ethylenic linkage or olefinic linkage.

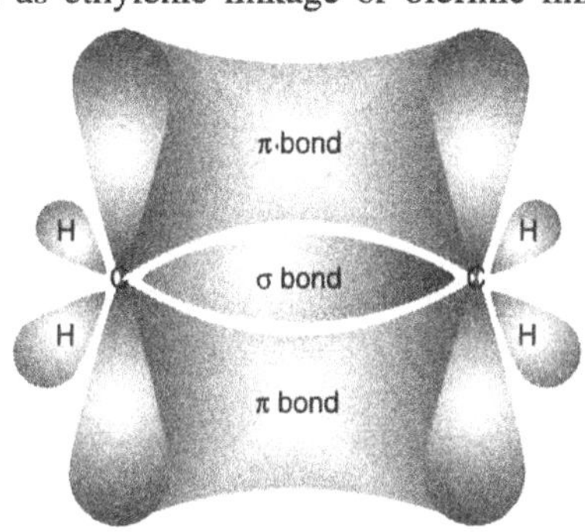

Structure of ethene molecule

NOMENCLATURE

ɑes of this class of compounds end with the suffix -ene. Alkenes constitute a ıologous series, as elucidated below:

Formula	*Common Name*	*IUPAC Name*
$CH_2 = CH_2$	Ethylene	Ethene
$CH_2 = CH - CH_3$	Propylene	Propene
$CH_2 = CH - CH_2 - CH_3$	Butylene	1-Butene
$CH_2 = CH - CH_2 - CH_2 - CH_3$	Amylene	1-Pentene

GENERAL METHODS OF PREPARATION

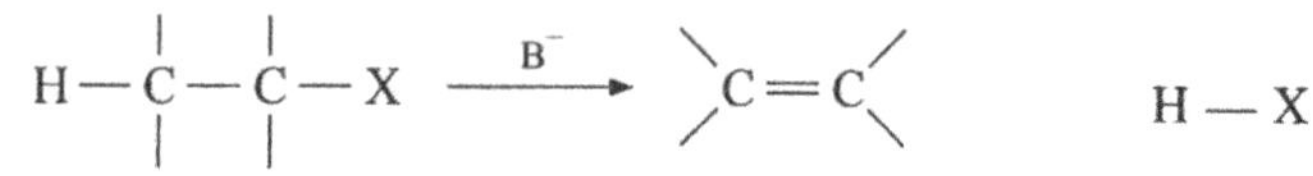

X = I, Br, Cl, (F)

$$R-CH(H)-CH_2(X) + \text{Alcoholic KOH} \xrightarrow{\Delta} R-CH=CH_2 + KX + H_2O$$

Alkyl halide — Alkene — X = Cl, Br or I

$$CH_3-CH(H)-CH_2(Br) + \text{Alcoholic KOH} \xrightarrow{\Delta} CH_3-CH=CH_2 + KBr + H$$

n-Propyl bromide — Propene

$$CH_3CH(Br)CH_2CH_3 \xrightarrow[\Delta]{\text{Alcoholic KOH}} CH_3CH_2CH=CH_2 + CH_3CH=CHC$$

2-Bromobutane — 1-Butene (20%) — 2-Butene (80%)

1. ***Dehydrohalogenation of Alkyl Halides*** Alkyl halides undergo dehydrohalogenati which is an example of elimination reaction. Dehydrohalogenation of alkyl halides i general reaction and is an excellent method for preparing alkenes. This reaction invol the removal of β-hydrogen and the leaving group (halogen) from adjacent carbon ato of an alkyl halide, by refluxing it with an alcoholic solution of base (potassium hydroxi sodium hydroxide, potassium ethoxide or sodium ethoxide). Therefore, dehydrohalogenati of alkyl halides to alkenes follows 1,2-elimination.

There are three fundamental events in these elimination reactions:

1. Removal of a proton
2. Formation of the carbon–carbon π bond
3. Existence of heterolytic dissociation of the covalent bond between carbon and t leaving group (halogen atom).

Reactivity of Alkyl Halides The ease of dehydrohalogenation of different halogens of the order iodides > bromides > chlorides. The ease of dehydrohalogenation of alk halides is: 3° alkyl halide > 2° alkyl halide > 1° alkyl halide.

Mechanism The dehydrohalogenation reaction involves cleavage of bonds (C — C — X) and formation of bonds (O — H and H — X, C = C). Depending on the relati timing of these events, different mechanisms are possible:

- *E1 reaction* Loss of the leaving group (LG) to form a carbocation, removal proton (H^+) and formation of carbon–carbon double (C = C) bond.
- *E2 reaction* Simultaneous proton (H^+) removal, carbon–carbon double (C = bond formation and loss of the leaving group (LG).

ınsaturation than the startıng materıals.

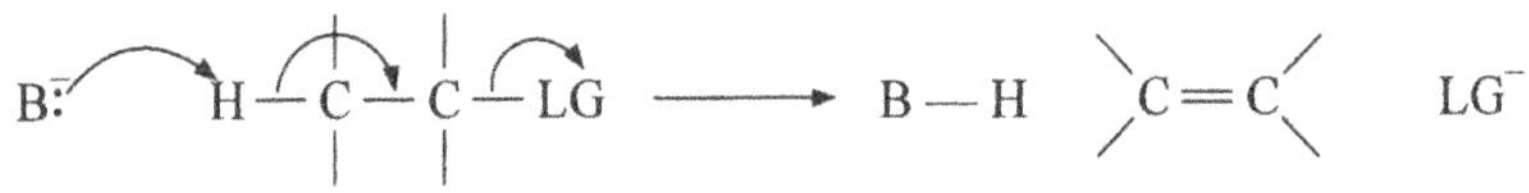

ˉig. 9.1 Simultaneous Removal of the Proton (H^+) by the Base, Loss of the Leaving Group (LG) and Formation of the π-Bond

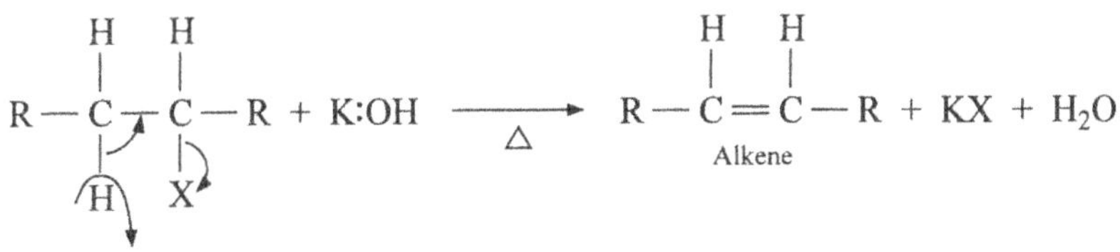

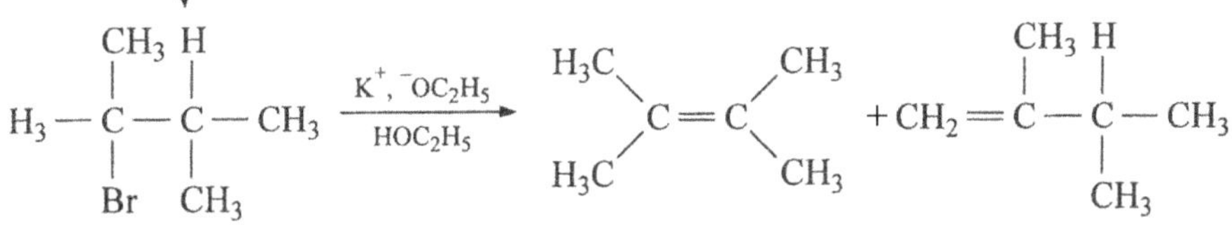

2-Bromo-2,3-dimethylbutane

2,3-Dimethyl-2-butene (Major product)

2,3-Dimethyl-1-butene (Minor product)

\ high concentration of a strong base in a relatively non-polar solvent is used to carry the E2 reaction. The combinations, such as sodium methoxide in methanol, sodium ›xide in ethanol, potassium isopropoxide in isopropanol, and potassium *tert*-butoxide *ert*-butanol or dimethyl sulphoxide (DMSO), are often used.

etics of E2 Reactions Studies have shown that the rate-determining step of E2 reaction ›lves a bimolecular collision. The rate of E2 reaction depends upon the concentration of ı the substrate (alkyl halide) and attacking reagent (base). This results in a rate law :ession:

$$R = k[\mathrm{R-X}][\mathrm{base}]$$

ʾhere is a smooth transition between the reactant and the product. Analogous to the reaction, no intermediate has been isolated or detected. Furthermore, no rearrangements ır under E2 conditions.

ctivity of alkyl halides towards E2 The order of reactivity of alkyl halides towards ıination bimolecular mechanism is tertiary alkyl halides > secondary alkyl halides > ıary alkyl halides. This is because branching at the carbon carrying the halogen increases oing from primary to secondary to tertiary alkyl halide. Now, greater the branching ter the number of β-hydrogens which can be attacked by the base and, therefore, ıer the probability of attack. Moreover, more branched an alkyl halide is more stable structure because of less E_a and more stability of transition state.

determining step (bond breaking is endothermic).

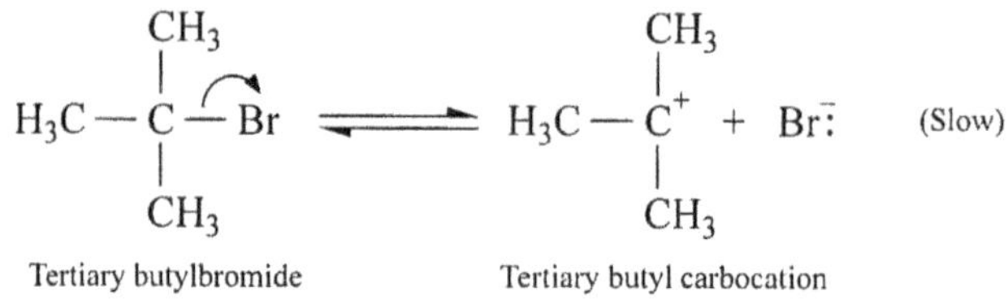

(b) In the *second* step of the reaction, deprotonation by a base from a carbon atoı (β) adjacent to the carbocation centre leads to the creation of the carbon–carbc double bond (C = C). It is an acid/base reaction.

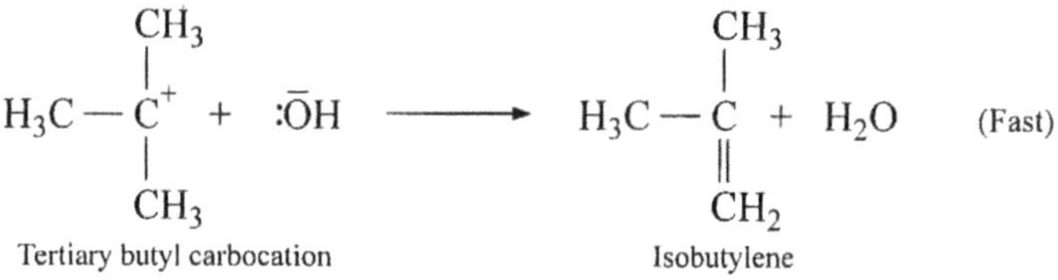

Since carbocation intermediates are formed during an E1, there is always the possibilit of rearrangements (e.g. 1,2-hydride or 1,2-alkyl shifts) to generate a more stable carbocatioı This is usually indicated by a change in the position of the alkene or a change in th carbon skeleton of the product when compared to the starting material, e.g. 3,3-dimethy 2-bromobutane forms 2,3-dimethyl-2-butene and 2,3-dimethyl-1-butene by E1 mechanisı through the intermediate formation of carbocation. This reaction involves rearrangemeı of carbocation.

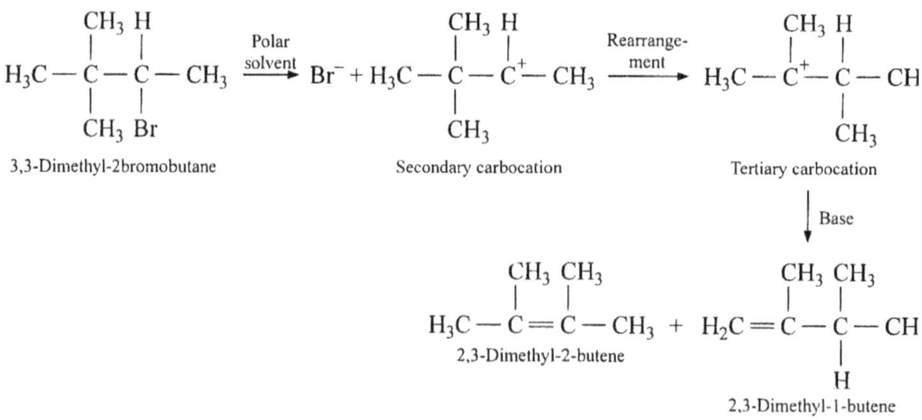

Kinetics of E1 Reactions The rate of E1 reaction depends upon the rate of slower stер i.e. the loss of leaving group (halide ion) to form carbocation. The rate of slower ste| (carbocation formation reaction) depends only on the concentration of the alkyl halide Hence the rate of E1 reaction depends upon the concentration of only alkyl halide. Thi results in a rate law expression:

entation of Dehydrohalogenation

tzeff's rule (Zaitsev rule) It is used to predict the orientation of dehydrohalogenation. ıe dehydrohalogenation of an alkyl halide can produce more than one alkene, then ɔrding to Saytzeff's rule, the main product is the highly substituted alkene. In other ·ds, the alkene having greatest number of alkyl groups attached to the doubly bonded ɔon atom predominates.

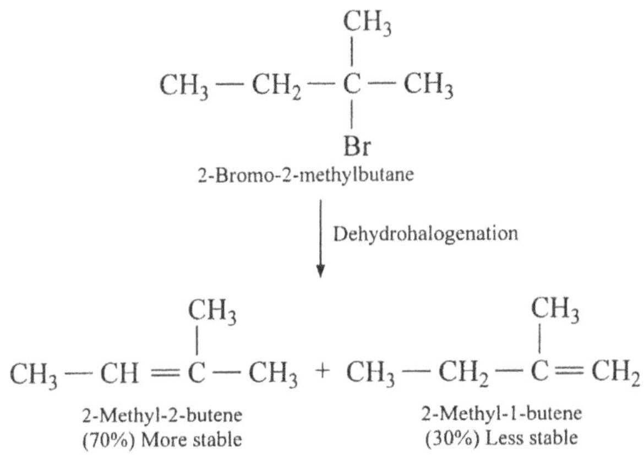

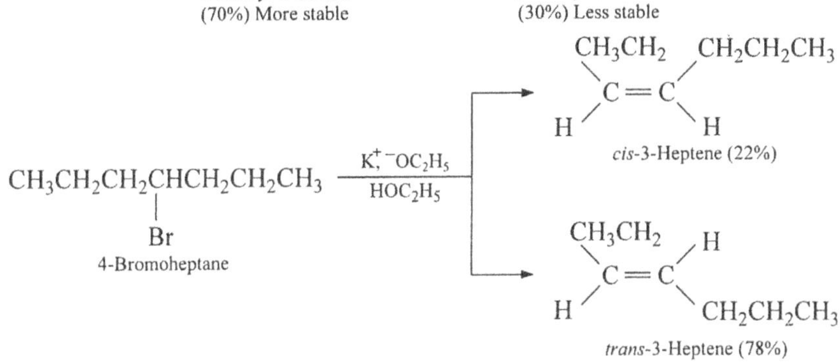

)f the two products (2-methyl-2-butene and 2-methyl-1-butene) 2-methyl-2-butene is e substituted hence it is the major product. This rule can be explained on the basis yperconjugation, because more stable alkene (more substituted one) has more number esonating structures.

rder of Stability of Alkenes The following is the order of stability of alkenes:

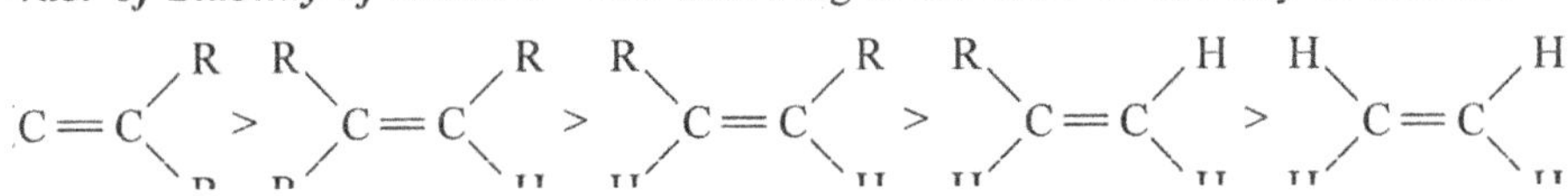

crowded β-carbon (secondary) atom. Instead, the base abstracts less crowded β-hydrog (primary) atom to form less-substituted alkene (Hofmann's product).

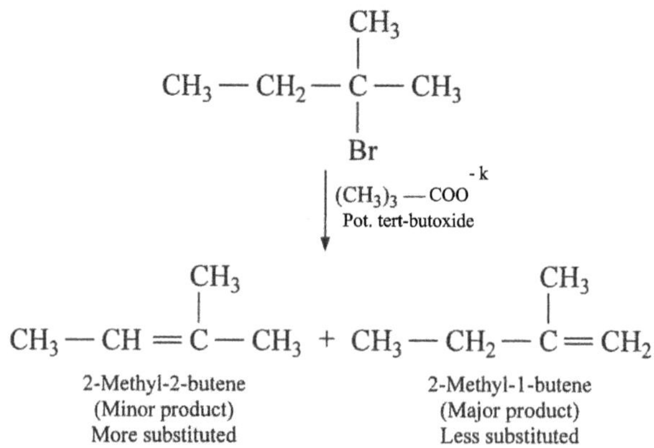

2. ***Dehydration of Alcohols*** Alcohols, by dehydration, i.e. elimination of a molecule water in presence of an acid (Lewis acid) and heat (200° C) yield alkenes. This is α,β-elimination reaction.

$$\underset{\substack{n\text{-Butanol} \\ \text{(Primary alcohol)}}}{CH_3CH_2CH_2CH_2OH} \xrightarrow{H_2SO_4} \underset{\text{2-Butene}}{CH_3CH = CHCH_3} + \underset{\text{1-Butene}}{CH_3CH_2CH = CH_2}$$

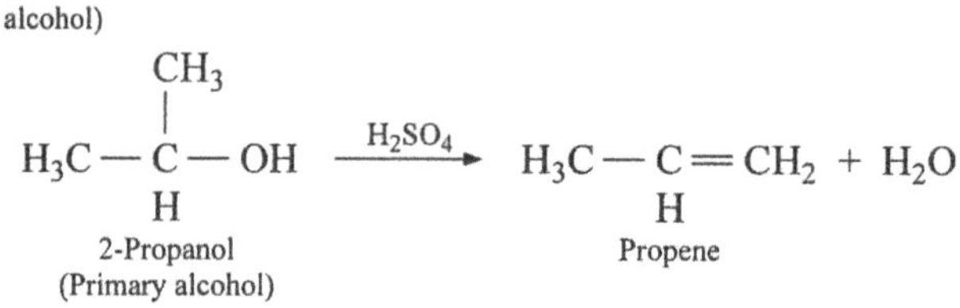

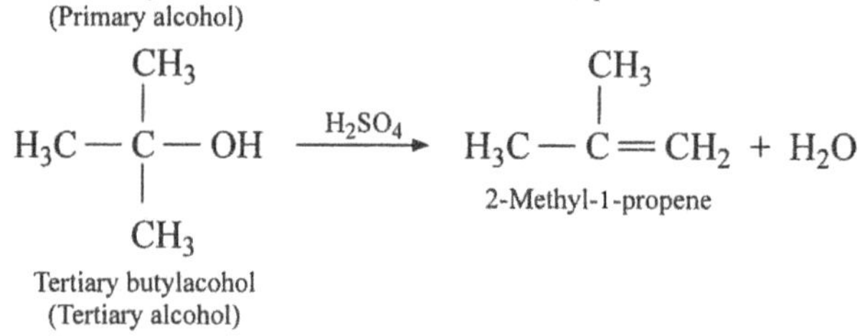

Mechanism Dehydration of alcohols takes place through the intermediate formation carbocation. This involves the following steps.

(i) *Formation of protonated alcohol*

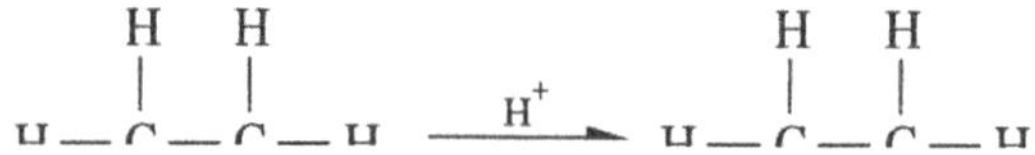

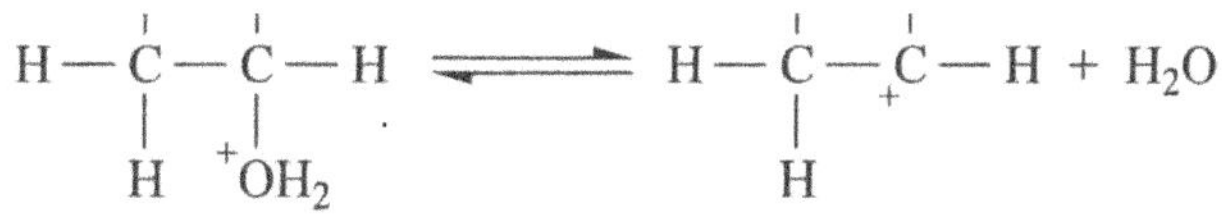

Protonated alcohol — Carbocation

(iii) *Formation of alkene by expulsion of a β-hydrogen atom*

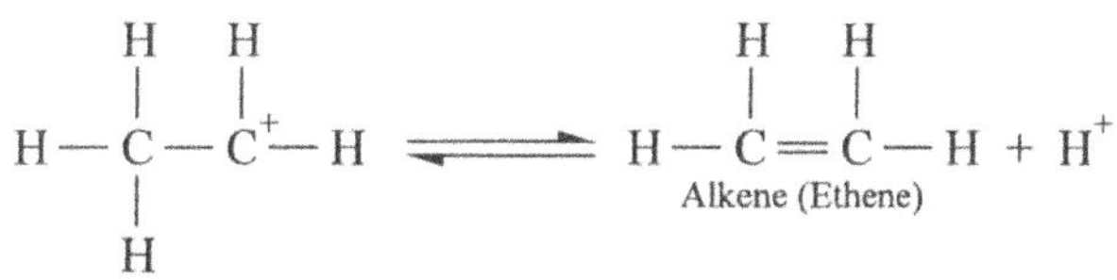

Carbocation — Alkene (Ethene)

ctivity The above mechanism is through the intermediate formation of carbocation. ice, the rate of elimination depends on the rate of formation of carbocation which in turn ends on the stability of carbocation. The rate of formation and stability of carbocation ows the sequence 3° carbocation > 2° carbocation > 1° carbocation. Therefore, the rate lehydration of alcohols follows the order 3° alcohol > 2° alcohol > 1° alcohol.

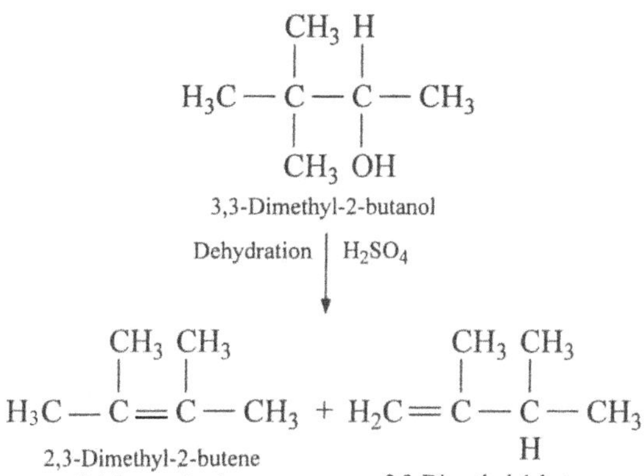

3,3-Dimethyl-2-butanol

Dehydration H_2SO_4

2,3-Dimethyl-2-butene (Major product) — 2,3-Dimethyl-1-butene (Minor product)

entation In *third* step of dehydration, hydrogen ion expels to form alkene. Whenever alkenes are formed, the major product is a more stable alkene. The more stable is the ne in which double bonded carbons are attached to more number alkyl groups. For nple, in dehydration of 3,3-dimethyl-2-butanol, two products are formed. Of these two lucts, 2,3-dimethyl-2-butene is the major product as it is more substituted than the other.

ehalogenation of Vicinal Dihalides A vicinal dihalide (a compound having two gens on adjacent carbon atoms) on heating with zinc in alcoholic solution gets ilogenated to form an alkene.

Alcohol

1,2-Dibromopropane

4. ***Controlled Reduction of Alkynes*** The controlled reduction of an alkyne to the alk stage may be brought with hydrogen in presence of a suitable catalyst (specially prepa palladium or nickel bromide) or with sodium in liquid ammonia.

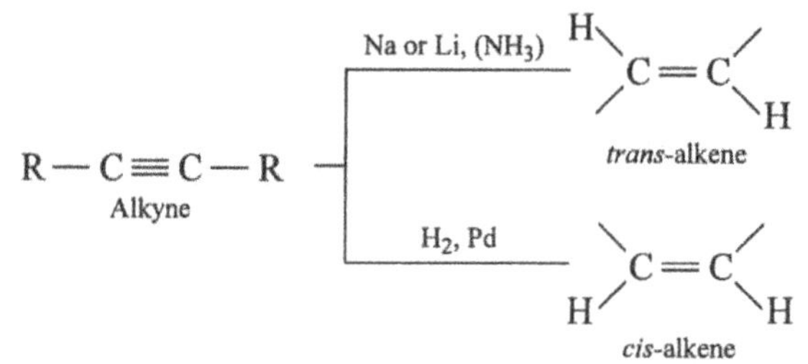

$$\underset{\text{2-Butyne}}{H_3C-C\equiv C-CH_3} \xrightarrow{H_2,\ Ni} \underset{\text{2-Butene}}{H_3C-\underset{H}{C}=CH-CH_3}$$

5. ***From Aldehydes or Ketones by Wittig Reaction*** Alkenes can also be prepared the reaction between aldehydes or ketones and phosphorus ylides. This reaction invol addition of nucleophilic organic group of ylides at electrophilic carbon of aldehydes ketones followed by elimination to form alkenes.

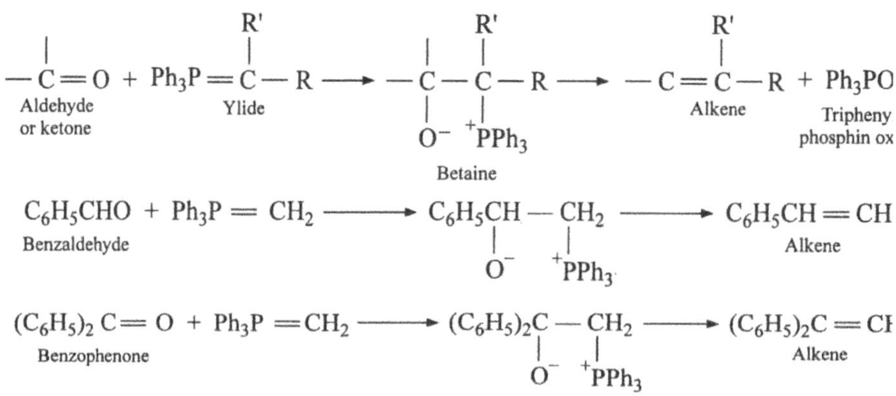

9.4 PHYSICAL PROPERTIES

1. The first three members of alkenes are gases, the next fourteen are liquids and higher members are solids.
2. The boiling points of alkenes increase regularly by increasing the number of carb atoms.
3. Alkenes are insoluble in water, but soluble in organic solvents like ether, benze

ıllowing chemical reactions

.5.1 Addition of Hydrogen

ı presence of finely divided catalyst such as platinum, palladium or nickel, hydrogen lds to alkenes to form alkanes. The addition of hydrogen is called hydrogenation. ydrogenation reactions are exothermic. The heat released in a hydrogenation reaction called the *heat of hydrogenation*. The catalyst decreases E_{act} by adsorbing the reactant olecules on its enormous surface and improves hydrogenation.

$$\underset{\text{Alkene}}{R-CH=CH-R} + H_2 \xrightarrow{\text{Ni}} \underset{\text{Alkane}}{RCH_2CH_2R}$$

$$\underset{\text{Ethene}}{H_2C=CH_2} + H_2 \xrightarrow{\text{Ni}} \underset{\text{Ethane}}{H_3C-CH_3}$$

Hydrogenation of an unsaturated compound proceeds by two different mechanisms. ıey are:

Heterogeneous Hydrogenation Heterogeneous hydrogenation is carried out with olecular hydrogen in presence of catalyst (Ni, Pt, Pd or Rh) that are insoluble in reaction edium. Catalytic hydrogenation results in the *cis*-addition of hydrogen to the double ınd, as this is the least hindered side of the molecule. Chemists proposed the following echanism for the reaction:

ep 1 The molecular hydrogen is adsorbed onto the metal surface. The relatively strong H — H sigma bond is broken and replaced with two weak metal—H bonds.

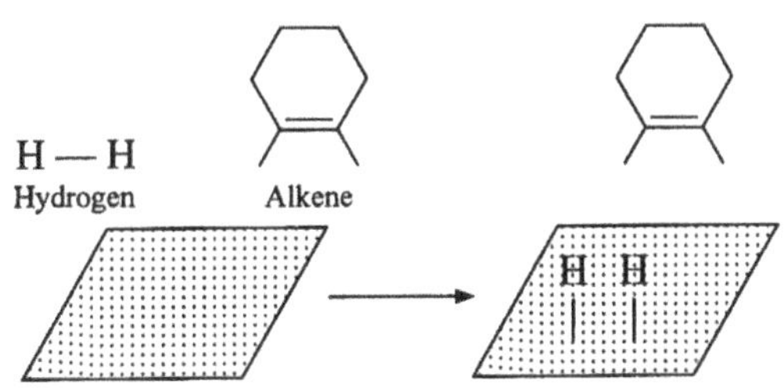

ɘp 2 The π bond of the alkene interacts with the metal catalyst weakening the bond. A hydrogen atom is transferred from the catalyst surface to one of the carbons of the double bond. Similarly, the second hydrogen atom is transferred from the catalyst surface forming the alkane. The two hydrogens add on to the same side of the alkene molecule hence the addition is termed as *syn*-addition.

The alkane is released from the catalyst's surface, allowing the catalyst to accept

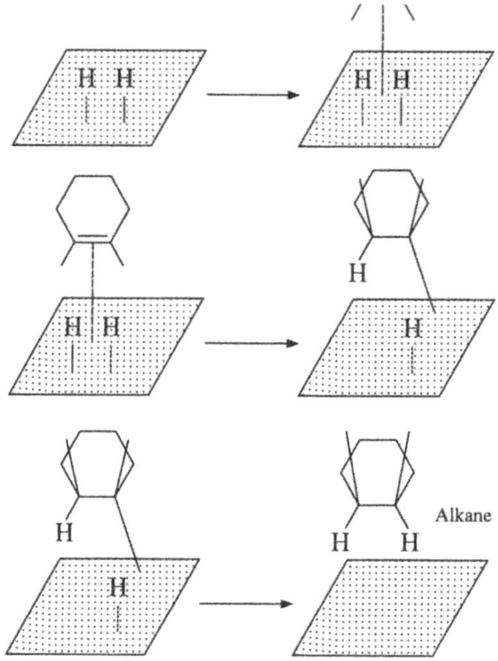

2. ***Homogeneous Hydrogenation*** Homogeneous hydrogenation is carried out in prese of soluble catalyst and molecular hydrogen. During the past three decades homogene hydrogenation has found widespread application in organic chemistry, including production of important pharmaceuticals, especially where a sophisticated degree selectivity is required, e.g. Wilkinson's Catalyst: $RhCl(PPh_3)_3$. The proposed mechani route is as follows:

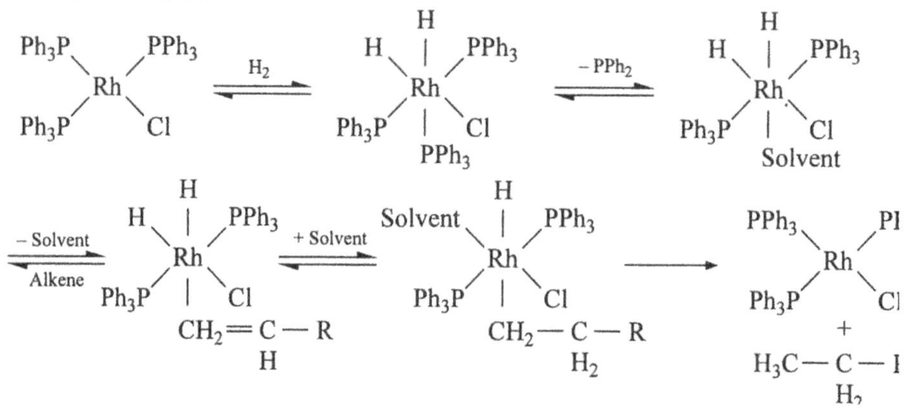

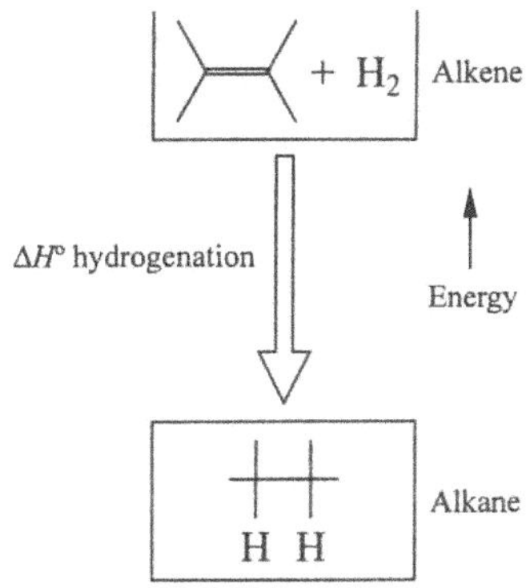

'he greater the heat of hydrogenation, the less stable the alkene. For example,

$$\text{I}_3\text{CH}_2\text{CH}=\text{CH}_2 + \text{H}_2 \xrightarrow{\text{Catalyst}} \text{CH}_3\text{CH}_2\text{CH}_2\text{CH}_3 \qquad \Delta H = -\,30.3\text{ kcal/mol}$$

1-Butene   Butane

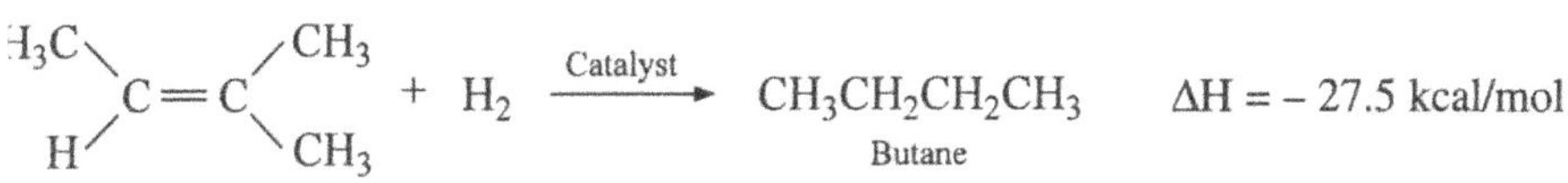

trans-2-Butene

-Butene evolves the greatest amount of heat than *trans*-2-butene, therefore, *trans*-2-ne is more stable.

2 Electrophilic Addition Reactions

most characteristic reaction of alkenes is the electrophilic addition reaction. An trophilic addition is an addition reaction in which an electron-rich molecule (alkene) tacked by an electrophile. Every alkene molecule contains a double bond. The double 1 consists of one strong sigma (σ) bond and the other weak pi (π) bond. Hence, in t of the chemical reactions addition occurs readily due to easy rupture of pi bond. *nes undergo electrophilic addition reactions.* In these reactions, the π bond of nes is dissociated and is replaced by two new σ-bonds.

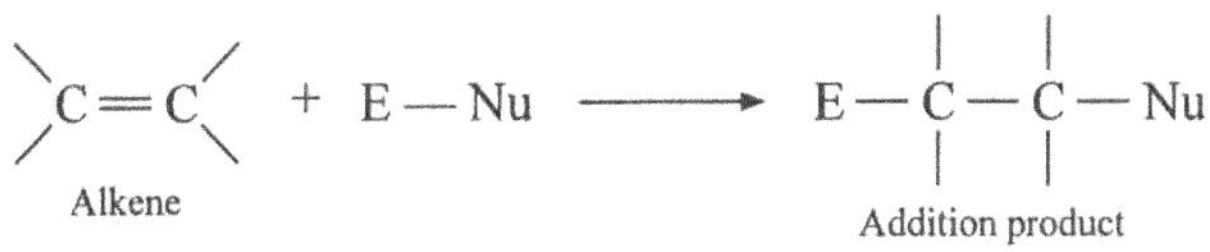

hanism The π electrons of the carbon–carbon double bond are less firmly held to carbon nuclei. Hence, carbon–carbon double bonds are electron-rich and are readily lable to any electron-seeking reagent, i.e. electrophilic reagents and free radicals. The

covalent bond with one carbon atom, whereas the other carbon atom ge positive charge. As a result a carbocation is formed.

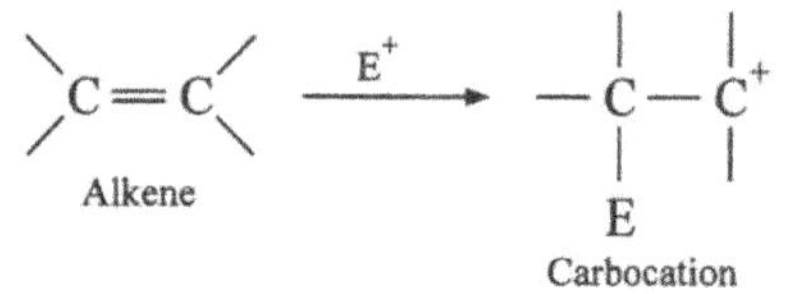

Step 3 The nucleophile generated in the first step now combines with the positi\ charged carbon to form an addition product.

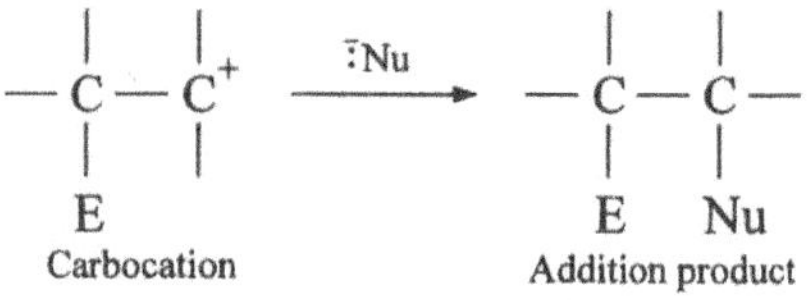

The electrophilic addition of alkenes is exemplified by the following reactions:

1. ***Addition of Hydrogen Halides*** Alkenes react with hydrogen halides (HCl, HBr or to form alkyl halides. The order of reactivity among the hydrogen halides with alke is HI > HBr > HCl > HF. The reason for the fastest reactivity of hydroiodic acid is du the weakest hydrogen–halogen bond (heterolytic bond dissociation energy values of HCl, HBr and HI are 568, 432, 366 and 298 kJ/mole, respectively. If the bond is weal it dissociates more readily and so the reaction is more likely to happen.

$$\underset{\text{Alkene}}{H_2C = CH_2} + \underset{\text{Hydrogen halide}}{H - X} \longrightarrow \underset{\text{Alkyl halide}}{H_3C - CH_2X} \quad \text{(HX = HF or HCl or HBr or H}$$

Mechanism (i) Hydrogen halides ionise to give a proton and a halide ion.

$$H - X \longrightarrow H^+ + X^-$$

(ii) Proton attacks one of the double-bonded carbon atom to form a more sta carbocation. If the structure permits, the carbocation undergoes rearrangeme

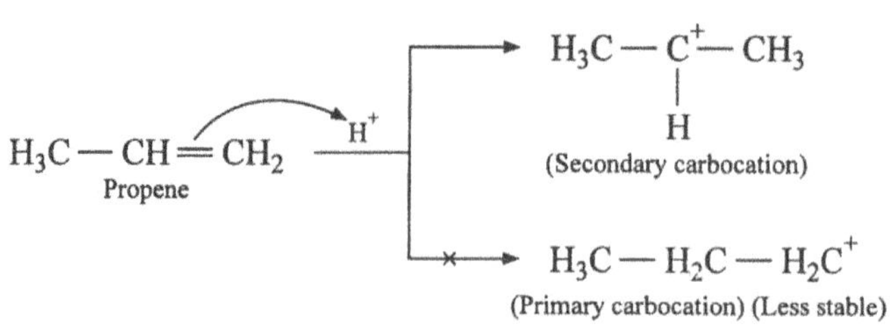

(iii) The halide ion attacks the more stable carbocation to give addition product.

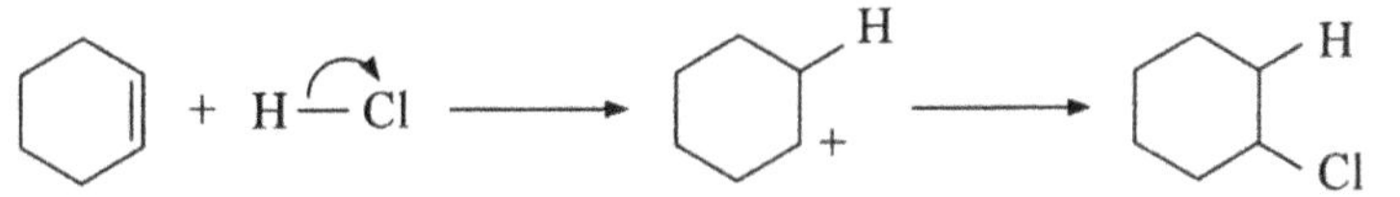

Cyclohexene Carbocation Chlorocyclohexane

rkovnikov's Rule When an unsymmetrical reagent (HCl, HBr, HI, H_2O, H_2SO_4, NOCl, X, etc.) adds to an unsymmetrical alkene, the positive part of the reagent becomes ched to the doubly bonded carbon atom that bears more number of hydrogen atoms s branched) and the negative part of the reagent attached to the carbon that bears er number of hydrogens (more branched).

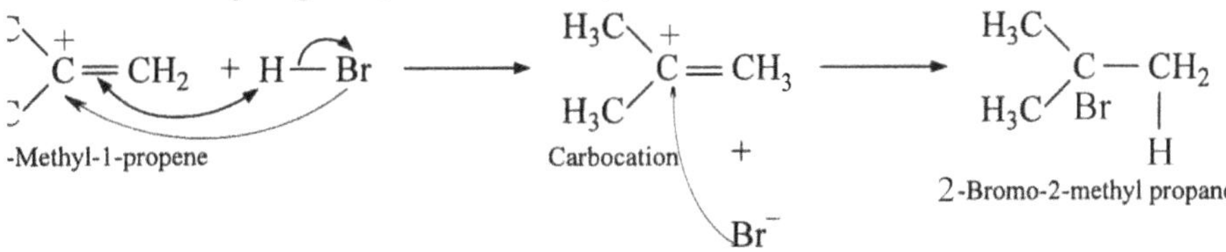

-Methyl-1-propene Carbocation 2-Bromo-2-methyl propane

ddition of Water (Hydration) Water adds to the more reactive alkenes in presence cids to yield alcohols. The components of water (hydrogen and hydroxyl group) are ed to the double bonded carbon atoms of alkene. This addition follows Markovnikov's ntation through the intermediate formation of carbocation. For example,

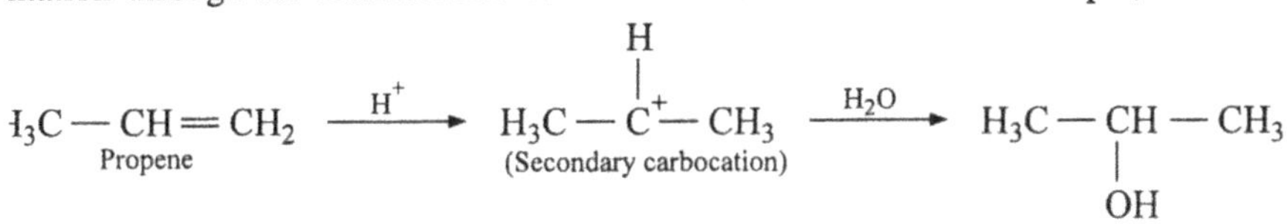

Propene (Secondary carbocation) Isopropanol

hanism This addition follows Markovnikov's orientation through the intermediate ation of carbocation. It involves the following steps:

) Protonation of the alkene to generate more stable carbocation.
) Attack of the nucleophilc water molecule on the electrophilic carbocation creates an oxonium ion.
) Deprotonation of oxonium ion by a base generates alcohol and regenerates the acid catalyst.

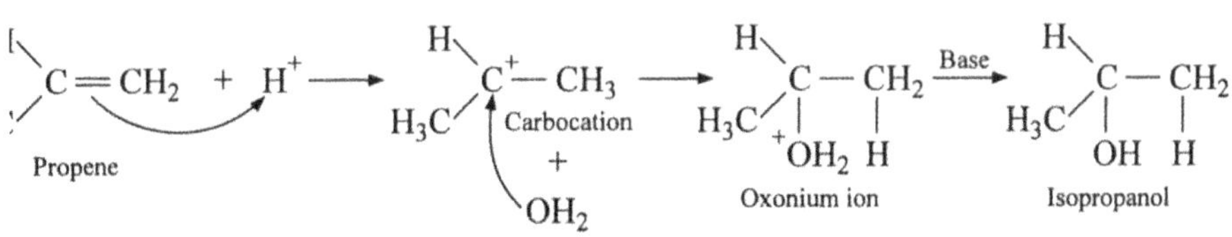

Propene Carbocation Oxonium ion Isopropanol

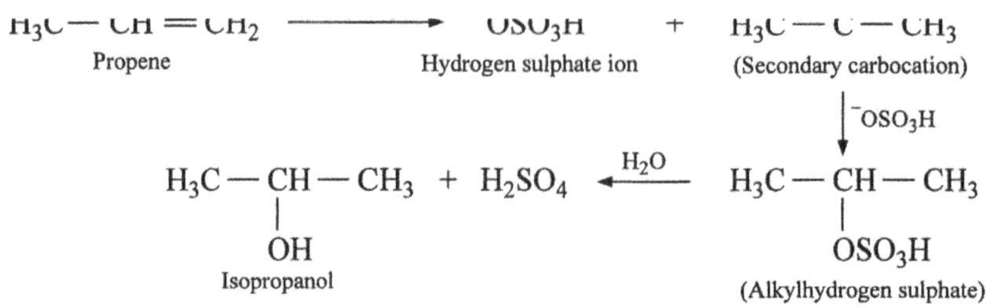

4. ***Addition of Hypohalous Acids*** Alkenes react with hypohalous acid (HOX) to form corresponding halohydrins. In case of unsymmetrical alkene, the addition takes place according to Markovnikov's rule (electrophile = X^+, nucleophile = ^-OH).

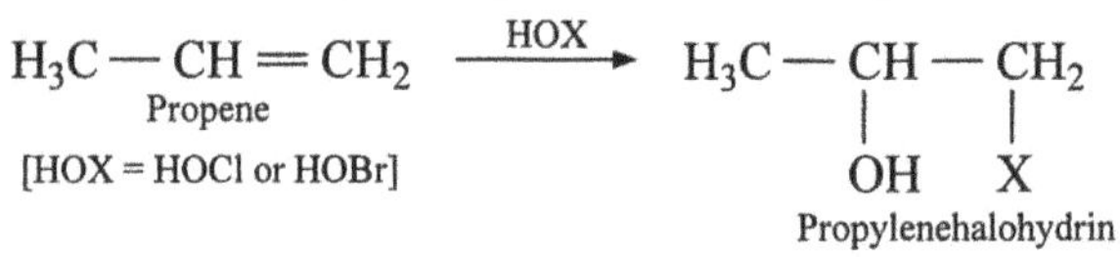

5. ***Addition of Nitrosyl Chloride*** Alkenes react with nitrosyl chloride or nitrosyl bromide to give crystalline nitrosohalides (electrophile = NO^+, nucleophile = X^-). This reaction is another example for electrophilic addition reaction.

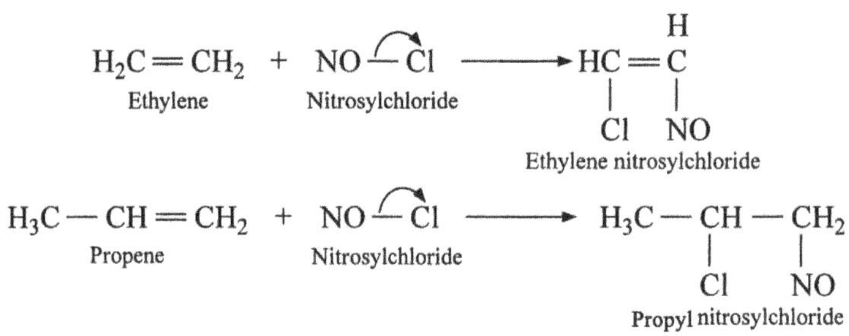

6. ***Addition of Alkanes (Alkylation)*** Alkenes can also add on alkanes in presence of acidic medium (HF, H_2SO_4, $AlCl_3$) to form higher alkanes. This reaction is believed to take place through electrophilic addition mechanism. The reaction is known as alkylation, which is commercially employed for the manufacture of 2,2,4-trimethyl pentane (aviation fuel).

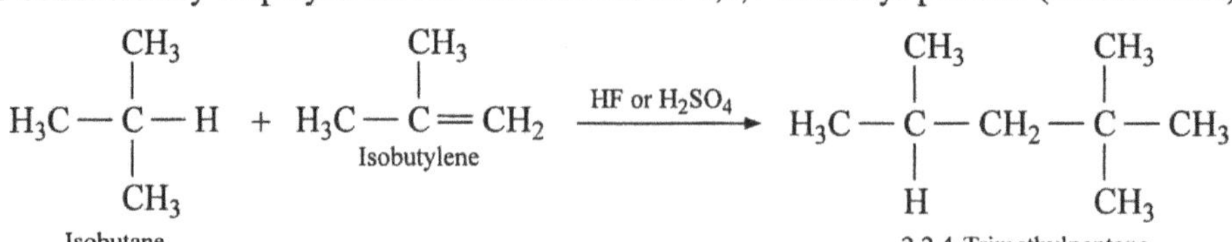

7. ***Addition of Alkenes*** Under suitable conditions (acidic conditions) two alkene molecules react with one another to form an alkene containing twice the number of carbon atoms

Isobutylene

2,4,4-Trimethyl-1-pentene   2,4,4-Trimethyl-2-pentene

Hydroboration–Oxidation Alkenes when treated with diborane $(BH_3)_2$ gives alkyl ranes which on oxidation yield alcohols.

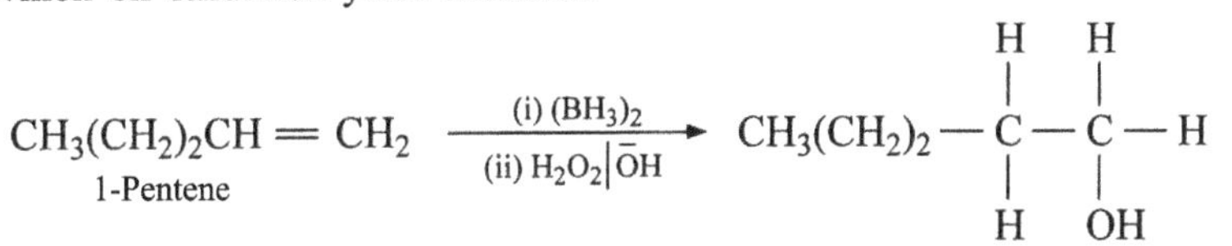

1-Pentene → 1-Pentanol

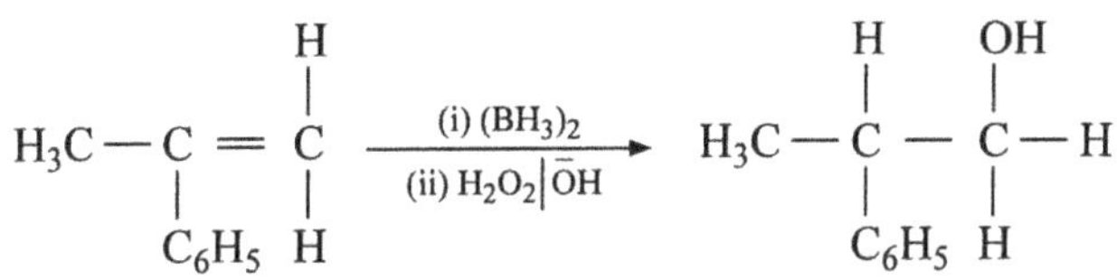

2-Phenyl-1-propene → 2-Phenyl-1-propanol

echanism Hydroboration–oxidation of alkenes is an electrophilc addition reaction. The ctrophile is electron-deficient boron atom of borane, which attacks the double bond of kene. The mechanism involves the following steps:

(i) *Hydroboration* The first step involves addition of hydrogen of BH_3 to one double bonded carbon and —BH_2 to the other. This reaction takes place through a 4-membered transition state.

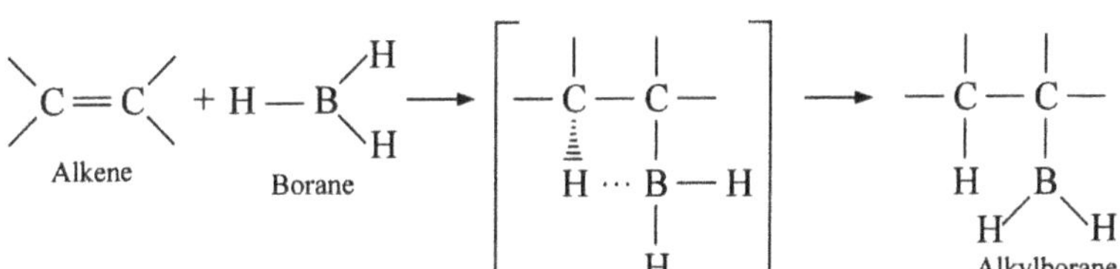

Alkene   Borane   Transition state   Alkylborane

(ii) *Oxidation* In second step, the obtained alkyl borane is oxidised with H_2O_2 in alkali to yield alcohols (boron is replaced by —OH).

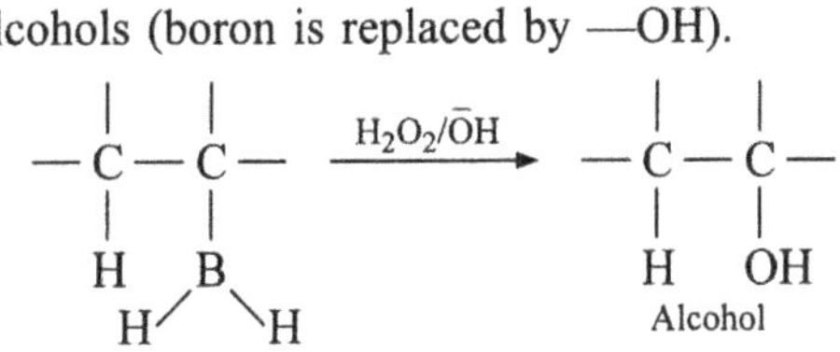

Alkylborane   Alcohol

The hydroboration–oxidation process gives products corresponding to anti-rkovnikov's addition because the steric bulk of the borane is enough to force it to add

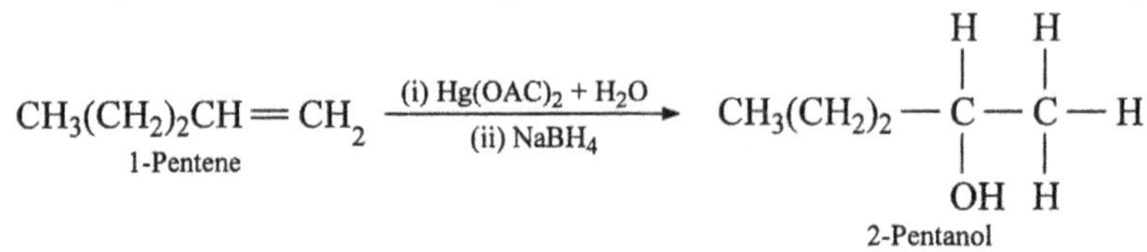

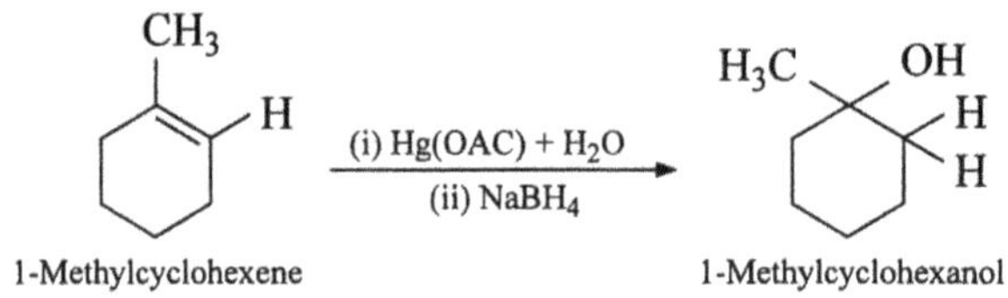

Mechanism Oxymercuration–demercuration of alkenes is an electrophilic addition reactio The electrophile is electron deficient mercury atom of mercuric acetate, which adds at th double bond of alkene. The mechanism involve the following steps:

(i) *Oxymercuration* In the first step, — OH and — HgOAC groups are added t the carbon-carbon double bond and produce hydroxy mercurial compound throug the intermediate formation of cyclic mercurinium ion.

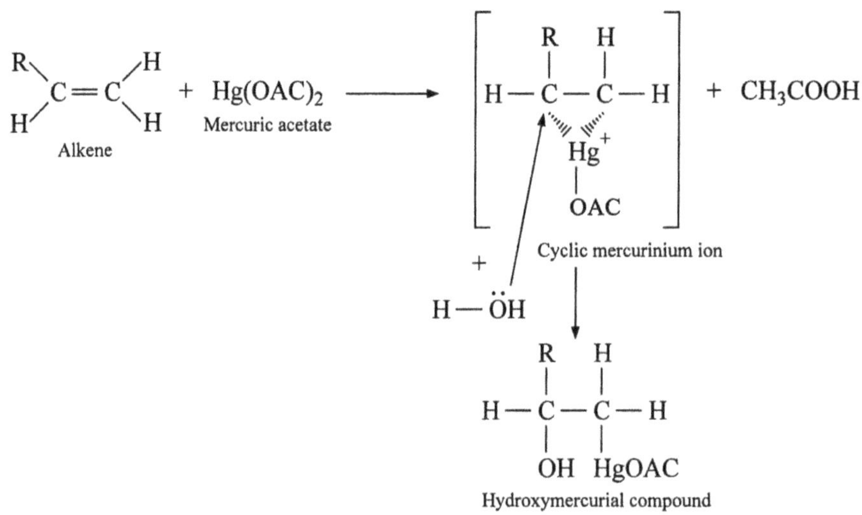

(ii) *Demercuration* In this step HgOAC is replaced by —H in presence of reducin agent ($NaBH_4$).

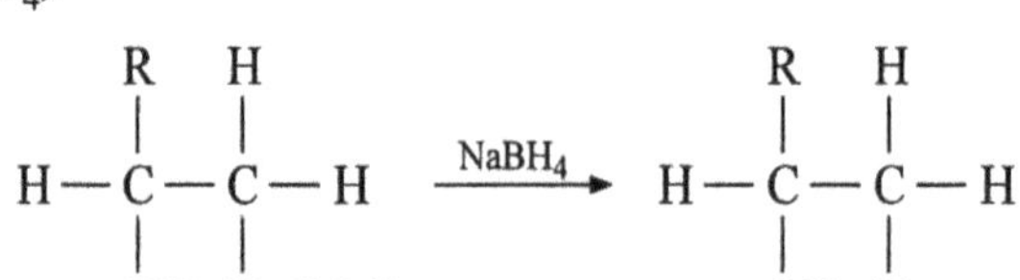

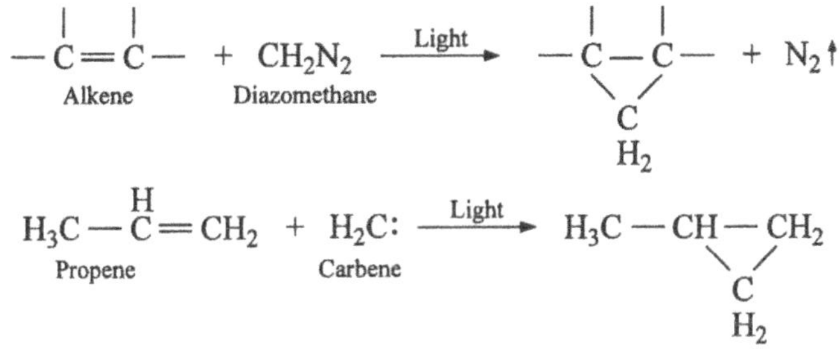

Гhe addition of a singlet carbene to a multiple bond is a stereoselective and a eospecific reaction.

Addition of Halogens Halogens add to alkenes to form vicinal dihalides. The order reactivity of halogens in the addition reactions to alkenes is fluorine > chlorine > mine > iodine. Addition of fluorine causes extensive cleavage of the molecule and ne gives unstable dihalides, hence chlorine or bromine is used in this reaction.

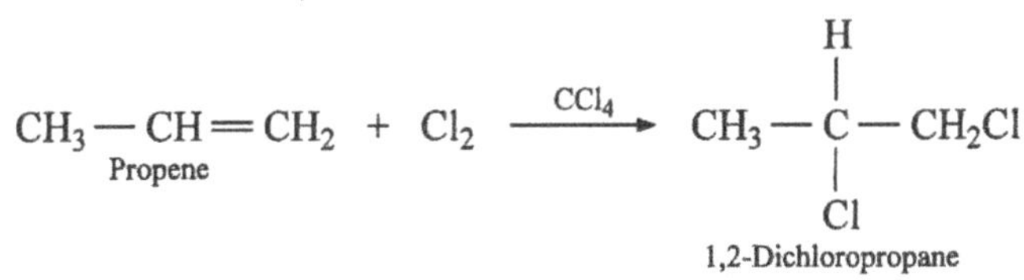

:hanism The addition of halogens to alkenes involves the formation of halonium ion :lic ion) hence no rearrangements occur. As the halogen molecule approaches the :ne and gets polarised, the positively polarised halogen forms a π-complex with ectrons of alkene. This complex undergoes heterolytic cleavage of halogen–halogen d to form halonium ion and a negative halide ion. Finally, the halide ion attacks one he carbon atoms of halonium ion to form the dihalide.

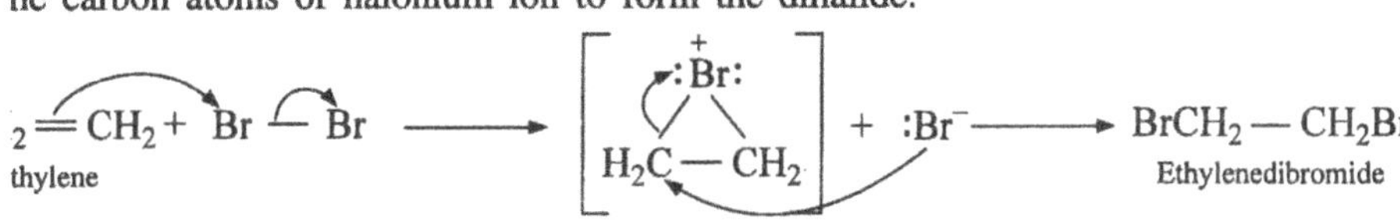

Bromonium ion (Cyclic halonium ion)

.3 Free-Radical Addition

enes undergo free-radical addition. The free radicals seek an electron from π electrons lkene. The free-radical addition of alkenes is exemplified by the addition of HBr to :nes in the presence of peroxide. The addition of HBr to an unsymmetrical alkene ɔws peroxide effect or *anti-Markovnikov's addition,* i.e. HBr adds to alkene in a manner osite to Markovnikov's rule. This phenomenon is known as *Kharasch peroxide effect,*

(a) Alkoxy free radical is generated.

$$RO - OR \longrightarrow 2RO\cdot$$

(b) Alkoxy free radical attacks, HBr to form bromine radical ($\cdot$Br) and alcohol.

$$RO\cdot + H - Br \longrightarrow ROH + \cdot Br$$

(c) Bromine radical ($\cdot$Br) attacks alkene to form most stable alkyl free radical.

$$Br\cdot + \underset{\text{Propene}}{H_3C - HC = CH_2} \longrightarrow \underset{\text{Secondary free radical}}{CH_3 - \dot{C}H - CH_3}$$

(d) The alkyl free radical reacts with H—Br to form anti-Markovnikov's addition produc

$$\underset{\text{Secondary free radical}}{H_3C - CH - CH_2Br} + H - Br \longrightarrow \underset{n\text{-Propylbromide}}{H_3C - CH_2 - CH_2Br} + Br\cdot$$

Peroxide effect does not apply to additions involving hydrogen flouride, hydroge iodide. The H—Cl bond (103 kcal/mole) is stronger than H—Br bond (87 kcal/mole) hence it cannot be cleaved by alkoxy free radical. The H — I bond (71 kcal/mole) is weaker tha H—Br bond because of lower bond dissociation energy, so it is cleaved by alkoxy fre radical but iodine atoms formed readily combines with each other to form iodine molecule because of high atomic weight.

4. ***Polymerisation*** Polymerisation is a process in which the simple molecules unite togethe to form large molecules. The simple compound from which polymer is obtained is calle a monomer. For example, thousands of ethane molecules join together to make polyethan or polythene.

$$H_2C{=}CH_2 \longrightarrow *\!\!-\!\!\left[CH_2 - CH_2 \right]_n\!\!-\!\!*$$

Propene polymerises to give polypropylene.

$$\underset{\displaystyle H}{\overset{\displaystyle CH_3}{\overset{|}{C}}}{=}CH_2 \longrightarrow *\!\!-\!\!\left[\underset{\displaystyle H}{\overset{\displaystyle CH_3}{\overset{|}{C}}} - \underset{H_2}{C} \right]_n\!\!-\!\!*$$

The number of molecules joining up is very variable, but is in the region of 2,000 t 20,000.

Conditions

Temperature	:	About 200° C
Pressure	:	About 2,000 atmospheres.
Initiator	:	A small amount of peroxide.

Mechanism Polymerisation of alkenes proceeds through free-radical mechanism, whicl involves the following steps.

(a) *Chain initiation*

H$_2$ H$_2$ H$_2$ H$_2$

c) *Chain termination*

$$\text{)}-(CH_2)_n^{\bullet} + {}^{\bullet}(CH_2)_n-OR \longrightarrow RO-(CH_2)_n-(CH_2)_n-OR$$

ubstitution Reactions All alkenes, except ethene, contain one or more alkyl groups :hed to one or both of the double bonded carbon atoms. These alkyl groups undergo ;titution reactions similar to alkanes. This type of reaction where substitution takes e at β-carbon atom with respect to the double bond is referred as *allylic substitution.* low concentration of bromine required for allylic substitution is released by N-nosuccinimide (NBS) slowly and steadily. N-bromosuccinimide has a weak nitrogen–nine bond that can be fragmented into radicals upon warming or exposure to visible t. The formed bromine atom replaces allylic C — H (σ) bond by C — Br bond. The ic substitution involves the following steps:

)

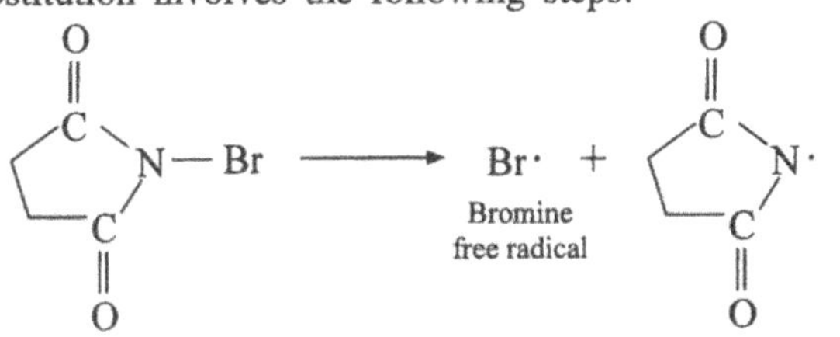

N-Bromosuccinimide

i) $CH_2{=}CH-CH_2-H + Br\cdot \longrightarrow CH_2{=}CH-\dot{C}H_2 + HBr$

Propene — Allyl radical

ii)

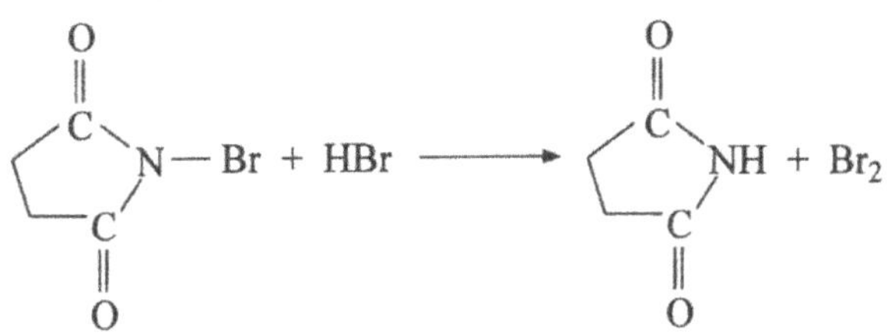

N-Bromosuccinimide — Succinimide

v) $CH_2{=}CH-\dot{C}H_2 + Br-Br \longrightarrow CH_2{=}CH-CH_2Br + Br\cdot$

Allyl radical — Allyl bromide

xidation Reactions Alkenes give a variety of products on oxidation with different ising agents.

(i) *Oxidation of alkenes with aqueous $KMnO_4$ solution* In alkenes, on treatment with a cold aqueous potassium permanganate solution, two hydroxyl groups are added to the double bonded carbon atoms to form vicinal glycols (1,2-dihydroxy compound). This reaction is commonly termed as hydroxylation. In this test

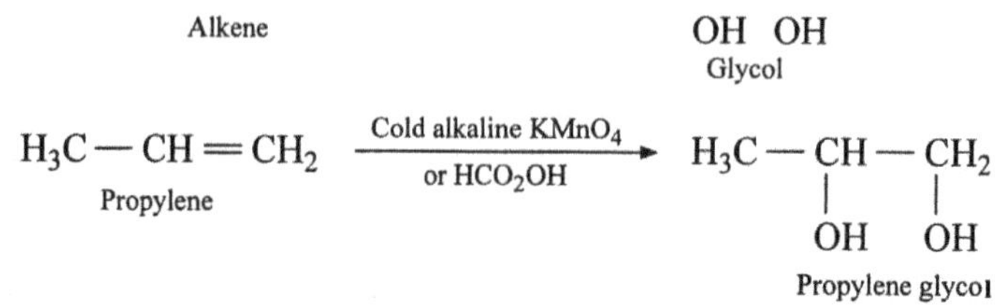

(ii) *Oxidation with peroxy acids (epoxidation)* Alkenes react with peroxyaci (peroxyacetic acid, peroxybenzoic acid) to form epoxides.

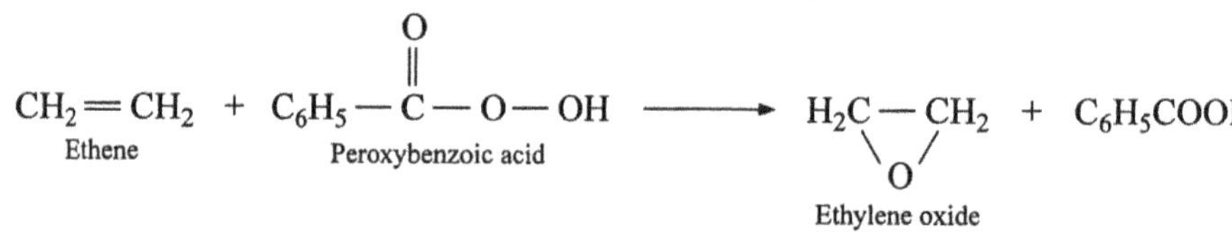

7. ***Cleavage Reactions*** In cleavage reactions the double bond is completely broken ar the alkene molecule changes into smaller fragments.

(i) *Ozonolysis* In ozonolysis, the double bond is cleaved with ozone. This reaction the most important of cleavage reactions, which involves addition of ozone to an alker to form ozonide that on hydrolysis yields one or more aldehydes or ketones. This methc is employed for locating the positions of double bond and identification of alkyl grouı present in an alkene.

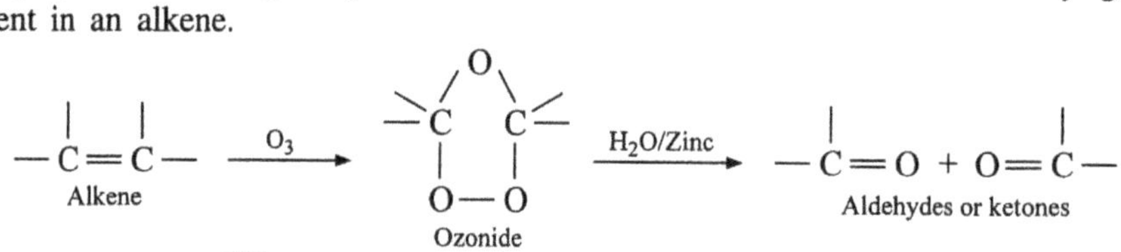

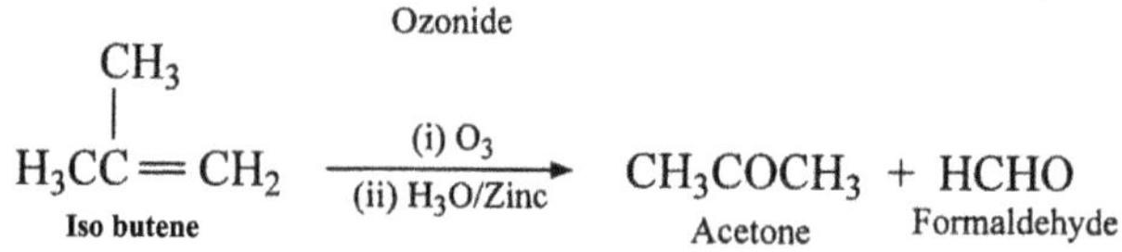

Mechanism

Step 1 The π-electrons act as the nucleophile, attacking the ozone at the electrophili terminal oxygen. A second C—O is formed by the nucleophilic oxygen attackin the other end of the C=C.

Step 2 The cyclic species called the malozonide rearranges to the ozonide.

Step 3 The ozonide decomposes to two carbonyl groups on reduction (usuall Zn/acetic acid).

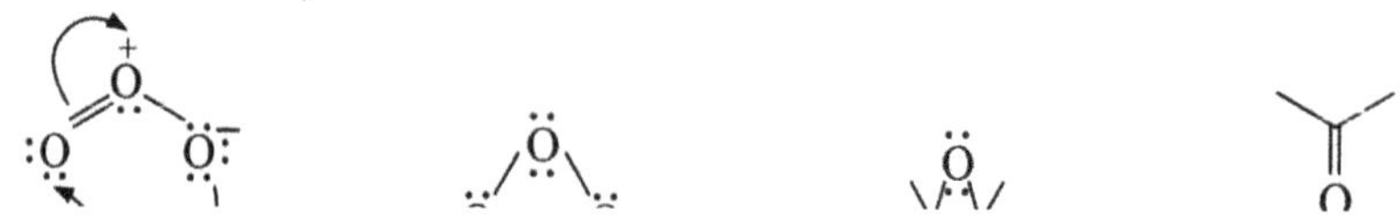

$$CH_3CH_2CH_2CH=CH_2 \longrightarrow CH_3CH_2CH_2COOH + CO_2$$

1-Pentene Butanoic acid

ombustion Alkenes are completely oxidised to CO_2 and water when burnt in air or gen.

$$CH_2=CH_2 + 3O_2 \longrightarrow 2CO_2 + 2H_2O + \text{energy}$$

PRACTICE QUESTIONS

(a) Enumerate and discuss various methods available for the preparation of alkenes.

(b) Suggest in each case the suitable alkylhalide that should be subjected to dehydrohalogenation to get the alkenes given below:

(i) Isobutylene
(ii) 2-Pentene
(iii) 2-Methyl-1-butene

(a) Give the structures of the alkenes expected from the dehydro-halogen of

(i) 1-Chloropentane
(ii) 2-Chloro-2,3-dimethyl butane
(iii) 3-Chloropentane

Predict the major product in each case.

(b) Formulate and explain the following conversions:

(i) *n*-Propyl alcohol to *n*-propane
(ii) Propene to *n*-propylbromide
(iii) 1,2-Dichlorobutane to 1-butene
(iv) Ethylene to ethylene glycol.

Formulate the reactions of ethylene with the following reagents, indicating the conditions and giving the structures and names of products:

(i) Br_2—H_2O
(ii) Conc. sulphuric acid
(iii) Hydrogen chloride
(iv) Acidified potassium permaganate
(v) Hypochlorous acid
(vi) Ozone

(a) 'Alkenes mainly undergo electrophilic addition reactions.' Substantiate the statement with suitable examples.

(b) Write Markovnikov's rule and anti-Markovnikov's rule. Explain with suitable examples.

(c) Write short notes on the importance of following reagents in the laboratory:

(i) Tollen's reagent
(ii) Bromine in CCl_4
(iii) Fehling's solution

Write the mechanism and products obtained when neopentyl alcohol is dehydrated by heating with conc. H_2SO_4.

(c) Elimination reaction

9. Account for the following:
   (a) Carbon–carbon double bond is shorter than carbon–carbon single bond.
   (b) An alkene is more reactive than alkane.
10. Give the mechanism of addition of hydrogen bromide on propylene, both in absence presence of peroxide.
11. How do you prepare the following?
   (a) Propylene from propyl chloride
   (b) Propane from propene
   (c) Propene from propanol
12. Dehydration of 2-propanol occurs in 75% H_2SO_4 at 100° C. Using curved arrows, write do all steps in a mechanism for the dehydration. Explain the essential role performed in alco dehydrations by the acid catalyst.
13. Outline all steps in a synthesis that would transform isopropyl alcohol [$CH_3CH(OH)CH$ into each of the following:
   (a) $(CH_3)_2CHCH(OH)CH_3$
   (b) $(CH_3)_2CHCH_2OH$
   (c) $(CH_3)_2CHCH(OH)CH(CH_3)_2$
14. The principal organic product formed in the reaction below is

$$CH_2 = CH(CH_2)_8COOH + HBr \text{ (in peroxide)}$$

U

HEMISTRY OF ALKYNES

.1 INTRODUCTION

cynes are unsaturated hydrocarbons that contain carbon–carbon triple bond having the ıeral formula of C_nH_{2n-2}. The carbon–carbon triple bond is the functional group of ynes, which determines their chemical reactivity. The carbon–carbon triple bond is made of one strong σ bond and two weaker π bonds. It has a total strength of 123 kcal/mole. erefore, the triple bond is stronger than the carbon–carbon double bond of an alkene and bon–carbon single bond of an alkane.

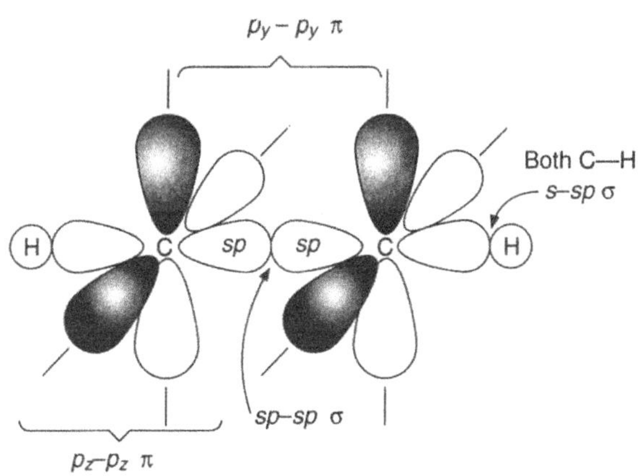

Orbital structure of ethyne

2 IUPAC NOMENCLATURE

(i) Determine the longest continuous chain of carbons that has the triple bond between two of its carbons. The chain does not necessarily have to be straight. The triple bond will be higher in priority than any simple alkyl or halide group, therefore the word root is derived by finding the longest chain which contains both atoms of the triple bond.

(ii) Number the carbons in the chain so that the triple bond between the carbons is

(v) The location of the triple bond is indicated by the number designated to the fi carbon atom of the triple bond.

(vi) There are two conventions in placing the number: the less common is to put t number between the root and suffix (e.g. prop-1-yne); the more common meth is to place the number before the word root (e.g. 1-propyne).

The names of alkynes are obtained by using suffix -yne instead of -ane of correspondi alkanes.

IUPAC Name	*Formula*
Ethyne (acetylene)	$HC{\equiv}CH$
Propyne	$HC{\equiv}CCH_3$
1-Butyne	$HC{\equiv}CCH_2CH_3$
1-Pentyne	$HC{\equiv}C(CH_2)_2CH_3$
1-Hexyne	$HC{\equiv}C(CH_2)_3CH_3$
1-Heptyne	$HC{\equiv}C(CH_2)_4CH_3$
1-Octyne	$HC{\equiv}C(CH_2)_5CH_3$
1-Nonyne	$HC{\equiv}C(CH_2)_6CH_3$
1-Decyne	$HC{\equiv}C(CH_2)_7CH_3$
2-Butyne	$CH_3C{\equiv}CCH_3$
2-Pentyne	$CH_3C{\equiv}CCH_2CH_3$

10.3 PREPARATION OF ALKYNES

10.3.1 Industrial Preparation of Acetylene

Simplest member of the alkyne family is acetylene. Traditionally, acetylene has been prepare by the action of H_2O on CaC_2 (calcium carbide) and CaC_2 is in turn prepared by th reaction between calcium oxide (obtained from limestone) and coke (obtained from coa at high temperatures (in electric furnace). This involves controlled, high-temperature parti oxidation.

$$\underset{\text{Coke}}{3C} + \underset{\text{Lime}}{CaO} \xrightarrow{2500^\circ C} \underset{\text{Calcium carbide}}{CaC_2} + CO$$

$$CaC_2 + 2H_2O \longrightarrow \underset{\text{Acetylene}}{H-C\equiv C-H} + Ca(OH)_2$$

10.3.2 Dehydrohalogenation of Alkyl Dihalides (Vicinal Dihalides)

It is an example for elimination reaction. A carbon–carbon triple bond is formed in th

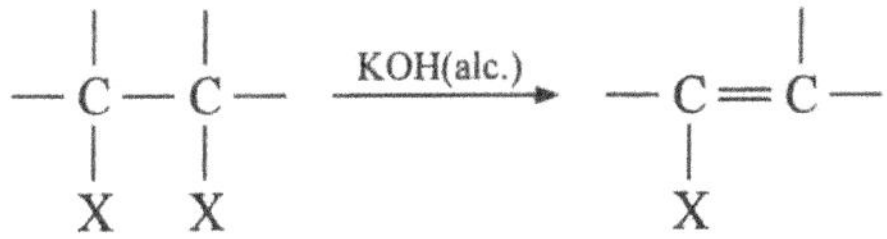

Alkyl dihalide Vinyl halide

(b) In the second step, a strong base ($NaNH_2$) is utilised to get an alkyne from vinyl halide by dehydrohalogenation.

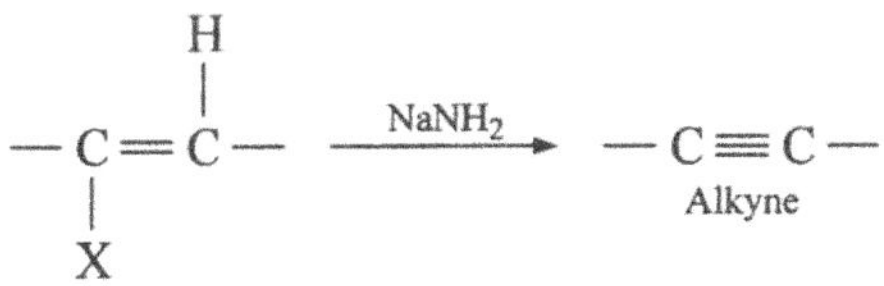

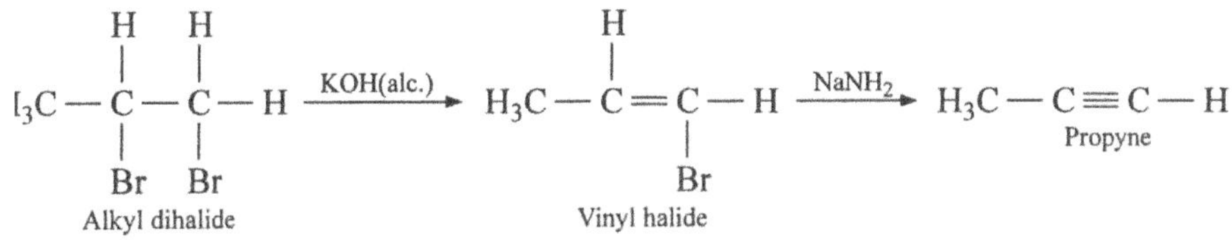

3.3 Reaction of Metal Acetylides with Alkyl Halides

s method is utilised to prepare larger alkynes from smaller alkynes. Acetylide anions powerful nucleophiles and are capable of displacing halide ion from primary alkyl des to get alkynes. In this reaction, the alkyl group becomes attached to the triple-ded carbon and thus a larger alkyne is generated.

$$\underset{\text{Alkyne}}{R-C\equiv C-H} + Na \longrightarrow \underset{\text{Sodium alkylide}}{R-C\equiv C\colon^{-}\ Na^{+}}$$

$$\underset{\text{Sodium alkylide}}{R-C\equiv C\colon^{-}\ Na^{+}} + R-Br \longrightarrow \underset{\text{Higher alkyne}}{R-C\equiv C-R} + NaBr$$

$$[_3-C\equiv C\colon^{-}\ Na^{+} + CH_3-Br \longrightarrow CH_3-C\equiv C-CH_3 + NaBr$$

3.4 Dehalogenation of Tetrahalides

etrahalide on removal of two halogen atoms in presence of zinc yields alkynes. This tion is severely limited by the fact that these halides are themselves prepared from the nes.

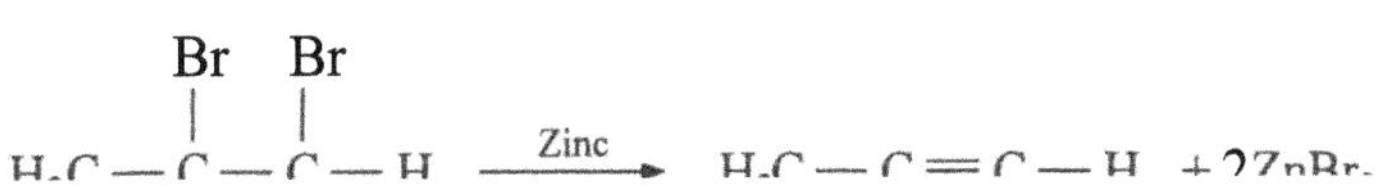

essentially the same as those of the alkanes and alkenes.

1. They are insoluble in water.
2. They are quite soluble in the usual organic solvents of low polarity (e.g. ligr ether, benzene, carbon tetrachloride, etc.).
3. They are less dense than water.
4. Their boiling points are very nearly the same as the boiling points of alkane: alkenes with the same carbon skeletons.
5. However, within the hamologue series the boiling points show the usual incre with increasing carbon number.

Table 10.1 Physical Properties of Alkynes

Name	*MP* (°C)	*BP* (°C)	*Density* (20° C)
Acetylene	– 82	– 75	–
Propyne	– 101.5	– 23	–
1-Butyne	– 122	91	–
1-Pentyne	– 98	40	0.695
1-Hexyne	– 124	72	0.719
1-Heptyne	– 80	100	0.733
1-Octyne	– 70	126	0.747
1-Nonyne	– 65	151	0.763
1-Decyne	– 35	182	0.770
2-Butyne	– 24	27	0.694
2-Pentyne	101	55	0.714

10.5 CHEMICAL PROPERTIES

The chemistry of alkynes is similar to alkenes in that both are formed by eliminat reactions, and the major chemical reactions are addition type. There are however so differences between alkynes and alkenes. The distinguishing feature of alkynes is presence of carbon–carbon triple bond that is made of a strong σ bond and two π bon Presence of π bonds in alkynes makes them to react with electrophilic reagents. The hybrid orbitals used in the formation of C≡C bond have greater *s* character and les effective size, the electron pairs in the triple bond are more firmly held by the carbon ato than in alkenes. Hence, the alkynes are less reactive than alkenes towards electroph reagents. Following are the major addition reactions.

1. ***Addition of Hydrogen*** Alkynes react with hydrogen in presence of catalyst form alkenes, which on further hydrogenation yield alkanes. Reduction of alkynes

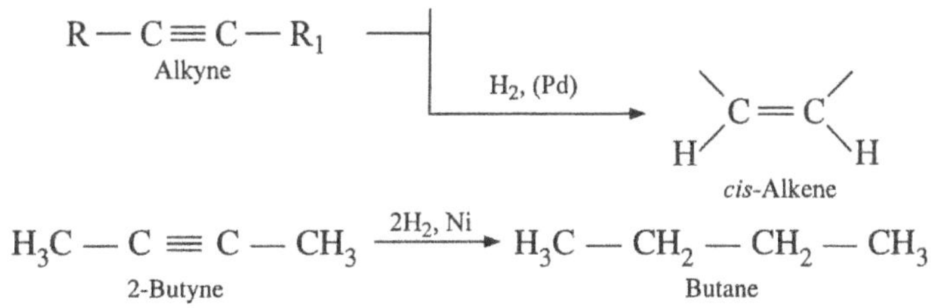

ıddition of Halogens Alkynes undergo addition with chlorine or bromine to form ıloalkenes or tetrahaloalkanes. The addition of halogens follows an electrophilic addition ıugh the intermediate formation of halonium ion.

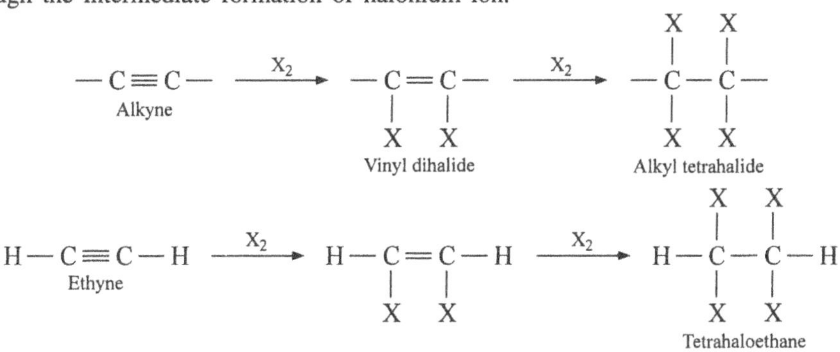

ddition of Hydrogen Halides Alkynes react with HCl and HBr to form haloalkenes ;eminal dihalides depending upon the amount of hydrogen halide used. Addition of rogen halides to alkynes is an electrophilic addition through the intermediate formation 'inylic cation, which is less stable than alkyl cation.

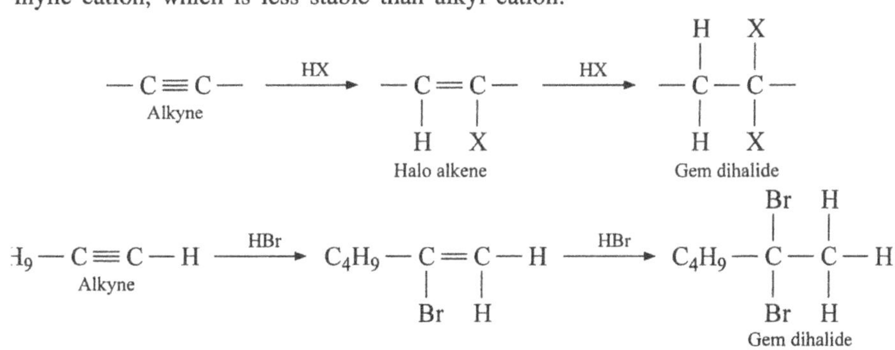

ıoth additions follow Markovnikov's rule (i.e. hydrogen atom of hydrogen halide ımes attached to the carbon atom that has the greater number of hydrogen atoms). resence of peroxides, HBr adds to alkynes by following anti-Markovnikov's addition.

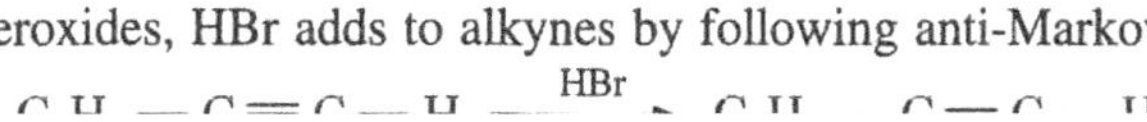

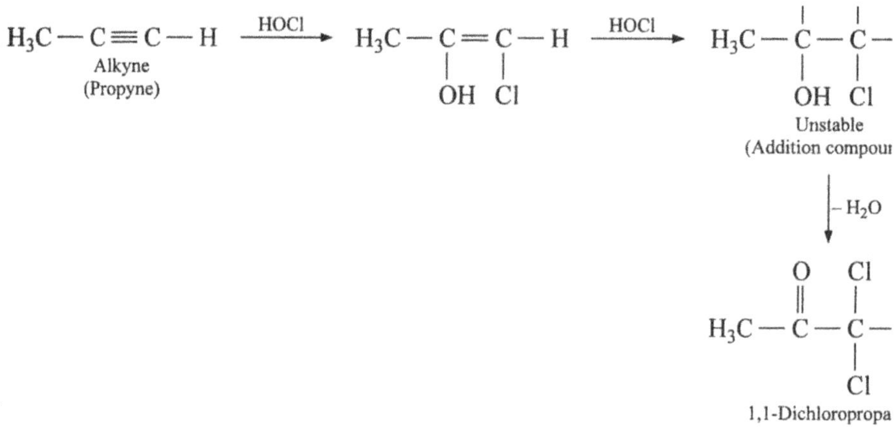

5. ***Addition of Water*** The addition of water to an alkyne occurs in presence of an ac catalyst (H_2SO_4 and $HgSO_4$). The initial product of hydration is an enol (vinyl alcoh produced if we use ethyne). Enols, being unstable isomerise to form keto compou except acetylene which exhibits aldehyde (keto-enol tautomerism).

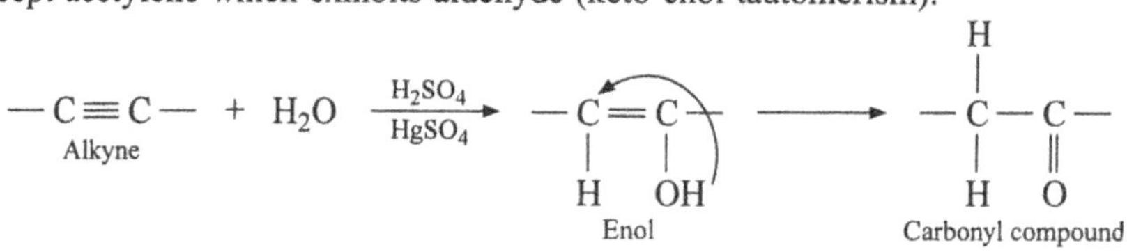

6. ***Nucleophilic Addition*** The electron pairs in the triple bond are more firmly held by carbon atoms. This decrease in reactivity of carbon–carbon triple bond with electrop reagents makes it suitable to react with nucleophilic reagents. The nucleophilic addi takes place in two steps. In the first step, the nucleophile attacks the alkyne to give vi carbanion. In the second step, the carbanion takes a proton to form the final product

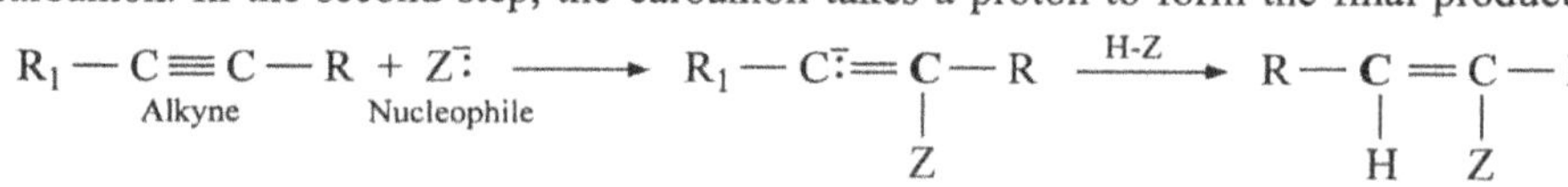

This reaction is exemplified by the addition of HCN and alcohol.

(i) *Addition of HCN* Alkynes react with hydrogen cyanide in presence of bari cyanide as catalyst by the following reaction.

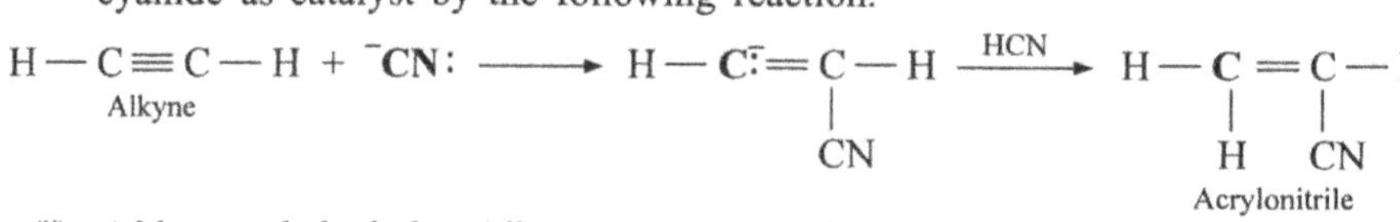

(ii) *Addition of alcohols* Alkynes react with alcohols to form unsaturated ethers the following nucleophilic addition reaction

$$\underset{\text{Alkyne}}{R_1-C\equiv C-R} \xrightarrow{\text{Alkaline } KMnO_4} R_1COOH + RCOOH$$

$$\underset{\text{Ethyne}}{H-C\equiv C-H} \xrightarrow{\text{Baeyer's reagent}} \underset{\text{Oxalic acid}}{\begin{matrix} COOH \\ | \\ COOH \end{matrix}}$$

$$R_1-C\equiv C-R \xrightarrow{O_3 + H_2O} R_1COOH + RCOOH$$

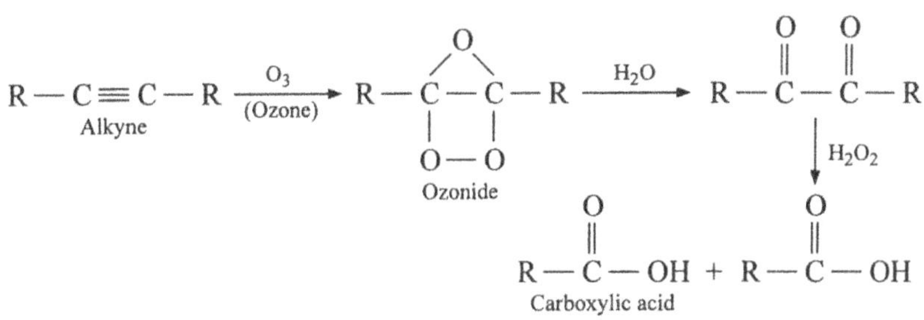

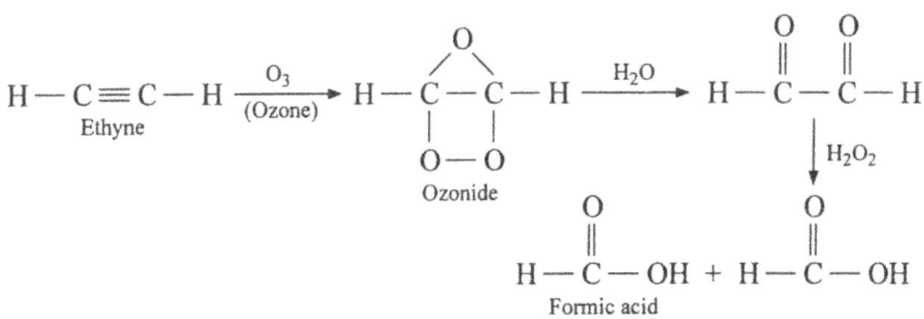

'olymerisation

(i) When acetylene is passed through a red-hot copper or quartz tube, it polymerises to benzene.

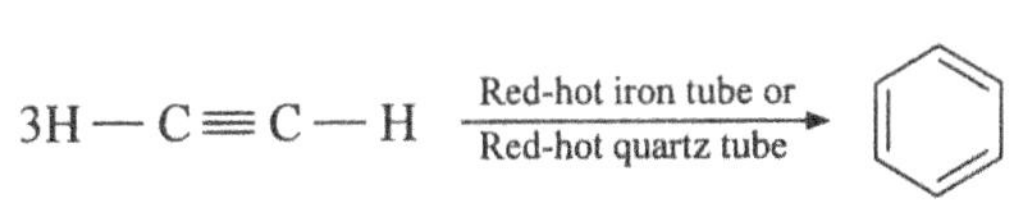

Benzene

ii) Two molecules of ethyne can be combined to produce vinyl ethyne, by passing the ethyne into a saturated solution of cuprous chloride in ammonium chloride.

form precipitates. Hence, this test can be utilised to differentiate terminal alkynes f internal alkynes.

$$\underset{\text{Ethyne}}{H-C\equiv C-H} \xrightarrow{Ag^+} \underset{\text{Silver acetylide}}{H-C\equiv CAg}$$

$$\underset{\text{Propyne}}{H_3C-C\equiv C-H} \xrightarrow{Cu^+} \underset{\text{Cuprous methylacetylide}}{H_3C-C\equiv CCu}$$

10. ***Acidity of Terminal Alkynes*** Due to the high degree of 's' character (the *sp* hy orbital is 50% '*s*' and 50% '*p*' in character) in the C—H bonds of terminal alkynes, alky are relatively acidic compared to other sp^3 and sp^2 hybridised hydrocarbons. The *s* ort is much more electronegative in character than a *p* orbital because it is smaller and closer to the nucleus.

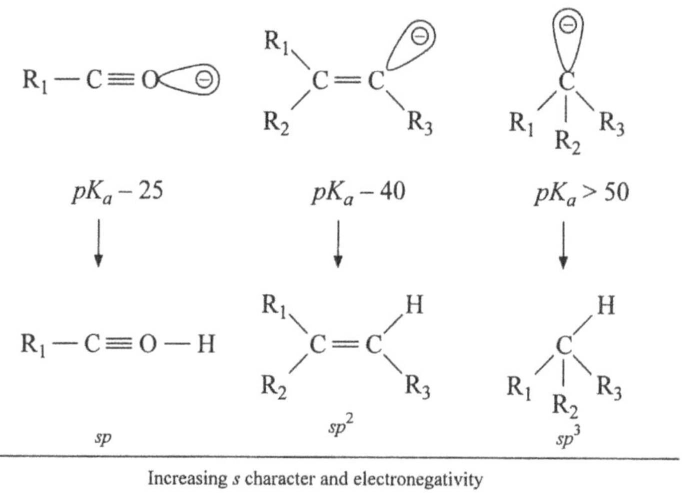

11. ***Combustion of Alkynes*** Acetylene burns with smoky flame in excess of air. Un controlled supply of air, it burns with a bright light, which is injurious to eyes. process is highly exothermic. Oxyacetylene flame is used for welding purposes and gi a temperature of about 3500° C.

$$\underset{\text{Ethyne}}{2C_2H_2} + 5O_2 \longrightarrow 4CO_2 + 2H_2O$$

$$\underset{\text{Butyne}}{2C_4H_6} + 11O_2 \longrightarrow 8CO_2 + 6H_2O$$

(i) Ethyne and ethane
(ii) 1-Butyne and 2-butyne
(iii) Acetylene and 2-butyne.

(b) Explain bonding in ethylene.

2. What are alkynes? Give any three methods to prepare alkynes. Give a brief account on electrophilic addition reactions of alkynes.

3. Write notes on:

(a) Acidity of alkynes
(b) Keto-enol tautomerism
(c) Ozonolysis of alkynes
(d) Polymerisation of alkynes
(e) Nucleophilic addition reactions of alkynes.

11

CHEMISTRY OF DIENES

Dienes are unsaturated hydrocarbons containing two carbon–carbon double bonds molecule and having the general formula C_nH_{2n-2}.

11.1 CLASSIFICATION OF DIENES

Dienes are classified depending upon the arrangement double bonds. They are of types.

1. ***Isolated Dienes*** Double bonds are separated by more than one single bond. double bond units occur separately (Fig. 11.1). The π systems are isolated from other by sp^3 hybridised centres. The result is that isolated dienes have reactivity is characteristic of simple alkenes, e.g.

$$H_2C=CH-CH_2-CH=CH_2$$

(1,4-Pentadiene)

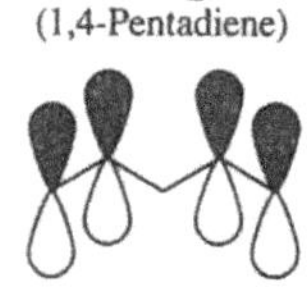

Fig. 11.1. An Isolated Diene

2. ***Cumulated Dienes*** Double bonds are present between successive carbon atoms. double bond units share a common *sp* hybridised C atom (Fig. 11.2). The result is cumulated dienes have reactivity more like simple alkynes. Note the relative spatial sitions of the two CH_2 units at the ends of the cumulated system, e.g.

$$H_3C-CH=C=CH_2$$

(1,2-Butadiene)

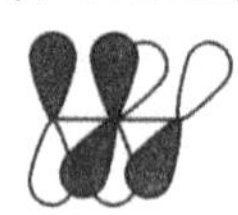

Fig. 11.2 A Cumulated Diene

3. ***Conjugated Dienes*** Double bonds are separated by a single bond. The double b units occur consecutively gives a continuous π system since the adjacent p orbitals

Fig. 11.3 A Conjugated Diene

.2 PREPARATION OF DIENES

ɜ following are more commonly employed methods.

Catalytic dehydrogenation of n-butane or 1-butene by passing over the catalyst O_3–Al_2O_3) at 600° C.

$$I_3CH_2CH_2CH_3 \xrightarrow[60°C]{\text{Catalyst}} CH_3CH_2CH=CH_2 \xrightarrow[600°C]{\text{Catalyst}} CH_2=CH-CH=CH_2$$

n-Butane 1-Butane 1,3-Butadiene

By the dehydration of 1,4-butanediol

$$\underset{\text{OH}}{CH_2}-CH_2-CH_2-\underset{\text{OH}}{CH_2} \xrightarrow[\text{Heat}]{H^+} CH_2=CH-CH=CH_2$$

1,4-Butanediol 1,3-Butadiene

By retro Diels–Alder reaction Retro Diels–Alder reaction is reverse of Diels–Alder ction. Dienes can be prepared by passing the vapours of cyclohexane over an alloy ickel and chromium (nichrome).

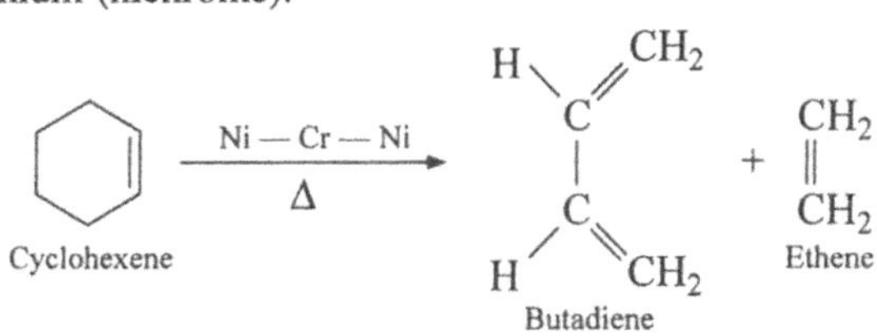

3 PROPERTIES OF DIENES

ɟeneral , dienes undergo electrophilic addition reactions in a manner similar to alkenes:

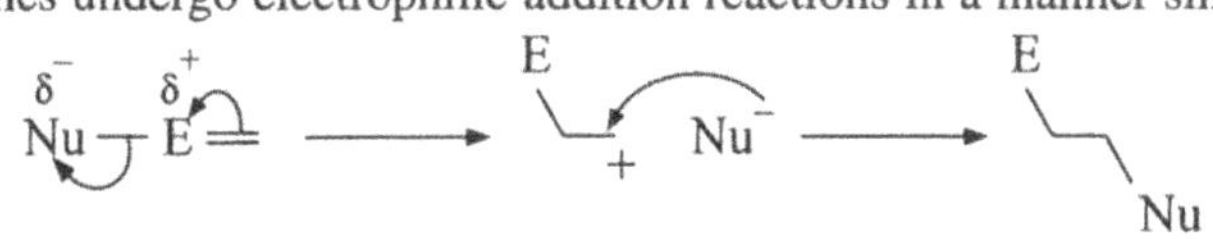

ʋever,

1. Conjugated dienes undergo addition but the proximity of the conjugated C=C influences the reactions.
2. Isolated dienes react just like alkenes.
3. Cumulated dienes react more like alkynes (both have *sp* hybridised C atoms).

ɟjugated dienes differ from simple alkenes in three ways:

1,3-Pentadiene	54.1

The stability of conjugated dienes is explained on the basis of the following fact

(i) The carbon–carbon single bond in 1,3-butadiene is formed as the result of overlap of an sp^2 orbital with another sp^2 orbital. Hence, this bond length is sho than a bond formed by overlap of sp^3–sp^2 orbitals. Shorter bonds are stronger, hence the molecule with conjugated double bonds is more stable.

$$CH_2{=}CH - CH{=}CH_2 \qquad\qquad CH_2{=}CH - CH_2 - CH{=}CH_2$$

Single bond formed by overlap of sp^2–sp^2 orbitals in 1,3-butadiene (Conjugated diene)

Single bonds formed by overlap of sp^3–sp^2 orbitals in 1,4-pentadiene (Isolated diene)

(ii) The second factor that causes conjugated diene to be more stable is *resonan* which means that the compound has delocalised electrons. The π electrons i conjugated double bond are not localised between two carbons but are delocalis The resulting delocalisation increases the molecular stability.
The delocalisation takes place due to overlapping of p orbital of a carbon at (C_2) with p orbitals of C_1 and of C_3 equally.

$$CH_2{=}CH - CH{=}CH_2 \leftrightarrow \overset{-}{C}H_2 - CH{=}CH - \overset{+}{C}H_2 \leftrightarrow \overset{+}{C}H_2 - CH{=}CH - \overset{-}{C}$$

Resonance contributing structures

$$\equiv$$

$$CH_2 \cdots CH \cdots CH \cdots CH_2$$

Resonance hybrid

(iii) The double bond units occur consecutively giving a continuous π system sir the adjacent p orbitals can all overlap with each other. The result is that con gated dienes reactivity differs to that of simple alkenes. The extra bonding int action between the adjacent π systems makes the conjugated dienes the m stable type of diene (see Fig. 11.3).

2. ***Conjugated Dienes undergo 1,4-Addition*** Dienes, like alkenes are nucleophiles b cause of the presence of electron density at π bonds hence they undergo electrophi addition reactions. The total quantity of reagent is two times to that for an alkene. F example, the reaction of 1,4-pentadiene (isolated diene) undergoes two independent a dition reactions with excess of reagent by following Markovnikov's rule.

$$\underset{\text{1,3-Butadiene}}{CH_2{=}CH - CH{=}CH_2} + Cl_2 \xrightarrow{CCl_4}$$

$$CH_2 - CH{=}CH - CH_2 + CH_2{=}CH - CH - CH_2$$

$$\underset{\text{1,4-Addition product}}{\underset{\displaystyle H}{CH_2} - CH = CH - \underset{\displaystyle Br}{CH_2}} + \underset{\text{1,2-Addition product}}{CH_2 = CH - \underset{\displaystyle Br}{CH} - \underset{\displaystyle H}{CH_2}} \leftarrow$$

If a conjugated diene (1,3-butadiene) reacts with a limited amount of electrophilic reagent, addition can occur at only one of the double bonds and two addition products. One ı 1,2-addition product that is formed by the addition of the reagent at 1- and 2-posi- ıs. The other is a 1,4-addition product, which is formed by the addition of the reagent 1- and 4-positions (1,4-addition or conjugated addition).

chanism (i) In the first step, proton of HBr adds to C-1(sp^2 carbon at the end of ıjugated system) which results in the formation of allylic cation. The allylic cation has › contributing resonance structures. The positive charge on the carbocation is not alised on C-2 and C-4 due to delocalisation of π electrons. Thus, allyl cation is more ɔle than even the tertiary carbocation hence formed preferentially.

$$'H_2 = CH - CH = CH_2 + H - Br$$

$$\longrightarrow CH_3 - \overset{+}{C}H - CH = CH_2 \xleftrightarrow{\text{An allylic cation}} CH_3 - CH = CH - \overset{+}{C}H_2$$

In the second step of the reaction, the bromide ion can attack either C-2 (direct addition) C-4 (conjugated addition) to form 1,2-addition product or 1,4-addition product.

$$\underset{\text{An allyic cation}}{CH_3 - \overset{+}{C}H - CH = CH_2 \longleftrightarrow CH_3 - CH = CH - \overset{+}{C}H_2} \xrightarrow{Br^-}$$

$$\underset{\text{1, 2-Addition product}}{CH_3 - \underset{\displaystyle Br}{CH} - CH = CH_2} + \underset{\text{1, 4-Addition product}}{CH_3 - CH = CH - \underset{\displaystyle Br}{CH_2}}$$

The distribution of the products depends on the reaction conditions as shown by the owing example:

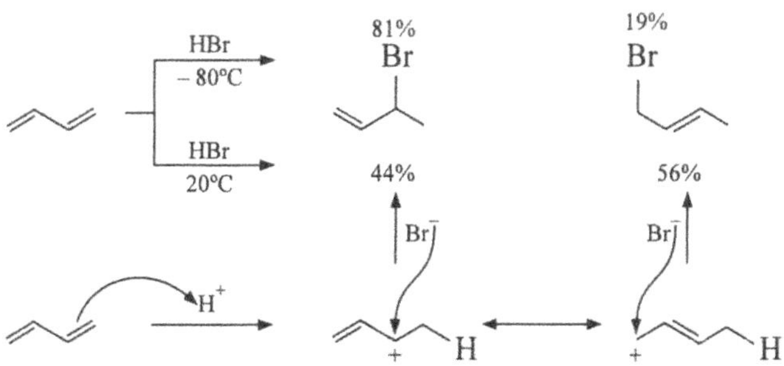

by drawing a potential energy diagram. Initially, the carbocation is formed, which re to yield 1,2-addition product faster than 1,4-addition product because the energy activation is lesser for 1,2-addition reaction than for 1,4-addition reaction. In the diagr the lower hill corresponds to the 1,2-addition reaction; hence, 1,2-addition produc formed faster than the 1,4-addition compound (Fig. 11.4).

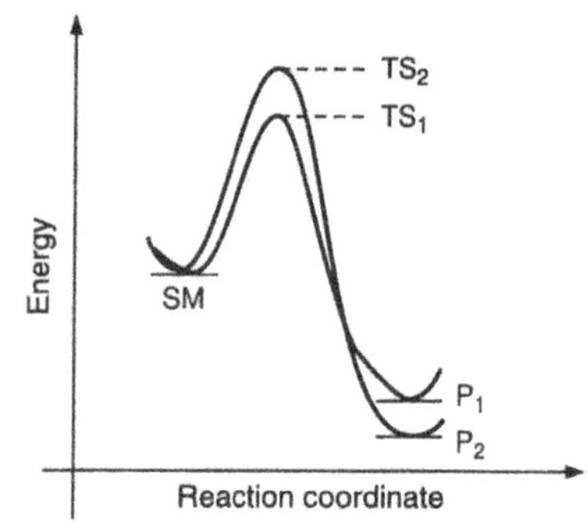

Fig. 11.4 Potential Energy Diagram of Addition Reaction

The 1,2-product is formed rapidly, but ionises rapidly. The 1,4-addition product is forr slowly but ionises even more slowly.

At low temperature, the reaction is under kinetic control (rate, irreversible conditic and the major product is that from fastest reaction, that of the bromide with the second cation.

At room temperature, the reaction is under thermodynamic control (equilibrium, reve ible conditions) and the major product is the more stable system (note the more hig substituted alkene).

(i) *Addition of halogens to dienes* Like the addition of hydrogen halides to conjuga dienes, halogens add to dienes via direct and conjugate addition pathways:

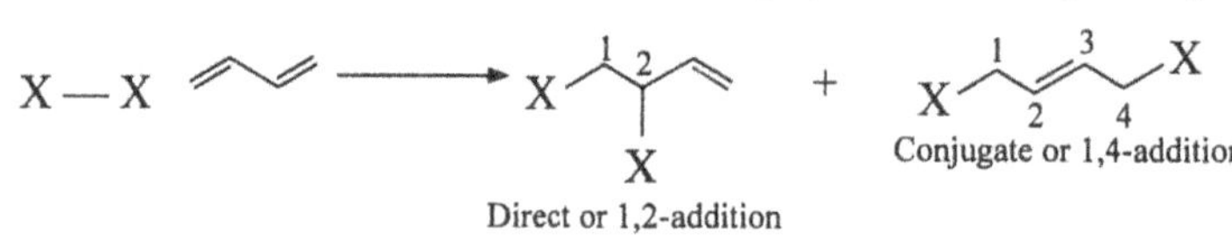

The major products are usually more stable, conjugate addition products with m stable E configuration of **C=C**.

(ii) *Free-radical addition* Conjugated dienes react with free radicals too. The fr radical reaction of the conjugated diene is again affected by resonance and, accordin we obtain the 1,2- and 1,4-products through the intermediate formation of free radical. T butadiene is added mainly in a 1,4-mode. The following steps are involved in the fr

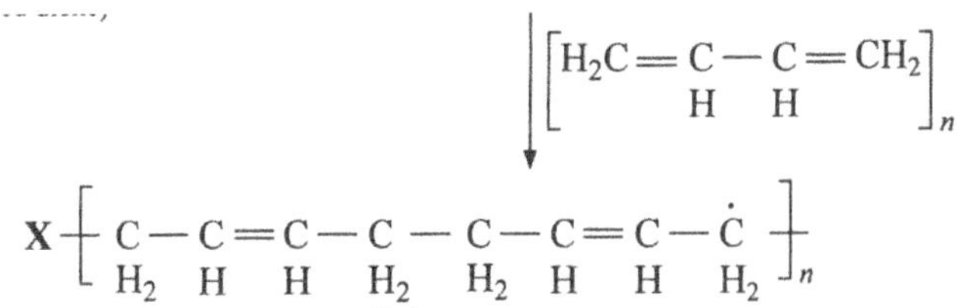

Polymer

BR (Styrene-Butadiene Rubber), for the manufacture of tyres is prepared by adding :e-radical initiator to a mixture of styrene and butadiene.

The Diels–Alder reaction The Diels–Alder reaction is an important reaction of con- ted dienes because it creates two new carbon–carbon bonds in the formation of a ic molecule. Hence, this reaction is also known as cycloaddition reaction.

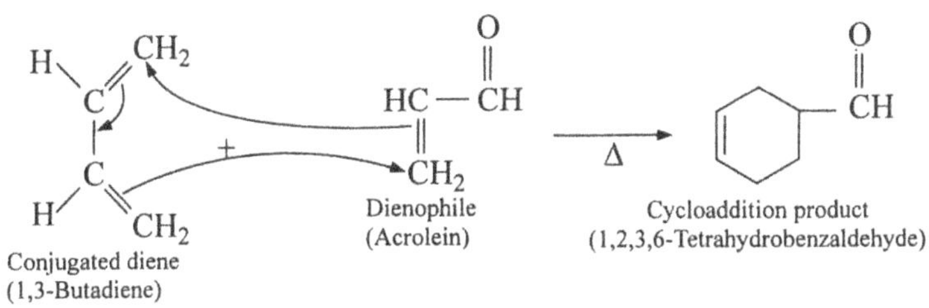

ı this reaction, a conjugated diene reacts with a compound containing a carbon– on double bond (dienophile). Dienophiles with electron-withdrawing groups bonded ıe of the sp^2-hybridised carbons are more reactive. The electron-withdrawing group rises the double bond, making the reaction easier to initiate. This reaction is more isely called as (4 + 2)-cycloaddition reaction because out of the 6π electrons involved e cyclic transition state, 4 come from the conjugated diene and 2 from the dienophile. reaction is usually thermodynamically favourable due to the conversion of two nds into two new stronger σ-bonds. The Diels–Alder reaction is a concerted process:

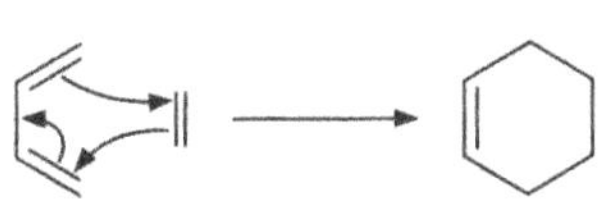

ue to the high degree of regio- and stereo-selectivity (due to the concerted mecha-) the Diels-Alder reaction is a very powerful reaction and is widely used in synthetic ıic chemistry.

PRACTICE QUESTIONS

Give neatly labelled structures and diagrams for any four:

2. Write short notes on:

   (a) Diels–Alder condensation
   (b) 1,4-addition

3. Account for the following:

   (a) Allyl cation is more stable than ethyl cation
   (b) Stability of conjugated dienes

4. What are dienes? Classify dienes with examples? Illustrate the chemical reactions of 1,3-Butadiene.
5. How do you prepare conjugated dienes? Explain electrophilic and free-radical addition mechanisms of conjugated dienes.
6. Explain why conjugated dienes undergo both 1,2 and 1,4 addition reactions.

ˉ2

·HEMISTRY OF CYCLOALKANES

cloalkanes (cyclo-paraffins) are saturated hydrocarbons in which the (sp^3) carbon at-
.s are joined by single covalent bonds to form a ring. They are also called alicyclic
npounds.

.1 NOMENCLATURE

ə IUPAC rules for naming cycloalkanes are as follows:

1. The name of an unsubstituted cycloalkane is obtained by attaching the prefix cyclo- to the name of the corresponding normal alkane having the same number of carbon atoms as in the ring.
2. Substituents, on the ring are named and numbers indicate their positions. The ring is numbered so that the carbons bearing the substituents will have the lowest numbers.

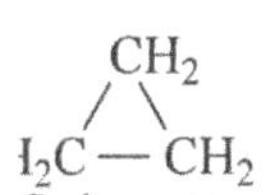
Cyclopropane

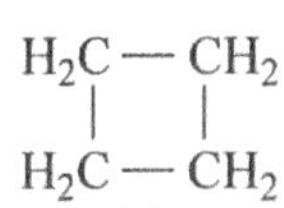
Cyclobutane

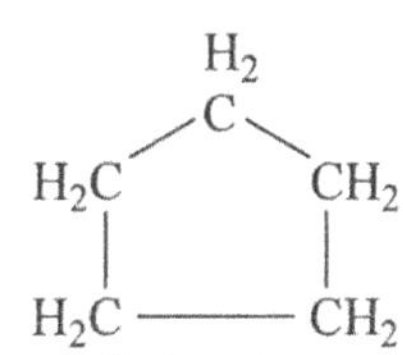
Cyclopentane

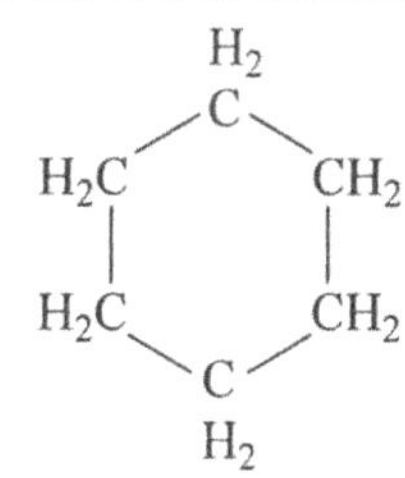
Cyclohexane

2 PREPARATION OF CYCLOALKANES

: following general methods are commonly used in the preparation of cycloalkanes:

From ω-Dihalides (Freunds Method) Dichloro or dibromo alkanes having terminal
ogen atoms (ω-dihalides) when treated with sodium or zinc produce cycloalkanes.

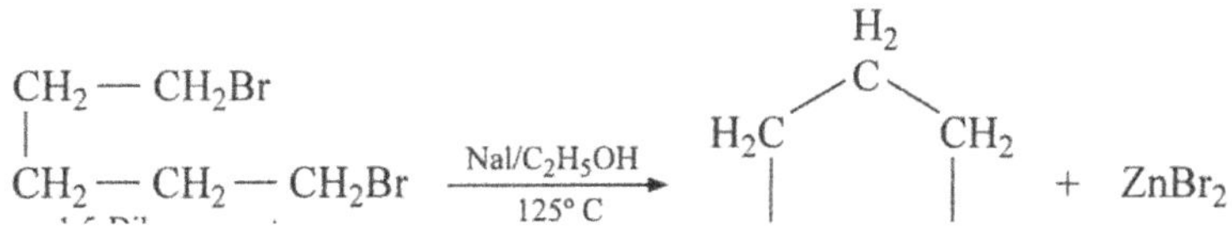

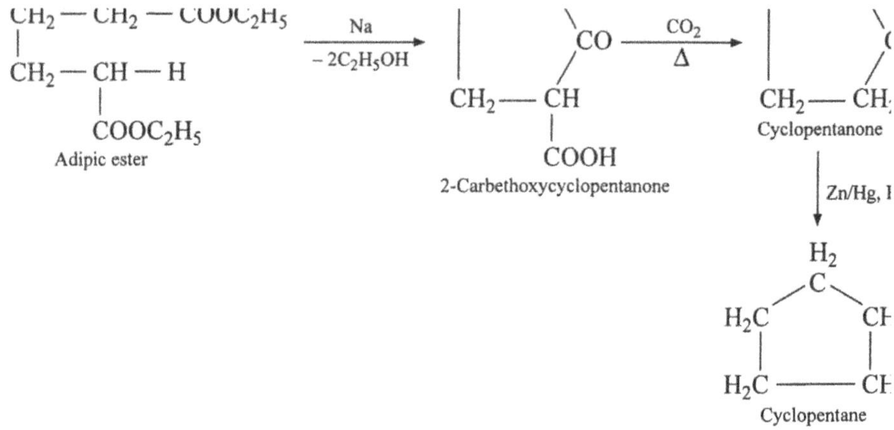

3. ***Addition of Methylene to Alkenes*** A good method to prepare cyclopropane deri tives involves the reaction between alkenes and methylene. This reaction is also refer to as cycloaddition.

$$\underset{\text{2-Butene}}{CH_3CH{=}CHCH_3} + \underset{\text{Diazomethane}}{CH_2N_2} \xrightarrow{\text{Light}} \underset{\text{1,2-Dimethylcyclopropane}}{CH_3\underset{\diagdown\ \diagup}{CH{-}CH}CHCH_3 \;(CH_2)}$$

4. ***Reduction of Unsaturated Cyclichydrocarbons*** Cycloalkanes can also be prepa by reduction of unsaturated hydrocarbons.

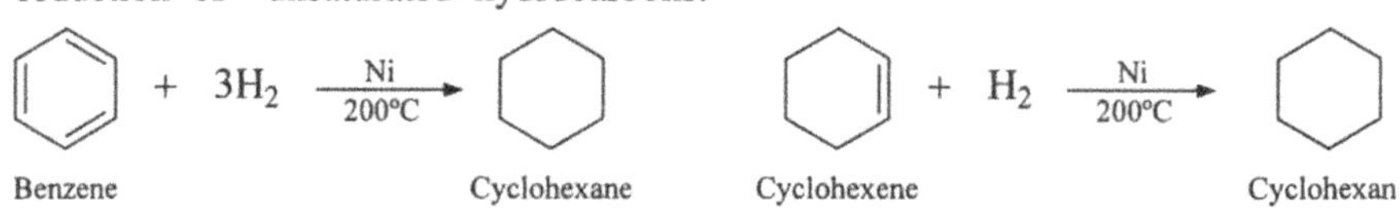

12.3 PHYSICAL PROPERTIES OF CYCLOALKANES

1. The first two members (cyclopropane and cyclobutane) are gases at room tempe ture. The higher members are colourless liquids with pleasant odour.
2. The M.P., B.P., and specific gravity show a gradual increase with the increase molecular weight. However, the B.P. and specific gravity of cycloalkanes are hig than those of isomeric alkenes and corresponding alkanes.
3. Cycloalkanes are insoluble in water, but soluble in alcohol and ether.

12.4 CHEMICAL PROPERTIES OF CYCLOALKANES

The general chemical behaviour of cycloalkanes is similar to open-chain hydrocarb

Cyclohexane Bromocyclohexane

3ut cyclopropane and cyclobutane react with chlorine or bromine (in the presence of :l$_3$ or $FeBr_3$) open the ring system and yield open-chain addition products.

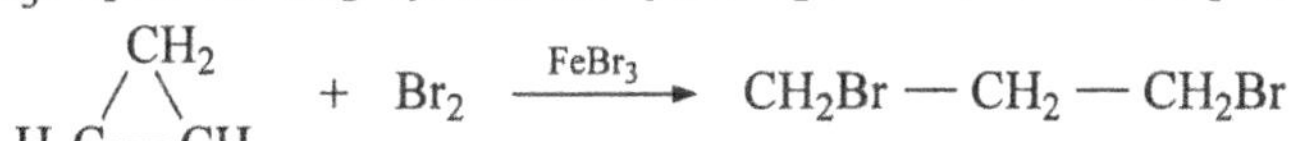

Cyclopropane 1,3-Dibromopropane

ʀeaction with Halogen Acids Higher cycloalkanes do not react with halogen acids cyclopropane reacts with halogen acids to form alkyl halides.

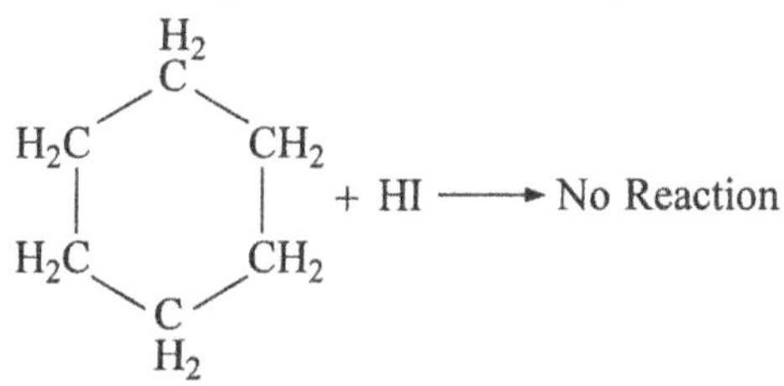

Cyclohexane

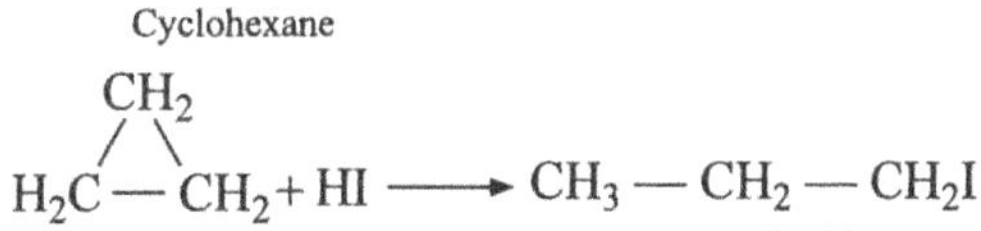

Cyclopropane *n*-Propyliodide

ʀeaction with Hydrogen Cyclopropane and cyclobutane give addition products on ing with hydrogen in the presence of catalyst (nickel) form open-chain addition lucts while higher cycloalkanes do not react.

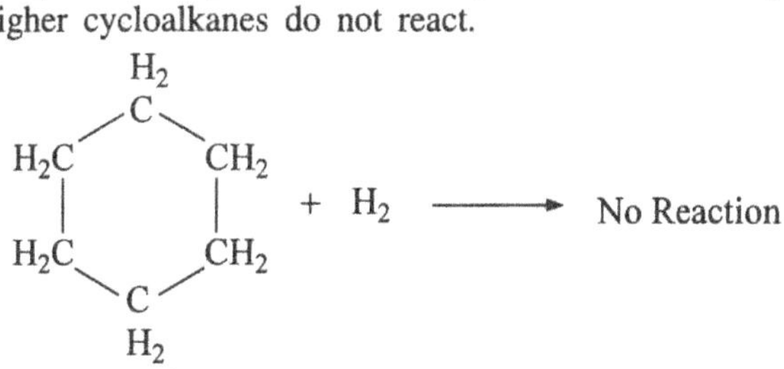

Cyclohexane

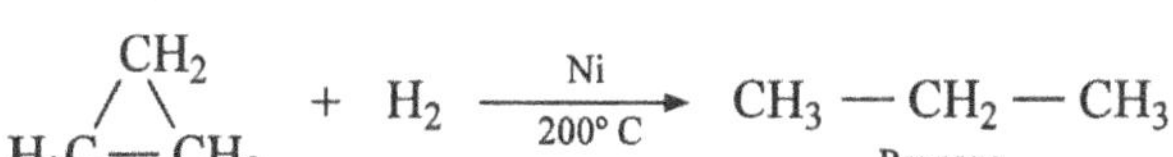

Propane

1. The normal bond angle between any two adjacent sp^3 carbon atoms in ring struc is 109°28′.
2. Any deviation (positive or negative) from the normal tetrahedral bond angle of 28′ during the formation of a ring produces a strain in the resultant molecule, w makes the molecule unstable.
3. The greater the deviation from the normal angle the greater is the strain and, th fore, the lesser is the stability. It may be noted however that the sign of devia makes no difference (see Fig. 12.1).
4. The strain is directly proportional to the distortion of the normal valency an
5. Bayer calculated angle strain of cycloalkanes of various ring sizes by following formula.

Angle strain = ½ [109° 28′ – Actual angle]

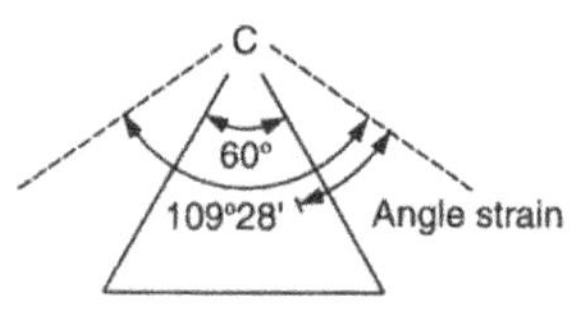

Fig. 12.1 Band Angle Strain in Cycloalkanes

6. The angle strain for various cycloalkanes are given in Table 12.1.

Table 12.1 Angle Strains for various Cycloalkanes

Cycloalkane	*Actual Bond Angle*	*Angle Strain*
Cyclopropane	60°	24.44°
Cyclobutane	90°	9.44°
Cyclopentane	108°	0.44°
Cyclohexane	120°	– 5.16°
Cycloheptane	128.34°	– 9.33°

Evidences of Baeyer Strain Theory

1. The Baeyer strain theory could explain the relative stabilities of cycloalkane u six carbon atom rings.
2. Baeyer strain theory could also account for the great reactivity of the ethyl bond. The double bond was considered as a two membered ring in which the a strain is + 54.44°. This large strain makes the alkenes more reactive.

Limitations Baeyer's theory failed to explain the following:

1. The ethylenic bond can be formed readily in spite of having such a large a strain.

posed. According to Sachse's theory, carbon atoms in 3- to 5-membered rings lie in same plane. But the carbon atoms in 6-membered and higher rings do not lie in the ie plane (they lie in different planes). Since the carbon atoms in 6-membered and higher ;s lie in different planes, the normal tetrahedral angle remains unaltered. Hence, there o angle strain in bigger rings and are stable, e.g. chair and boat forms are two strainless ;s of cyclohexane which are interconvertible (Fig. 12.2).

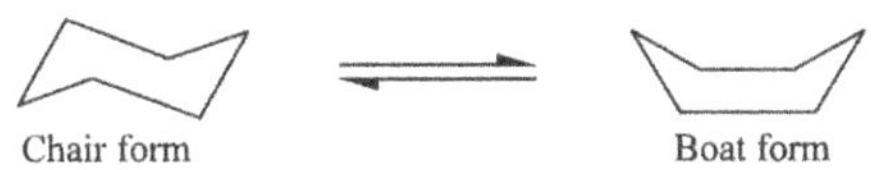

Fig. 12.2 Two Strainless Rings of Cyclohexane – Chain and Boat Conformations

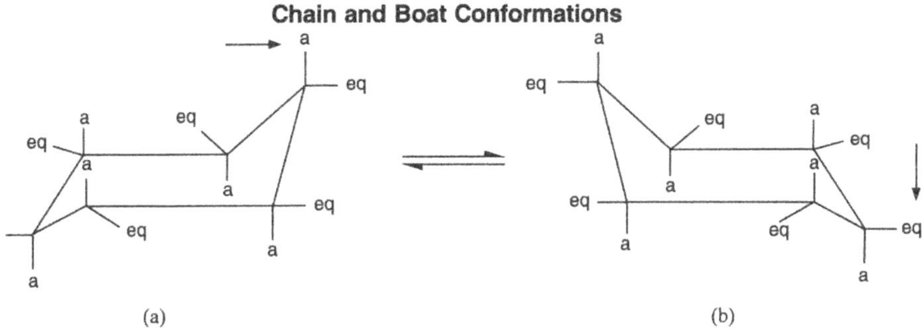

Fig. 12.3 Ring Flip of Cyclohexane

;achse's theory of strainless rings was further supported and elaborated by Mohr [8) to cover the compounds containing two rings fused together. The bigger rings are er difficult to synthesise even though there is no angle strain in these. This is pri- ily due to the fact that two ends of the chain of atoms must come close together for closure to take place. If the chain undergoing ring closure is long, there are relatively er chances of the two ends coming close enough for the ring to be formed. But once ı rings are formed they are quite stable.

PRACTICE QUESTIONS

What are cycloalkanes? Give two methods to prepare cycloalkanes.
Carbon–carbon bonds in cyclopropane are weaker than the carbon–carbon bonds in propane. Explain this on the basis of molecular orbital theory.
Explain the Baeyer's strain theory of cycloalkanes.
Explain Sachse–Mohr's theory of strainless rings.
Write the conformation of cyclohexane. Mention the stable isomer. Justify your answer.
What happens when cyclopropane reacts with:
(a) H_2/Ni at 100°C

13

CHEMISTRY OF ALKYL HALIDES

13.1 INTRODUCTION

Organic halogen compounds are obtained by replacing one or more hydrogen: hydrocarbons by halogen atoms. The halogen derivatives of alkanes are known as *a halides*, which are obtained by the replacement of one or more hydrogen atoms of alk: with halogen atoms like fluorine, chlorine, bromine or iodine, e.g. CH_3Cl (methyl chlori C_2H_5Cl (ethyl chloride) and so on.

13.2 CLASSIFICATION

Halogen derivatives can be categorised into two types, depending upon the natur hydrocarbon. These are:

1. ***Halogen Derivatives of Saturated Hydrocarbons*** These compounds are derived replacing one or more hydrogen atoms from saturated hydrocarbons by correspon number of halogen atoms (fluorine, chlorine, bromine or iodine). Monohalogen derivat have the general formula $C_nH_{2n+1}X$. Depending upon the number of halogen at present, the halogen derivatives are classified as mono-, di-, tri-, tetra-, etc., accordin having one, two, three, four, etc., halogen atoms respectively.

Monohalogen derivatives of alkanes are called as alkyl halides or haloalkanes. A halides are further classified as

(i) *Primary alkyl halides* When the carbon atom containing halogen atom is linke only one carbon atom.

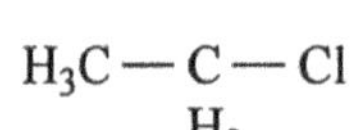

Chloroethane

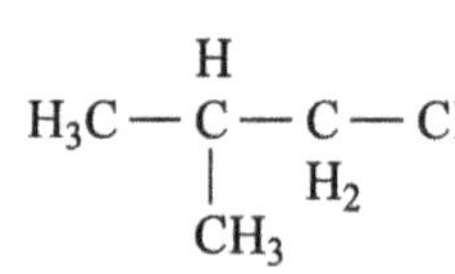

1-Chloro-2-methylpropane

(ii) *Secondary alkyl halides* When the carbon atom containing halogen atom is lin to two carbon atoms.

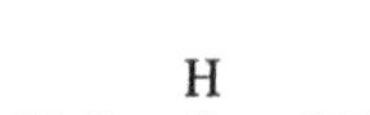

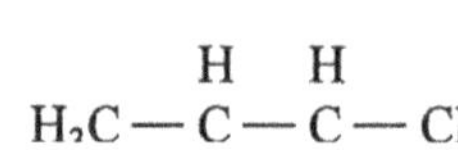

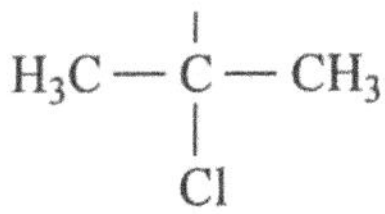

2-Chloro-2-methylpropane

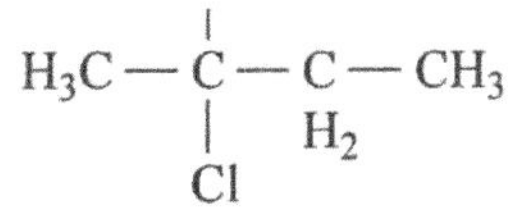

2-Chloro-2-methylbutane

Halogen Derivatives of Unsaturated Hydrocarbons These are of two types:

Alkenyl halides If the halogen atom is present over alkene hydrocarbons, the nohaloderivatives have general formula $C_n H_{2n-1} = X$ (where X = F, Cl, Br or I). These also called as alkenyl halides.

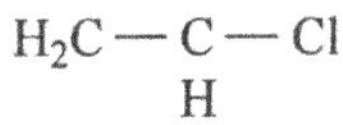

Chloroethene
(Vinyl chloride)

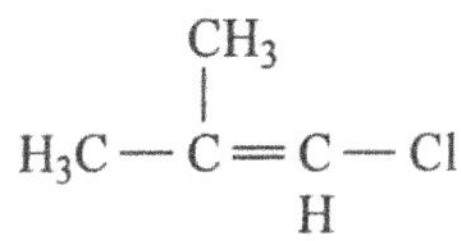

1-Chloro-2-methyl-prop-1-ene

Alkynyl halides If the halogen atom is present over alkyne hydrocarbons, the nohaloderivatives have general formula $C_n H_{2n-3}$ X (where X = F, Cl, Br or I). These also called as alkynyl halides.

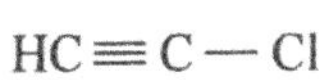

Chloroethyne

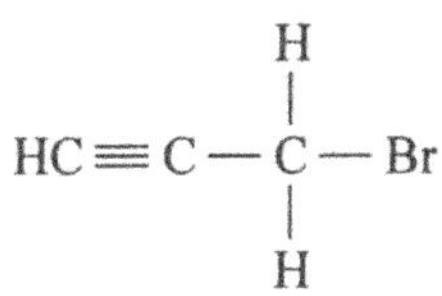

2-Bromoprop-1-yne

3 NOMENCLATURE OF ALKYL HALIDES

rivial System According to common or trivial system, monohaloderivatives are named lkyl halides.

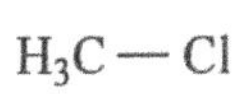

Methyl chloride

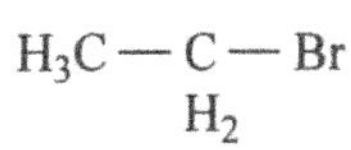

Ethyl bromide

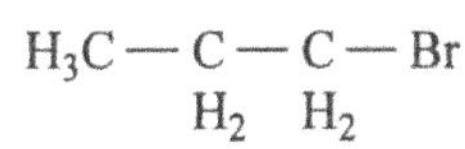

n-Propyl bromide

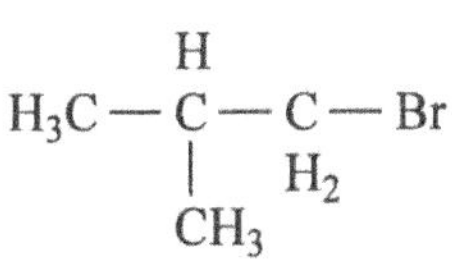

Isobutyl bromide

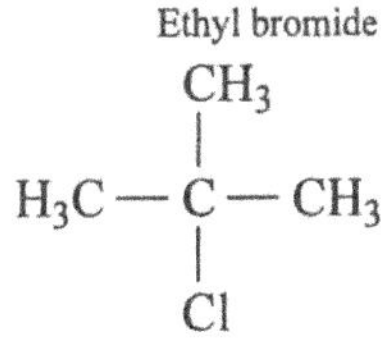

Tertiarybutyl chloride

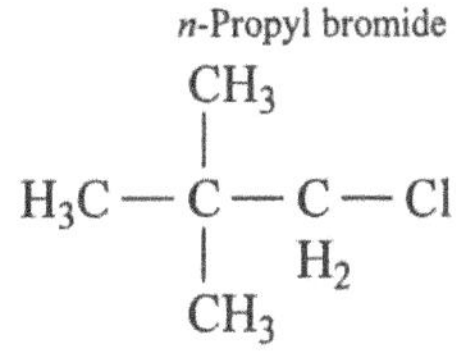

Neopentyl chloride

UPAC System According to IUPAC system, the monohaloderivatives are named as alkanes.

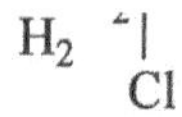

2-Chlorobutane

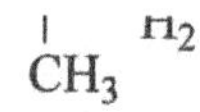

1-Chloro-2,2-dimethylpropane

(ii) If the different halogen atoms are present in a chain then we write th alphabetically and also counting will be done from that side by which halo; (bromine) gets the least possible position followed by chlorine, fluorine ; iodine alphabetically.

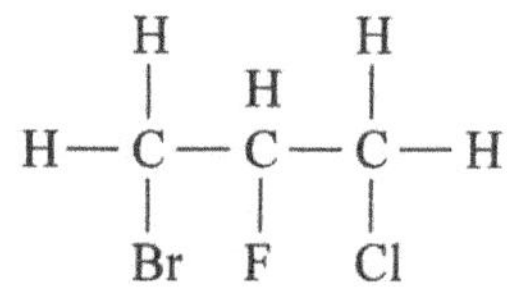

1-Bromo-3-chloro-2-fluoropropane

13.4 ISOMERISM IN ALKYL HALIDES

Structural isomerism of alkyl halides are of two types:

(i) *Chain isomerism* Chain isomerism arises due to the difference in arrangement carbon atoms of the alkyl radical in different possible chains.

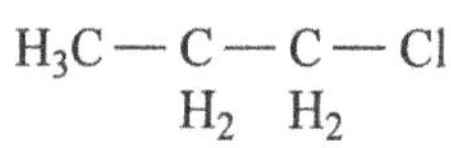

1-Chloropropane

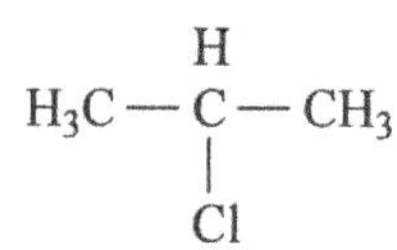

2-Chloropropane

(ii) *Position isomerism* Position isomerism arises due to the difference in position halogen atom in the carbon chain.

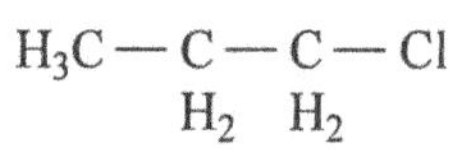

1-Chloropropane

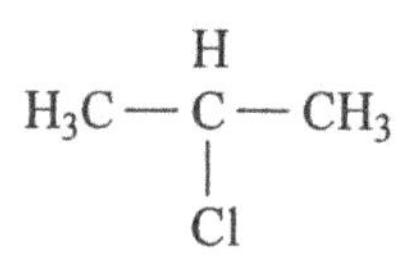

2-Chloropropane

13.5 METHODS TO PREPARE ALKYL HALIDES

The following are the most widely used methods to prepare alkyl halides:

1. ***Halogenation of Alkanes*** When alkanes are treated with chlorine or bromine presence of ultraviolet light or at 350°–400° C, alkyl chlorides/alkyl bromides are form

$$\underset{\text{Methane}}{CH_4} \xrightarrow[350°–400° C]{Cl_2,\ \text{UV light or}} \underset{\text{Methyl chloride}}{CH_3Cl}$$

$$\underset{\text{Methane}}{CH_4} \xrightarrow[350°–400° C]{Br_2,\ \text{UV light or}} \underset{\text{Methyl bromide}}{CH_3Br}$$

Addition of Hydrogen Halides to Alkenes and Alkynes Alkyl halides may be prepared the addition of hydrogen halides HX (X = Cl, Br or I) to alkenes or alkynes in dark, room temperature. The addition of HX follows Markovnikov's rule. This reaction is an ample of electrophilic addition.

$$\underset{\text{Alkene}}{RCH{=}CH_2} + HX \longrightarrow \underset{\text{Alkyl halide}}{RCH(X){-}CH_3}$$

$$\underset{\text{Propene}}{CH_3{-}CH{=}CH_2} + HCl \longrightarrow \underset{\text{2-Chloropropane}}{CH_3{-}CHCl{-}CH_3}$$

$$\underset{\text{Ethyne}}{CH{\equiv}CH} + HCl \longrightarrow \underset{\text{Vinyl chloride}}{CH_2{=}CHCl} \xrightarrow{HCl} \underset{\text{1,1-Dichloroethane}}{CH_3{-}CHCl_2}$$

From Alcohols Alcohols give alkyl halides on reaction with hydrogen halides (HCl HBr), phosphorous halides (PX_5 or PX_3) or thionyl chloride ($SOCl_2$).

$$\underset{\text{Alcohol}}{R{-}OH} \xrightarrow{HX \text{ or } PH_5 \text{ or } PX_3} \underset{\text{Alkyl halide}}{R{-}X}$$

$$\underset{n\text{-Propanol}}{CH_3CH_2CH_2{-}OH} \xrightarrow{HCl/ZnCl_2} \underset{n\text{-Propylchloride}}{CH_3CH_2CH_2{-}Cl} + H_2O$$

$$\underset{\text{Ethanol}}{CH_3CH_2{-}OH} + PCl_5 \longrightarrow \underset{\text{Ethylchloride}}{CH_3CH_2{-}Cl} + POCl_3 + HCl$$

$$\underset{\text{Ethanol}}{CH_3CH_2{-}OH} + SOCl_2 \longrightarrow \underset{\text{Ethylchloride}}{CH_3CH_2{-}Cl} + SO_2 + HCl$$

Halogen Exchange This method is particularly useful for the preparation of alkyl ides. It involves the interaction of the corresponding chloride or bromide with sodium ide in acetone. (This reaction is known as Finkelstein reaction.)

$$\underset{\text{Alkylchloride}}{RCH_2Cl} + NaI \longrightarrow \underset{\text{Alkyliodide}}{RCH_2I} + NaCl$$

From Silver Salts of Carboxylic Acids (Hunsdiecker Method) Alkyl halides have o been produced by the decomposition of silver salts of fatty acids by chlorine or mine.

gases or low boiling liquids. The higher members, above C-6, are liquids and tho above C-12 are solids.

2. Although the alkyl halides are polar compounds they are incapable of formi hydrogen bonds, hence they are insoluble in water (lower molecular weig compounds are soluble in H_2O) but freely soluble in ether, benzene, chloroform, et

13.7 CHEMICAL PROPERTIES OF ALKYL HALIDES

The alkyl halides are highly reactive compounds. Because of their easy availability ar very reactive nature, alkyl halides can be transformed into a large variety of compound The following are some of their important chemical reactions.

13.7.1 Nucleophilic Substitution of Alkyl Halides

This is one of the most important reactions of alkyl halides. In this reaction, an alkyl halic reacts with a nucleophile, resulting in displacement of the halide ion. Nucleophilic, substitutic reactions occur when an electron-rich species (the nucleophile) reacts at an electrophil saturated carbon atom, attached to an electronegative group (the leaving group).

$$R - X + :Nu \longrightarrow R - Nu + :X^-$$

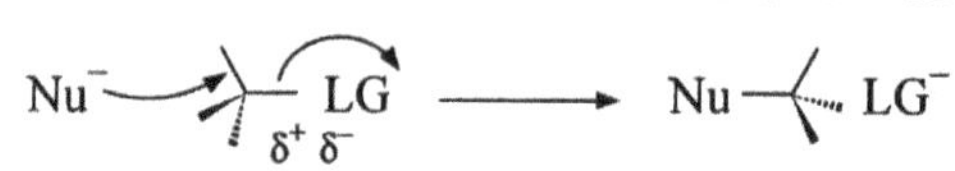

The most common nucleophiles are $:OH^-$, OR'^-, $:^-C\equiv CR'^-$, $:CN^-$ and neutral molecul (containing a non-bonding electron pair such as NH_3, amines, water, alcohol, etc.). Th following are various examples of nucleophilic substitution reactions of alkyl halides:

R:X	+	$:OH^-$	$\longrightarrow$ R:OH + $:X^-$	Alcohols
R:X	+	$:OR'^-$	$\longrightarrow$ R:OR′	Ethers
R:X	+	$^-:C\equiv CR'$	$\longrightarrow$ $R:C\equiv CR'$	Alkynes
R:X	+	R′-Metal	$\longrightarrow$ R:R′	Alkanes
R:X	+	$:I^-$	$\longrightarrow$ R:I	Alkyl iodides
R:X	+	$:CN^-$	$\longrightarrow$ R:CN	Alkyl nitriles
R:X	+	$H_2O:$	$\longrightarrow$ R:OH	Alcohols
R:X	+	$:NH_3$	$\longrightarrow$ $R:NH_2$	Primary amines
R:X	+	$:NH_2R'$	$\longrightarrow$ R:NHR′	Secondary amines
R:X	+	:NHR′R″	$\longrightarrow$ R:NR′R″	Tertiary amines
R:X	+	$:SH^-$	$\longrightarrow$ R:SH	Thiols
R:X	+	$:SR'^-$	$\longrightarrow$ R:SR′	Thioethers

ırbon. Although the carbon–iodine bond does not have permanent dipole, the bond is ısily polarised by the approaching nucleophile.

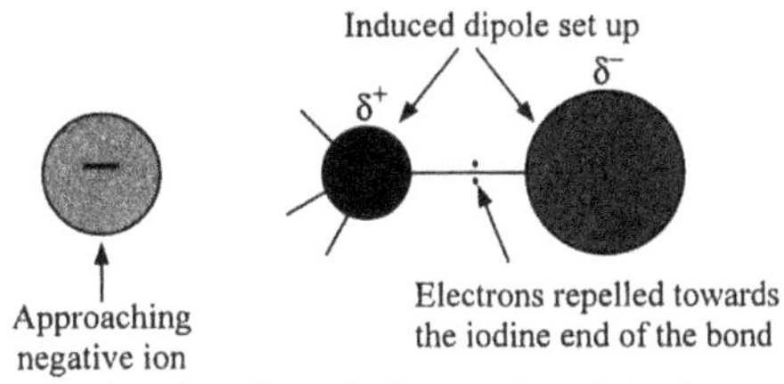

Therefore, the electron pair of carbon–halogen, bond is drawn more towards halogen, sulting in development of partial +ve charge on carbon and partial –ve charge on halogen. onsequently, when an alkyl halide is treated with a nucleophile, the latter attacks the ırbon (attached to halogen) and displaces the halogen as halide ion. There are two ndamental events in a nucleophilic aliphatic substitution reaction:

(i) Formation of the new sigma bond between a nucleophile and an electrophilic carbon.
(ii) Heterolytic dissociation of the sigma bond occurs between the leaving group (halogen) and carbon.

Depending on the relative timing of bond dissociation and bond formation, the following 'o mechanisms are possible:

1. Bimolecular nucleophilic substitution (S_N2)
2. Unimolecular nucleophilic substitution (S_N1)

Bimolecular Nucleophilic Substitution (S_N2) Technically, this mechanism is called a $_N2$ mechanism; S stands for substitution, N for nucleophilic, and the 2 is because two olecules collide at the critical point in the reaction.

echanism This mechanism can be illustrated by considering the hydrolysis of methyl omide by hydroxyl ions.

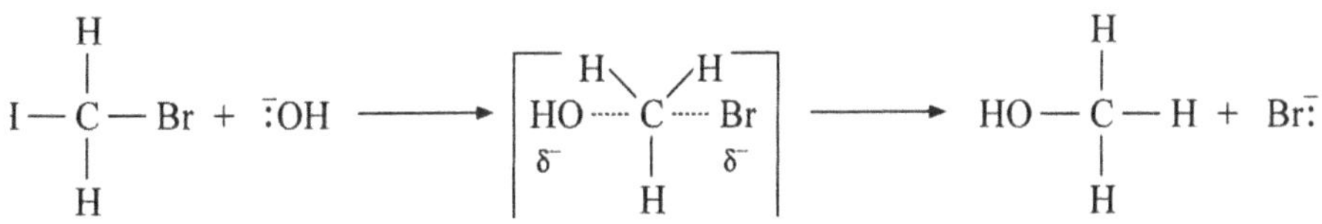

According to this mechanism the reaction occurs in a single step. The pair of electrons the nucleophile (hydroxyl anion) will be strongly attracted to the electrophilic carbon +), and will move towards it, beginning to make a coordinate bond. In the process, the ectrons in the carbon-halogen (bromine) will be pushed even closer towards the halogen making it increasingly negative. The movement goes on until the nucleophile is firmly ached to the carbon, and the halogen (bromine) has been expelled as a halide ion aving group). Therefore, attack of nucleophile (hydroxyl ion) at carbon and loss of

opportunities for a nucleophile to collide with an alkyl halide molecule. The rate of reaction will increase proportionately as the alkyl halide concentration is made hig Similarly, an increase in the nucleophile concentration will result in a proportionate incre in the rate. This shows that the rate of reaction should depend on the concentratioı both the reagents. So the reaction is said to follow second-order kinetics. This can summarised in the rate equation:

$$R = k[RX]\,[OH^-]$$

(ii) *Energy considerations of* S_{N^2} *reaction* The S_{N^2} reaction has a very simple reac energy diagram because the reaction is concerted. Figure 13.1 shows the reaction ene diagram. The left side of the reaction energy diagram, where the energy is the low represents nucleophile and alkyl halide (methyl bromide) prior to the beginning of reaction. The right side of the reaction energy diagram, where the energy is almost as l represents leaving group (bromide ion) and substitution product at the end of the react The centre of the diagram, where the energy is the highest, represents the transition st S_{N^2} reaction proceeds with no intermediate but has a single transition state.

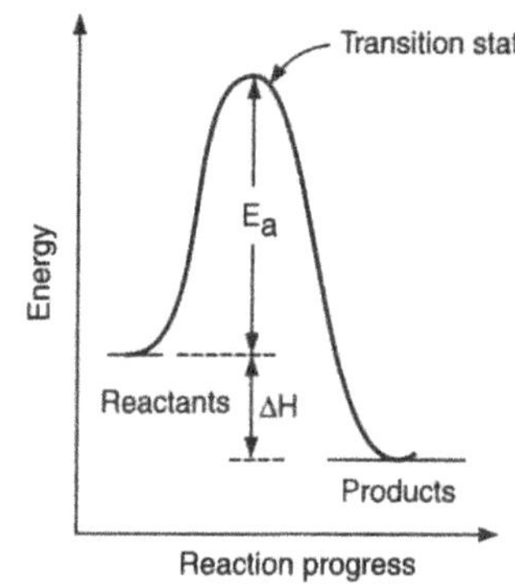

Fig. 13.1 The Reaction Energy Diagram in a Bimolecular Nucleophilic Substitution

As the reaction process goes forward, the energy required for heterolytic bc dissociation is obtained from bond formation between a carbon and a nucleopł (Fig. 13.2). At the transition state there is roughly a half-bond between the carbon a the nucleophile and a half-bond between the carbon and leaving group (halogen). T transition state is pentavalent and is quickly transformed into the final products. Si the energy is maximum at transition state, any slight movement will cause it to decrea either to go back to reactants or to go on to products. Figure 13.3, depicting transit state during the course of S_{N^2} reacts, is the key to understand the characteristics of

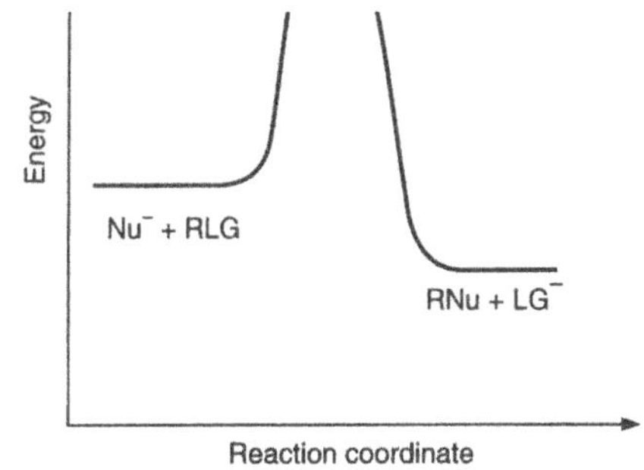

Fig. 13.2 Energy Diagram of a S_{N^2} Reaction

he energy required to boost the nucleophile and the alkyl halide to the transition state gy level is called the activation energy. The activation energy (E_a) comes from the :tive collisions. If the activation energy is low, the reaction will be fast and if the 'ation energy is high the reaction will be slow.

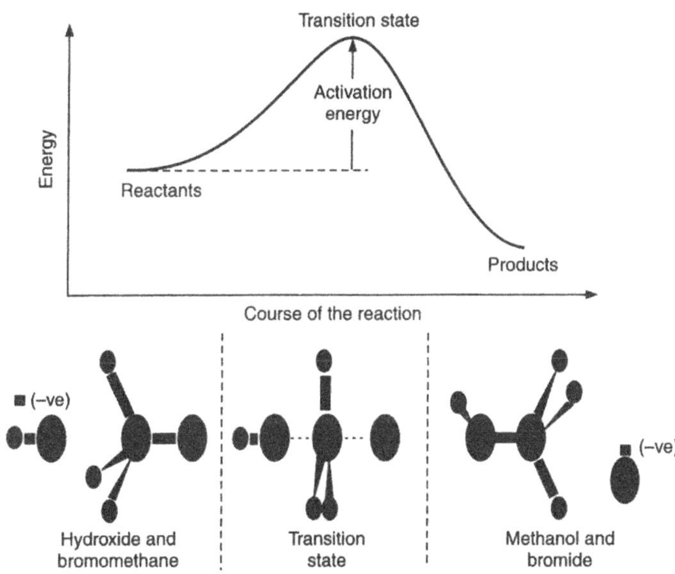

Fig. 13.3 Energy Diagram of S_N2 reaction

Stereochemistry and stearic hindrance of S_{N^2} *reaction* The nucleophile (hydroxyl attacks the carbon on the side opposite to leaving group (bromine) because the king nucleophile cannot approach the methyl bromide molecule from any other side o repulsion by the negatively polarised halogen (bromine). This is referred as *backside*

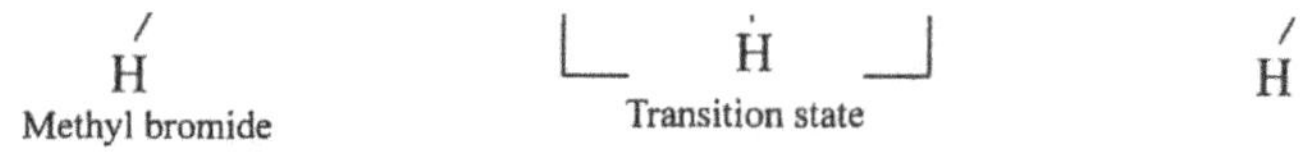

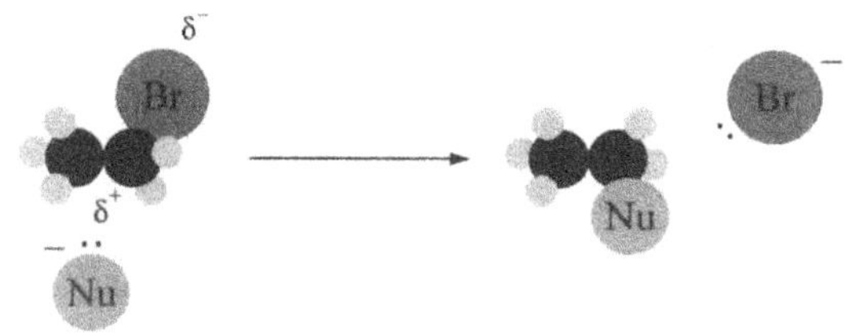

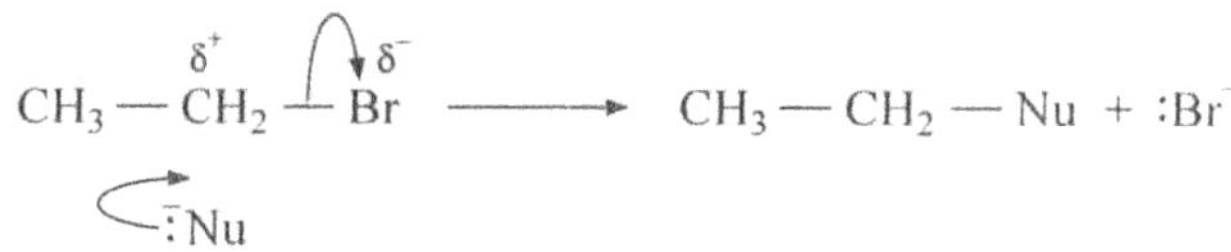

The nucleophile occupies a position opposite to that previously occupied by –Br. the configuration of product is opposite to that of alkyl halide. The reaction in which configuration of a product is opposite to that of the reactant is said to take place v inversion of configuration. S_{N^2} reactions proceeding with complete inversion configuration of substitution product to starting reactant is an inherent and consis characteristic of the S_{N^2} mechanism. Consequently, if we determine that a nucleoph substitution reaction proceeds with inversion of configuration, we conclude that mechanism is S_{N^2}.

Examples

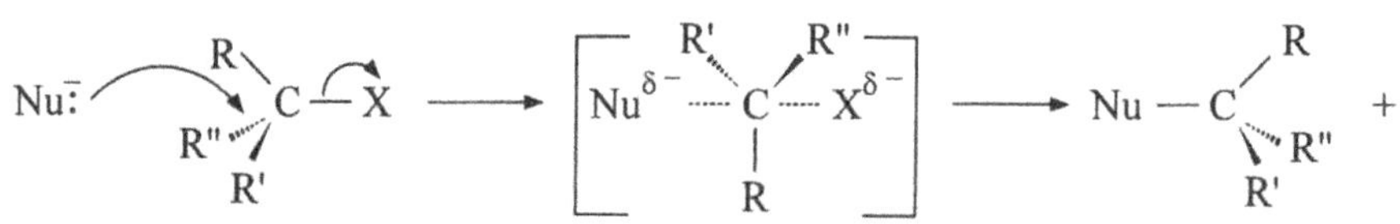

Factors Influencing the Rates of S_{N^2} Reactions

(i) *Nature of alkyl group in alkyl halides* To compare the reactivity of alkyl halide: is necessary to study the effect of size of groups attached to the carbon carrying halogen atom. In the reaction of methyl bromide with a nucleophile, the reactant and product contain tetrahedral carbon. But in the transition state the carbon is pentavale When the hydrogen atoms in methyl bromide are successively replaced by larger grou such as CH_3 and C_2H_5, there is an increased crowding. This gives rise to strong n bonded interactions in transition state because five groups attached to the same carb As a result E_a rises and the rate of reaction slows down. Therefore, the order of reacti of alkyl halides towards S_{N^2} is methyl halides > 1° alkyl halides > 2° alkyl halides >

	H	H	CH_3	CH_3
$sec^{-1} mole^{-1}$ litre	2140	170	4.7	–
k_{rel}	12.59	1.00	0.028	–

Nature of leaving group in alkyl halide A leaving group is an atom or a group of ns that is displaced as stable species taking with it the bonding electrons. Typically, leaving group is an anion or a neutral molecule. The ease of elimination of leaving ıp depends upon its nucleophilicity, i.e. weaker the nucleophilicity, the better would the leaving group.

Table 13.1 Degree of Nucleophilicity of various Nucleophile

Excellent	TsO^-, NH_3
Very good	I^-, H_2O
Good	Br^-
Fair	Cl^-
Poor	F^-
Very poor	^-OH, $^-NH_2$, ^-OR

herefore, the order of reactivity of alkyl halides is RI > RBr > RCl > RF.

Nature of solvent The rates of S_N2 reactions, generally increased considered when reactions are carried out in polar aprotic solvents (DMF, DMSO, DMA). These solvents ate cations preferably because their negative ends orient around the cation and donate ıared electron pairs to vacant orbitals of the cation. But the positive centres of these ents are well shielded from any interaction with anions. Polar aprotic solvents (polar no ability to be hydrogen-bond donor) have the following characteristic features:

. These solvents have dipoles due to polar bonds.
. They do not have H atoms that can be donated into a H-bond.
. Anions are not solvated by polar protic solvents and are 'naked' and reaction is not inhibited. For example:

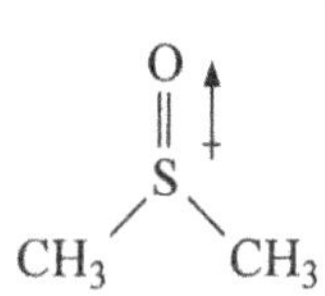
Dimethylsulphoxide

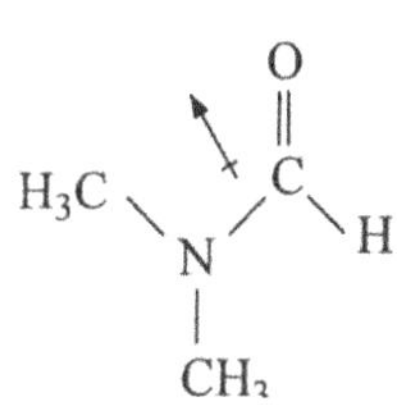

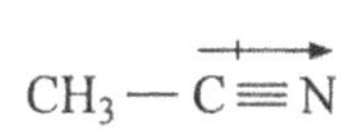
Acetonitrile

	Moment (μ)	Constant (ε)	Rate	
CH_3OH	2.87	33	1	protic
H_2O	1.84	78	7	protic
DMSO	3.96	49	300	aprotic
DMF	3.82	37	2,800	aprotic
CH_3CN	3.92	38	5,000	aprotic

(iv) *Nature of nucleophile* The rates of S_N2 reactions depend on both the concentratic and the identity of the attacking nucleophile. Increasing the concentration of tl nucleophile increases the rate of an S_N2 reaction.

2. ***Unimolecular Nucleophilic Substitution*** (S_N1) Technically, this mechanism is calle an S_N1 mechanism; S stands for substitution, N for nucleophilic, and the 1 signifies th single molecular species influence the reaction rate.

Mechanism The nucleophilic unimolecular substitution (S_N1) reaction is explained t considering the reaction between tertiary alkyl halide, such as *t*-butyl chloride and nucleophile like $:OH^-$.

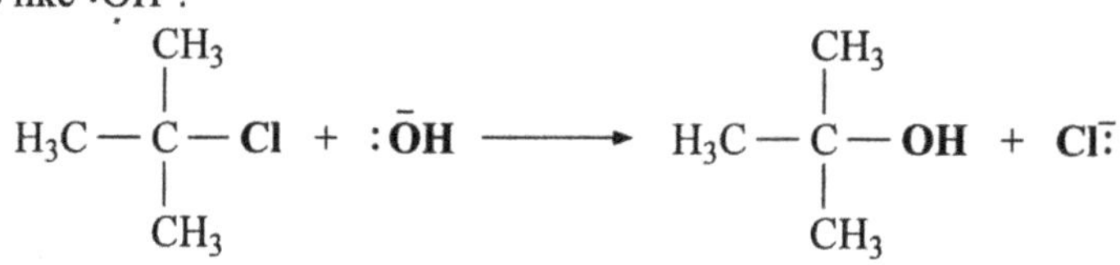

Tertiarybutylchloride Tertiarybutylalcohol

This reaction occurs in two stages:

(i) *Formation of carbocation* The first step involves heterolytic dissociation of alk halide to carbocation. This is a slow step.

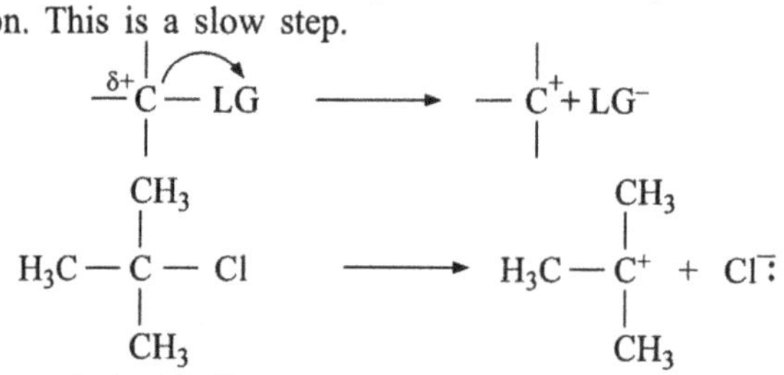

(Slov

Tertiarybutylchloride Tertiarybutyl carbocation

The energy required to dissociate the carbon–halogen bond is supplied by:

(a) Solvolysis of carbocation by polar aprotic solvent (i.e. the formation of ion–dipol interactions between the two kinds of partially developed ions and the solvent).

(b) Stabilisation of carbocation due to the flow of electrons from the alkyl grour to the positively charged carbon atom.

(ii) *Reaction of carbocation with nucleophile* The pair of electrons on the nucleophil is strongly attracted towards the positive carbon atom and moves towards it to create new sigma bond. Once the carbocation is formed it rapidly combines with nucleophile t form product. The second step is fast.

Tertiarybutyl carbocation Tertiarybutyl alcohol

-urther, the reactions taking place by $S_N{}^1$ mechanism may undergo rearrangement of ›ocation (1,2-hydride or 1,2-alkyl shifts) to form a more stable carbocation whenever sible.

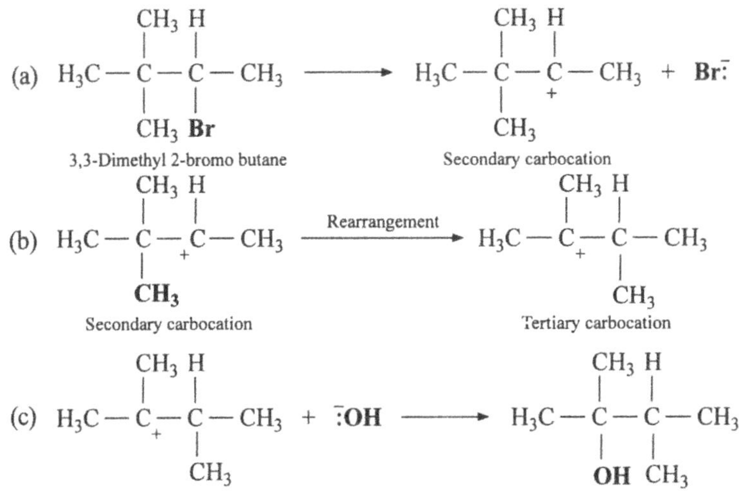

(a) 3,3-Dimethyl 2-bromo butane → Secondary carbocation + Br^-

(b) Secondary carbocation → (Rearrangement) Tertiary carbocation

(c) Tertiary carbocation + ^-OH → 2,3-Dimethyl-2-butanol

Kinetics of $S_N{}^1$ *reaction* The rate of $S_N{}^1$ reaction depends upon the rate of the first w) step, i.e. the loss of a leaving group (halide ion) to form a carbocation. Hence, the of $S_N{}^1$ reaction depends upon the concentration of only alkyl halide.

$$R = k[RX]$$

'herefore, $S_N{}^1$ reaction is said to be unimolecular reaction and the rate of reaction ›ws first-order kinetics.

Energy considerations of $S_N{}^1$ *reaction* $S_N{}^1$ is a multi-step reaction that proceeds ı an intermediate (I) and several transition states (TS_1 and TS_2 in Fig. 13.4).

ǝeneral Case

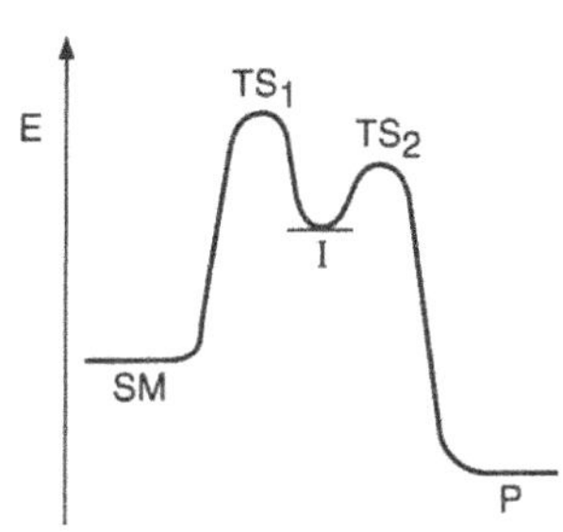

carbocation (dispersal of positive charge by electron releasing groups) should also stabi transition state and improve the rate of overall reaction.

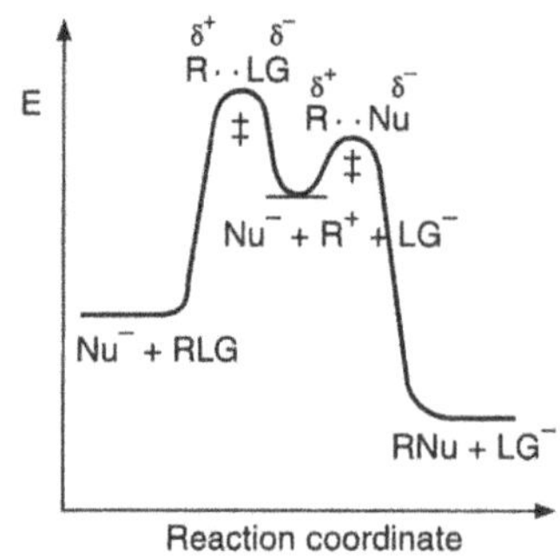

Fig. 13.5 The Mechanics of Energy Consideration in S_N1 Reaction

(v) *Stereochemistry of* S_{N^1} *reaction* S_{N^1} reaction proceeds through the intermed formation of carbocation. The carbocation formed in the first step is planar because central positively charged carbon atom is sp^2 hybridised. In this reaction, the leav group leaves before the nucleophile attacks. This means the nucleophile is free to att either side of the planar carbocation. If a nucleophile attacks the side from which bromide ion left, the product will have the same relative configuration as the reactant it attacks the opposite side, the product will have the inverted configuration.

(a)

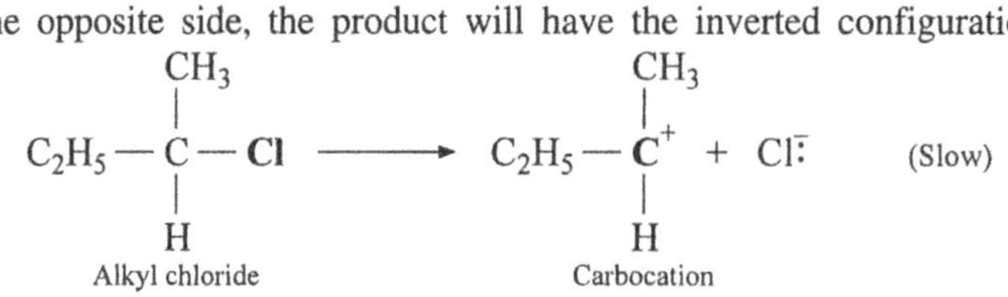

(b)

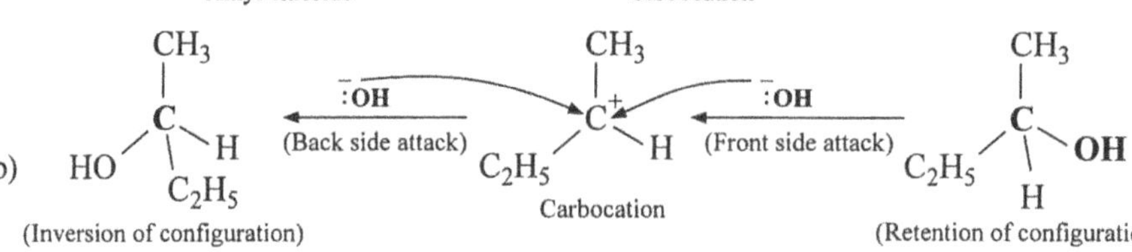

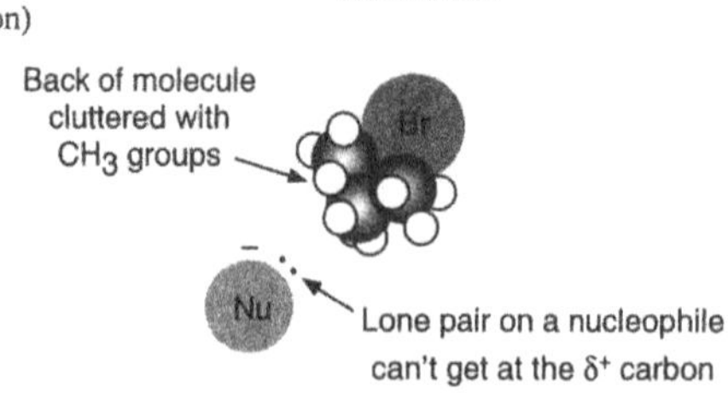

In reactions involving optically active alkyl halides, an equal amount of two stereiosom

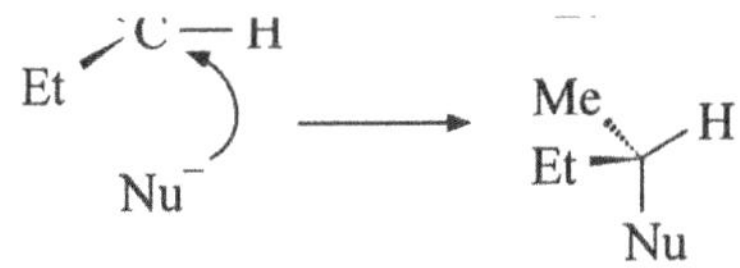

Notice that the products are mirror images

Factors influencing the rates of S_N1 reactions

(a) *Structure of the substrate* In an S_N1 reaction, the rate determining step is the loss of the leaving group to form the intermediate carbocation. The primary factor that determines the reactivity of organic substrates in an S_N1 reaction is the relative stability of carbocation that is formed. The more stable the carbocation is, the easier it is to form, and faster will be the S_N1 reaction. Hence, the order of reactivity of alkyl halides towards S_N1 is tertiary alkyl halides > secondary alkyl halides > primary alkyl halides.

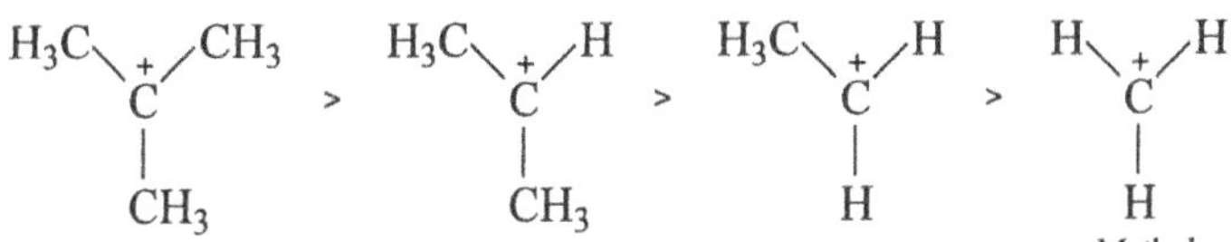

3° 2° 1° Methyl

(b) *Nature of the nucleophile* Since the nucleophile does not participate in the rate-determining step of an S_N1 reaction, the rates of S_N1 reactions are unaffected by either the concentration or the identity of the nucleophile.

(c) *Nature of the solvent* In an S_N1 reaction, the intermediate is a carbocation. Polar protic solvents (water, methanol, ethanol) will greatly increase the rate of ionisation of an alkyl halide, stabilises the transition state by solvation which improves the carbocation formation. The characteristic features of polar protic solvents (polar and ability to be H-bond donor) are:

- They have dipoles due to polar bonds.
- They have H atoms that can be donated into a H-bond. Basicity is also usually measured in water.
- Anions will be solvated by polar protic solvents due to H-bonding, inhibiting their ability to function.

For example, for an S_N1 reaction, the polarity and ability of the solvent to stabilise the intermediate carbocation is of paramount importance, as shown by the relative rate data for the solvolysis of tertiarybutyl chloride (see Table 13.3).

Table 13.3 Relative Rate Data for Solvolysis of Tertiarybutyl Chloride

Solvent	*Dipole Moment (μ in debye)*	*Dielectric Constant (ε)*	*Relative Rate*

by lowering energy of activation and thus improves the rate of reaction. order of reactivity of alkyl halides is RI > RBr > RCl > RF.

13.7.2 Dehydrohalogenation of Alkyl Halides

Alkyl halides undergo dehydrohalogenation, which is an example of elimination reacti Dehydrohalogenation of alkyl halides is a general reaction and is an excellent method preparing alkenes. This reaction involves the removal of β-hydrogen and the leav group (halogen) from adjacent carbon atoms of an alkyl halide on refluxing it with alcoholic solution of base (potassium hydroxide, sodium hydroxide, potassium ethox or sodium ethoxide). Therefore, dehydrohalogenation of alkyl halides to alkenes follc 1,2-elimination.

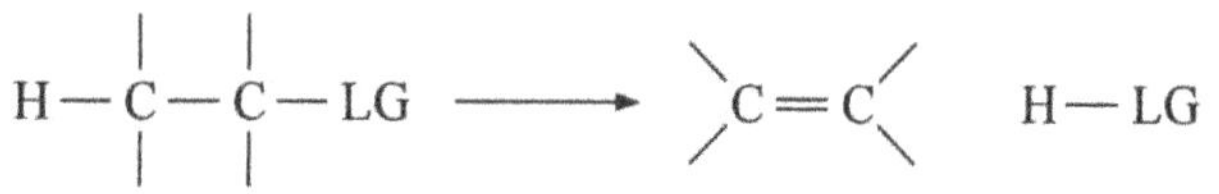

$$\underset{\text{Alkyl halide}}{R-\underset{H}{CH}-\underset{X}{CH_2}} + \text{Alcoholic KOH} \xrightarrow{\Delta} \underset{\text{Alkene}}{R-CH=CH_2} + KX + H_2O$$

(X = Cl, Br or I)

$$\underset{n\text{-Propyl bromide}}{CH_3-\underset{H}{CH}-\underset{X}{CH_2}} + \text{Alcoholic KOH} \xrightarrow{\Delta} \underset{\text{Propene}}{CH_3-CH=CH_2} + KX + H_2($$

$$\underset{\text{2-Bromobutane}}{CH_3\underset{Br}{CH}CH_2CH_3} \xrightarrow[\Delta]{\text{Alcoholic KOH}} \underset{\text{1-Butene (20\%)}}{CH_3CH_2CH=CH_2} + \underset{\text{2-Butene (80\%)}}{CH_3CH=CHCH}$$

There are three fundamental events in these elimination reactions:

1. Removal of a proton
2. Formation of the carbon–carbon π bond
3. Occurrence of heterolytic dissociation of the covalent bond between carbon and t leaving group (halogen atom)

Dehydrohalogenation of alkyl halide yields only one product in some cases where more than one in others depending upon the structure of alkyl halide.

$$\underset{\text{2-Bromobutane}}{CH_3\underset{Br}{CH}CH_2CH_3} \xrightarrow[\Delta]{\text{Alcoholic KOH}} \underset{\text{1-Butene (20\%)}}{CH_3CH_2CH=CH_2} + \underset{\text{2-Butene (80\%)}}{CH_3CH=CHCH_3}$$

- *E1 reaction* Loss of the leaving group (LG) to form a carbocation, removal of proton (H^+) and formation of carbon–carbon double (C = C) bond.
- *E2 reaction* Simultaneous proton (H^+) removal, carbon–carbon double (C = C) bond formation and loss of the leaving group (LG).

limination Bimolecular Mechanism The term E2 stands for 'elimination bimolecular' ı E2 reaction, a base removes a proton from a β-carbon adjacent to the carbon bonded ıe halogen. As the proton is removed, the electrons between hydrogen and carbon e towards the carbon (α) bonded to the halogen and forms a π bond. The halogen ı leaves alkyl halide molecule as halide ion (leaving group) by taking bonding electrons it. The product of an E2 elimination reaction has one more degree of unsaturation the starting materials.

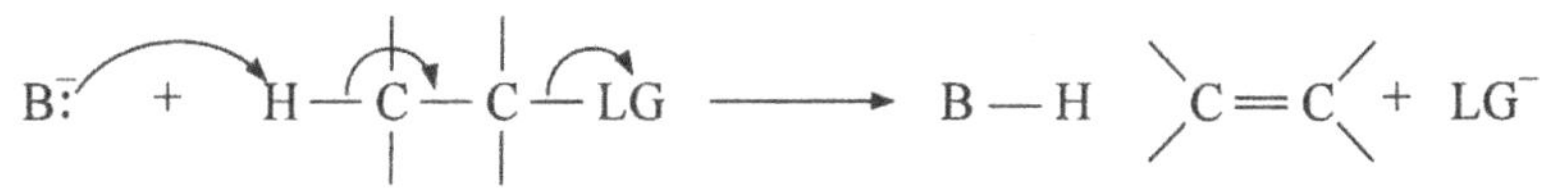

g. 13.6 Simultaneous Removal of the Proton (H^+) by the Base Loss of the Leaving Group (LG), and Formation of the π bond in an E2 Reaction

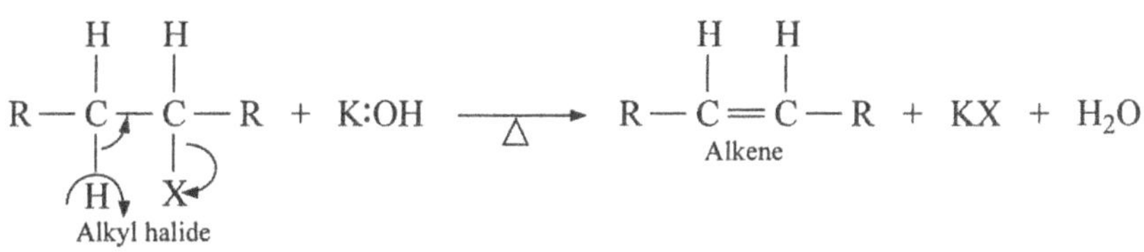

high concentration of a strong base in a relatively non-polar solvent is used to carry he E2 reaction. Such combinations as sodium methoxide in methanol, sodium ethoxide hanol, potassium isopropoxide in isopropanol, and potassium *tert*-butoxide in *tert*-ıol or dimethyl sulphoxide (DMSO) are often used.

inetics of E2 reactions Studies have shown that the rate-determining step of E2 ion involves a bimolecular collision. The rate of E2 reaction depends upon the entration of both the substrate (alkyl halide) and attacking reagent (base). This results rate law expression:

$$R = k\,[R - X][\text{base}]$$

here is a smooth transition between the reactants and the product. Analogous to the eaction, no intermediate has been isolated or detected. Furthermore, no rearrangements r under E2 conditions.

Iydrogen isotope effect with E2 reactions The hydrogen effect is an effect that alters hydrogen atoms with deuterium atoms in the organic substrate. This would only be notice if the rate-determining step involves the breaking of a carbon–hydrogen bond which is tl E2 path. If we compare the dissociation rate of 2,2 di-duetero-1-chloropropane with th of 1-chloropropane, we would find that the dissociation rate of the deuterated substra would be lesser as compared to the rate of the non-deuterated substrate. We say th eliminations following the E2 path will exhibit a hydrogen isotope effect. Indeed, we ca tell whether the elimination is following this path or some other path such as E1 path

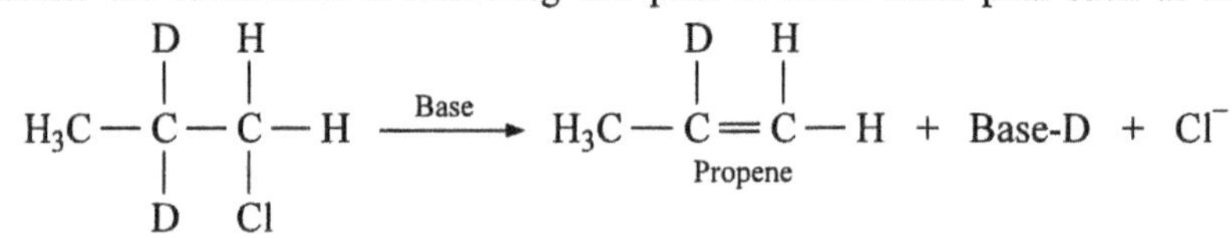

2,2-Diduetero-1-chloropropane

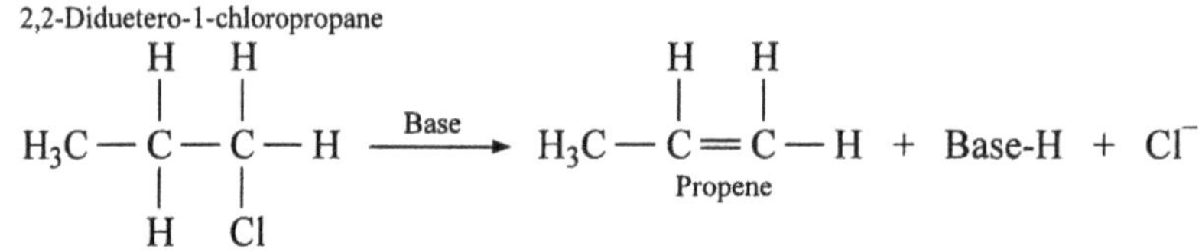

1-Chloropropane

(iii) *Stereochemistry* E2 reactions occur most rapidly when the H — C bond an C — LG bonds involved are co-planar, most often at 180° or anti-periplanar. This sets u the σ bonds that are broken in the correct alignment to become the π bond. Experiment evidence indicates that the five atoms involved in the E2 elimination reaction must lie i the same plane (the anti-periplanar conformation). This conformation is necessary for th orbital overlap that must occur for the π bond to be generated in the alkene. The *sp* hybridised atomic orbitals on carbon, which comprise the C — H and C — X σ bonc broken in the reaction, develop into the *p* orbitals comprising the σ bond of the alken formed. For example, in cases where *cis*- or *trans*-alkenes can be formed, the reactio exhibits stereoselectivity, and the more stable *trans*-isomer is the major product.

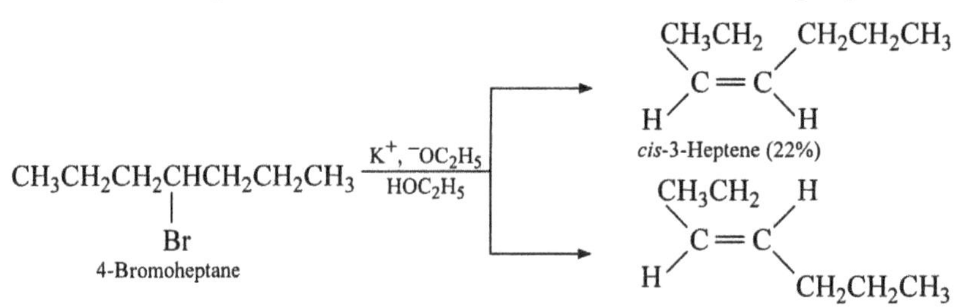

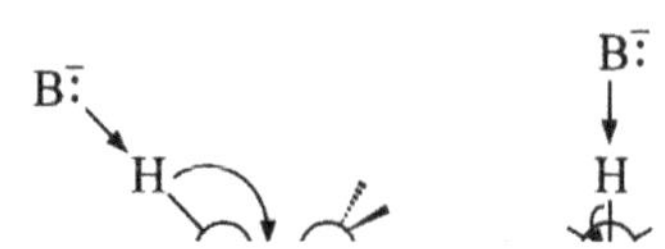

s, the base removes a less hindered β-hydrogen atom, leading to a predominance of thermodynamically *less stable (terminal) alkene* in the product mixture. This type of lt is often referred to as anti-Zaitsev or Hofmann elimination. Thus, in the reaction bromo-2,3-dimethylbutane, the 2,3-dimethyl-1-butene would be the major product (anti-sev) if the conditions involve use of a bulkier base.

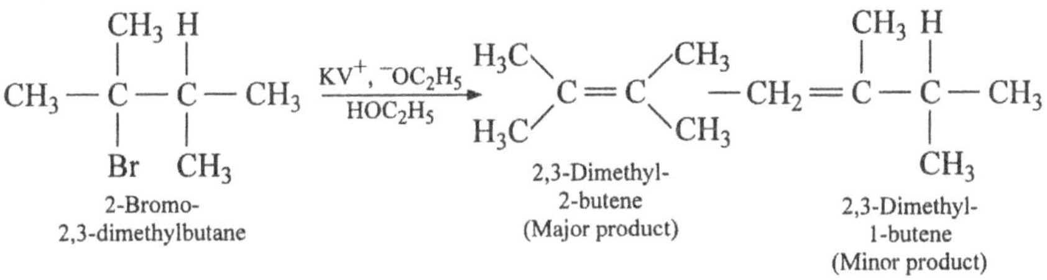

he periplanar arrangements are illustrated in the Newman projections in Fig. 13.8.

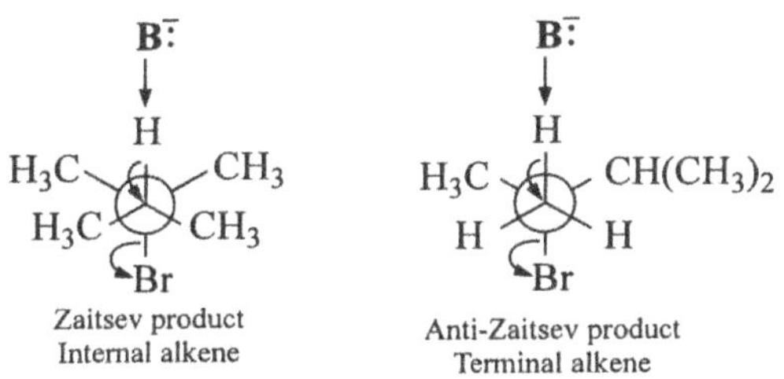

ig. 13.8 Two Anti-periplanar Conformations of 2-Bromo-2,3-dimethylbutane

ehydrohalogenation of alkyl halides in the presence of strong base (E2) is often mpanied by the formation of substitution (S_{N^2}) products.

$$CH_3CH_2CH_2Br + KOH \longrightarrow CH_3CH_2 = CH_2 + CH_3CH_2CH_2OH$$

n-Propylbromide — Propene (Elimination product) — *n*-Propanol (Substitution product)

Reactivity of alkyl halides towards E2 The order of reactivity of alkyl halides towards ination bimolecular mechanism is tertiary alkyl halides > secondary alkyl halides > ary alkyl halides. This is because branching at the carbon carrying the halogen increases oing from primary to secondary to tertiary alkyl halide. Now greater the branching er the number of β-hydrogens which can be attacked by the base and therefore, er the probability of attack. Moreover, more branched alkyl halide is more stable use of less E_{act} and more stability of transition state.

limination Unimolecular Reaction Technically, this mechanism is called an E1 anism; E stands for elimination, and the 1 signifies single molecular species that ence the reaction rate. An E1 reaction pathway is a multi-step process with the wing two critical steps:

Tertiarybutylbromide Tertiarybutyl carbocation

In the *second step* of the reaction, deprotonation by a base from a carbon atom (β adjacent to the carbocation centre leads to the creation of the carbon–carbon doubl bond (C = C). It is an acid/base reaction.

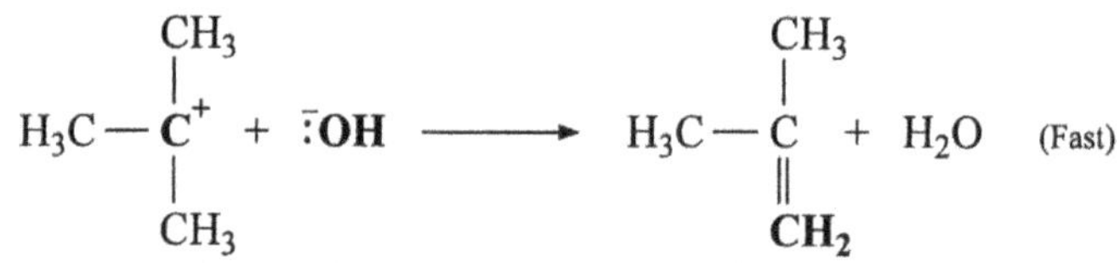

Tertiarybutyl carbocation Isobutylene

Since carbocation intermediates are formed during an E1, there is always the possibilit of rearrangements (e.g. 1,2-hydride or 1,2-alkyl shifts) to generate a more stable carbocatio This is usually indicated by a change in the position of the alkene or a change in th carbon skeleton of the product when compared to the starting material.

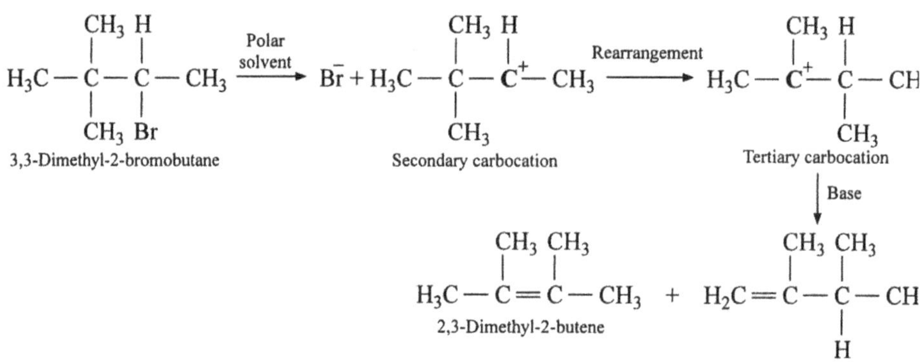

3,3-Dimethyl-2-bromobutane Secondary carbocation Tertiary carbocation 2,3-Dimethyl-2-butene 2,3-Dimethyl-1-butene

(i) *Kinetics of E1 reactions* The rate of E1 reaction depends upon the rate of slowe step, i.e. the loss of leaving group (halide ion) to form carbocation. The rate (carbocatio formation reaction) depends only on the concentration of the alkyl halide. Hence, the rat of E1 reaction depends upon the concentration of only alkyl halide. This results in a rat law expression:

$$R = k\,[RX]$$

Therefore, E1 reaction is said to be unimolecular reaction and the rate of reactio follows first-order kinetics. An E1 reaction is analogous to S_N1 reaction and hence a weal base and a protic polar solvent (H_2O, ROH) favour E1 reaction. Generally, tertiary an secondary alkyl halides follow this mechanism because primary alkyl halides encounte difficulty in forming primary carbocations.

(ii) *Orientation of dehydrohalogenation Saytzeff's rule (Zaitsev rule)* It is used t predict the orientation of dehydrohalogenation. If the dehydrohalogenation of an alky

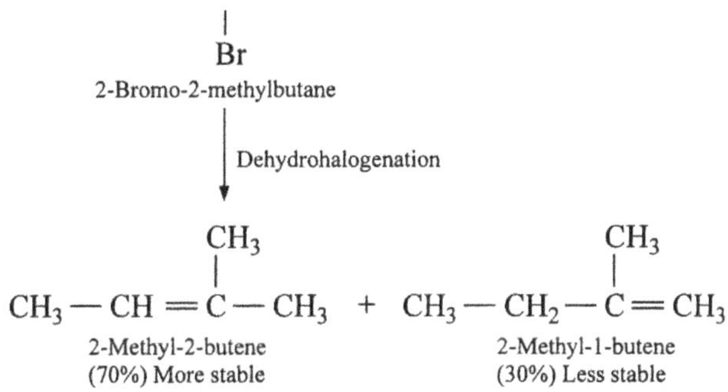

Of the two products (2-methyl-2-butene and 2-methyl-1-butene) 2-methyl-2-butene is ore substitued hence it is the major product. This rule can be explained on the basis hyperconjugation, because more stable alkene (more substituted one) has more number resonating structures.

i) *Order of stability of alkenes* The following is the order of stability of alkenes:

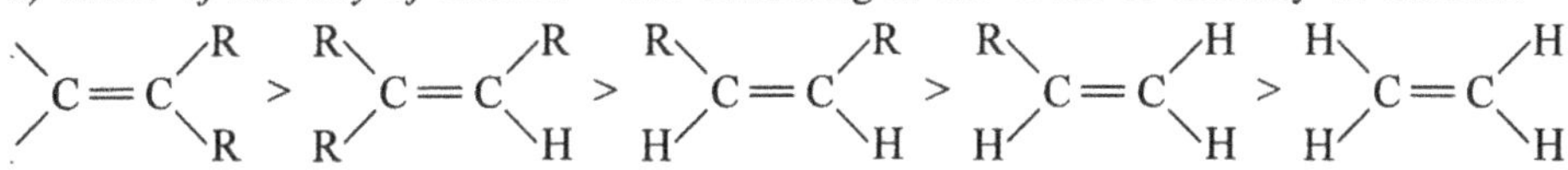

Hofmann rule When dehydrohalogenation is carried out with a bulkier base (potassium tertiary butoxide) in tertiary butyl alcohol solvent the major product is less substituted, which is contrary to Saytzeff's rule. This rule is known as Hoffmann's rule and the product (less substituted) is Hofmann's product. The reason for this unusual behaviour is steric bulk of the base, which is difficult to remove β-hydrogen atom from greater crowded β-carbon (secondary) atom. Instead the base abstracts less crowded β-hydrogen (primary) atom to form less substituted alkene (Hofmann's product).

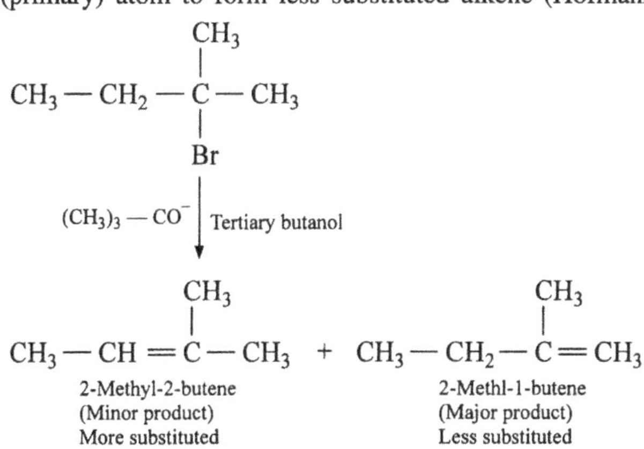

.7.3 Reduction of Alkyl Halides

$$\underset{\text{Ethylchloride}}{C_2H_5 - Cl} \longrightarrow \underset{\text{Ethane}}{C_2H_5 - H}$$

13.7.4 Grignard Reagent Formation

The Grignard reaction is a versatile and popular technique for making carbon–cart bonds and building elaborate carbon frameworks. The Grignard reagent is an organometa compound – a compound with a bond between carbon and a metal that has much coval character. The metal is usually magnesium but lithium is also used and makes more react reagents. The Grignard reagent is made from the direct reaction of magnesium with alkyl halide in alcohol-free anhydrous ether solvent. Notice that aryl halides (ArX) a vinyl halides that are inert to nucleophilic substitution are reactive in this Grignard reacti

Grignard reagent is an extremely reactive reagent and has the approximate composit of $R - Mg^+X^-$. It undergoes decomposition in air, moisture, carbon dioxide. Hence, i usually prepared in situ, in an inert atmosphere (nitrogen atmosphere).

$$RCH_2^{\delta-} - Mg^{\delta+}X$$

$$\underset{\text{Alkyl halide}}{R - X} + Mg \xrightarrow{\text{Anhydrous alcohol-free ether}} \underset{\text{Alkylmagnesium halide}}{R - MgX}$$

$$\underset{\text{Methyl chloride}}{CH_3 - Cl} + Mg \xrightarrow{\text{Anhydrous alcohol-free ether}} \underset{\text{Methylmagnesium halide}}{CH_3 - MgCl}$$

This α-carbon of Grignard reagent consequently has significant nucleophilic charact The Grignard reagent reacts well as a nucleophile with any electrophilic atom or gro as a target. The setup for the experiment is shown in Fig. 13.9. It is crucial that t equipment for this experiment is dry.

Preparation of a solution of phenylmagnesium bromide in ether All apparatus a reagents must be absolutely dry. The Grignard reagent is prepared in a dry 100-ml reacti flask fitted with a Claisen adapter. To one arm of the Claisen adapter fit a rubber septu To the other arm of the Claisen adapter fit a reflux condenser. A calcium chloride dryi tube is fitted at the top of the condenser. Have a cold water bath standing by in ca the reaction becomes too vigorous. Add approximately 0.15 g of magnesium metal to t flask. Add 1.5 ml of dry ether and 0.25 ml of bromobenzene to the magnesium. Add o or two small crystals of iodine to clean the surface of the magnesium and initiate t reaction with bromobenzene. Soon the mixture should start boiling. (Use the water ba if the reaction gets too vigorous.) Add an additional 1 ml of ether through the rubb septum. As the magnesium is consumed, the reaction will begin to slow. At this poi warm the mixture to reflux (use warm water bath) for an additional 15–20 minutes or un

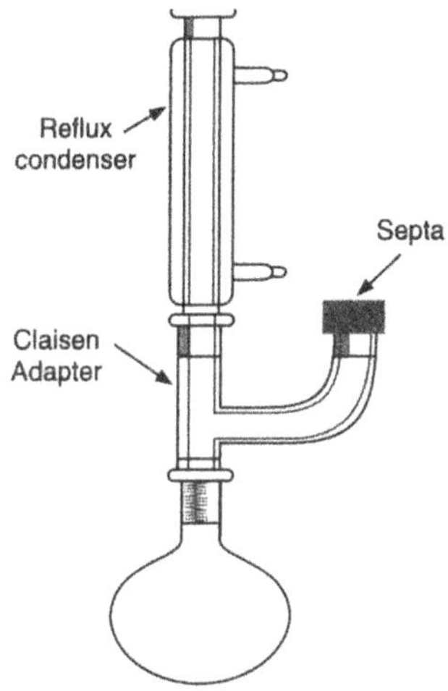

Fig. 13.9 Experimental Setup for Preparation of Grignard Reagent

S_N1 vs S_N2 REACTION: A SUMMARY

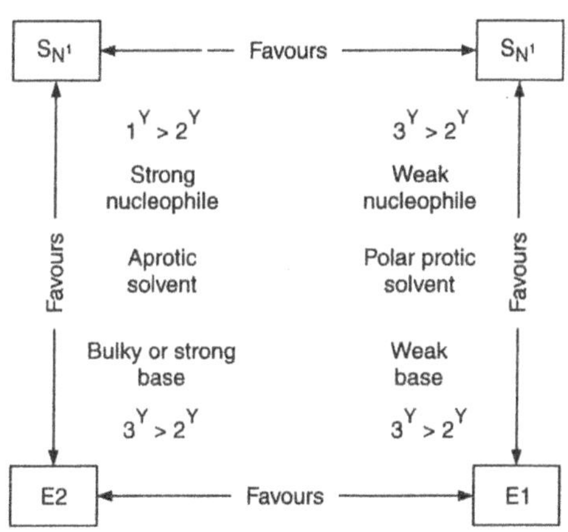

S_N1	S_N2
A two-step mechanism	1. A one-step mechanism
Rate of reaction depends on concentration of alkyl halide	2. Rate of reaction depends on concentration of alkyl halide and nucleophile
It is a unimolecular reaction	3. It is a bimolecular reaction
S_N1 reaction proceeds with	4. S_N2 reaction proceeds with inversion of

alkyl halide > primary alkyl halide > methyl halides	> secondary alkyl halide > tertiary alkyl halide
7. S_N1 reaction favoured by polar solvents	7. S_N2 reaction favoured by non-polar solv
8. S_N1 reaction can occur with weak bases	8. S_N2 reaction requires strong base

13.9 E1 vs E2 REACTION: A SUMMARY

E1	*E2*
1. A two-step mechanism	1. A one-step mechanism
2. Rate of reaction depends on concentration of alkyl halide	2. Rate of reaction depends on concentratioı alkyl halide and nucleophile
3. It is a unimolecular reaction	3. It is a bimolecular reaction
4. Rearrangement occurs	4. Rearrangement does not occur
5. Rate of reaction depends on structure: tertiary alkyl halide > secondary alkyl halide > primary alkyl halide > methyl halides	5. Rate of reaction depends on structure: tert alkyl halide > secondary alkyl halide > primary alkyl halide > methyl halides
6. E1 reaction favoured by polar solvents	6. E2 reaction favoured by aprotic solvents
7. E1 reaction can occur with weak bases	7. E2 reaction requires strong bases

13.10 IMPORTANT PHARMACEUTICAL COMPOUNDS

1. ***Ethyl Chloride (C_2H_5Cl)*** Ethyl chloride is prepared by passing dry hydrogen chlor gas into absolute alcohol in presence of $ZnCl_2$

$$\underset{\text{Ethyl alcohol}}{C_2H_5OH} + HCl \xrightarrow{ZnCl_2} \underset{\text{Ethyl chloride}}{C_2H_5Cl} + H_2O$$

Uses

1. It is used as a general anaesthetic and refrigerant.
2. It is used as ethylating agent in the preparation of tetraethyl lead, ethyl cellulo

2. ***Chloroform ($CHCl_3$)*** Chloroform is prepared by distilling ethyl alcohol with bleachi powder and water. The available chlorine of bleaching powder serves as oxidising a chlorinating agent. This involves the following steps:

(i) Bleaching powder on hydrolysis gives chlorine and calcium hydroxide.

$$CaOCl_2 + H_2O \longrightarrow Cl_2 + Ca(OH)_2$$

(ii) Ethyl alcohol reacts with chlorine and produces acetaldehyde.

$$CH_3CH_2OH + Cl_2 \longrightarrow CH_3CHO + 3HCl$$

(iv) Chloral reacts with chlorine to produce chloroform

$$CH_3CHO + 3Cl_2 \longrightarrow 2CHCl_3 + Ca(HCOO)_2$$

Uses

1. It is used as a general anaesthetic.
2. It is used as solvent for fats and oils.

3. ***Iodoform* (CHI$_3$)** Iodoform is a yellow crystalline solid and is prepared by adding iodine solution slowly with shaking to acetone in alkali. It is used as an antiseptic.

$$\underset{\text{Acetone}}{H_3C-\overset{\overset{\displaystyle O}{\|}}{C}-CH_3} + 3I_2 + 4NaOH \longrightarrow \underset{\text{Sodium acetate}}{CH_3COONa} + 3NaI + H_2O + \underset{\text{Iodoform}}{CHI_3}$$

4. ***Carbon Tetrachloride* (*CCl$_4$*)** Carbon tetrachloride is a colourless liquid, which boils at 77°C. It is prepared by chlorination of methane.

$$CH_4 + 4Cl_2 \longrightarrow CCl_4 + 4HCl$$

Uses

1. It is used as an operating fluid for refrigerators and air-conditioning equipment,
2. It is also used as anthelmenthic.

5. ***Vinyl Chloride*** Vinyl chloride is a colourless gas, which is prepared by controlled addition of HCl to acetylene in presence of mercury salts as catalysts.

$$HC\equiv CH + HCl \xrightarrow{Hg2+} H_2C=CH_2-Cl$$

6. ***Dichloromethane*** Natural sources of dichloromethane include oceanic sources, macroalgae, wetlands, and volcanoes. It is also called as methylene chloride, methylene bichloride. Methylene chloride is a clear, colorless, nonflammable, volatile liquid chlorinated hydrocarbon with a sweet, pleasant odor.

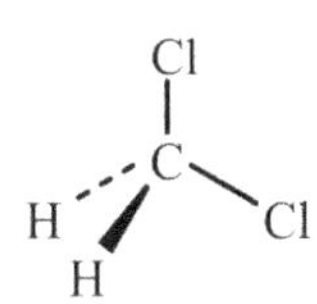

Uses

1. Dichloromethane is a chlorinated hydrocarbon that has been used as an inhalation anesthetic.
2. Methylene chloride is predominantly used as a solvent in paint strippers and removers.

3. It is used as an extraction solvent for spice oleoresins, hops, and for the removal of caffeine from coffee.

7. ***Tetrachloroethylene*** It is chlorinated hydrocarbon and is a potential carcinogen. Tetrachloroethylene is a colorless, volatile, nonflammable, liquid, chlorinated hydrocarbon with an ether-like odor.

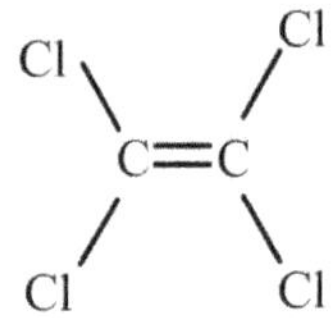

Uses

1. Tetrachloroethylene is used for dry cleaning and textile processing, as a chemical intermediate, and for vapor degreasing in metal-cleaning operations.
2. Exposure to this substance irritates the upper respiratory tract and eyes and causes neurological effects as well as kidney and liver damage.

8. ***Trichloroethylene*** Trichloroethylene is a clear colorless volatile liquid having a chloroform- like odor and is slightly soluble in water. It also called as ethinyl trichloride or trichloroethene. Trichloroethylene is highly volatile inhalation anesthetic.

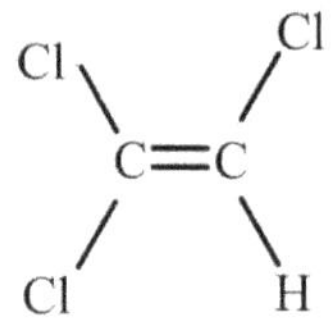

Uses

1. Trichloroethylene is used mainly as a degreaser for metal parts.
2. Trichloroethylene was used in the past as a general anesthetic.
3. Trichloroethylene is also used as an extraction solvent for greases, oils, fats, waxes, and tars, a chemical intermediate in the production of other chemicals, and as a refrigerant.

PRACTICE QUESTIONS

1. Give the mechanism, stereochemistry and kinetics of SN^1 and SN^2 reactions for the hydrolysis of alkyl halides.
2. Explain the mechanisms of the two major pathways of nucleophilic substitution. Undergone by alkyl halides giving kinetic and stereochemical evidences. Discuss the effect or experimental conditions on these mechanisms.

3. (a) What are the salient features of SN^1 and SN^2 reactions? Explain with suitable examples, the mechanism of these reactions.

   (b) Write the balanced equations for the reaction of ethyl chloride with (i) KCN, (ii) AgCN, (iii) aq.KOH, (iv) Dry Ag_2O

4. (a) Write about the stereochemistry of SN^1 and SN^2 reactions.

   (b) What is the influence of substituents on the course of SN^1 and SN^2 reactions.

   (c) Write four important reactions of alkyl halides emphasizing their utility.

5. What are organometallic compounds? How are they prepared? How can ethyl magnesium bromide be used for the synthesis of (a) l-butanol, (b) 2-butanol, (c) dimethyl carbinol, (d) propionic acid and (e) propionaldehyde?

6. Discuss SN^1 and SN^2 reaction mechanism for the hydrolysis of primary and tertiary alkyl halides.

7. Explain the following:

   (a) Tertiary carbonium ion is more stable than methyl carbonium ion.

   (b) Ethanol is not useful as a solvent in the Grignard reaction of ethyl iodide on acetone.

   (c) Treatment of alkyl halides with aqueous alkali gives alcohols while alcoholic alkali gives olefins.

8. A primary alkyl halide (A) C_4H_9Br is reacted with hot alcoholic KOH to give compound (B). Compound (B) is reacted with HBr to give an isomer of (A), (C). When (A) was reacted with sodium it gave compound produced when *n*-butyl bromide was reacted with sodium. Identify (A), (B), (C) and (D). Write equations for all the reactions.

9. Give a comparative account of elimination and substitution reactions.

10. What are alkyl halides? Classify alkyl halides with examples? Explain various methods to prepare alkyl halides.

14

ALCOHOLS

Alcohols are hydroxy derivatives of hydrocarbons having the general formula of R—OH. These are formed by replacement of one, two or more hydrogen atoms of hydrocarbons by a corresponding number of hydroxyl groups (—OH). The hydroxyl group of alcohol is not to be confused with the hydroxide ion, which is negatively charged oxygen bonded to hydrogen. The hydroxyl group is electrically neutral. It represents the position in an molecule where the chemical change takes place.

14.1 CLASSIFICATION OF ALCOHOLS

Alcohols are classified according to number of hydroxyl groups present in a molecule.

1. ***Monohydric Alcohols*** Alcohols with one hydroxyl group are known as monohydric alcohols.

$H_3C—OH$
Methanol

$H_3C\,H_2C—OH$
Ethanol

$H_3C\,H_2C\,H_2C—OH$
Propanol

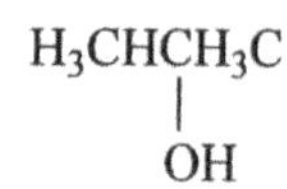
Propan-2-ol

Monohydric alcohols can be classified further as primary, secondary or tertiary according as the hydroxyl group attached to a primary, secondary or tertiary carbon atom.

$H_3CCH_2—OH$
Ethyl alcohol
(Primary alcohol)

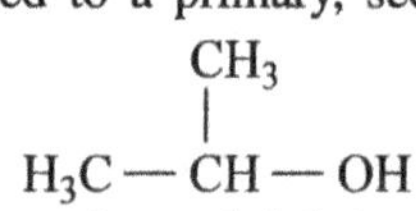
Isopropyl alcohol
(Secondary alcohol)

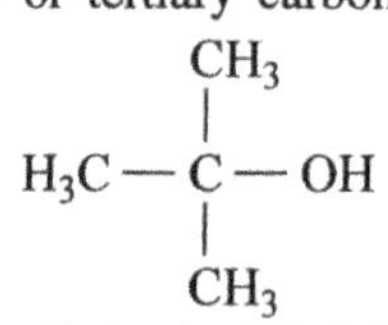
Tertiary butyl alcohol
(Tertiary alcohol)

2. ***Dihydric Alcohols*** Alcohols with two hydroxyl groups (—OH) are dihydric alcohols (diols).

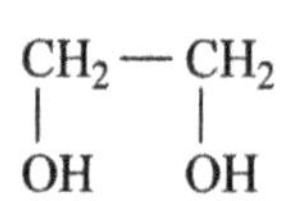
Ethylene glycol

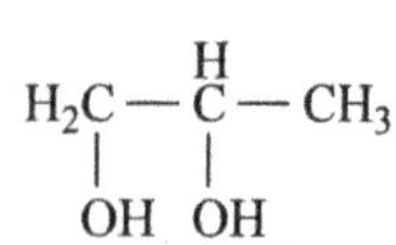
Propylene glycol

3. ***Trihydric Alcohols*** Alcohols containing three hydroxyl groups (—OH) are known as trihydric alcohols (triols).

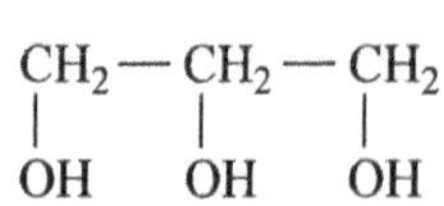
Glycerol
(Trihydric alcohol)

4. ***Polyhydric Alcohols*** Alcohols with four or more hydroxyl groups are called polyhydric alcohols (polyols).

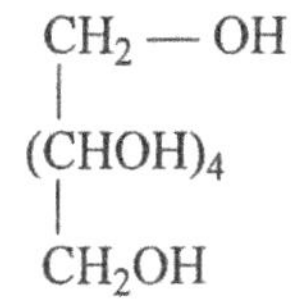

Sorbitol
(Polyhydric alcohol)

14.2 NOMENCLATURE OF ALCOHOLS

According to IUPAC system, alcohols are called alkanols. The following rules are followed:

1. Identify the longest continuous chain of carbons in which the hydroxyl group(s) are attached to one of the carbons in the chain.
2. Number the carbon chain to give the lowest number to the carbon attached with hydroxyl group (—OH).
3. Identify and locate the other branches on the chain so that they are named alphabetically and their carbon number is hyphenated onto the front of the name. If more than one of the same group is present use the Greek prefix (*di* = 2, *tri* = 3, etc.) attached to the branch name.
4. After all the branches have been named and located, attach the carbon number that is attached to the hydroxyl group onto the alkane name (associated with the number of carbons found in the continuous chain in step 1).
5. Drop 'e' on the alkane name and attach the characteristic IUPAC ending 'ol' to the rest of the alkane name.
6. Other substituents, if any, are numbered, named and placed as prefixes in alphabetical order.

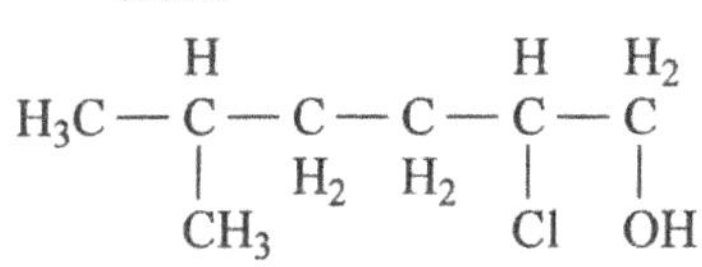

2-Chloro-5-methyl-1-hexanol

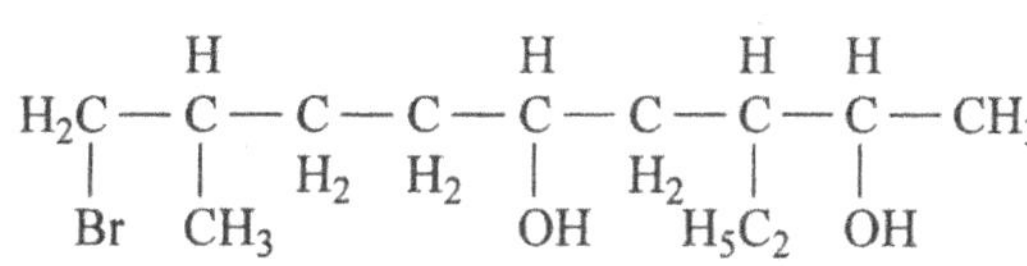

9-Bromo-3-ethyl-2,5-nonanediol

14.3 ISOMERISM IN ALCOHOLS

The alcohols exhibit chain, position and functional isomerism.

1. ***Chain Isomerism*** This isomerism is due to difference in the structure of the chain. For example, *n*-butyl alcohol and isobutyl alcohol.

$$CH_3 - CH_2 - CH_2 - CH_2 - OH \qquad CH_3 - CH\,(CH_3) - CH_2 - OH$$

n-Butyl alcohol   Isobutyl alcohol

2. ***Position Isomerism*** This isomerism is due to difference in the position of hydroxyl group when the carbon chain is same. For example, *n*-butyl alcohol and isopropyl alcohol.

$CH_3 — CH_2 — CH_2 — OH$ $CH_3 — CH(OH) — CH_3$

n-Propyl alcohol   Isopropyl alcohol

3. ***Functional Isomerism*** Alcohols also exhibit functional isomerism with ethers. Ethyl alcohol (C_2H_5OH) and dimethyl ether ($CH_3 — O — CH_3$) are functional isomers, propanol (C_3H_7OH) and ethyl methyl ether ($C_2H_5 — O — CH_3$) are functional isomers.

14.4 PREPARATION OF ALCOHOLS

The following methods are used to prepare alcohols.

1. ***Hydrolysis of Alkyl Halides*** Alkyl halides on hydrolysis with aqueous alkali or silver oxide suspended in water yield alcohols. In this method 1°, 2° and 3° alcohols can be prepared. This reaction involves nucleophilic substitution of alkyl halides (S_N1 or S_N2). The method suffers from the drawback that dehydrohalogenation may take place to produce simultaneously an alkene. This shortcoming is overcome by using either aqueous potassium carbonate or moist silver oxide for hydrolysis.

$$\underset{\text{Alkyl halide}}{R—X} + \bar{O}H \longrightarrow \underset{\text{Alcohol}}{R—OH} + X^-$$

$$\underset{\text{Alkyl halide}}{R—X} + AgOH \longrightarrow \underset{\text{Alcohol}}{R—OH} + AgX$$

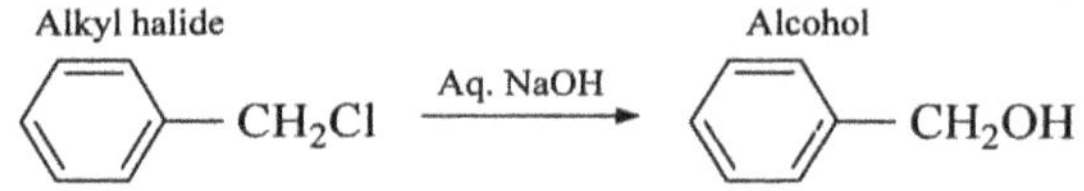

Benzyl chloride   Benzyl alcohol

2. ***Oxymercuration–Demercuration of Alkenes*** Alkenes react with mercuric acetate in presence of water to give hydroxymercurial compounds, which on reduction with $NaBH_4$ yield alcohols. This reaction follows Markovnikov's orientation through the intermediate formation of cyclic mercurinium ion, which is comparable to carbocation. Oxymercuration–demercuration proceeds without rearrangements because the intermediate is a cyclic ion.

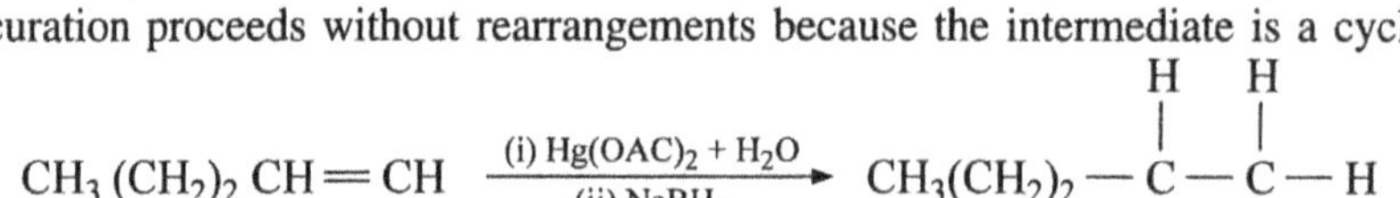

1-Pentene   2-Pentanol

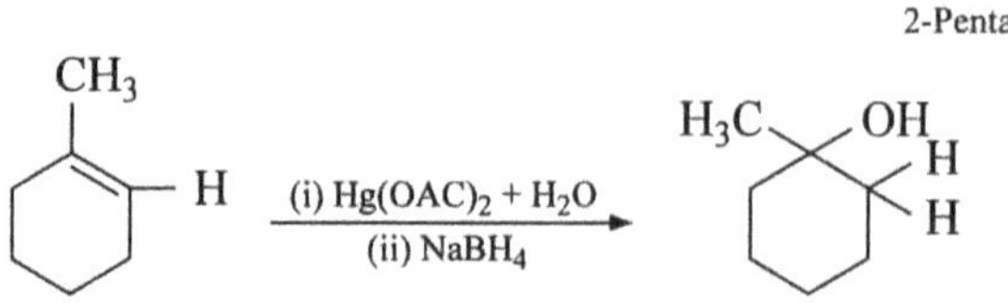

1-Methylcyclohexene   1-Methylcyclohexanol

Mechanism Oxymercuration-demercuration of alkenes is an electrophilic addition reaction. The electrophile is an electron-deficient mercury atom of mercuric acetate, which adds at the double bond of alkene. The mechanism involves the following steps:

(i) *Oxymercuration* In the first step, —OH and —HgOAC groups are added to the carbon–carbon double bond and produce hydroxymercurial compound through the intermediate formation of cyclic mercurinium ion.

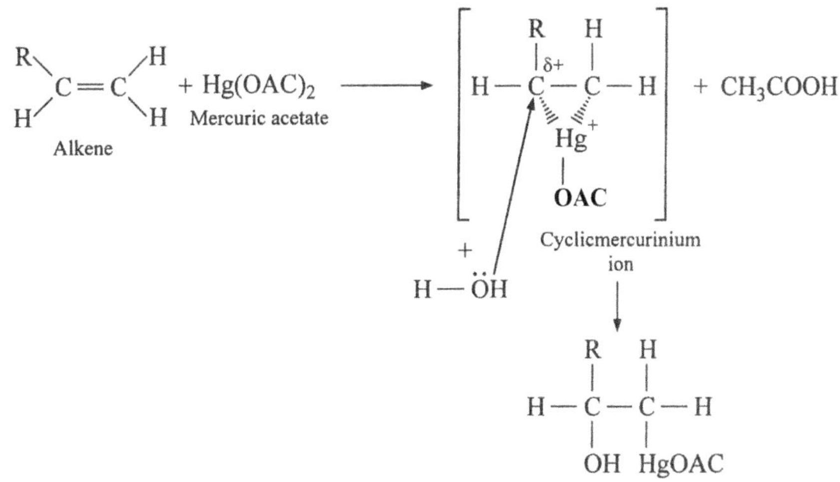

Alkene + Mercuric acetate → Cyclicmercurinium ion + CH_3COOH → Hydroxymercurial compound

(ii) *Demercuration* In this step, HgOAC is replaced by —H in presence of reducing agent ($NaBH_4$).

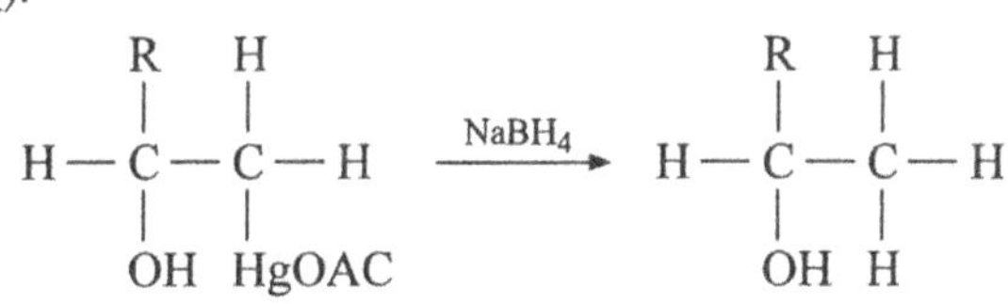

Hydroxymercurial compound → Alcohol

3. ***Hydroboration–Oxidation of Alkenes*** Alkenes when treated with diborane $(BH_3)_2$ gives alkyl boranes which on oxidation yield alcohols.

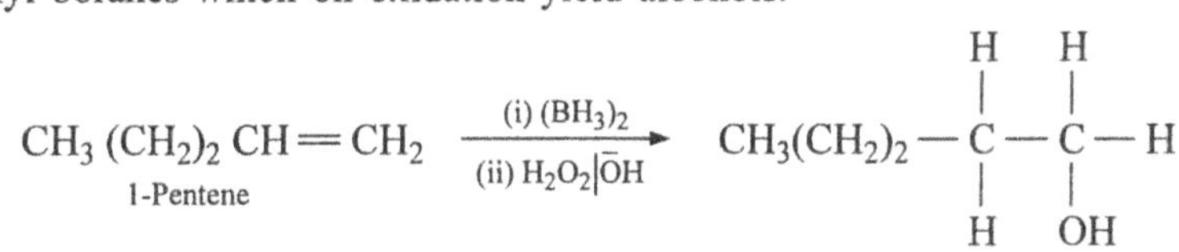

1-Pentene → 1-Pentanol

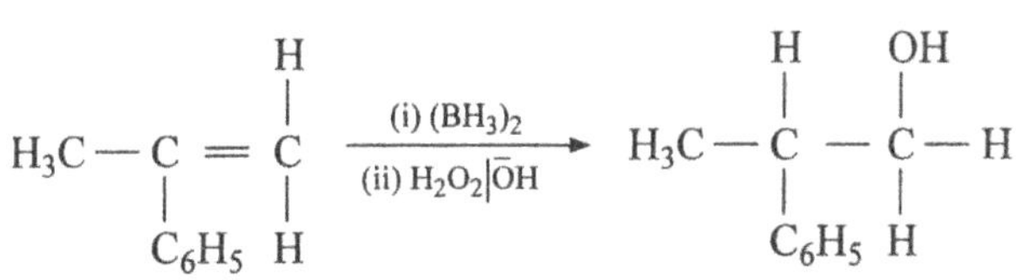

2-Phenyl-1-propene → 2-Phenyl-1-propanol

Mechanism Hydroboration–oxidation of alkenes is an electrophilic addition reaction. The electrophile is electron deficient boron atom of borane which attacks the double bond of alkene. The mechanism involve the following steps:

(i) *Hydroboration* The first step involves addition of hydrogen of BH_3 to one double-bonded carbon and $—BH_2$ to the other. This reaction takes place through a 4-membered transition state.

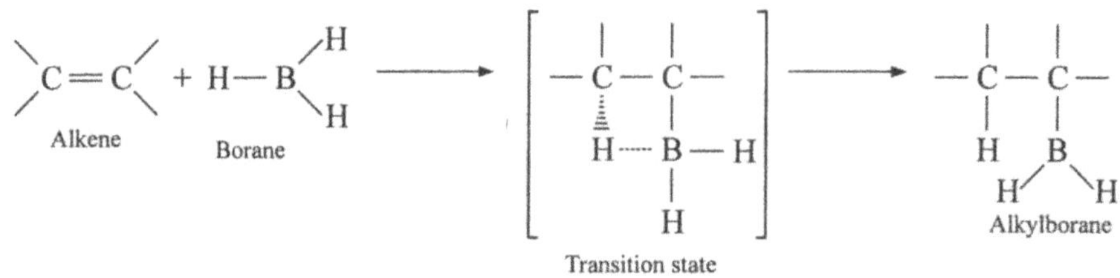

(ii) *Oxidation* In second step, the obtained alkyl borane is oxidised with H_2O_2 in alkali to yield alcohols (boron is replaced by —OH).

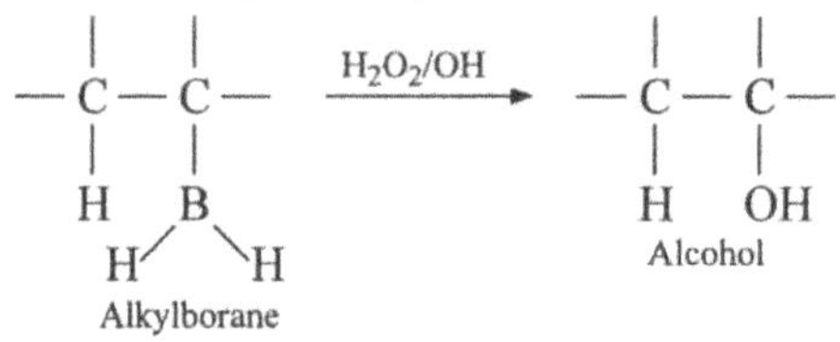

The hydroboration–oxidation process gives products corresponding to anti-Markovnikov's addition because the steric bulk of the borane is enough to force it to add to the less sterically hindered side. This reaction proceeds without rearrangements.

4. ***From Grignard Reagent*** Grignard reagent reacts with aldehydes and ketones in dry ether followed by acidification to give alcohols. This reaction involves nucleophilic addition of organic group (alkyl or aryl) of Grignard reagent to electrophilic carbonyl carbon of aldehydes or ketones to form magnesiumalkoxide, which on treatment with acidified water, yield alcohols.

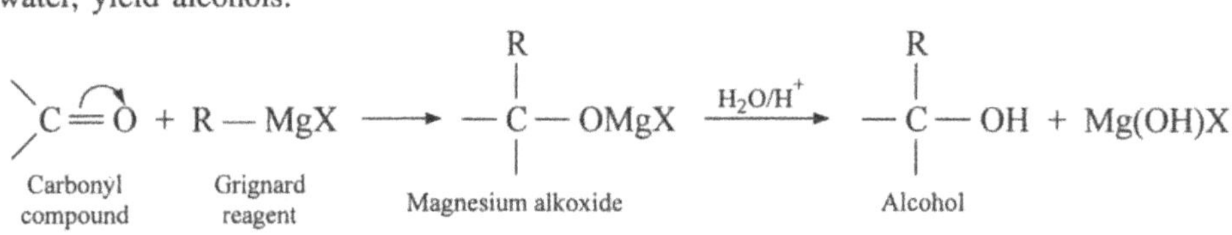

Formaldehyde gives primary alcohol on reaction with Grignard reagent, which is followed by hydrolysis with acidified H_2O, whereas higher aldehydes give secondary alcohol. All ketones react with Grignard reagent and produce tertiary alcohol.

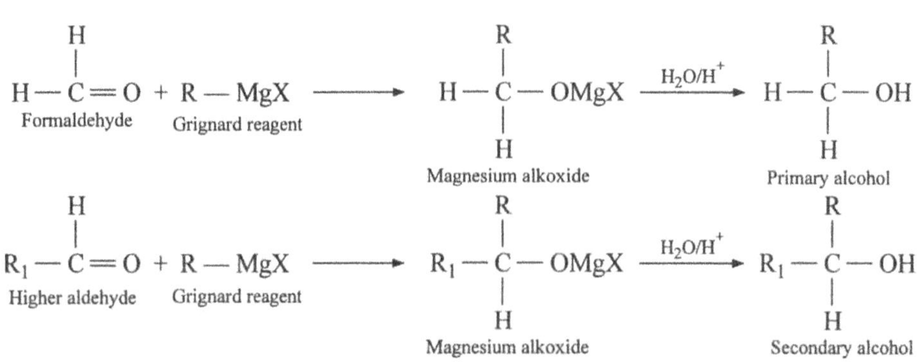

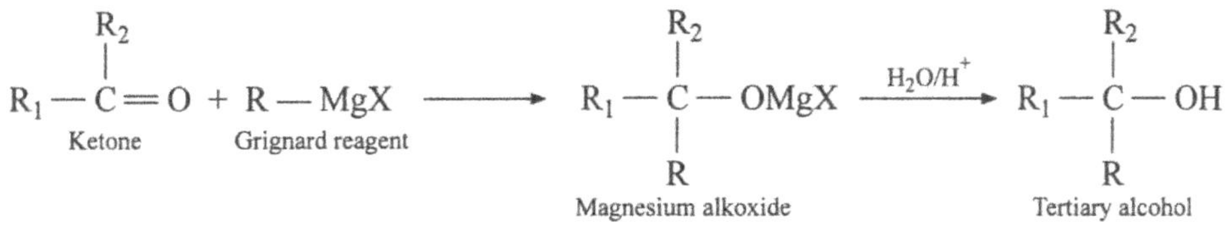

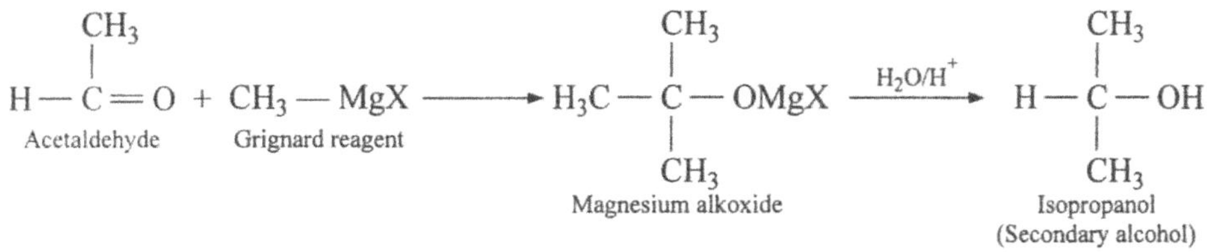

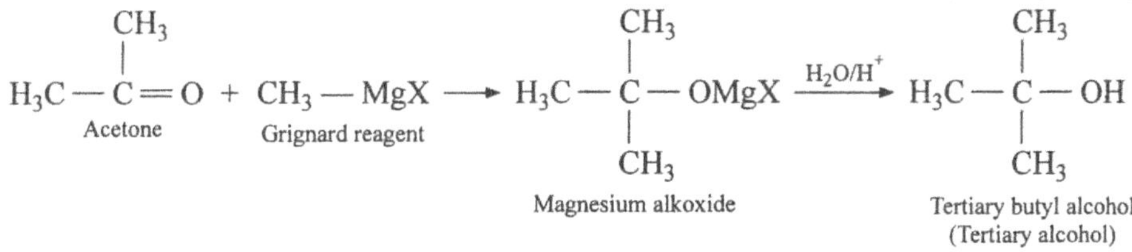

5. ***Reduction of Carbonyl Compounds*** The carbonyl group of aldehydes and ketones can be reduced to primary and secondary alcohols, respectively, in presence of hydrogen gas and metal catalyst (Pt, Pd or Ni) or chemical reducing agents ($LiAlH_4$, $NaBH_4$ or aluminium isopropoxide).

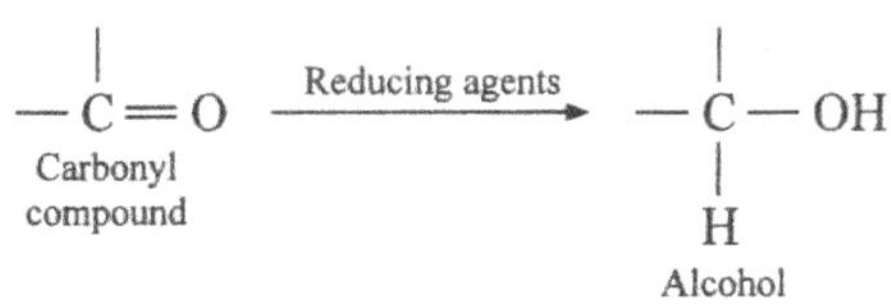

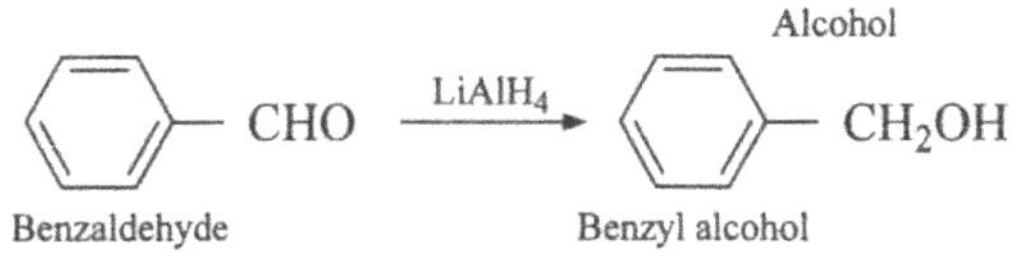

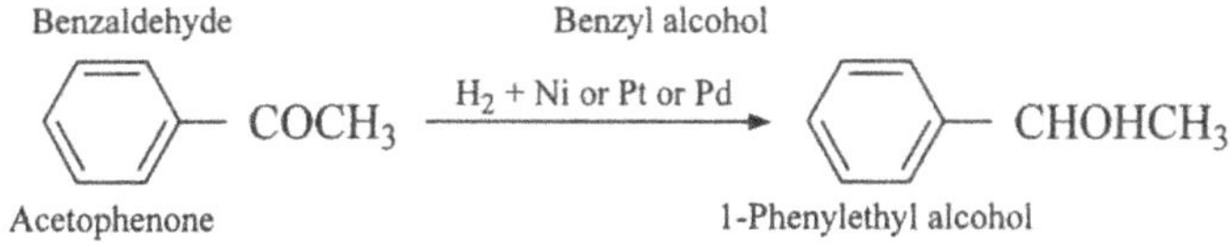

The reduction of aldehydes or ketones to the corresponding alcohols with aluminium isopropoxide in isopropanol is known as Meerwein–Pondorf–Verley reduction (which is the reverse of the Oppenauer oxidation).

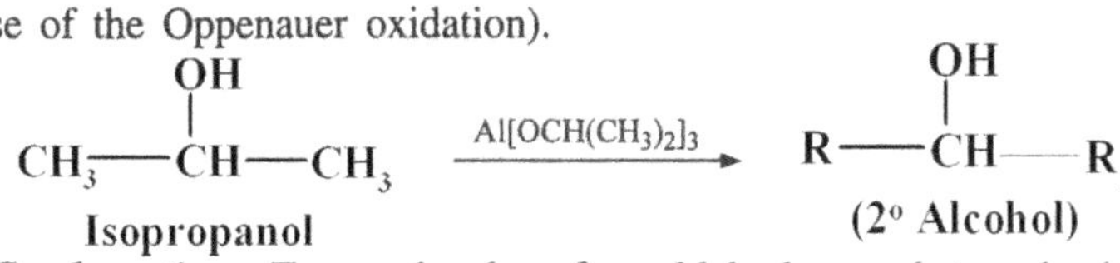

6. ***Aldol Condensation*** Two molecules of an aldehyde or a ketone having α-hydrogen atoms, undergo self-condensation in presence of dilute base or dilute acid at room

temperature to form product called aldol (β-hydroxy aldehyde or ketone). Hence, this reaction is known as aldol condensation.

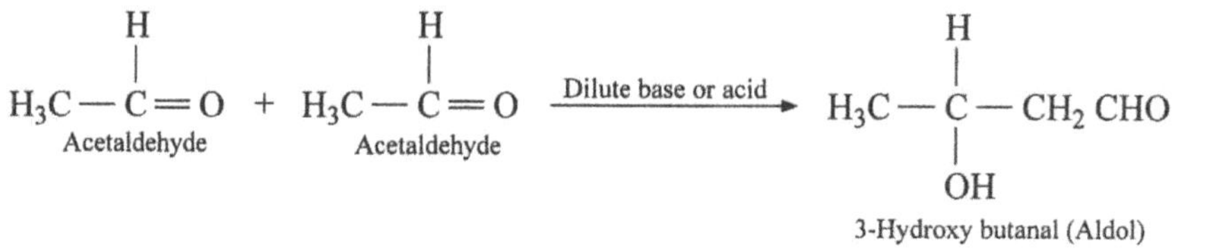

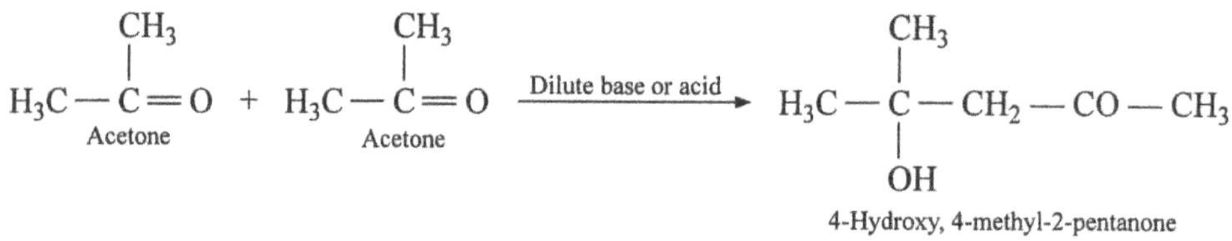

Mechanism The base (:OH^-) abstracts hydrogen from α-carbon of carbonyl compound to form carbanion.

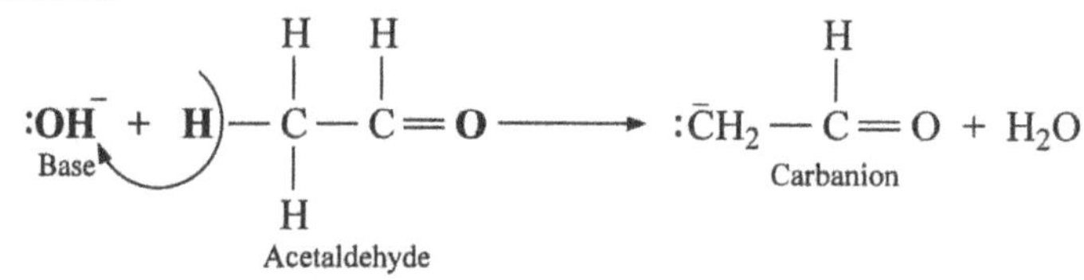

The nucleophilic carbanion attack carbonyl carbon of second molecule to form an anion, which picks up a proton from water to form aldol.

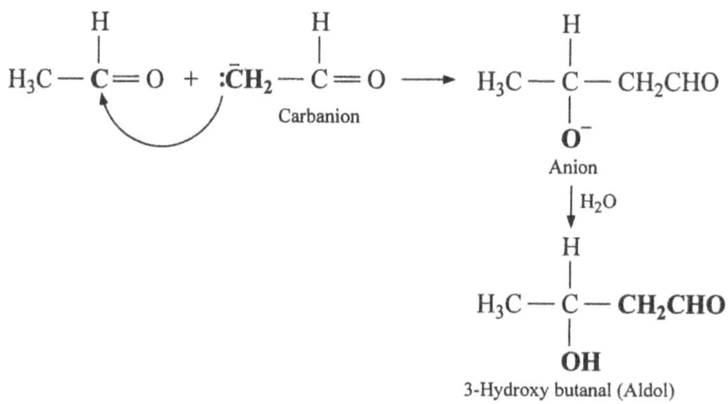

7. ***Reduction of Carboxylic Acids*** Carboxylic acids can be reduced by $LiAlH_4$ to form primary alcohols.

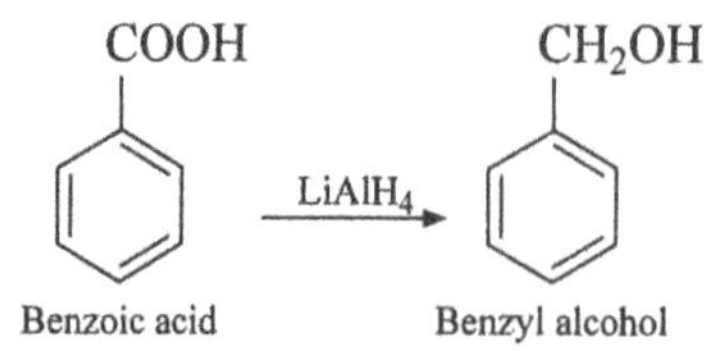

8. ***Hydroxylation of Alkenes*** Vicinal glycols (1,2-dihydroxy compounds) are prepared from alkenes on treatment with a cold aqueous potassium permanganate solution. This

reaction is commonly termed as hydroxylation, during which two hydroxyl groups are attached to double-bonded carbon atoms of alkene.

$$\underset{\text{Alkene}}{>C=C<} \xrightarrow[\text{or } HCO_2OH]{\text{Cold alkaline } KMnO_4} \underset{\text{Glycol}}{-\underset{OH}{\underset{|}{C}}-\underset{OH}{\underset{|}{C}}-}$$

$$\underset{\text{Propylene}}{H_3C-CH=CH_2} \xrightarrow[\text{or } HCO_2OH]{\text{Cold alkaline } KMnO_4} \underset{\text{Propylene glycol}}{H_3C-\underset{OH}{\underset{|}{CH}}-\underset{OH}{\underset{|}{CH_2}}}$$

14.5 INDUSTRIAL MANUFACTURE OF ETHYL ALCOHOL

At industrial scale, ethyl alcohol is prepared from molasses by fermentation process. Molasses is the dark brown-coloured mother liquor left after the crystallisation of cane sugar from concentrated sugar cane juice. Molasses contains about 50% uncrystallisable cane sugar, glucose and fructose. Molasses is diluted with water so that it contains 10% sugar. Requisite quantities of ammonium salts (ammonium sulphate and phosphate) are added which act as substrate for the growth of yeast.

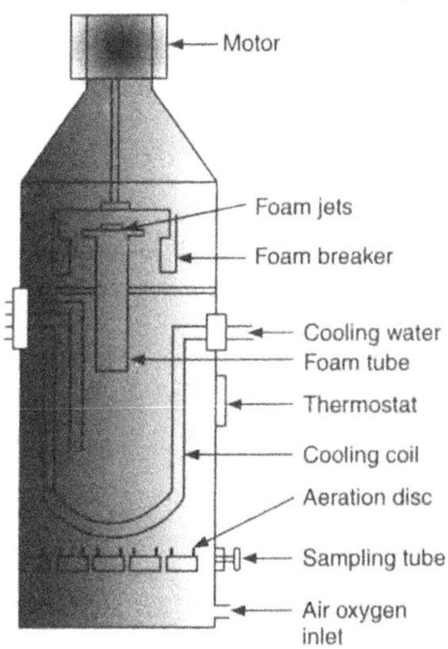

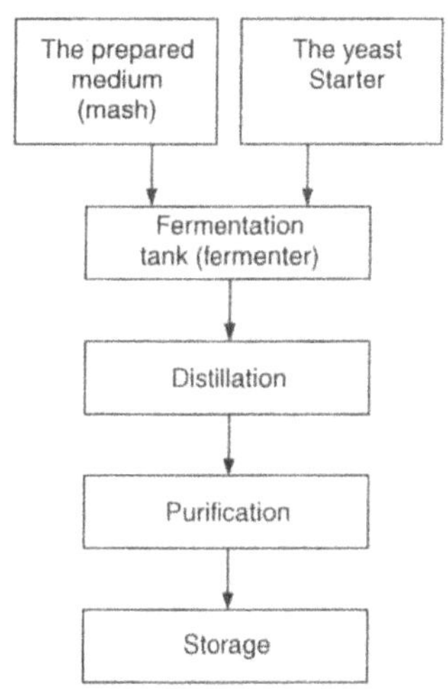

The solution is now transferred to a fermentation tank and yeast is added to it. The temperature is maintained at 30°C and kept for 2 to 3 days. Yeast is the source of enzymes which act as catalysts. In the first step, cane sugar is converted into glucose and fructose by the enzyme *invertase*.

$$C_{12}H_{22}O_{11} + H_2O \xrightarrow{\text{Invertase}} \underset{\text{Glucose}}{C_6H_{12}O_6} + \underset{\text{Fructose}}{C_6H_{12}O_6}$$

In the second step, enzyme *zymase* converts glucose and fructose into ethyl alcohol.

$$C_6H_{12}O_6 \xrightarrow{\text{Zymase}} \underset{\text{Ethyl alcohol}}{2H_3CCH_2-OH} + CO_2$$

The liquor so produced in fermentation tank is technically called wash. It contains a large quantity of water, small quantities of higher alcohols, acids and glycerol besides 10–15% ethyl alcohol. The wash is then subjected to fractional distillation to obtain 96% alcohol. This is commercially known as rectified spirit. The remaining 4% of water is removed by using quick lime or magnesium ethoxide to make absolute alcohol.

14.6 INDUSTRIAL MANUFACTURE OF METHYL ALCOHOL

Methanol is manufactured by a method different from that used in the preparation of other alcohols. The naphtha fraction obtained from the distillation of crude petroleum is used as a raw material for the manufacture of methanol. When naphtha is reacted with a high steam ratio, under pressure and at high temperature, synthesis gas of low methane content is obtained. Most of the carbon from the naphtha is converted to carbon monoxide and carbon dioxide which can be removed from the gaseous mixture to leave hydrogen of high purity.

$$\underset{}{C} + H_2O \xrightarrow{1000^\circ C} \underset{\text{Carbon monoxide}}{CO} + \underset{\text{Hydrogen}}{H_2}$$

When a mixture of hydrogen and carbon monoxide in the ratio 2 : 1 is passed over a catalyst (e.g. a mixture of zinc oxide and chromium oxide) under high pressure and at high temperature, methanol is formed.

$$CO + 2H_2 \xrightarrow{400^\circ C} \underset{\text{Methanol}}{CH_3OH}$$

Uses of methanol Methanol is an important industrial material and it is used

1. in the manufacture of formaldehyde,
2. as a solvent in the paint and varnish industry, and
3. as an anti-freeze in car radiators.

14.7 PHYSICAL PROPERTIES OF ALCOHOLS

1. The alcohols are colourless, neutral compounds with a characteristic smell.
2. The lower alcohols are liquids while higher ones are colourless, waxy solids.
3. The alcohols exhibit the phenomenon of hydrogen bonding due to binding of hydrogen atom to a highly electronegative element such as oxygen. The covalent bond between oxygen and hydrogen is unequally shared and results in a dipole. These dipoles induce electrostatic forces of attraction between molecules of alcohol. As a result alcohols exist in the form of associated molecules and thus exhibit high melting and boiling points.

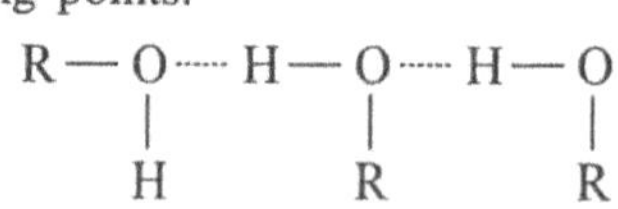

4. Branching will tend to decrease the boiling point since a more symmetrical molecule will have less London Dispersion forces and more hydrocarbon branching around

the carbinol carbon results in the hydrogen bonding of fewer molecules and, therefore, the compound can be vapourised at a lower temperature, e.g. 1-butanol, 3-methyl-1-propanol, 2-butanol, and 2-methyl-2-propanol boils at 118°C, 108°C, 100°C, and 83°C, respectively.

5. Due to the existence of hydrogen bonding between the molecules of alcohols, the boiling points of alcohols are higher than those of hydrocarbons or ethers of comparable molecular weights.
6. The lower alcohols are highly soluble in water but the solubility decreases with the increase in molecular weights. Alcohols with four or more carbons have a much lower water solubility. The high solubility of lower alcohols is due to the formation of intermolecular hydrogen bonds with water. The polar water molecules are attracted to the hydroxyl group by hydrogen bonding that occurs between the hydrogens of the water molecules and the oxygen of the alcohol. In case of lower alcohol molecules the water can more easily surround alcohol molecules thus effectively separating them from one another. This is called *solvation* and alcohol molecule is easily encapsulated in a water cage. The high molecular weight alcohol molecules require more water.

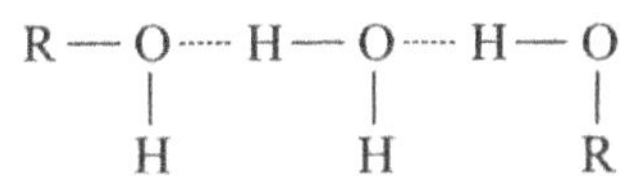

14.8 CHEMICAL PROPERTIES OF ALCOHOLS

1. ***Acidity of Alcohols*** Alcohols are capable of losing the hydrogen atom and thereby act as an acid. The acidity of alcohols is very much comparable to that of water. That is, both water and most alcohols have pK_as in the range of 15–16 (pK_a of alcohol =15; pK_a of water =14).

$$\text{HOH} + \text{CH}_3\text{O}^{\ominus} \rightleftharpoons {}^{\ominus}\text{OH} + \text{CH}_3\text{OH}$$

Water and alcohols have about the same acidity, which also means that hydroxide ion and alkoxide ions have approximately the same base strength.

2. ***Reaction with Metals*** Alcohols react with active metals like sodium, potassium, magnesium and aluminium to liberate hydrogen and form metal alkoxides. This reaction suggests that alcohols are acidic in nature. The general order of reactivity in this type of reactions is primary alcohol > secondary alcohol > tertiary alcohol.

$$\underset{\text{Alcohol}}{\text{ROH}} + \underset{\text{Metal}}{\text{M}} \longrightarrow \underset{\text{Metal alkoxide}}{\text{RO}^-\text{M}^+} + \text{H}\uparrow$$

$$\underset{\text{Ethyl alcohol}}{2\text{CH}_3\text{CH}_2\text{OH}} + \underset{\text{Sodium}}{\text{Na}} \longrightarrow \underset{\text{Metal alkoxide}}{\text{CH}_3\text{CH}_2\text{O}^-\text{Na}^+} + \text{H}_2\uparrow$$

3. ***Reaction with Grignard Reagent*** Alcohols react with Grignard reagents to produce hydrocarbons. In this reaction, active hydrogen of alcohol reacts with nucleophilic organic group of Grignard reagent and yields alkane and magnesium salt of alcohol.

$$\underset{\text{Alcohol}}{ROH} + \underset{\text{Grignard reagent}}{R'MgX} \longrightarrow \underset{\text{Alkane}}{R'X} + ROMgX$$

$$\underset{\text{Methyl alcohol}}{CH_3OH} + \underset{\text{Grignard reagent}}{CH_3MgX} \longrightarrow \underset{\text{Methane}}{CH_4} + CH_3OMgX$$

4. ***Dehydration of Alcohols*** Alcohols by dehydration, i.e. elimination of a molecule of water in presence of an acid (Lewis acid) and heat (200°C) yield alkenes. This is an α, β-elimination reaction.

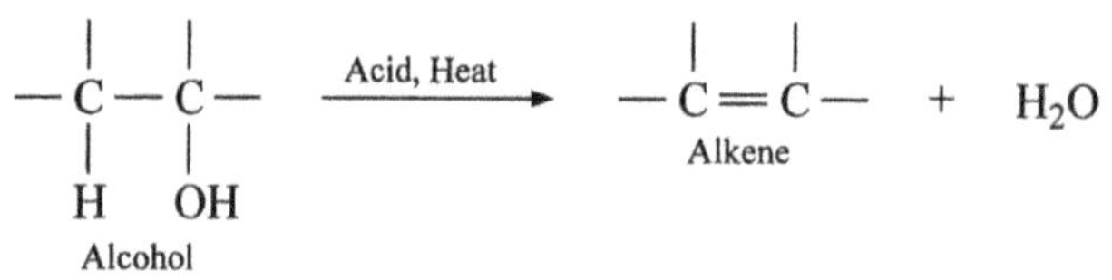

$$\underset{n\text{-Butanol}}{CH_3CH_2CH_2CH_2OH} \xrightarrow[200^\circ C]{H_2SO_4} \underset{\text{2-Butene}}{CH_3CH{=}CHCH_3} + \underset{\text{1-Butene}}{CH_3CH_2CH{=}CH_2}$$

5. ***Reaction of Alcohols with Hydrogen Halides*** Alcohols react with hydrogen halides to yield alkyl halides and water. The reaction is carried out either by passing the dry hydrogen halide gas into the alcohol or by heating the alcohol with concentrated aqueous acid. The reactivity of alcohols toward HX is in the order of allyl, benzyl > 3° > 2° > 1° < CH_3. The reaction is catalysed by acids.

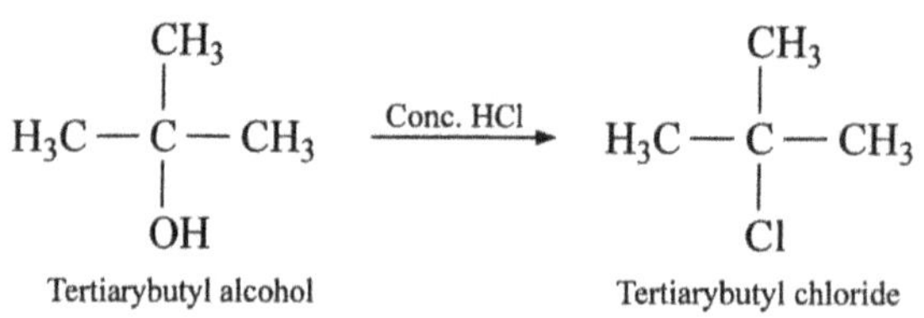

Mechanism This reaction takes place by nucleophilic substitution. The mechanism of the substitution reaction depends on the structure of the alcohol. Tertiary and secondary alcohols undergo S_N1 reaction.

$$\underset{\text{Alcohol}}{ROH} + HX \rightleftharpoons \underset{\text{Protonated alcohol}}{R\overset{+}{O}H_2} + X^-$$

$$\underset{\text{Protonated alcohol}}{R\overset{+}{O}H_2} \rightleftharpoons \underset{\text{Carbocation}}{R^+} + H_2O$$

$$\underset{\text{Carbocation}}{R^+} + X^- \longrightarrow \underset{\text{Alkyl halide}}{RX}$$

Primary alcohols cannot undergo S_N1 reactions because 1° carbocations are unstable hence they undergo S_N2 mechanism.

$$[\overset{\delta^-}{X} \cdots R \cdots \overset{\delta^+}{O}H_2] \longrightarrow \underset{\text{Alkyl halide}}{X{-}R} + H_2O$$

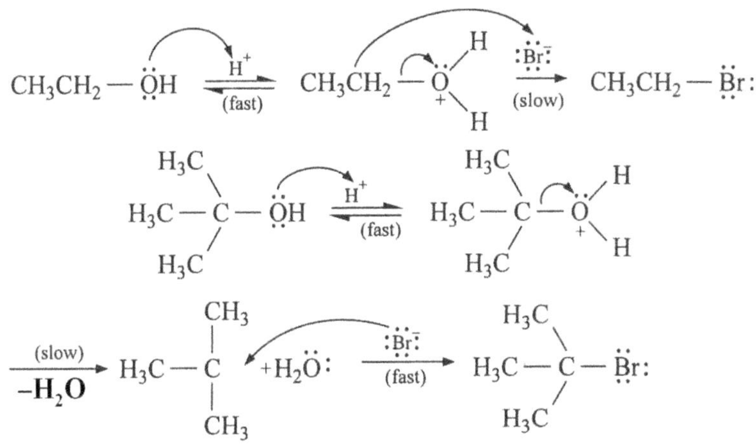

6. ***Oxidation of Alcohols*** Alcohols undergo oxidation. The product formed by oxidation of an alcohol depends upon the type of alcohol (1°, 2° or 3°). The reagents commonly used for the oxidation of alcohols are acidic solutions of potassium permanganate, sodium dichromate, sodium chromate or chromic anhydride. These oxidising agents oxidise primary alcohols to aldehydes. The reaction, however, does not stop at the aldehyde, the aldehyde is further oxidised to a carboxylic acid.

$$\underset{\text{Ethyl alcohol}}{CH_3CH_2OH} \xrightarrow[H_2SO_4]{Na_2Cr_2O_7} \underset{\text{Acetaldehyde}}{CH_3CHO} \xrightarrow{\text{Further oxidation}} \underset{\text{Acetic acid}}{CH_3COOH}$$

The oxidation of primary alcohol can be stopped at the aldehyde formation level by using a milder oxidising agent (pyridinium chlorochromate) or by contact with copper metal at high temperatures.

$$\underset{\text{Primary alcohol}}{RCH_2OH} \xrightarrow[\text{or Cu, Heating}]{\text{Pyridinium chlorochromate}} \underset{\text{Aldehyde}}{RCHO}$$

Secondary alcohols are oxidised to ketones by using oxidising agents or by heating with copper.

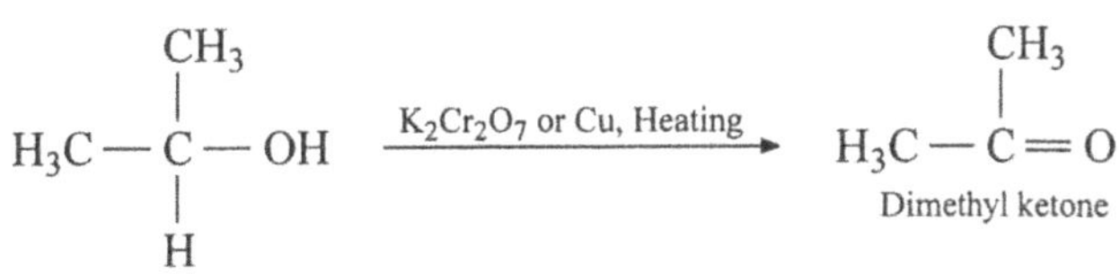

Tertiary alcohols are not at all oxidised under alkaline conditions.

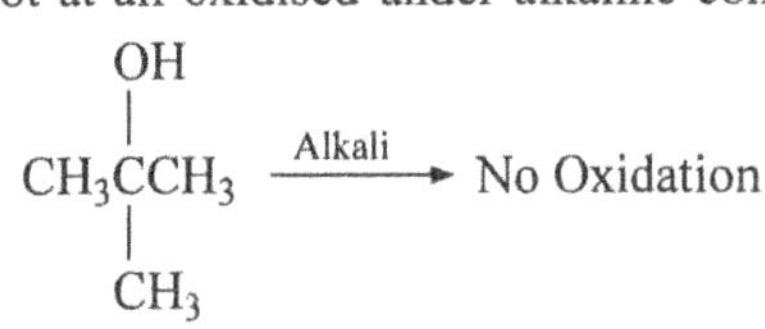

7. ***Reaction with Phosphorous Trihalides*** Alcohols can also be converted into alkyl halides using phosphorous tribromide (PBr_3), phosphorous trichloride (PCl_3) or thionyl

chloride ($SOCl_2$). These reagents convert the alcohol into an intermediate with a leaving group that is readily displaced by a halide ion.

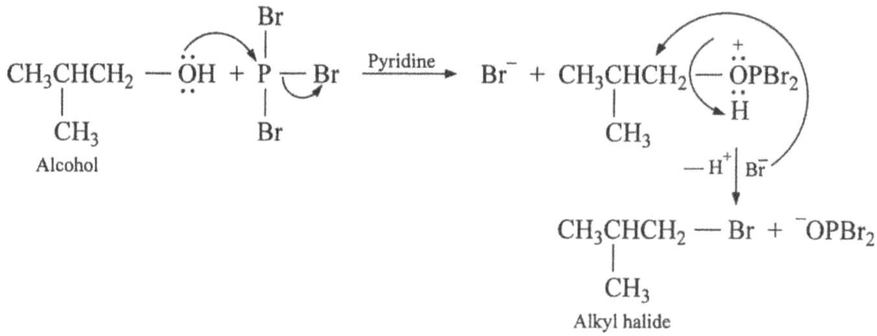

8. ***Reaction with Sulphonyl Chloride*** When alcohol reacts with a sulphonyl chloride (para-toluene sulphonyl chloride or methane sulphonyl chloride) a sulphonate ester is formed.

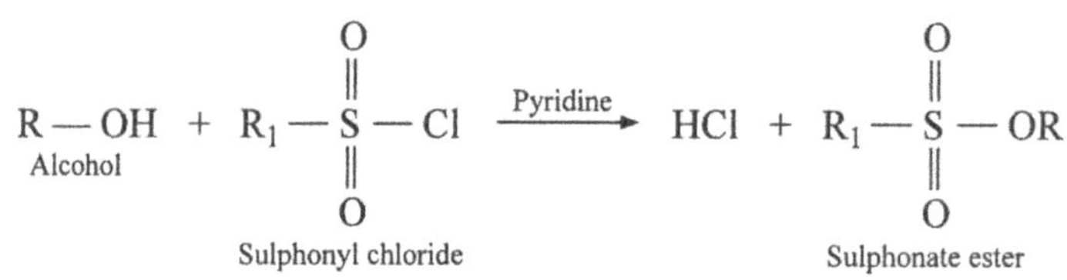

9. ***Reaction with Acids*** Alcohols react with organic acids to form esters. The reaction is reversible and is carried out in the presence of concentrated sulphuric acid or dry hydrogen chloride. This reaction is known as *esterification*. Inorganic acids such as nitric acid, too react with alcohols to form esters.

$$\underset{\text{Alcohol}}{R-OH} + \underset{\text{Carboxylic acid}}{R'CO-OH} \xrightleftharpoons{H^+} \underset{\text{Ester}}{R'COOR} + H_2O$$

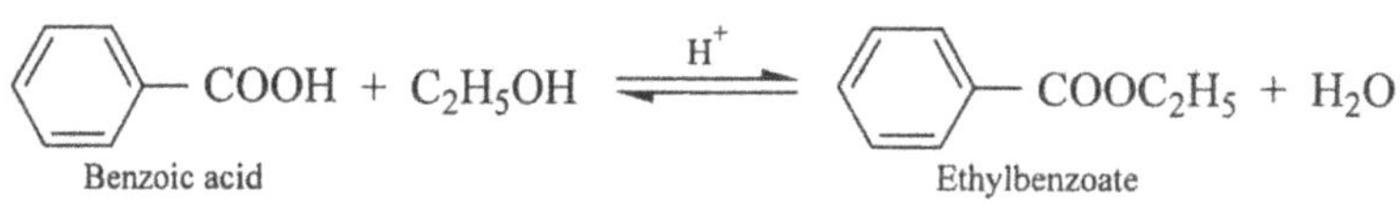

14.9 CHEMICAL DISTINCTION AMONG PRIMARY, SECONDARY AND TERTIARY ALCOHOLS

The following tests are used to distinguish three classes of alcohols from one another:

1. ***Lucas Test*** This test involves treating the alcohol with Lucas reagent (mixture of concentrated hydrochloric acid and anhydrous zinc chloride). Appearance of cloudiness in the reaction mixture due to formation of alkyl chloride indicates the conversion of alcohol into alkyl chloride. Tertiary alcohol develops cloudiness immediately, secondary alcohol reacts within five minutes while a primary alcohol does not react at room temperature.

$$\underset{\text{Alcohol}}{ROH} + HCl \xrightarrow{ZnCl_2} \underset{\text{Alkyl chloride}}{RCl} + H_2O$$

$$\underset{\text{Propan-2-ol}}{H_3CH\underset{\underset{OH}{|}}{C}H_3C} + HCl \xrightarrow{ZnCl_2} \underset{\text{2-Chloropropane}}{H_3CH\underset{\underset{Cl}{|}}{C}H_3C} + H_2O$$

$$\underset{\text{Tertiarybutylalcohol}}{H_3C-\overset{\overset{CH_3}{|}}{\underset{\underset{CH_3}{|}}{C}}-OH} + HCl \xrightarrow{ZnCl_2} \underset{\text{Tertiarybutyl chloride}}{H_3C-\overset{\overset{CH_3}{|}}{\underset{\underset{CH_3}{|}}{C}}-Cl} + H_2O$$

2. ***Victor Meyer's Test*** The given alcohol is treated with phosphorus and iodine to form alkyl iodide. The alkyl iodide is then treated with silver nitrite to get the corresponding nitroalkane. The nitroalkane is finally treated with nitrous acid and made alkaline. The formation of blood-red colouration shows the original alcohol is primary, a blue colouration indicates the secondary alcohol while the solution remains colourless in case of tertiary alcohol.

$$\underset{\text{Primary alcohol}}{RCH_2OH} \xrightarrow{P + I_2} RCH_2I \xrightarrow{AgNO_2} RCH_2NO_2 \xrightarrow{HNO_2} \underset{\text{Nitrolic acid}}{R-\overset{\overset{NOH}{\|}}{C}-NO_2}$$

(Develops blood-red colour with alkali)

$$\underset{\text{Secondary alcohol}}{R_2CHOH} \xrightarrow{P + I_2} R_2CHI \xrightarrow{AgNO_2} R_2CHNO_2 \xrightarrow{HNO_2} \underset{\text{Pseudo nitrile}}{R_2\overset{\overset{NO}{|}}{C}-NO_2}$$

(Develops blue colour with alkali)

$$\underset{\text{Tertiary alcohol}}{R_3COH} \xrightarrow{P + I_2} R_3CI \xrightarrow{AgNO_2} R_3CNO_2 \xrightarrow{HNO_2} \text{No reaction}$$

3. ***Oxidation Test*** The basis of this test is that different alcohols give different products on oxidation. A primary alcohol gives an aldehyde and then the corresponding acid containing the same number of carbon atoms as the original alcohol. Secondary alcohols form ketones containing the same number of carbon atoms but on further oxidation of ketones form acids containing lesser number of carbon atoms. Tertiary alcohols are resistant to oxidation.

$$\underset{\text{Ethyl alcohol}}{CH_3CH_2OH} \xrightarrow[H_2SO_4]{Na_2Cr_2O_7} \underset{\text{Acetaldehyde}}{CH_3CHO} \xrightarrow{\text{Further oxidation}} \underset{\text{Acetic acid}}{CH_3COOH}$$

$$\underset{\text{Secondary alcohol}}{R-\overset{\overset{R_1}{|}}{\underset{\underset{H}{|}}{C}}-OH} \xrightarrow{K_2Cr_2O_7\ \text{Cu, Heating}} \underset{\text{Ketone}}{R-\overset{\overset{R_1}{|}}{C}=O}$$

14.10 PHARMACEUTICAL COMPOUNDS

1. *Methyl alcohol* Methyl alcohol occurs is also called as methanol, carbinol or wood spirit. It acquired the name **"wood alcohol"** because it was produced as a byproduct of the destructive distillation of wood. It is a light, volatile, colorless, flammable liquid with a distinctive odor very similar to that of ethanol. The molecular formula of methanol is CH_3OH. Methanol is manufactured by the reaction between carbon monoxide and hydrogen in the presence of copper chromite catalysts.

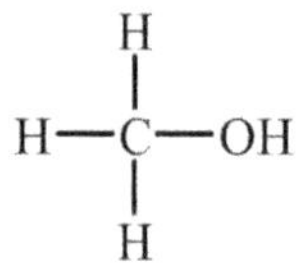

Uses

1. Methanol is primarily used as an industrial solvent for inks, resins, adhesives and dyes.
2. It is also used as a solvent in the manufacture of cholesterol, streptomycin, vitamins, hormones, and other pharmaceuticals.
3. Methanol is also used as an antifreeze for automotive radiators, an ingredient of gasoline (as an antifreezing agent and octane booster), and as fuel for picnic stoves. Methanol is also an ingredient in paint and varnish removers.

Methanol is also used as an alternative motor fuel.

2. *Absolute Alcohol or Dehydrated Alcohol* Absolute alcohol contains 99.4% v/v or 99% w/w of ethanol. This can be prepared commercially by azeotropic distillation of ethanol and benzene mixture. Absolute alcohol is available as clear, colourless, mobile, volatile liquid. It is inflammable and boils at 78°C. It is miscible with water, ether and chloroform.

Absolute alcohol is mainly used as a chemical agent, but it has also been used for the local relief of pain in neuralgias and in carcinomas. It is also used as pharmaceutical aid (solvent).

3. *Dilute Alcohol* This alcohol contains 49% v/v of ethanol.

4. *Rectified Spirit or Denatured Alcohol* Rectified spirit or denatured alcohol is ethanol that has been renderd unfit for drinking and by adding certain substances is used for industrial and pharmaceutical purposes. A common practice is to add about 4% of methyl alcohol together with traces of pyridine and some colouring agents. Hence, this alcohol is also called as denatured alcohol which is obtained free from excise duty. This alcohol contains 90% v/v ethanol.

Rectified spirit is widely used in the preparation of a variety of pharmaceutical preparations including spirits, tinctures, and fluid extracts.

5. *Chlorbutanol* Chlorbutanol is a colourless, crystalline solid derivative of tertiary butyl alcohol. Chlorbutanol is prepared by mixing acetone with chloroform in presence of solid potassium hydroxide. Chlorbutanol has characteristic camphor-like odour. It is freely soluble in ethanol, ether, chloroform and slightly soluble in water. Chlorbutanol is used as a hypnotic and sedative.

$$\underset{\text{Acetone}}{(CH_3)_2CO} + \underset{\text{Chloroform}}{CHCl_3} \longrightarrow \underset{\text{Chlorbutanol}}{(CH_3)_2(CCl_3)\text{-}OH}$$

6. *Glycerine* Glycerine is a colourless trihydric alcohol. This can be obtained by the hydrolysis of oils and fats with alkali. Glycerine is available as clear, colourless, odourless, syrupy liquid. It is very hygroscopic and is miscible with water and ethanol. Glycerine is used as a lubricant, laxative and humectant.

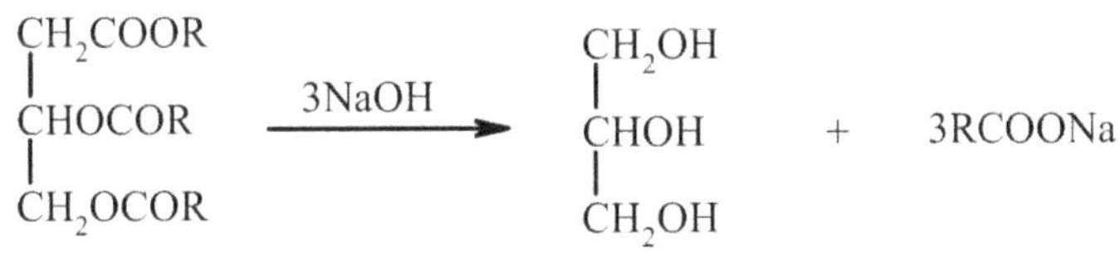

7. *Nitroglycerine* Nitroglycerine is a triester of glycerol and nitric acid. It is a colourless oily liquid and is prepared by adding glycerine slowly to a mixture of nitric acid and sulphuric acid at 200° C. Nitroglycerine has sweet, burning taste and is soluble in-organic solvents but slightly soluble in water. It is used in the treatment of angina pectoris and in the preparation of explosives.

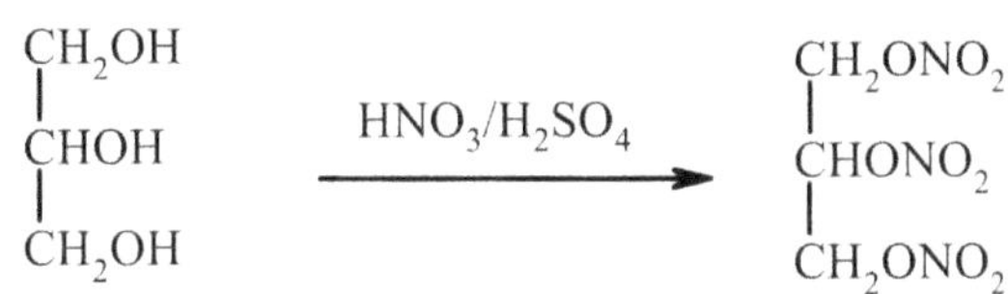

8. *Benzyl Alcohol* Benzyl alcohol is produced naturally by many plants and is commonly found in fruits and tea leaves. It is also found in a variety of essential oils including jasmine, hyacinth, and ylang-ylang. It is also called as phenyl methanol or phenyl carbinol. Benzyl alcohol is a colorless liquid with a mild pleasant aromatic odor which boils at 205 °C. Molecular formula of benzyl alcohol is C_7H_8O, it is synthesized by oxidation of toluene to form benzoic acid followed by esterification with methanol to produce methyl benzoate which on further hydrogenation yield benzyl alcohol.

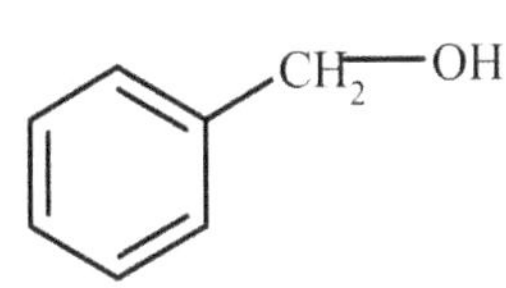

Uses

1. Benzyl alcohol is used as a bacteriostatic preservative at low concentration in intravenous medications, cosmetics and topical drugs.
2. 5% Benzyl alcohol is used effectively for treating lice.

9. ***Atenolol*** Chemically atenolol is (2-[4-[2-hydroxy (isopropylamino)propoxy]phenyl] acetamide. It is a β_1-selective (cardioselective) adrenoreceptor-blocking agent. The most straightforward method of preparing atenolol involves the reaction of 4-hydroxy-phenyl acetamide with epichlorhydrin, followed by the addition of isopropylamine at elevated temperatures for a long period of time.

(i) (a) 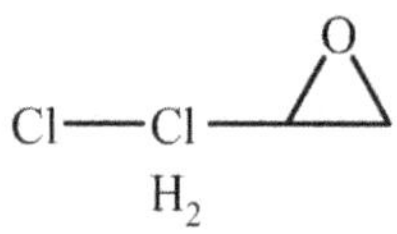

(b) Benzyltrimethylammonium chloride

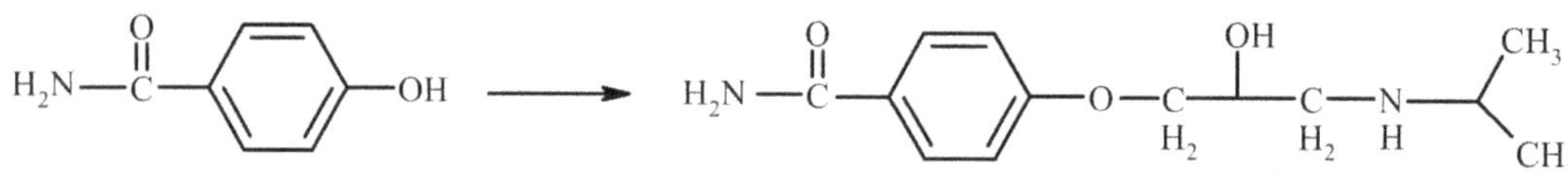

4-Hydroxyphenylacetamide

Atenolol

(ii) (a) 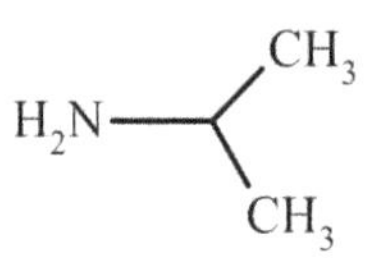

(b) H_2O

Atenolol is available as colourless powder. It is insoluble in ethanol and sparingly soluble in water. Atenolol is used as β-adrenoreceptor antagonist.

10. ***Cetostearyl Alcohol*** Cetostearyl alcohol is a mixture of solid aliphatic alcohols, mainly stearyl and cetyl alcohols, obtained by the reduction of appropriate fatty acids. It contains not less than 90% of stearyl and cetyl alcohols and not less than 40% of stearyl alcohol.

Cetostearyl alcohol is available as a colourless or cream-coloured unctuous mass or almost white flakes or granules with a faint characteristic odour. It melts between 49° and 56° C to a clear colourless or pale-yellow liquid. Practically, it is insoluble in water but soluble in ether.

Uses

1. Cetostearyl alcohol is used in creams, ointments, and other tropical preparations as a stiffening agent and an emulsion stabiliser.
2. It is also used to improve the emollient properties of paraffin ointments.

11. ***Mannitol*** Mannitol is a hexahydric alcohol related to mannose. It is isomeric with sorbitol. Commercially, mannitol is prepared from glucose or mannose by electrolytic or catalytic reduction.

Mannitol is available as a colourless crystalline powder, or granules with a sweet taste. Mannitol crystallised from alcohol possesses orthorhombic needles. It melts at 166°C. Mannitol is soluble in water (1 in 6 ml of water), very sparingly soluble in alcohol and practically insoluble in ether.

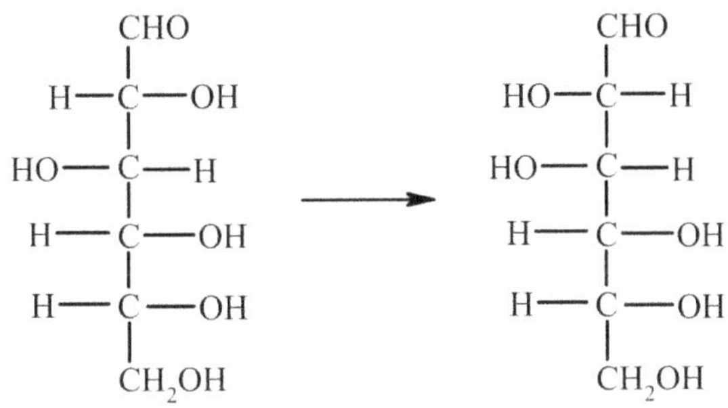

Glucose → Mannose

Uses

1. Mannitol is used (by intravenous infusion) as an osmotic diuretic.
2. It is used as filler for conventional tablets.
3. Mannitol is widely used as an excipient to prepare chewable tablets because of its negative heat of solution, its sweetness and its mouth feel.

12. *Sorbitol* Sorbitol was first isolated from the juice of Mountain Ash Berry *(Sorbus Americana),* in 1872, by the French chemist, Joseph Boressingault. Nowadays, it is prepared by high-pressure hydrogenation with copper-chromium or nickel catalyst or by electrolytic reduction of glucose.

Sorbitol is available as colourless, crystalline, odourless, hygroscopic powder. Sorbitol has a pleasant, cooling, sweet taste and has approximately 50-60% the sweetness of sucrose.

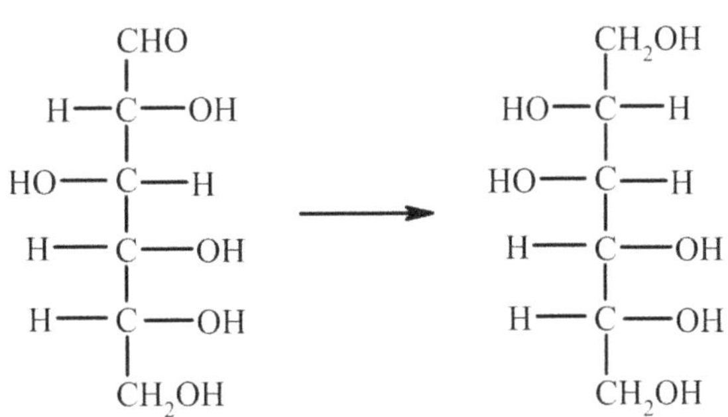

Glucose → Sorbitol

Uses

1. Sorbitol is widely used as an excipient in pharmaceutical formulations. It is used as a dilutent in tablet formulations.

2. It is used extensively in cosmetics and food products.
3. Sorbitol is used in injectable and topical preparations.
4. Therapeutically, sorbitol is used as an osmotic laxative.

13. *Propylene Glycol* Propylene glycol, also called propane 1,2-diol, is a synthetic organic compound with the chemical formula $C_3H_8O_2$. It is a viscous, colorless and nearly odorless liquid but possesses a faintly sweet taste. Chemically it is classed as a diol and boils at 188.2 ^oC.

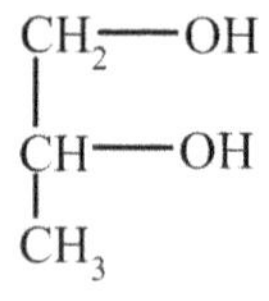

Uses

1. It is an effective humectant.
2. It is a solvent for fragrances and preservatives.
3. It can be used as an emulsifier or co-surfactant.
4. It can be used as a preservative due to its antifungal and antimicrobial properties.
5. It is frequently used in deodorants and antiperspirants.
6. It is found in hand cleansers and disinfecting gels.
7. It is a common additive in shaving creams and gels.

14. *Dimercaprol* Dimercaprol is 2,3-dimercaptopropand. Dimercaprol is a sulphur analogue of glycerin. It is prepared from allyl alcohol by the following chemical reactions.

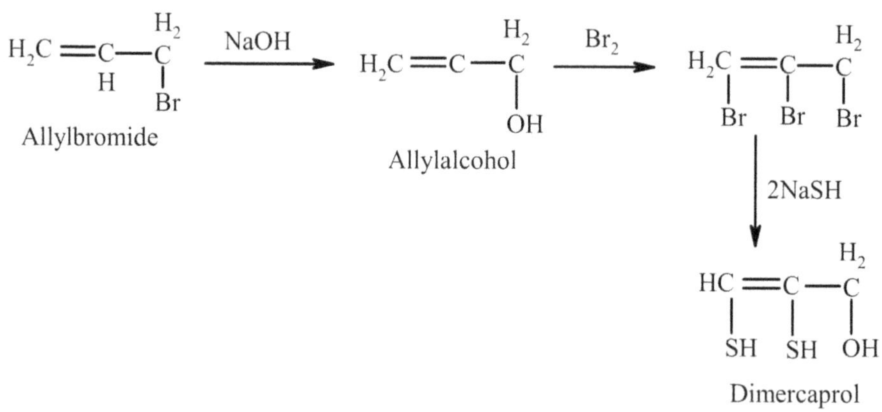

Dimercaprol is a colourless liquid having characteristic onion-like odour.

Use Dimercaprol is used as an antidote for arsenical poisoning.

15. *Menthol* Menthol occurs in peppermint oil. It is a low melting (43°C), colourless solid and is optically active. The molecular formula of menthol is $C_{10}H_{20}O$. Menthol is prepared from Pulegone or menthone by reduction.

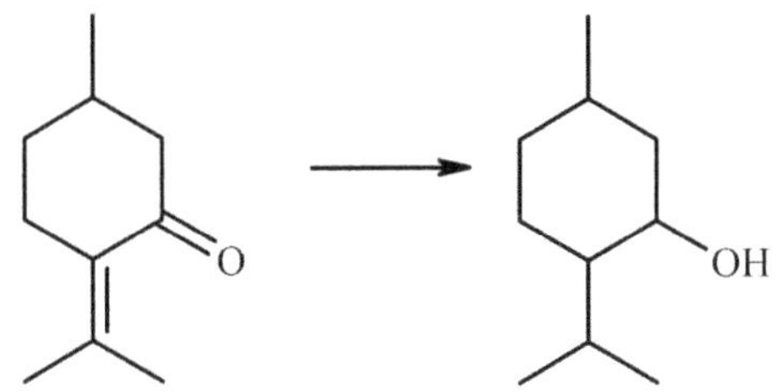

Uses

1. Menthol is used as conter-irritant to relieve local irritations.
2. It has anti-pruritic effect.
3. Menthol has been used for the relief of headache, neuralgia and nasalcongestion.

16. *Salbutamol* Salbutamol is an adrenergic agent. It is an amino alcohol derivative. Chemically, salbutamol is 1-(4-hydroxy-3-hydroxymethylphenyl)-2-(tertiarybutylamino) ethanol.

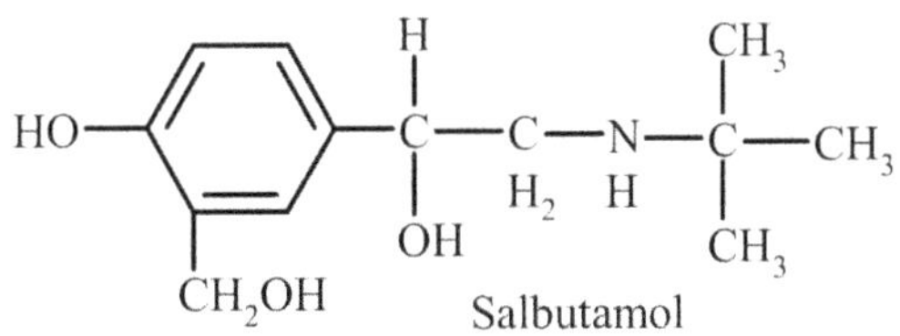

Salbutamol

Salbutamol is prepared from 4-hydroxy-3-hydroxymethylbenzaldehyde by acetylation with acetic anhydride followed by treatment with tertiary butyl cyanide and reduction.

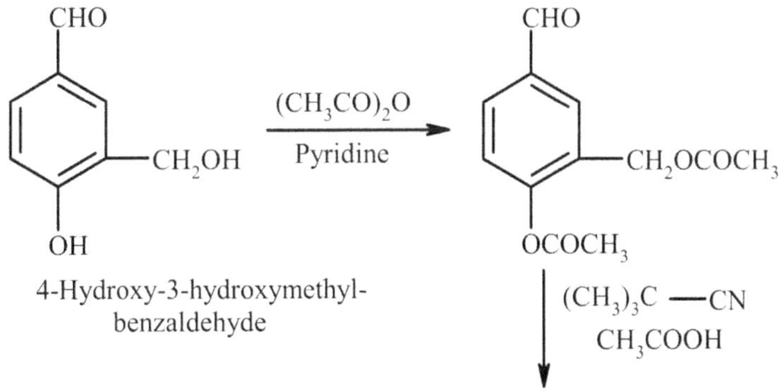

4-Hydroxy-3-hydroxymethyl-benzaldehyde

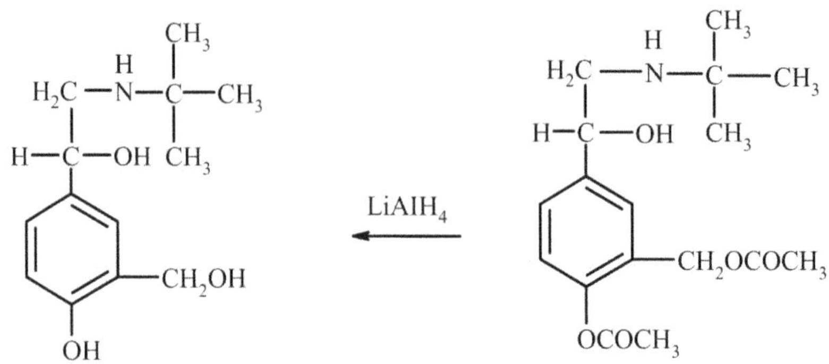

Salbutamol

Salbutamol is a colourless crystalline powder. It melts at 156°C. Salbutamol is soluble in water, alcohol and slightly soluble in ether.

Uses

1. Salbutamol is a sympathomimetric agent.
2. It is used as a bronchodialator.
3. It is used for prevention of premature labour.

PRACTICE QUESTIONS

1. (a) Explain and give equations for the methods of preparation of primary, secondary and tertiary alcohols by using Grignard reagent as one of the reactions.
   (b) 0.6 g of a saturated primary alcohol A on reaction with excess of metallic sodium liberated 224 ml of hydrogen gas at STP. Determine the molecular formula and structure of A. Also, write the isomer of A if any.
2. (a) Ethyl alcohol is having high boiling point and high water solubility than dimethylether. Justify the statement.
   (b) Neopentyl alcohol when treated with hydrochloric acid gives tertiary pentylchloride but not neopentylchloride. Comment.
   (c) How do you effect the following conversions:
      (i) Acetone to tertiary butylalcohol
      (ii) *n*-propanol to isopropanol
      (iii) Ethanol to *n*-propanol
      (iv) Ethanol to chloroform
3. How will you distinguish the following pairs of compounds in the laboratory:
   (a) *n*-Propyl alcohol and isopropyl alcohol
   (b) Ethyl alcohol and *t*-butyl alcohol
   (c) Methyl alcohol and ethyl alcohol
4. Compound (A) of molecular formula $C_4H_{10}O$ reacts with Leuca's reagent in 5 minutes. On oxidation, it gives a compound B of molecular formula C_4H_2O. Compound B gives an organe- red precipitate with 2,4-DNP reagent but fails to give Tollen's test and Fehling's test. On treatment with iodine in sodium hydroxide solution. Compound B

gives iodoform and sodium propionate. What are compounds A and B? Explain all the reactions mentioned.

5. (a) Write various methods of preparation of alcohols.
   (b) What is the reactivity of different classes of alcohols during dehydration? Justify your answer with a suitable example.
6. Name the reagents and explain the chemistry involved in the following conversions:
   (a) Ethanol to aldohol
   (b) Ethanol to butan-l-ol
7. Give the method of preparation and uses of:
   (a) Chlorbutol
   (b) Atenolol
   (c) Nitroglycerine
   (d) Mannitol
   (e) Sorbitol
   (f) Dimercaprol
   (g) Menthol
8. Give the uses of:
   (a) Chlorobutol
   (b) Dimercaprol
   (c) Cetostearyl alcohol
   (d) Atenolol
9. Define and classify monohydric alcohols with examples? Discuss the oxidation of different types of alcohols?
10. Write notes on:
    (a) Aldol condensation
    (b) Oxymercuration-demercuration
    (c) Hydroboration-oxidation
    (d) Dehydration of alcohols
    (e) Meerwein-Pondorf-Verley reduction
    (f) Mechanism of Lucas test
11. Very briefly explain why we would expect many similarities in reactions of alcohols and water.

15

CHEMISTRY OF ETHERS AND EPOXIDES

15.1 INTRODUCTION

Ethers are a class of organic compounds containing a C—O—C linkage. They have the general formula of R—O—R. The two R groups may be identical (symmetrical ethers) or different (unsymmetrical ethers). Both R groups may be alkyl or aryl or one may be alkyl and the other may be aryl. For example,

$CH_3 — O — CH_3$	Dimethyl ether (Methoxy methane)
$CH_3 — O — C_2H_5$	Ethyl methyl ether (Methoxyethane)
$C_2H_5 — O — C_2H_5$	Diethyl ether (Ethoxyethane)
$C_6H_5 — O — CH_3$	Methylphenyl ether or Anisole (Methoxybenzene)
$C_6H_5 — O — C_6H_5$	Diphenyl ether (Phenoxybenzene)

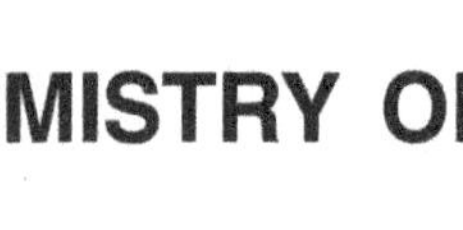

2-Methoxy-2-methylpropane
tert-butyl methyl ether

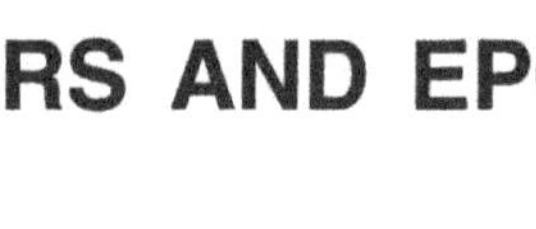

4-Ethoxy-2-methyl-1-hexene

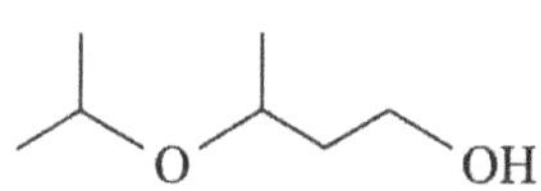

3-Isopropoxy-1-butanol

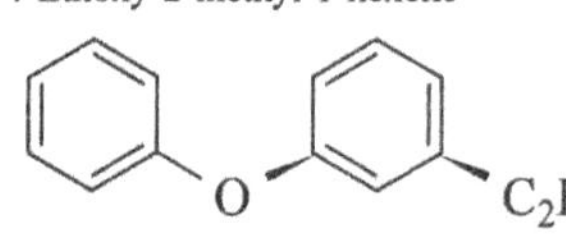

cis-1-Ethyl-3-phenoxycyclohexane

Many simple ethers are symmetrical, in that the two alkyl substituents are the same. These are named as 'dialkyl ethers'. Examples are: $CH_3CH_2OCH_2CH_3$, diethyl ether (sometimes referred to as ether), and $CH_3OCH_2CH_2OCH_3$, ethylene glycol dimethyl ether (glyme).

15.2 NOMENCLATURE OF ETHERS

According to IUPAC system, ethers are considered as alkoxy (—OR) derivatives of hydrocarbons. In case of unsymmetrical ethers, the R group having the larger number

Alkyl Group	*Name*	*Alkoxy Group*	*Name*
CH_3 —	Methyl	CH_3O —	Methoxy
CH_3CH_2 —	Ethyl	CH_3CH_2O —	Ethoxy
$(CH_3)_2CH$ —	Isopropyl	$(CH_3)_2CHO$ —	Isopropoxy
$(CH_3)_3C$ —	tert-Butyl	$(CH_3)_3CO$ —	tert-Butoxy
C_6H_5 —	Phenyl	C_6H_5O —	Phenoxy

CH_3—O—C_2H_5 Ethyl methyl ether (Methoxyethane)

C_6H_5—O—CH_3 Methylphenyl ether or Anisole (Methoxybenzene)

of carbon atoms is chosen as the parent hydrocarbon while the other group along with oxygen is taken as alkoxy group.

15.3 FUNCTIONAL ISOMERISM

This isomerism is due to the presence of different functional groups in compounds having the same molecular formula. For example, the molecular formula C_2H_6O represents two compounds

$$\underset{\text{Ethanol}}{CH_3CH_2OH} \quad \text{and} \quad \underset{\text{Dimethyl ether}}{H_3C-O-CH_3}$$

These compounds have different physical and chemical properties due to the presence of different functional groups.

15.4 GENERAL METHODS OF PREPARATION

Ethers may be prepared by the following methods.

1. ***Acid Catalysed Intermolecular Dehydration of Alcohols*** When an excess of alcohol is heated with concentrated H_2SO_4 at 135°C, two moles of the alcohol lose one mole of water to form symmetrical ether. Diethyl ether is prepared in the laboratory and on the large scale by heating a mixture of ethyl alcohol and concentrated sulphuric acid at 135°C on a sand bath. The ether obtained in this way contains water, alcohol and sulphurous acid, from which it must be freed. It is, therefore, washed by shaking in a separating funnel with a small quantity of dilute sodium hydroxide solution. The ether obtained after washing is dried with small pieces of anhydrous calcium chloride.

$$\underset{\text{Alcohol}}{R-OH} \xrightarrow[135°C]{H_2SO_4} \underset{\text{Ether}}{R-O-R} + H_2O$$

$$\underset{\text{Ethyl alcohol}}{C_2H_5-OH} \xrightarrow[135°C]{H_2SO_4} \underset{\text{Diethyl ether}}{C_2H_5-O-C_2H_5} + H_2O$$

At temperatures from 110° to 130°C, an S_N2 reaction of the alcohol conjugate acid leads to an ether product. At higher temperatures (over 150°C) E2 elimination takes place.

$$2CH_3CH_2-OH + H_2SO_4 \xrightarrow{130°C} CH_3CH_2-O-CH_2CH_3 + H_2O$$

$$CH_3CH_2-OH + H_2SO_4 \xrightarrow{150°C} CH_2=CH_2 + H_2O$$

Mechanism This reaction involves an initial protonation of one molecule of the alcohol followed by an S_N2 type of substitution on another alcohol molecule.

$$\underset{\text{Ethyl alcohol}}{C_2H_5-OH} \xrightarrow{H^+} \underset{\text{Protonated alcohol}}{C_2H_5-\overset{+}{O}H-H} \longrightarrow \underset{\text{Ethyl carbocation}}{{}^+C_2H_5} + H_2O$$

$$\underset{\text{Ethyl carbocation}}{{}^+C_2H_5} + C_2H_5-OH \longrightarrow \underset{\text{Protonated ether}}{C_2H_5-\overset{+}{O}(C_2H_5)-H} \longrightarrow \underset{\text{Diethyl ether}}{C_2H_5-O-C_2H_5} + H^+$$

This preparation of ethers is rather severely limited to primary alcohols, secondary and tertiary alcohols, which lead to form alkenes (elimination products).

2. ***Williamson's Synthesis*** This is the most important and widely used method to prepare both symmetrical and unsymmetrical ethers. This is carried out by treating an alkyl halide with sodium alkoxide or sodium phenoxide. This reaction involves nucleophilic substitution of alkoxide or phenoxide for the halogen of alkyl halide. To prepare methyl ethers, methyl sulphate is used instead of methyl halides.

$$\underset{\text{Sodium alkoxide}}{R'ONa} + \underset{\text{Alkyl halide}}{RX} \longrightarrow \underset{\text{Ether}}{R'-O-R} + NaX$$

$$\underset{\text{Sodium ethoxide}}{C_2H_5ONa} + C_2H_5I \longrightarrow \underset{\text{Diethyl ether}}{C_2H_5-O-C_2H_5} + NaI$$

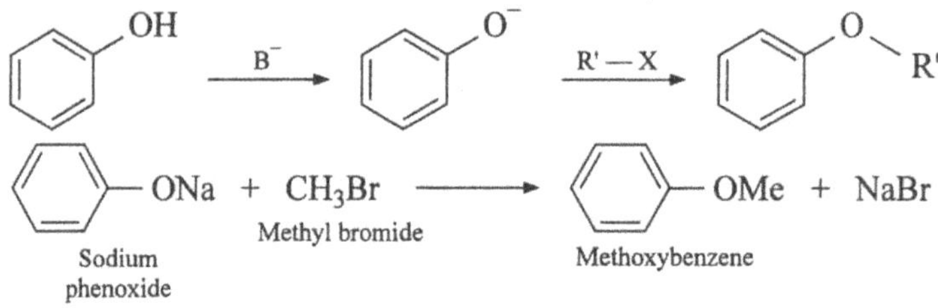

15.4.1 Reaction Type: Nucleophilic Substitution

Mechanism *Williamson ether synthesis* proceeds by an S_N2 reaction of an alkoxide nucleophile with an alkyl halide. Reactions 1 and 2 below are two examples of this procedure. Since alkoxide anions are strong bases, the possibility of a competing E2 elimination must always be considered. Thus, Reaction 1 gives a better and cleaner yield of benzyl isopropyl ether than does Reaction 2, which generates considerable elimination product.

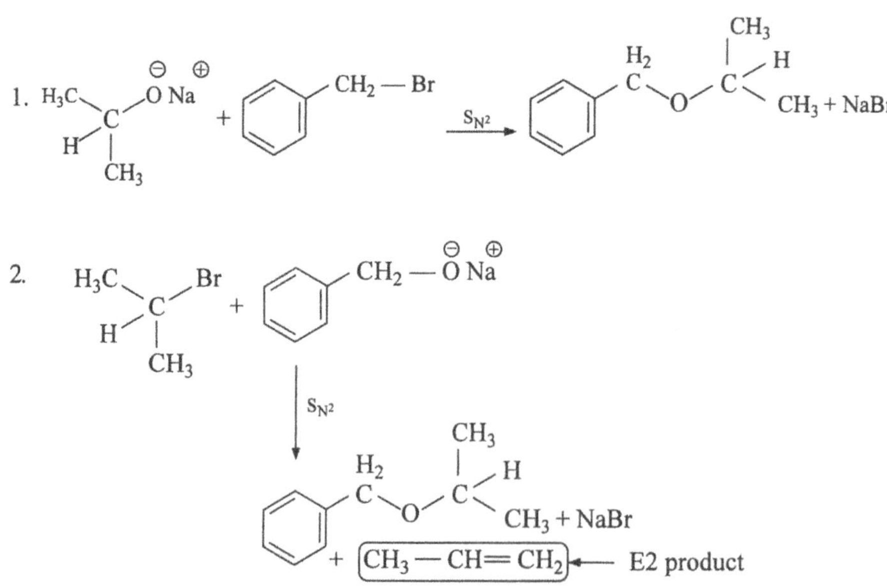

3. 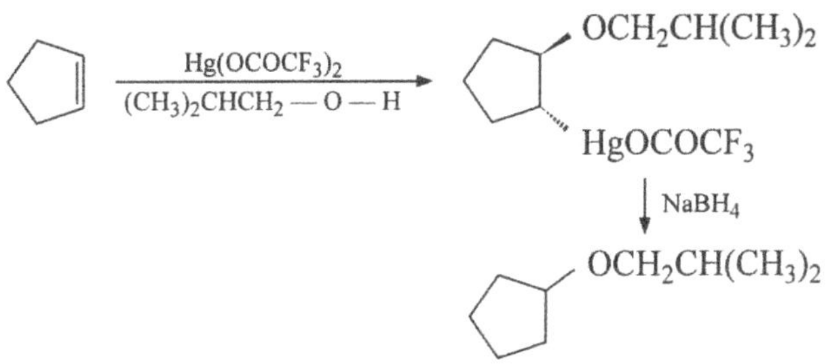

4. 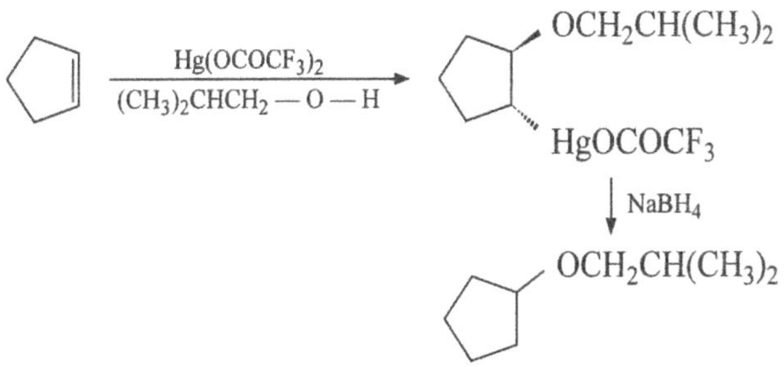

Limitations

- Aryl halides are not used in this method to prepare alkyl aryl ethers because a halogen atom attached to an aromatic ring cannot be replaced by a nucleophile.
- Diaryl ethers cannot be prepared by Williamson's synthesis.
- Elimination can also take place as a competing reaction to substitution.

15.5 PHYSICAL PROPERTIES OF ETHERS

1. The ethers are highly non-polar, non-associated substances. Their melting and boiling points are very close to those of hydrocarbons.
2. Ethers are highly inflammable and have relatively high vapour pressures, so they constitute a significant fire hazard.
3. Simple ethers on exposure to air, they react slowly with oxygen to form highly explosive unstable peroxides.
4. Ethers are non-associated substances, they cannot form hydrogen bonds with water and so do not show any tendency to dissolve in water.
5. They are freely soluble in hydrocarbons, halohydrocarbons. However, sometimes ethers dissolve in strongly acidic solvents (H_2SO_4, HI) due to formation of oxonium ion.

15.6 CHEMICAL PROPERTIES OF ETHERS

Ethers are widely used as solvents for a variety of organic compounds and reactions, suggesting that they are relatively unreactive themselves. Indeed, with the exception of the alkanes, cycloalkanes and fluorocarbons, ethers are probably the least reactive, common class of organic compounds. The inert nature of the ethers relative to the alcohols is undoubtedly due to the absence of the reactive O—H bond. The ethereal oxygen is a highly unreactive group, consequently ethers are inert-compounds that closely resemble hydrocarbons in reactions. They are inert in alkali, aqueous acids and with oxidising and reducing agents. However, ethers undergo the following reactions:

1. ***Formation of Oxonium Salts*** Ethers dissolve in concentrated strong mineral acids by forming oxonium salts (ethers behave as weak bases).

$$\underset{\text{Ether}}{R-O-R} + H_2SO_4 \longrightarrow \underset{\text{Dialkyloxonium hydrogen sulphate}}{R-\underset{\displaystyle H}{\overset{}{O}}-R\,HS\bar{O}_4}$$

$$\underset{\text{Diethyl ether}}{C_2H_5-O-C_2H_5} + H_2SO_4 \longrightarrow \underset{\text{Diethyloxonium hydrogen sulphate}}{C_2H_5-\underset{\displaystyle H}{\overset{+}{O}}-C_2H_5HS\bar{O}_4}$$

2. ***Cleavage by Acids*** The most common reaction of ethers is cleavage of the C—O bond by strong acids. This may occur by S_N1 or E1 mechanisms for 3°-alkyl groups or by an S_N2 mechanism for 1°-alkyl groups. On heating with concentrated acids (HI), the ether linkage cleaves to form an alcohol or phenol and an alkyl halide. In presence of excess of HI, the alcohol formed reacts with HI to form alkyl halide. The order of reactivity of halogen acids is HI > HBr > HCl.

$$R'OH + HI \longrightarrow R'I + H_2O$$

$$R-O-R' + HI \longrightarrow RI + R'OH$$

$$\underset{\text{Diethyl ether}}{C_2H_5-O-C_2H_5} + HI \longrightarrow \underset{\text{Ethyl iodide}}{C_2H_5I} + C_2H_5OH$$

Mechanism Cleavage of ethers with HI or HBr occurs by nucleophile substitution (S_N1 pathway). The leaving group of ether in these reactions is ^-OR.

15.7 EPOXIDES

Epoxides are cyclic ethers with three-membered rings. In IUPAC nomenclature, epoxides are termed as oxiranes, for example

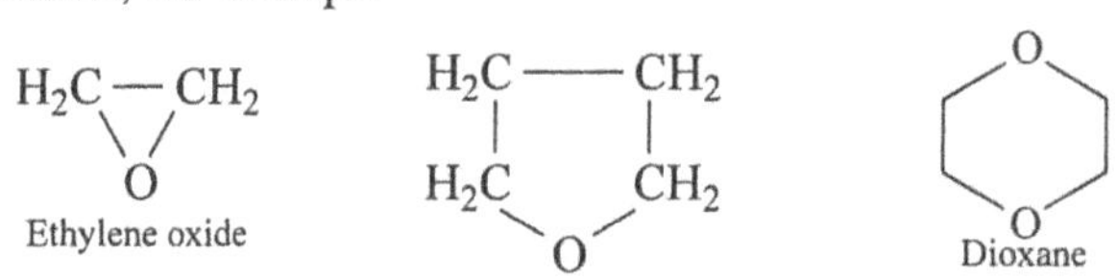

Ethylene oxide   Tetrahydrofuran   Dioxane

1. ***Preparation of Epoxides*** The most widely used method to prepare epoxides involves treatment of alkene with an organic peroxy acid (peroxybenzoic acid). This process is called epoxidation. During this reaction, the peroxy acid transfers an oxygen atom to the alkene to form epoxide.

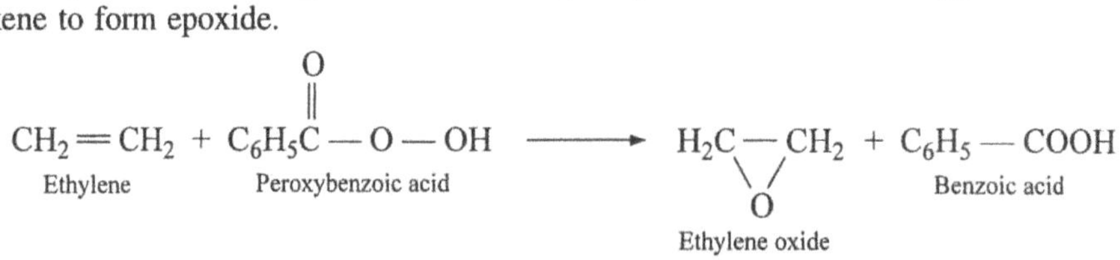

2. ***Reactions of Epoxides*** Three-membered ring epoxides are more reactive than ethers because of the strain in three-membered rings. Epoxides undergo the following reactions:

(i) *Acid catalysed ring-opening reactions* An epoxide is converted by an acid into protonated epoxide, which can undergo an attack, by a number of nucleophilic reagents including weak nucleophile like water.

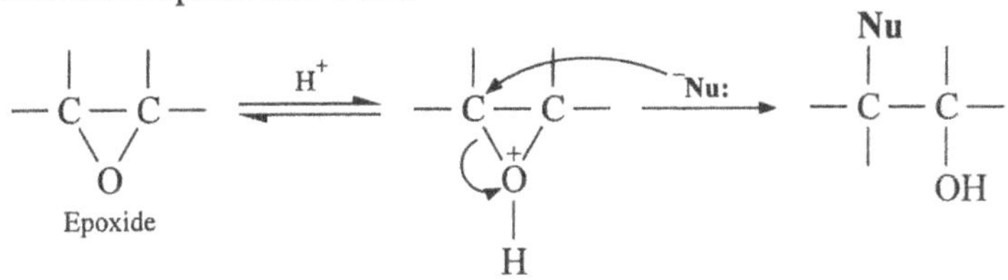

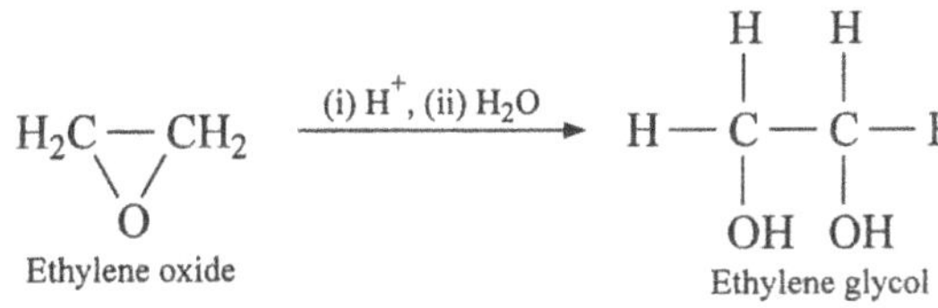

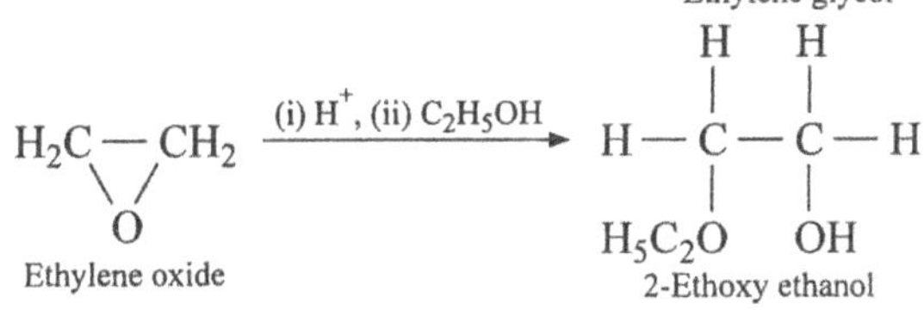

(ii) *Base-catalysed ring-opening reactions* Epoxides are cleaved by nucleophilic reagents due to the strain in the ring system. They are cleaved by the nucleophiles like hyroxide ion, phenoxide ion, alkyde ion, etc., e.g.

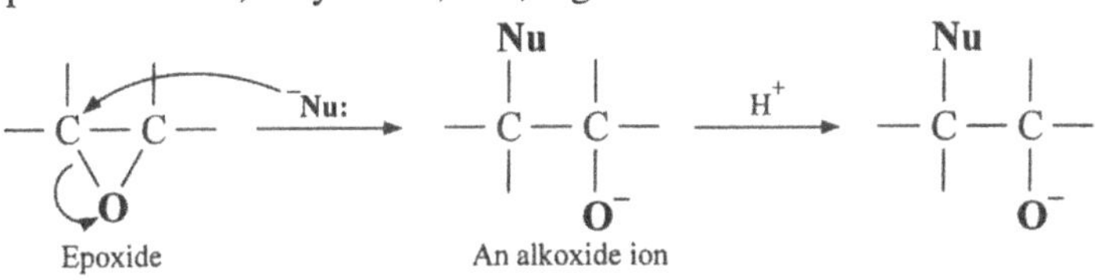

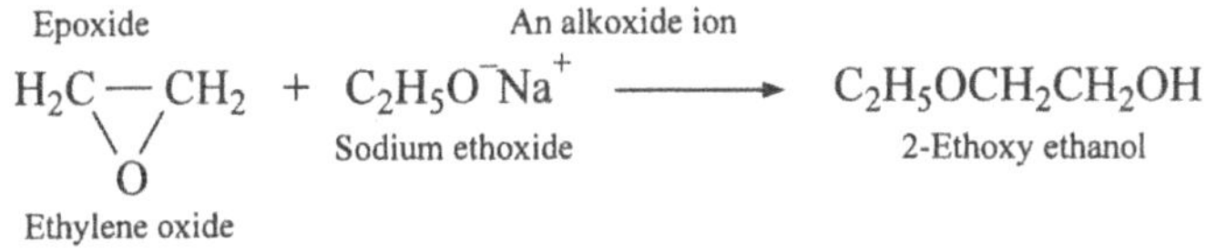

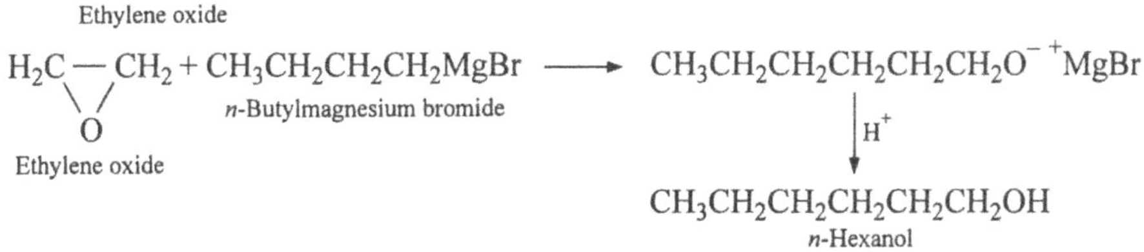

15.8 PHARMACEUTICAL COMPOUNDS

1. ***Diethyl Ether*** Diethyl ether was the first compound to be used as an anaesthetic by an American doctor. In 1846, James Simpson popularised the use of ether as an anaesthetic in surgical operations. It is prepared in the laboratory and on a large scale by heating a mixture of ethyl alcohol and concentrated H_2SO_4 which is purified with sodium hydroxide followed by drying on anhydrous calcium chloride.

$$R - OH \xrightarrow[135°C]{H_2SO_4} R - O - R + H_2O$$

$$C_2H_5 - OH \xrightarrow[135°C]{H_2SO_4} C_2H_5 - O - C_2H_5 + H_2O$$

Properties

(i) Diethyl ether is a colourless, volatile, highly inflammable liquid, having sweet burning taste and a characteristic adour.

(ii) The anaesthetic ether should be stored in well-closed, light-resistant containers in a cool place.

(iii) Stabilisers like sodium pyrogallate, hydroquinoul, or propyl gallate are added to anaesthetic ether.

Uses

1. It is a safe general anaesthetic.
2. It is inexpensive.

2. ***Guaiphenesin*** Guaiphenesin is an ether. Chemically, it is 3-(2-methoxyphenoxy) propane-1,2-diol. Guaiphenesin is available as colourless, crystalline powder. It is slightly soluble in water.

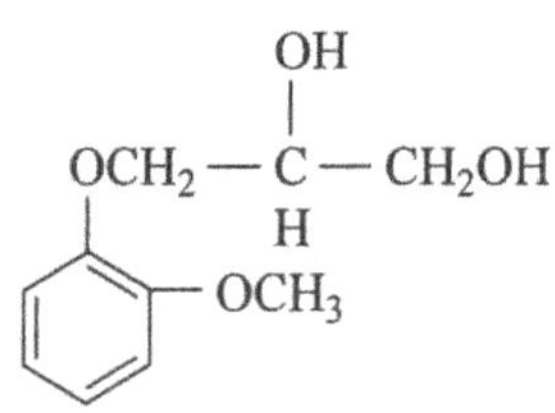

Guaiphenesin is used as an expectorant.

PRACTICE QUESTIONS

1. Consider the structure of ethyl methyl ether ($CH_3OCH_2CH_3$). What is the hybridisation of the oxygen atom, and the approximate C—O—C bond angle?
2. (a) Give three important methods of preparation of diethyl ether.
   (b) What happens when diethyl ether is treated with
      (i) Cold HI, and
      (ii) Boiling HI?
3. Write short notes on:
   (a) Williamson synthesis
   (b) Epoxides
4. Write structure, properties and uses of:
   (a) Diethyl ether
   (b) Guaiphenesin
5. Explain why ethers weakly reactive in comparison to alcohols.

16

CHEMISTRY OF BENZENE AND AROMATICITY

16.1 INTRODUCTION

The word arene is used to denote a group of compounds that are aromatic hydrocarbons. These organic compounds were classified as aromatic because all of these had a (in Greek *aroma* means smell) characteristic smell. In the earlier days of development of organic chemistry, the division between aromatic and aliphatic compounds was on the basis of smell whereas in later years, the emphasis shifted to chemical reactivity.

16.2 STRUCTURE

1. ***Molecular Formula*** The molecular formula of benzene as found by elemental composition and molecular weight determination is C_6H_6. Since benzene contains six hydrogen atoms less than the corresponding alkane, i.e. hexane (C_6H_{14}), it should be a highly unsaturated compound.

2. ***Chemical Behaviour*** Benzene behaves in the most remarkable manner in its chemical reactions unlike aliphatic unsaturated compounds. The typical reactions of benzene are the substitution reactions and not the addition reactions, as discussed below.

(i) *Substitution reactions* Benzene readily undergoes a number of characteristic substitution reactions such as:

(a) *Halogenation*

$$\underset{\text{Benzene}}{C_6H_6} + Cl_2 \xrightarrow{FeCl_3} \underset{\text{Chlorobenzene}}{C_6H_5 — Cl} + HCl$$

(b) *Nitration*

$$\underset{\text{Benzene}}{C_6H_6} + HNO_3 \xrightarrow{H_2SO_4} \underset{\text{Nitrobenzene}}{C_6H_5NO_2}$$

(c) *Sulphonation*

$$\underset{\text{Benzene}}{C_6H_6} + H_2SO_4 \longrightarrow \underset{\text{Benzenesulphonic acid}}{C_6H_5SO_3H}$$

(d) *Friedel–Crafts reaction*

$$\underset{\text{Benzene}}{C_6H_6} + \underset{\text{Alkylchloride}}{RCl} \xrightarrow{\text{Anhydrous } AlCl_3} \underset{\text{Alkylbenzene}}{C_6H_5 — R} + HCl$$

(ii) *Failure to undergo some typical addition reactions* Benzene does not undergo many addition reactions characteristic of aliphatic unsaturated compounds. These are:

- It does not decolourise $KMnO_4$ solution
- It does not decolourise bromine in the dark
- It does not add on halogen acids.

(iii) *Occurrence of some addition reactions* Under drastic conditions, benzene undergoes some addition reactions.

(a) *Addition of hydrogen*

$$\underset{\text{Benzene}}{C_6H_6} + 3H_2 \xrightarrow[\text{High pressure}]{150°\text{–}200°C} \underset{\text{Cyclohexane}}{C_6H_{12}}$$

(b) *Addition of halogens*

$$\underset{\text{Benzene}}{C_6H_6} + 3Cl_2 \xrightarrow{\text{Sunlight}} \underset{\text{Benzenehexachloride}}{C_6H_6Cl_6}$$

(c) *Benzene forms a triozonide on ozonolysis*

$$\underset{\text{Benzene}}{C_6H_6} + O_3 \longrightarrow \underset{\text{Benzenetriozonide}}{C_6H_6O_3}$$

3. ***Isomer Number*** (i) Benzene yields only *one mono substitution product* (C_6H_5Y). For example, only one bromobenzene (C_6H_5Br) and only one nitrobenzene ($C_6H_5NO_2$) are known to exist. This fact clearly indicates that all the six hydrogen atoms of benzene are equivalent to one another. A number of structures, as shown here, were proposed for benzene from time to time.

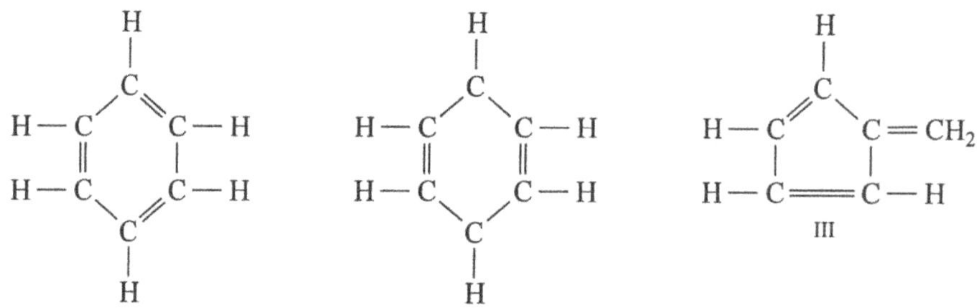

I II III

$$\underset{\text{IV}}{H_3C\,C{\equiv}C{-}C{\equiv}CCH_3} \qquad \underset{\text{V}}{CH_2{=}CH{-}C{\equiv}CCH{=}CH_2}$$

Now, Structure V is rejected since it would yield two isomeric monobromo derivatives (1-bromo, 2-bromo derivatives) – *all hydrogens are not equivalent.* Similarly, Structures II and III are unsatisfactory while I and IV among others, are still possibilities.

(ii) Benzene yields 3 *isomeric disubstitution* products ($C_6H_4Y_2$ or C_6H_4YZ). The disubstitution products of benzene can exist in three isomeric forms (i.e. *ortho*, *meta* and *para* forms), e.g. 3-dichloro benzenes, three bromo phenols have been obtained. This fact further limits our choice of a structures, for example, Structure IV must now be rejected.

(iii) At first glance, Structure I (proposed by *Kekule*) seems to be consistent and conforms to this new fact, i.e. we can expect three isomeric dibromo derivatives, viz., 1,2; 1,3 and the 1,4 dibromo compounds:

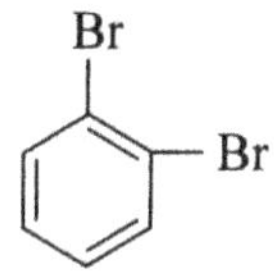

1,2-Dibromobenzene

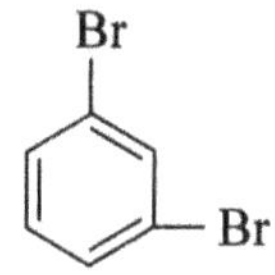

1,3-Dibromobenzene

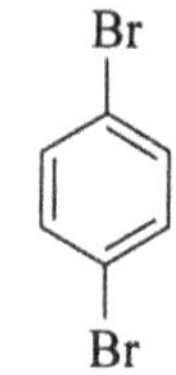

1,4-Dibromobenzene

The only formula which received general support was the hexagonal formula, i.e. Structure I proposed by Kekule (1865). It showed all the hydrogen atoms to be equivalent and, therefore, justified the formation of one monosubstituted benzene. Moreover, it could also explain the addition of three molecules of hydrogens or halogens to benzene.

(iv) But *Ladenburg* (1869) objected to Kekule's structural formula on the grounds that it should yield *four disubstituted derivatives:* two ortho derivatives, one meta and one para as shown here:

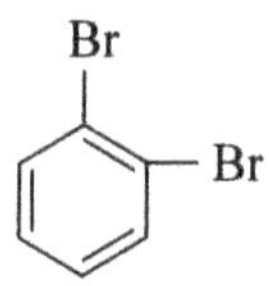

1,2-Dibromobenzene
(Ortho isomer)

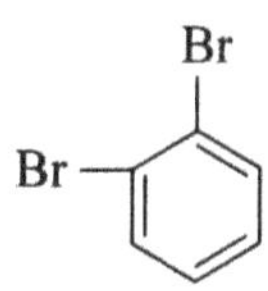

1,6-Dibromobenzene

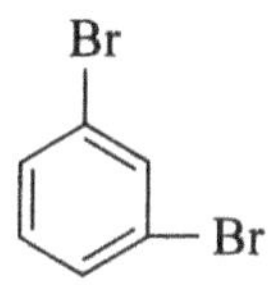

1,3-Dibromobenzene
(Meta isomer)

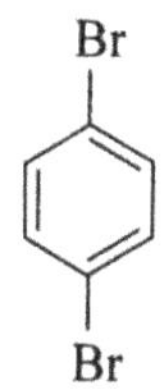

1,4-Dibromobenzene
(Para isomer)

It may be noted that the two ortho structures shown above differ in the positions of the substituents relative to the double bond.

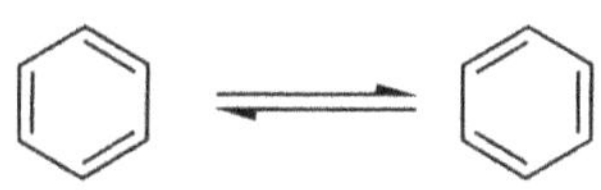

VI VII
Kekule structure

(v) Kekule overcame this difficulty by suggesting that the double bonds were not static but in a state of rapid oscillation between two forms, i.e. Structures VI and VII, as shown here.

Due to oscillation of double bonds, the two ortho disubstituted derivatives could not be distinguished from one another.

4. ***Stability of Benzene*** Benzene is 1,3,5-cyclohexatriene. We would predict benzene to liberate approximately 85.8 kcal/mol (3 × 28.6) when it is hydrogenated. When benzene is experimentally hydrogenated, only 49.8 kcal/mol is released. This difference between the amount of heat evolved and that calculated on the basis of Kekule structure is called *resonance energy*. Thus, benzene is stable by 36 kcal/mol.

The stability of benzene can be demonstrated by comparing the experimentally determined heats of hydrogenation of cyclohexenes. Benzene, cyclohexene, and cyclohexadiene all give cyclohexane upon catalytic hydrogenation. Hydrogenation of cyclohexene to cyclohexane releases 120 kJ/mol. Theoretically, reduction of cyclohexadiene should release 2 × 120 or 240 kJ/mol. This is the value obtained with 1,4-cyclohexadiene but is 8 kJ/mol more than the heat of hydrogenation of 1,3-cyclohexadiene. The difference is attributed to the delocalisation of electrons in the conjugated diene system. Benzene, according to its Kekule structure should have a heat of hydrogenation of 3 × 120 or 360 kJ/mol. The actual value of – 208 kJ/mol reveals an energy difference of 152 kJ/mol! This is the resonance stabilisation energy of benzene.

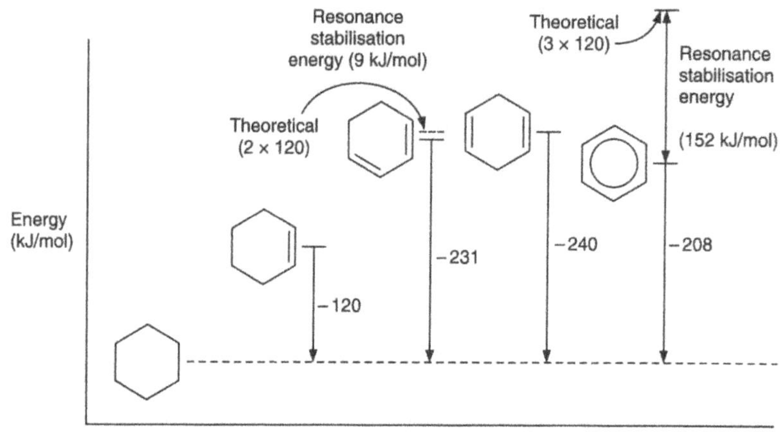

5. ***Valence-Bond Theory or Resonance Theory*** To overcome the objections raised against the Kekule structures and to account for all the known facts regarding benzene, the resonance theory has been suggested. According to this theory, the structure of benzene is considered to be resonance hybrid of two Kekule structures that are interconvertible by electron shifts.

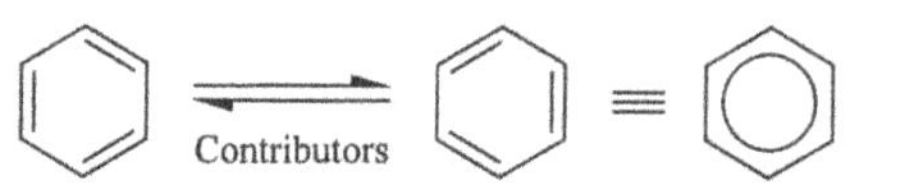

VI VII Resonance hybrid

The Kekule Structures VI and VII meet the condition for resonance, i.e. structures that differ only in the arrangement of electrons. Benzene is a hybrid of VI and VII since VI and VII are exactly equivalent and hence the same stability and make equal contribution to the hybrid. The stabilisation due to resonance should be large (36 kcal). The six bond lengths are identical (i.e. 1.39Å) because of the same resonance phenomenon. The high stability of benzene is also due to existence of resonance phenomenon. The 36 kcal resonance energy is responsible for new set of properties, i.e. aromatic properties.

6. ***Molecular Orbital Theory*** The molecular orbital theory gives a good picture for the structure of benzene. This theory was derived from X-ray and spectroscopic data. In benzene each carbon is bonded to three other atoms, so it uses sp^2 hybrid orbitals. These lie in the same plane as that of the carbon nucleus and are directed towards the corners of an equilateral triangle. If we arrange the six carbons and six hydrogens of benzene to permit maximum overlap of these orbitals, it attains the following structure:

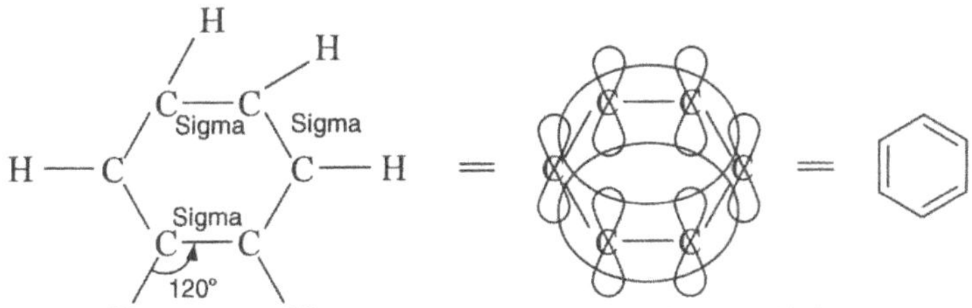

Each carbon atom has a *p* orbital perpendicular to the ring

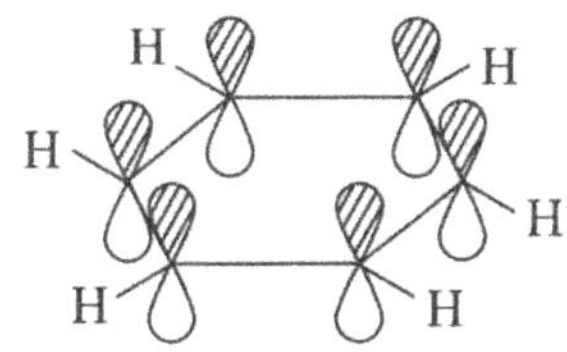

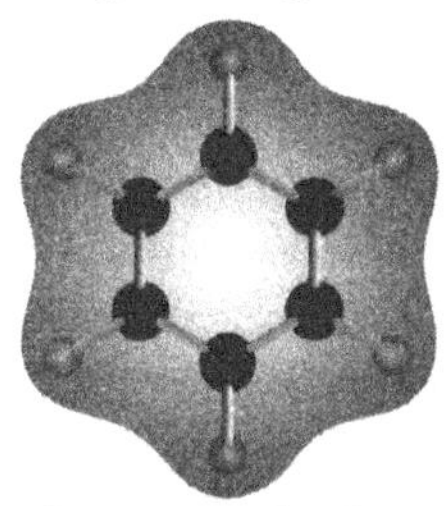

Thus, the benzene molecule is *planar, regular hexagon* with all the six carbon atoms lying in the same plane. Each bond orbital is cylindrically symmetrical about the line joining the atomic nucleus and hence these bonds are designated as σ bonds. However, the molecule is not yet complete still there are six electrons to be accounted. In addition to the three orbitals already used, each carbon atom has a fourth orbital, i.e. a p_z orbital. The unused orbitals on each carbon of benzene overlap with one another to form π bonds. It is obvious from the structures written above that p_z orbital can overlap with both adjacent p_z orbitals. Thus, *continuous π-molecular orbital* is formed. There are two continuous π-molecular clouds, i.e. one is above the plane and the other is below the plane. The electrons involved in the continuous π-molecular orbital are called *delocalised* electrons.

16.3 PREPARATION

1. ***From Coal Tar*** Benzene is obtained in large scale from light oil fraction (this fraction contains benzene, toluene, xylene, thiophene and phenol) of coal-tar distillation. This fraction is first treated with H_2SO_4 to remove basic substances including thiophene. The acid layer is separated and the remaining oil is washed with sodium hydroxide to remove phenol and acidic substances. The alkali layer is also removed, the remaining oil layer is washed with water and subjected to fractional distillation. The fraction obtained at 170°C temperature is cooled in a freezing mixture to get crystals of benzene. Benzene still contains small amounts of *thiophene as impurity*, which is removed by treating benzene layer repeatedly with H_2SO_4 (thiophene reacts with sulphuric acid to form thiophene sulphate) and pure benzene is obtained by redistillation.

2. ***From Acetylene*** When acetylene is passed through a red-hot copper or quartz tube acetylene polymerises to benzene.

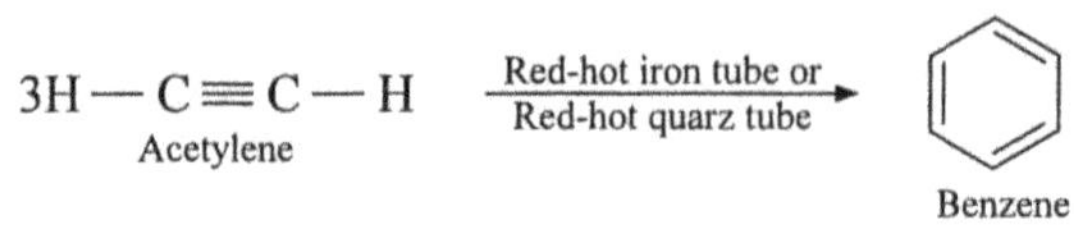

16.4 PHYSICAL PROPERTIES

1. Benzene is a colourless liquid which is immiscible in water but miscible in non-polar organic solvents.
2. It has a characteristic odour.
3. It is an inflammable liquid.
4. It burns with sooty flame.
5. It boils at 80°C and melts at 5.5°C.
6. It is carcinogenic.

16.5 CHEMICAL REACTIONS

Benzene readily undergoes aromatic substitution reactions rather than addition due to the stability of the aromatic ring system that would be destroyed during addition reactions. The term aromatic substitution refers to the substitution of an atom, generally hydrogen or a group attached to the carbon of the benzene ring, by another group. Benzene ring has an electron-rich π cloud which is attacked by electrophiles, hence it undergo electrophilic aromatic substitution reactions.

16.5.1 Electrophilic Aromatic Substitution

The most important characteristic reactions of benzenoid arenes are the electrophilic aromatic substitution reactions in which the resonance-stabilised ring is preserved. It can be explained as follows:

Above and below the plane of benzene ring, there is a cloud of π-electrons. Because of resonance, these π-electrons are more involved in holding together carbon nuclei. In comparison of σ-electrons, these π-electrons are loosely held and are available to electrophiles. Thus, benzene ring serves as a source of electrons and the compounds that it reacts are deficient in electrons, i.e. electrophilic reagents. These typical reactions are known as *electrophilic aromatic substitution reactions.* These substitution reactions are nitration, halogenation, sulphonation and Friedel–Crafts reactions.

General Mechanism of Electrophilic Aromatic Substitution The electrophilic aromatic substitution reactions involve the replacement of hydrogen atom of an aromatic ring by an electrophile.

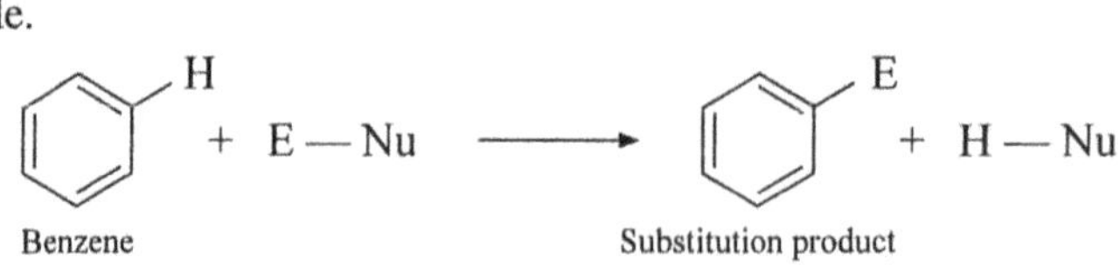

All electrophilic substitution reactions follow the same 3-step mechanism:

Step 1 Formation of an electrophile The electrophiles are either +ve ions (E^+) or some other electron-deficient species with a large partial +ve charge, that is

$$E - Nu \ + \ Catalyst \longrightarrow E^+ \ + \ Nu - Catalyst$$

Step 2 The electrophile attacks aromatic ring to give an arenium ion Electrophiles attack the π system of C_6H_6 to form an arenium ion. In Step 2 the electrophile takes two electrons of the six electron π system to form a σ bond to one carbon atom of the C_6H_6 ring. Formation of this bond interrupts the cyclic system of π-electrons. In the formation of arenium ion the carbon that forms a bond to the electrophile becomes sp^3 hybridised and, thus, no longer has an available *p* orbital. Now, only five carbon atoms of the ring are still sp^2 hybridised and still have *p* orbital. The four π-electrons of the arenium are delocalised through these five *p* orbitals.

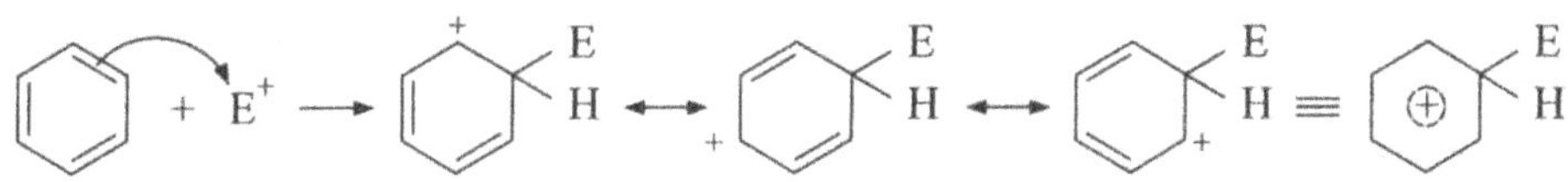

Benzene

Arenium ion (Sigma complex)

Resonance stabilised arenium ion

Step 3 Removal of proton from arenium ion to give the product In Step 3, the arenium ion loses a proton from the carbon atom that bears the electrophile. The two electrons that bonded this proton to carbon become a part of the π system. The carbon atom that bears the electrophile becomes sp^2 hybridised again, and a benzene derivative with six fully delocalised π-electrons is formed.

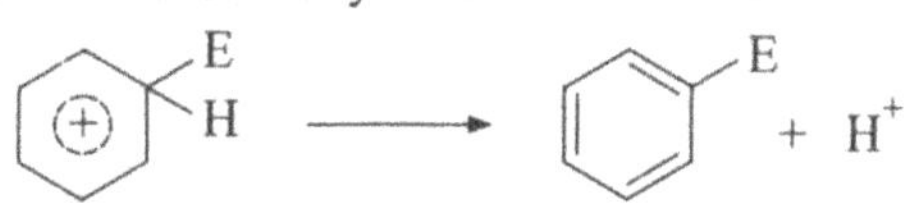

Resonance stabilised arenium ion

Substitution product

There is firm experimental evidence that the arenium ion is a true intermediate in electrophilic substitution reactions.

1. ***Nitration*** When benzene is treated with a mixture of conc. H_2SO_4 and HNO_3 at 50°–60°C for an hour, nitrobenzene is formed. The mechanism of this reaction is given below:

(i) *Generation of an electrophile* This step generates nitronium ion. The reaction is an acid–base reaction.

$$HNO_3 \ + \ 2H_2SO_4 \longrightarrow H_3O^+ \ + \ 2HSO_4^- \ + \ NO_2^+$$

However, solutions of stable nitronium ion salts like nitronium perchlorate ($NO_2^+ClO_4^-$) and nitronium fluoborate ($NO_2^+BF_4^-$) in nitromethane or acetic acid have been found to nitrate aromatic compounds smoothly in high yield at room temperature.

(ii) *The nitronium ion attacks benzene ring to form arenium ion* In the second step, nitronium ion attacks one of the carbon atoms of benzene through covalent bond by utilising π-electrons of benzene. This leads to form an arenium ion that is represented by the following resonance structure.

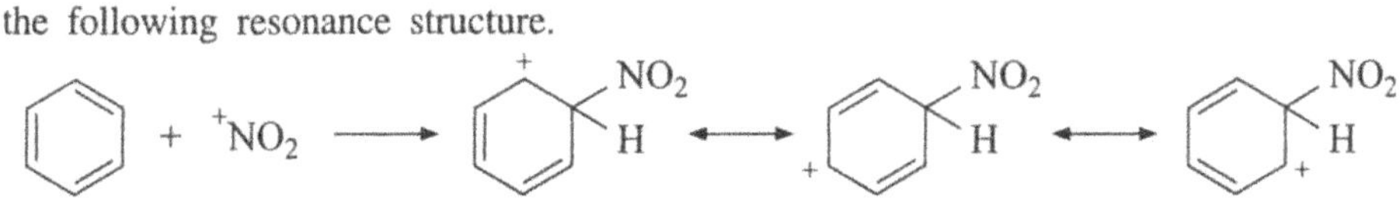

Benzene

The actual ion must be a resonance stabilised one.

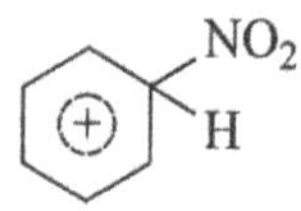

Resonance hybrid

(iii) *The arenium ion loses a proton to form nitrobenzene*

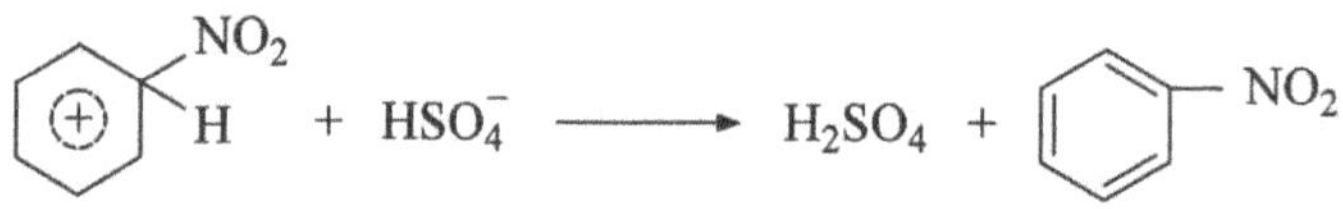

Arenium ion

Nitrobenzene

2. ***Sulphonation*** When benzene is warmed with H_2SO_4 at 50°C, it forms benzene sulphonic acid. This process involves replacement of hydrogen atom by a sulphonic acid (—SO_3H) group.

Mechanism

(i) *Generation of an electrophile* (SO_3)

$$H_2SO_4 + H_2SO_4 \rightleftharpoons SO_3 + H_3O^+ + HSO_4^-$$

(ii) *The electrophile* (SO_3) *attacks benzene ring to form resonance stabilised arenium ion*

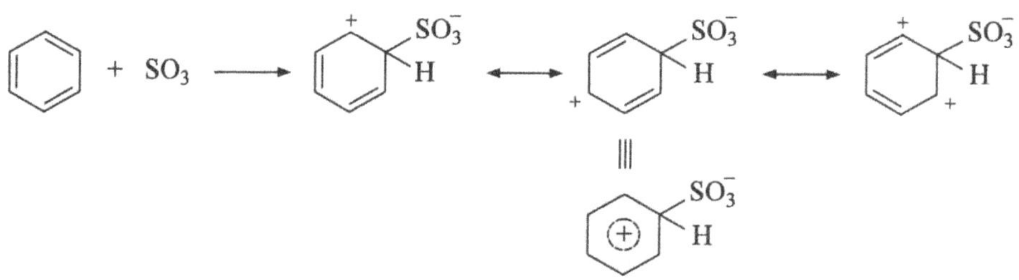

Resonance stabilised arenium ion

(iii) *Arenium ion loses a proton*

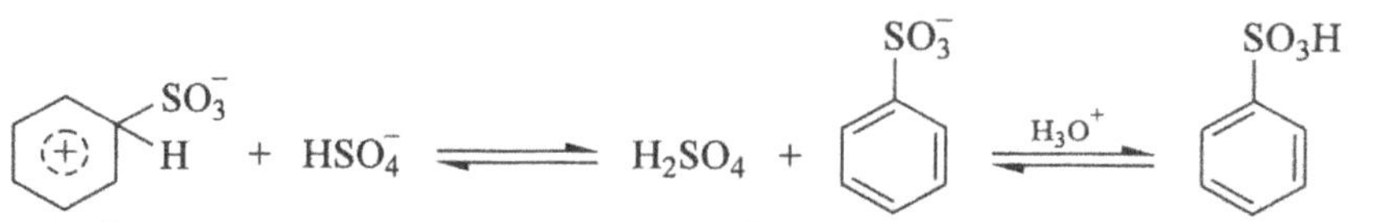

Arenium ion

Benzenesulphonate ion

Benzenesulphonic acid

3. ***Halogenation*** When benzene is treated with halogens (Cl_2 or Br_2) in presence of a Lewis acid ($FeCl_3$ or $FeBr_3$) it forms halobenzene.

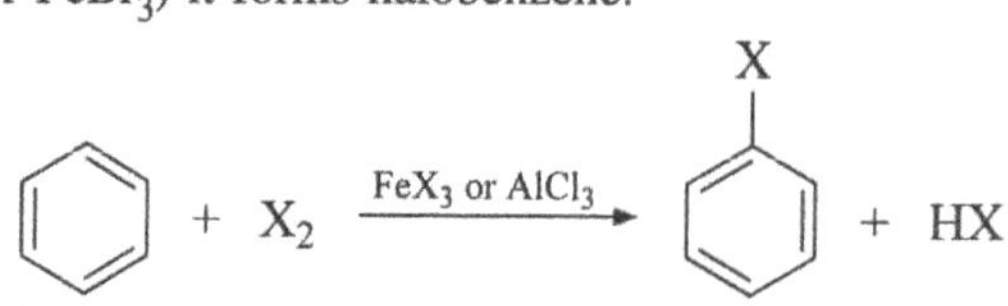

Benzene

Halobenzene

Mechanism

(i) *Generation of an electrophile*

$$X - X \ + \ FeX_3 \longrightarrow FeX_4^- \ + \ X^+$$

(ii) Electrophile (**X^+**) attacks benzene ring to form resonance-stabilised arenium ion.

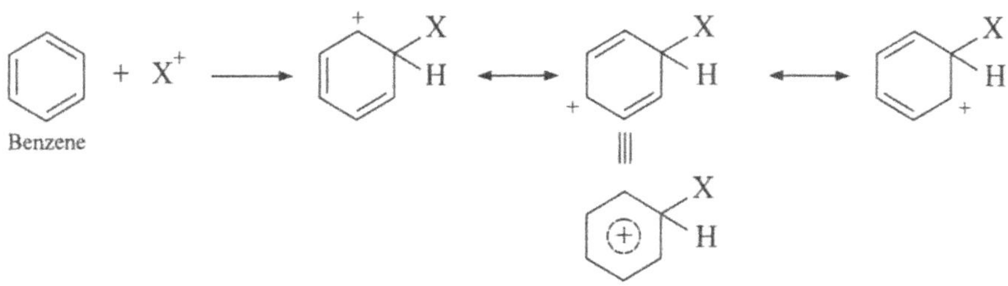

(iii) Arenium ion loses a proton to form halobenzene

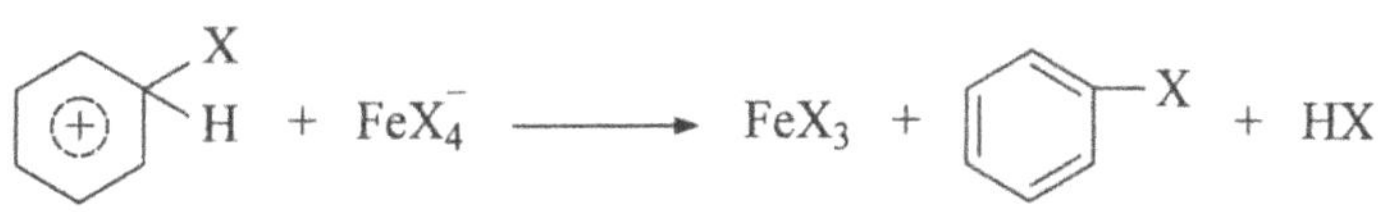

Resonance stabilised areanium ion — Halobenzene

4. ***Friedel–Crafts Alkylation*** Charles Friedel, a French chemist and James Mason Craft, an American, discovered this reaction in 1877. In this reaction, an alkyl halide reacts with an aromatic compound in the presence of a Lewis Acid catalyst (BF_3, $AlCl_3$, $AlBr_3$), often $AlCl_3$. This reaction is known as Friedel–Crafts alkylation.

For example, benzene reacts with 2-chloropropane in the presence of aluminium trichloride to form 2-phenylpropane.

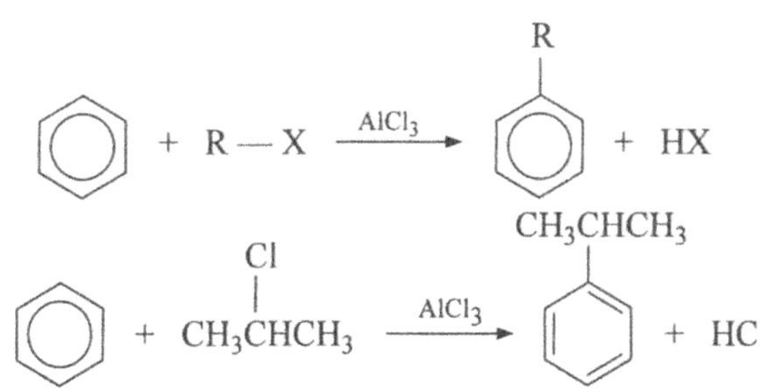

Mechanism

(i) *Generation of an electrophile*

$$R - X \ + \ AlCl_3 \longrightarrow AlCl_4^- \ + \ R^+$$

(ii) *The electrophile attacks benzene ring to form resonance-stabilised arenium ion.*

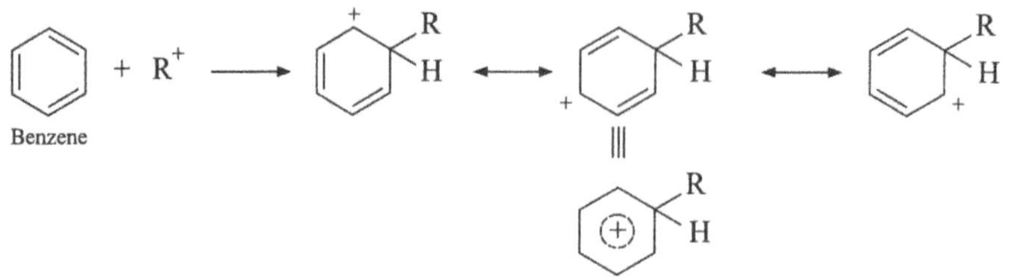

Resonance stabilised arenium ion

(iii) *Arenium ion loses proton to form alkyl benzene.*

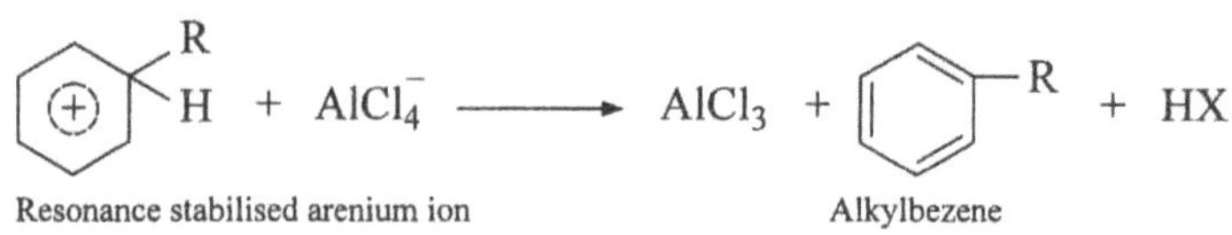

Limitation With primary halides, the electrophile is a 1° carbocation, which usually undergoes rearrangement to give a more stable 2° or 3° carbocation. For example, the reaction of 1-chloropropane with benzene gives 2-phenylpropane as the major product not 1-phenylpropane.

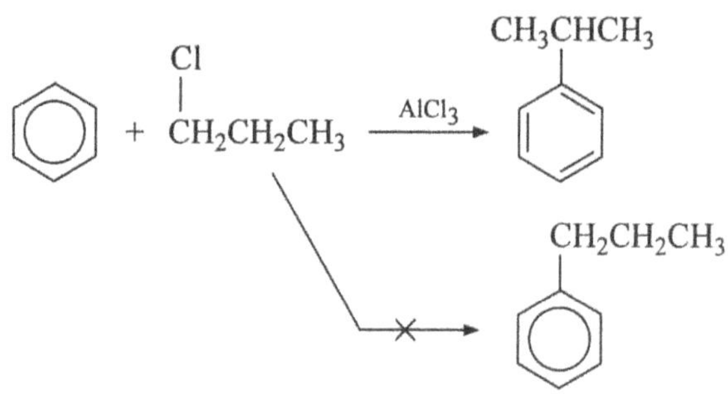

Rearrangement of intermediate electrophile occurs by a shift of a hydrogen atom.

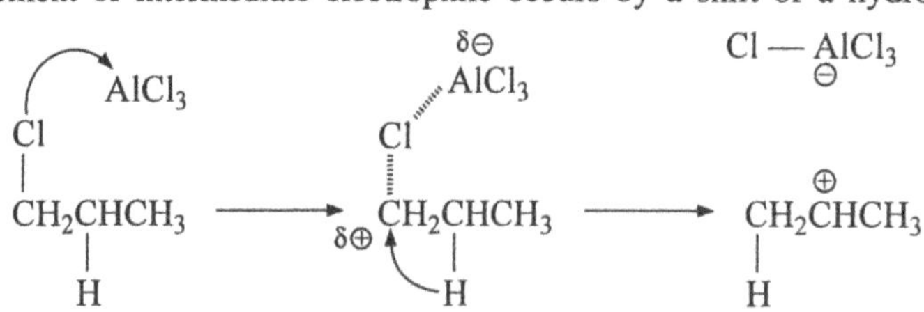

5. ***Friedel–Crafts Acylation*** When benzene is treated with acid chloride in presence of a Lewis acid (catalyst), it forms acyl benzene. This is known as Friedel–Crafts acylation.

$$ArH + R{-}C(Cl){=}O \xrightarrow{AlCl_3} R{-}C(Ar){=}O + HCl$$

Mechanism

(i) *Generation of an electrophile*

$$\underset{\text{Acyl chloride}}{RCOCl} + AlCl_3 \longrightarrow \underset{\text{Acylium ion}}{R{-}\overset{O}{\overset{\|}{C}}{\oplus}} + AlCl_4^-$$

(ii) *The electrophile (acylium ion) attacks benzene ring to form arenium ion.*

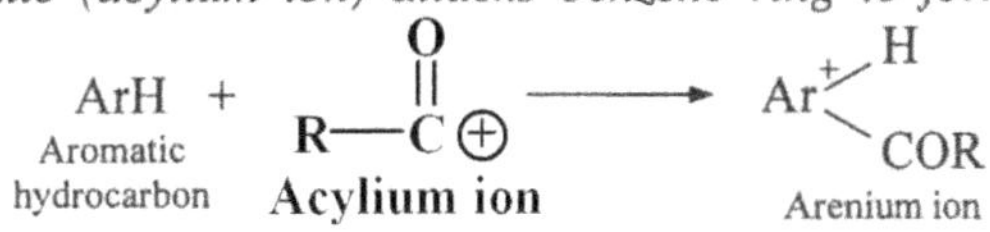

(iii) *Arenium ion loses a proton to give acyl benzene.*

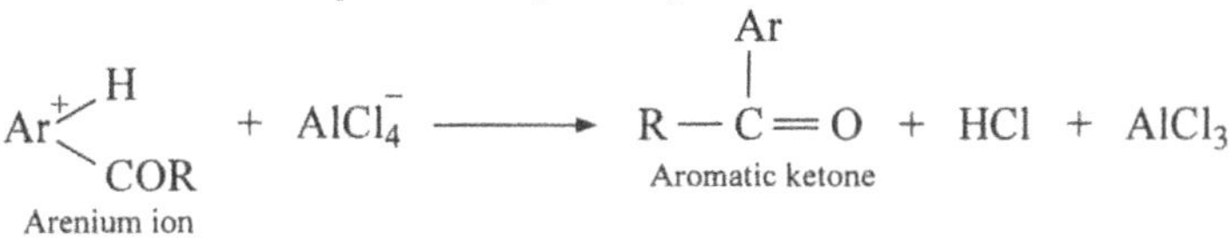

Importance of Friedel–Crafts Reactions

- Alkyl benzenes can be prepared.
- Acyl benzenes can also be synthesised.

Limitations of Friedel–Crafts Reactions

- Arylhalides cannot be used in place of alkyl halides.
- Substrates, like nitro benzene, cannot be alkylated due to deactivating influence of nitro group.
- Aniline and other aromatic amines fail to undergo this reaction due to the formation of complex between base and Lewis acid.

16.6 ELECTROPHILIC AROMATIC SUBSTITUTION REACTIONS OF SUBTITUTED BENZENES

When an electrophilic reagent attacks a monosubstituted aromatic ring, the group already attached to the ring determines the reactivity and also orientation of substitution.

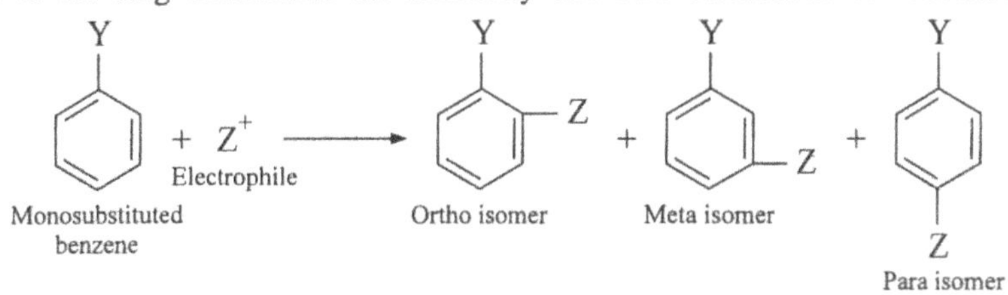

On the basis of these two characteristics (reactivity and orientation), various substituents have been divided into the following categories:

1. ***Activating and Ortho-, Para-directing Groups*** Activating groups make the benzene ring more reactive towards electrophilc substitution. These substituents orient the incoming substituent toward ortho or para position, e.g. $—NH_2$, —NHR, $—NR_2$, —OH, —OR, —NHCOR, —OCOR, —R, —Ar, $—CH{=}CR_2$.

2. ***Deactivating and Meta-directing Groups*** Deactivating groups makes the ring less reactive than benzene towards electrophilic substitution. These substituents direct the second substituent to the meta position, e.g. —CHO, —COR, —COOR, —COOH, —COCl, $—C \equiv N$, $—SO_3H$, $—{}^+NH_3$, $—{}^+NH_2R$, $—{}^+NHR_2$, $—{}^+NR_3$, $—{}^+NO_2$.

3. ***Deactivating and Ortho-, Para-directing Groups*** These substituents make the benzene ring less reactive towards electrophilic substitution but direct the second substituent towards ortho position, e.g. —F, —Cl, —Br, —I.

16.6.1 Activation and Deactivation

Monosubstituted benzene, like benzene, undergoes electrophilic substitution due to the presence of delocalised π-electron sextet. The rate-determining step of an electrophilic aromatic substitution is attack of an electrophile on the nucleophilic aromatic ring. Therefore, increase in the electron density of the benzene ring results in increase in its nucleophilicity and thus improves the electrophilic substitution reaction. The substituents that withdraw electrons from the ring will decrease the rate of electrophilic substitution due to withdrawal of electrons from benzene ring.

Table 16.1 lists common aromatic substituents according to their effect on reactivity and orientation in electrophilic substitution reactions. Note that ortho, para directors may be activating or deactivating but all meta directors are deactivating groups.

Table 16.1 Common Aromatic Substituent

Ortho, Para Directors		*Meta Directors*
Activating Groups	*Deactivating Groups*	*Deactivating Groups*
	• F	• — NO_2
Strongly activating	• Cl	• — CN
• — NH_2	• Br	• — CO_2H
• — OH		• — SO_3H
	• I	
		• — C=O
Moderately activating		
• — OCH_3		
• — $NHCOCH_3$		
Weakly activating		
• — C_6H_5		
• alkyl		

There are two ways by which substituents can donate or withdraw electrons from benzene ring. These are (i) inductive effect, and (ii) resonance effect.

1. ***Inductive Effect*** In this effect, the electrons in the *bond that attach substituent to the ring* may move either towards the benzene ring or away from the benzene ring than the electrons that bond a hydrogen to the ring. Donation of electrons through σ bond is called inductive electron donation, e.g. alkyl substituents donate electrons by inductive effect than hydrogen. Withdrawal of electrons through σ bond is called inductive electron withdrawal, e.g. —$^{+}NH_3$ group withdraws by inductive effect.

2. ***Resonance Effect*** If a substituent has a pair of non-bonded electrons on the atom directly attached to the benzene ring, these electrons can be delocalised into the ring through *p* orbital overlap. Such substituents donate electrons by resonance, e.g. NH_2, OH, etc.

If a substituent attached to the benzene ring by an atom, which is doubly or triply bonded to a more electronegative atom, the π-electrons of the ring can be delocalised onto the substituents and such substituents withdraw electrons by resonance, e.g. C=O, C≡N, NO_2.

The *activating substituent donate electrons* to benzene ring either by *inductive effect or by resonance effect,* stabilises intermediate arenium ion, thus decrease E_a and improves electrophilic aromatic substitution. The *deactivating groups, on the other hand, withdraw electrons* from benzene ring by *inductive or resonance effect and destabilise intermediate arenium ion*, thus increases E_a, thereby decrease electrophilic aromatic substitution.

16.6.2 Orientation

The substituents already attached to benzene determine the location of the new substituent.

All the activating substituents including halogens direct an incoming electrophile to the ortho and para positions. Similarly, when monosubstituted benzene containing an electron-withdrawing group is subjected to electrophilic substitution, *m*-isomer is predominant.

16.6.3 Influence of Activating (Ortho-, Para-directing) Substituents

The carbocation formed due to ortho and para attack is hybrid of four structures, whereas hybrid of only three structures is formed during meta attack. Therefore, the resonance hybrid carbocation formed during ortho and para attack is more stable because it requires less E_a in rate-determining step. The contributing forms ID and IIID are particularly more stable contributing forms because *every carbon atom has octet configuration.*

Ortho Attack

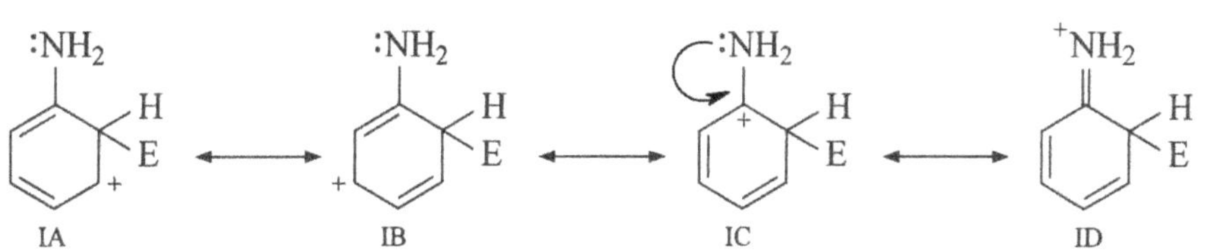

Meta Attack

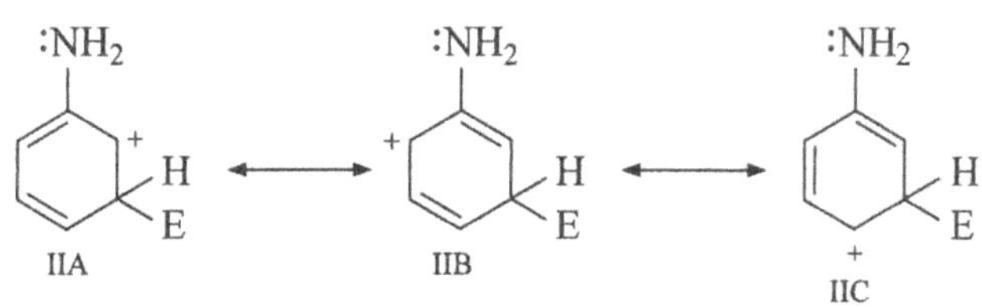

Para Attack

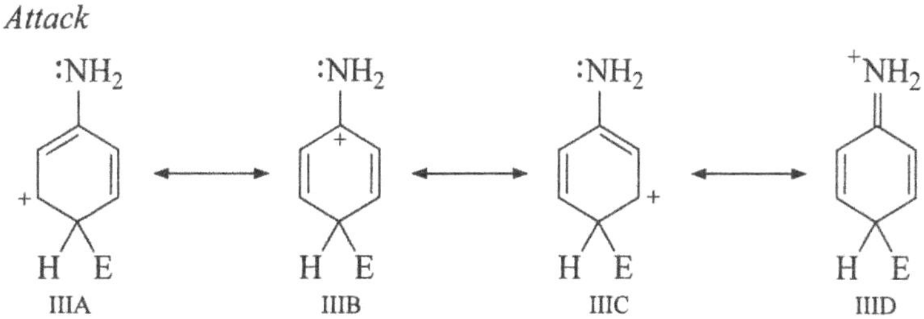

No such corresponding form is possible for the meta isomer. The positive charge in forms I and III are spread over a larger area including the substituent hence they also lower the energy in comparison to the meta isomers. All these lead to the conclusion that substituents having an unshared electron pair, situated on the atom attached to the ring, would always give stable carbocation and also activate the reaction.

The arenium ions, which are stabilised due to the inductive effect, are those where the substituent is an alkyl radical. They also activate the ring and give ortho and para substitution. The various resonance hybrids are as follows when methyl group is a substituent.

The resonance structures (IC and IIIB) of ortho and para attack possess positive charge on carbon atom to which methyl group is bonded. These structures are more stable due to greater electron-releasing inductive effect than any other. Hence, they make greater contribution to the resonance hybrid of ortho, para attack than meta attack.

Ortho Attack

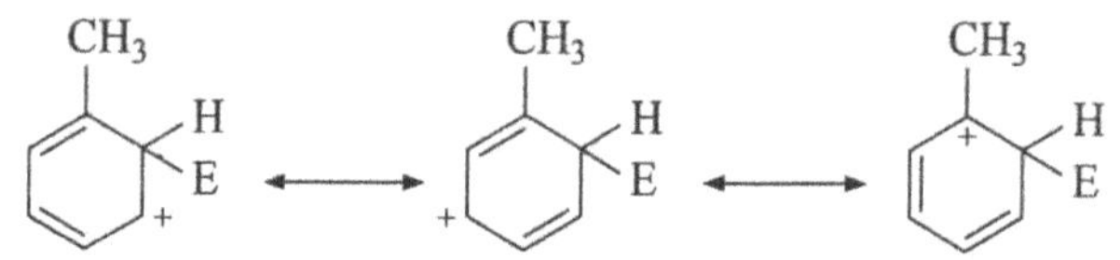

IA IB IC

Meta Attack

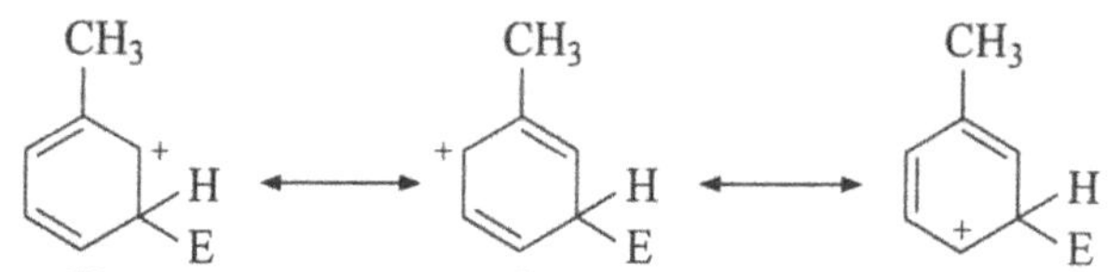

IIA IIB IIC

Para Attack

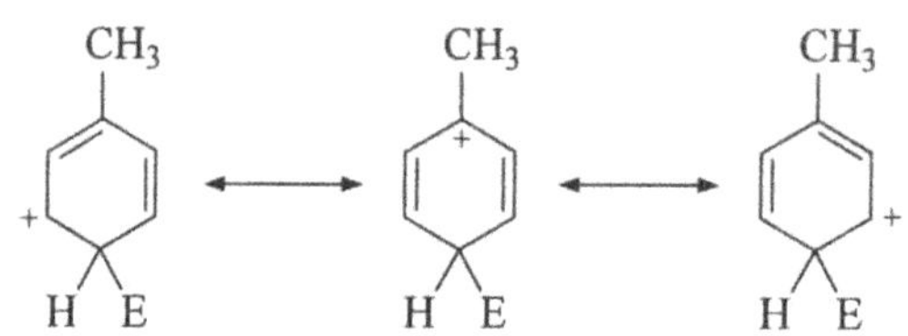

IIIA IIIB IIIC

16.6.4 Influence of Deactivating (Meta-directing) Substituents (except Halogens)

The electron-withdrawing substituents destabilise the arenium ion (intermediate) because of the presence of positive charge on the atom attached with the ring. So substitution takes place less readily and ring is deactivated. To understand preferably substitution at meta position to other positions, the following resonance structures formed from ortho, meta and para attack are to be considered:

Ortho Attack

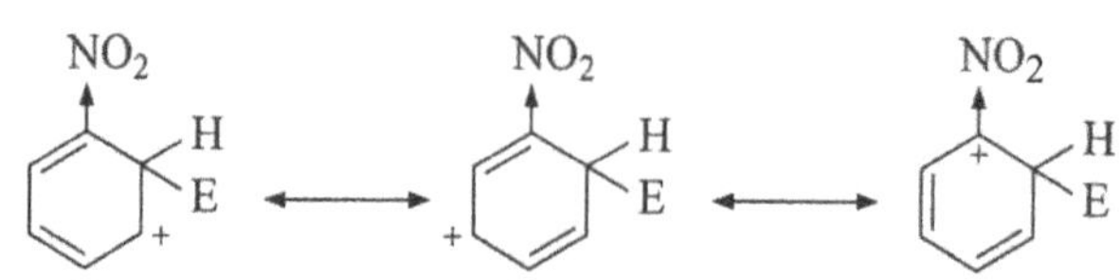

IA IB IC

In these hybrid structures all positions including the meta, are less reactive than unsubstituted benzene ring. Of these forms, IC and IIIB are particularly unstable because positive charge is located directly on the carbon carrying the electron-withdrawing substituent. So the arenium ions from ortho and para substitution are hybrids of only two structures while from meta substitution is a hybrid of three structures. So substitution occurs preferentially at the meta position relative to benzene. We can say that *inductive withdrawal of electrons reinforced by resonance deactivates the ring.*

Meta Attack

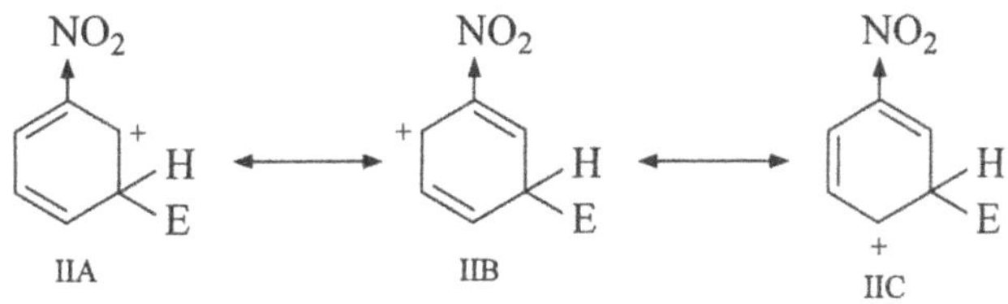

Para Attack

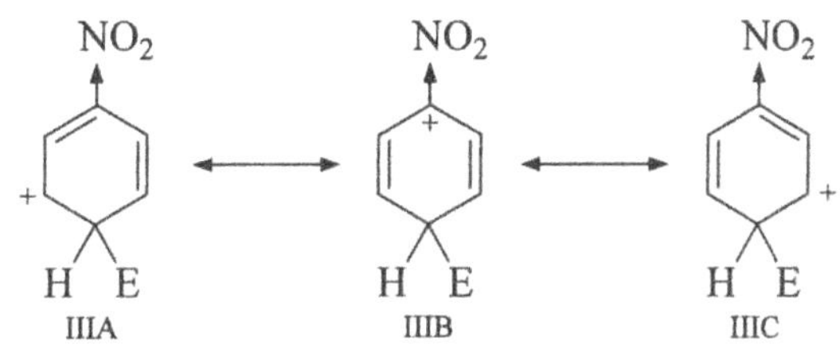

16.6.5 Influence of Deactivating but Para-Directing Groups

The influence of halogens was anomalous for long time, because chlorine, bromine and iodine being electron-withdrawing deactivate the nucleus when attached to the ring, but still lead to predominantly ortho-para substitution. Fluorine is least deactivating and flurobenzenes show reactivity comparable to benzene itself. The resultant of these effects can be understood by considering the contributing forms obtained from ortho, para and meta attack.

Ortho Attack

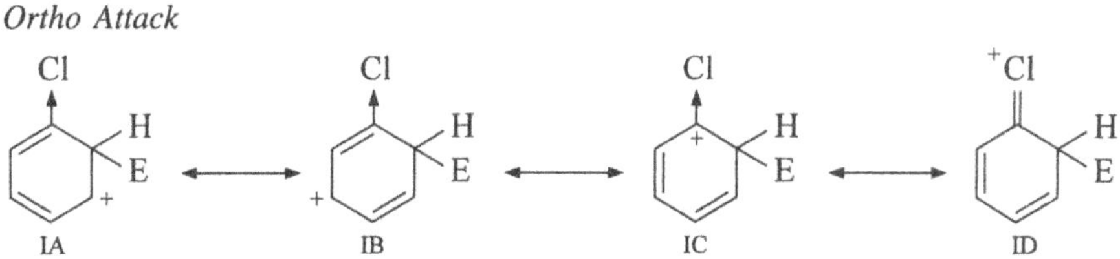

Structures ID and IIID have been obtained due to mesomeric effect. Therefore, in halobenzene the inductive and mesomeric effects are opposed to each other. But in the inductive effect, which is stronger, there is a withdrawal of electrons from the ring and hence deactivation of the ring. Therefore, the halobenzene although gives substitution reactions but the rate is slower.

Of the various canonical forms in ortho and para attack, Structures IC and IIIB are most unstable while ID and IIID are most stable and make great contribution towards ortho and para substitution. No such comparable structure is obtained during meta attack. So ortho and para substitution occurs even though the nucleus is deactivated. Therefore, the arenium ions from ortho and para substitution are more stable than those form the meta substitution. This is why ortho, para substitution occurs in preference to meta substitution. So in *halobenzenes* we find that the *rate of substitution is controlled by the stronger inductive effect while orientation is controlled by the weaker mesomeric effect.*

Meta Attack

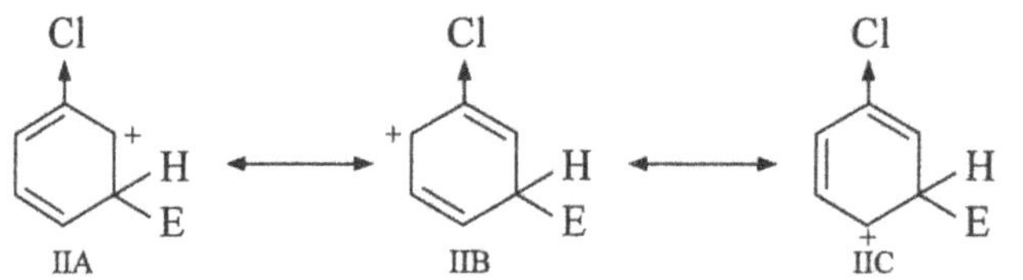

Para Attack

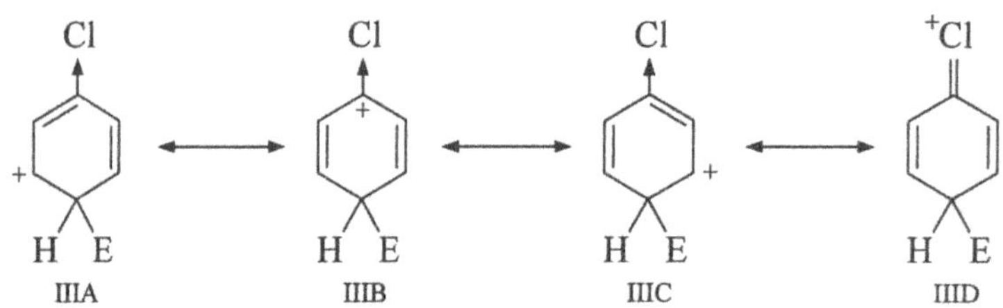

16.7 AROMATICITY

Benzene and several other compounds including hydrocarbon anions and cations are aromatic. Possessing of aromatic character by a compound is aromaticity. The following are various conditions for aromaticity:

(i) The compound structure must be cyclic.
(ii) The cyclic ring system or systems must be planar.
(iii) Each atom in the ring must be sp^2 hybridised and have an unhybridised p orbital. The unhybridised porbital overlap to give continuous ring of delocalised π-electrons.
(iv) The compound should follow Hückel's rule which states that the total number of π-electrons must be $(4n + 2)$ where $n = 0, 1, 2, 3, \ldots$ For example,

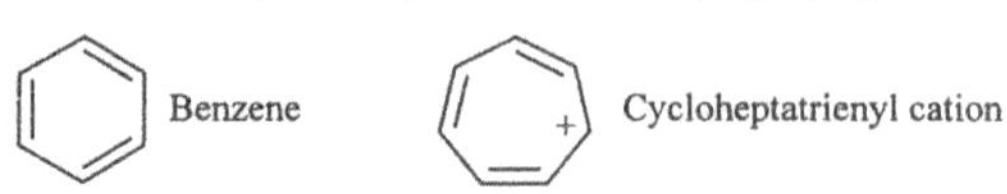

Cyclobutadiene meets the first two criteria but has only four π-electrons so it is not aromatic. 1,3,5-Cyclooctatriene is not planar and contains six π-electrons and is not aromatic. Benzene with its six π-electrons meets all three criteria and is aromatic.

Hückel's rule also applies to polycyclic compounds. Naphthalene and azulene both have 10 continuous π-electrons in a planar molecule and are aromatic.

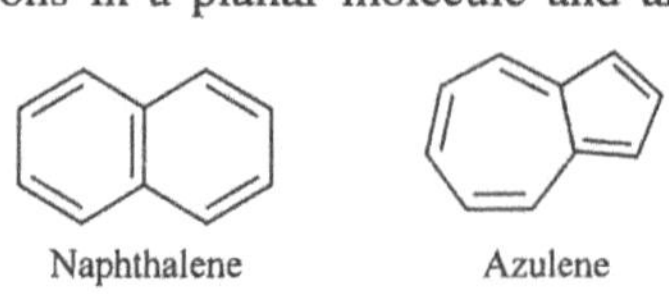

16.8 ANTI-AROMATICITY

A planar, cyclic, conjugated species which are less stable than corresponding acyclic unsaturated species are called anti-aromatic. They have $4n$ π-electrons, e.g. 1,3-cyclobutadiene (n = 1) is anti-aromatic and unstable in spite of having alternate double and single bonds.

Anti-aromatic compound undergoes addition reactions and also positive Bayer's test and bromine-water test.

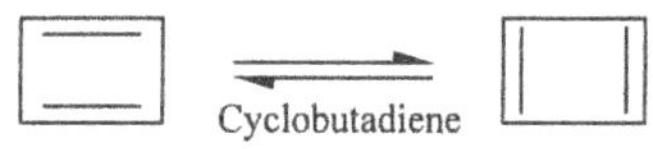

Cyclobutadiene

To be anti-aromatic, a compound should have the following characteristics:

1. Be cyclic and have a closed loop of electrons and a flat structure.
2. Must contain an even pair of electrons, $4n$ p-electrons.

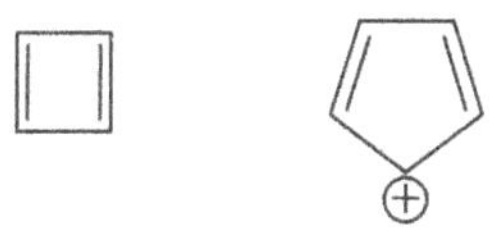

Both anti-aromatic

PRACTICE QUESTIONS

1. What do you understand by the terms 'resonance' and 'resonance energy'? Discuss Kekule's structure of benzene. What is Hückel's rule?
2. How do you elucidate the structure of benzene?
3. t-Pentyl benzene is the major product of the reaction of benzene in the presence of BF_3 with 2-methyl-1-butanol. Account for the formation.
4. (a) Write the mechanism of nitration of benzene.
   (b) Benzene undergoes electrophilic substitution but not addition.
   (c) Why polysubstitution is a complicating factor in Friedel–Crafts alkylation as against nitration?
5. Discuss importance of electrophilic aromatic substitution with suitable examples and also the mechanism involved in the example.
6. Complete the following reduction schemes stating the products and any essential conditions.

$$C_6H_6 + O_2 \longrightarrow$$

7. An aromatic bromo compound on Friedel–Crafts reaction with ethyl chloride and $AlCl_3$ gave B (C_8H_9B). B on oxidation with permanganate gave an acid C. 0.1005 g of C was neutralised by 5 ml of decinormal alkali. Suggest possible structures for A, B and C. (At. Wt. of Br = 80).
8. Define aromaticity and explain the solubility of aromatic compounds in terms of the orbital picture and the Hückel's rule. Mention the typical reactions of such compounds and explain the mechanism of any one of the reactions.
9. Give the methods of preparation and uses of:
   (a) Dicophane
   (b) Gammexane

10. Write short notes on:
    (a) Friedel–Crafts alkylation
    (b) Friedel–Crafts acylation
    (c) Anti-aromaticity
    (d) Aromaticity
11. (a) What do you understand by activating and deactivating groups in electrophilic substitution of benzene? Give two examples each.
    (b) Write the mechanism of nitration and halogenation of benzene.
12. Give three sources for generating electrophiles capable of substituting activated aromatic rings along with suitable equations.
13. (a) Explain why methyl and halogens are ortho, para-directing while nitro group is meta-directing.
    (b) Give the names and structures of three electrophiles capable of substitution only strongly activated aromatic rings.
14. Outline a synthesis for the following products with the given starting reactant.

	Starting Reactant	*Product*
(a)	Benzene	*m*-Chlorobenzoic acid
(b)	Benzene	*tert*-Butyl benzene
(c)	Benzene	*n*-Butyl benzene
(d)	Benzene	1-*tert*-Butyl-4-chlorobenzene
(e)	Benzene	*p*-Bromobenzoic acid
(f)	Toluene	2-Bromo-4-nitrotoluene
(g)	Toluene	2,4,6-Trinitrotoluene (TNT)
(h)	Aniline	2,4,6-Tribromoaniline

17

CHEMISTRY OF ARYL HALIDES

17.1 INTRODUCTION

Aryl halides are aromatic halogen compounds in which the halogen is directly attached to a carbon atom of an aromatic ring. They have the general formula of Ar—X, where Ar is a phenyl (or) a substituted phenyl (or) some other aryl group (e.g. naphthyl).

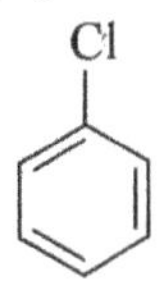

Chlorobenzene

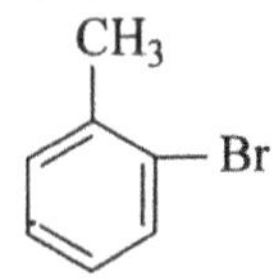

o-Bromotoluene

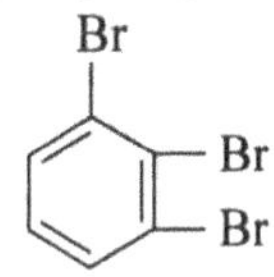

1,2,3-Tribromobenzene

17.2 SYNTHESIS OF ARYL HALIDES

The following methods are used to prepare aryl halides:

1. ***By Halogenation of Aromatic Hydrocarbons*** Aromatic hydrocarbons, on *electrophilic aromatic substitution* with halogens yield aryl halides.

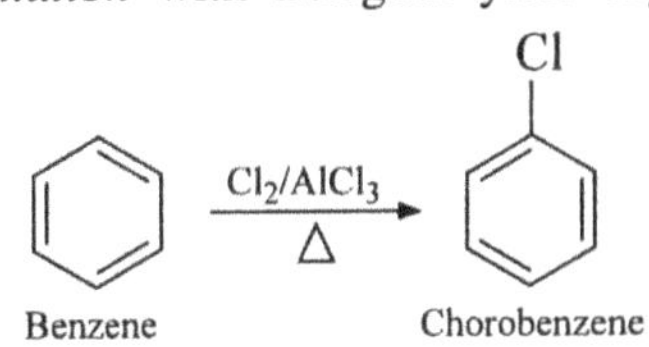

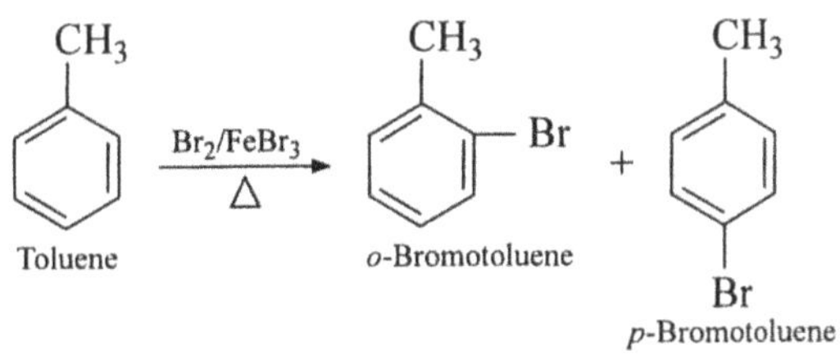

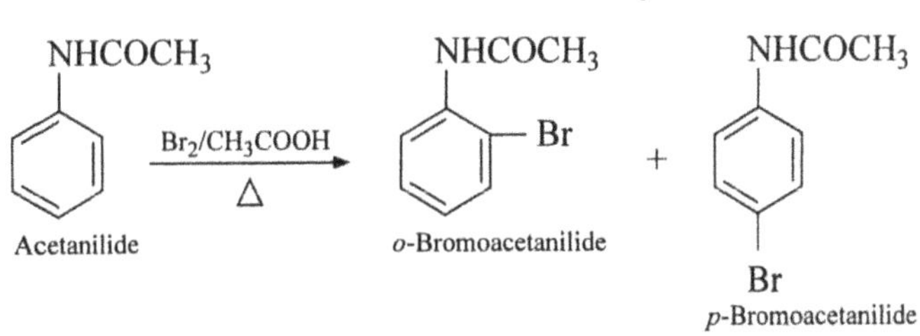

This reaction involves through the formation of arenium ion and involves following steps.

(i) *Generation of an electrophile*

$$X-X + FeX_3 \longrightarrow FeX_4^- + X^+$$

(ii) *The electrophile attacks benzene ring to form resonance-stabilised arenium ion.*

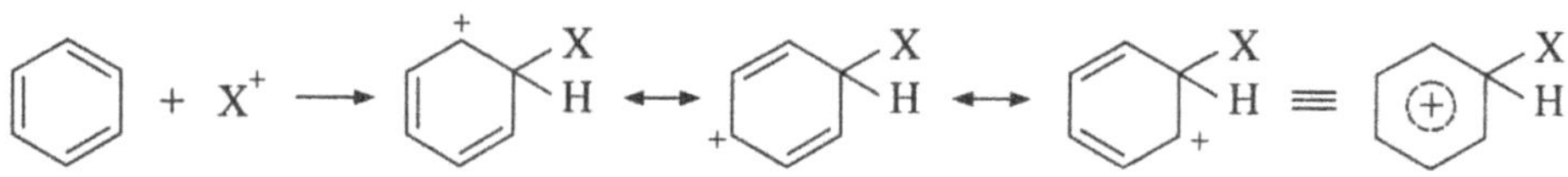

(iii) *Arenium ion loses a proton to form halobenzene*

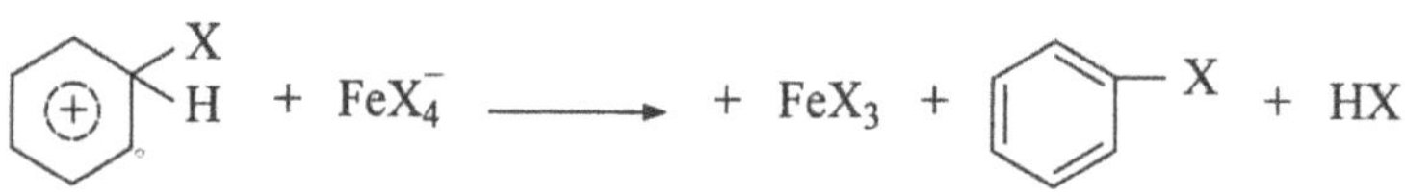

Resonance-stabilised arenium ion — Halobenzene

2. ***From Diazonium Salts*** When an aqueous solution of a diazonium salt is treated with potassium halide or potassium cyanide in presence of metallic copper powder, the diazonium group is replaced to yield a halo or cyano derivative. This reaction is known as *Gattermann reaction*.

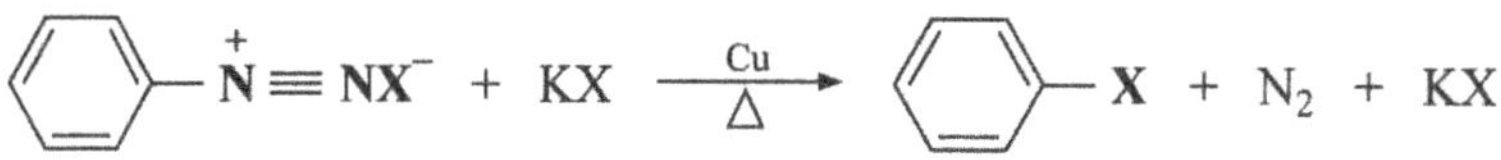

Diazonium halide
(X = hologen or cyano group) — Halo- or cyano-benzene

3. ***Hunsdiecker Reaction*** This reaction involves heating of a silver salt of a carboxylic acid with halogens to get aryl halides.

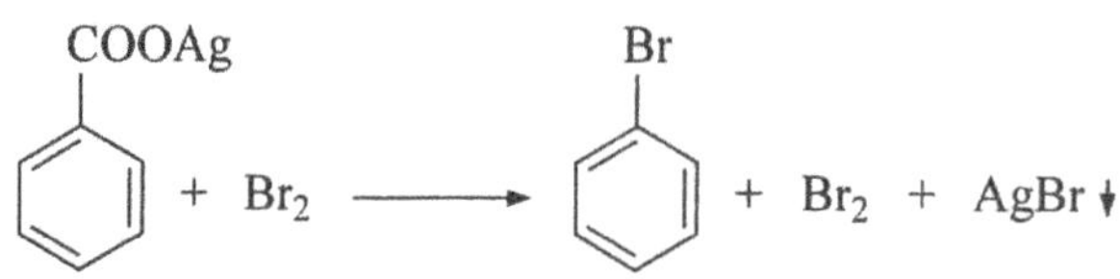

Bromobenzene

17.3 PHYSICAL PROPERTIES

1. They are insoluble in water and soluble in organic solvents.
2. The aryl halides are denser than water and most of these have pleasant smell.

17.4 CHEMICAL PROPERTIES

The aryl halides are less reactive than alkyl halides due to the stronger and shorter carbon–halogen bond in aryl halides. The following are some of the important reactions of aryl halides:

1. ***Formation of Grignard Reagent*** Organomagnesium compounds, frequently called Grignard reagents, are prepared by adding an aryl halide to magnesium shavings in diethyl ether (or) THF solvent.

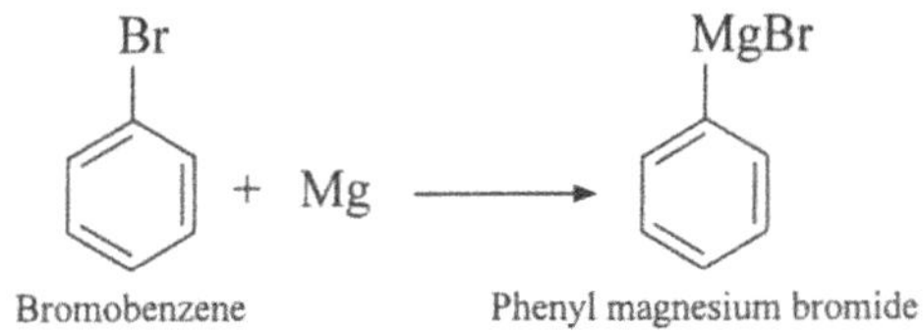

2. ***Wurtz–Fittig Reaction*** Aryl halides react with alkyl halides in presence of sodium metal to yield alkyl benzenes.

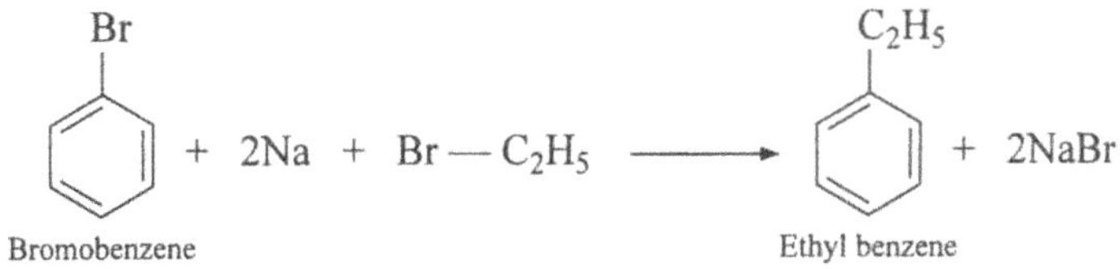

3. ***Nucleophilic Aromatic Substitution*** Aryl halides undergo nucleophilic substitution with great difficulty hence drastic conditions are required (strong nucleophile, high temperature). However, aryl halides undergo nucleophilic substitution readily if the aromatic ring contains electron-withdrawing substituents like —NO_2, —NO or —CN at ortho or para position to halogens. The low reactivity of aryl halides towards nucleophilic substitution is attributed to the following:

(i) *Delocalisation of electrons by resonance* Aryl halide is a hybrid of the following structures:

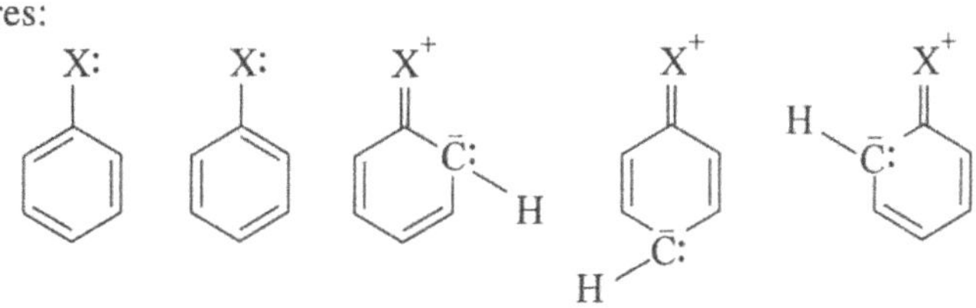

Resonance contributors of an aryl halide

The carbon–halogen bond is stronger than a single covalent bond because it is in between a double bond and a single covalent bond.

(ii) sp^2 hybridised carbon in aryl halides. The bond between carbon–halogen is shorter and stronger and the molecule is more stable.

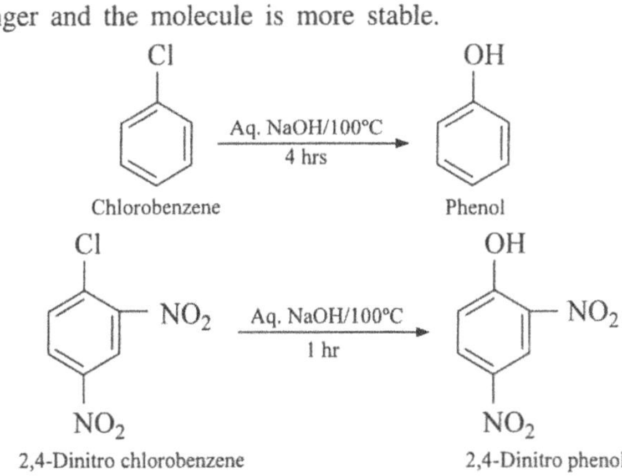

Mechanism The following mechanisms have been suggested for aromatic nucleophilic substitution.

(i) *Intermediate carbanion mechanism* This mechanism involves two steps:

- Formation of carbanion by the addition of nucleophile to the substrate. The carbanion is stabilised by resonance. This step is slow hence is rate determining.

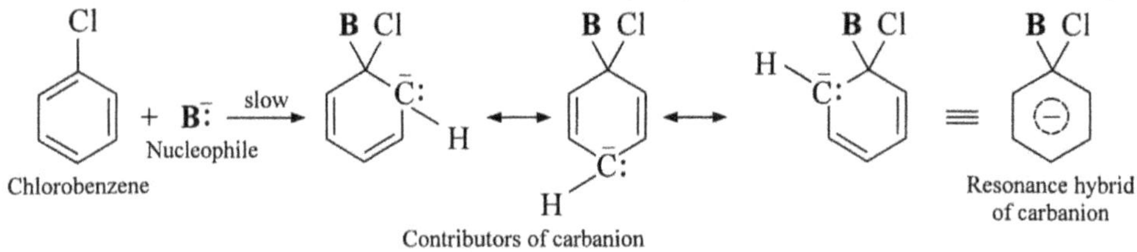

- Elimination of original substituent (halogen) as anion from carbanion to form nucleophilic substitution product.

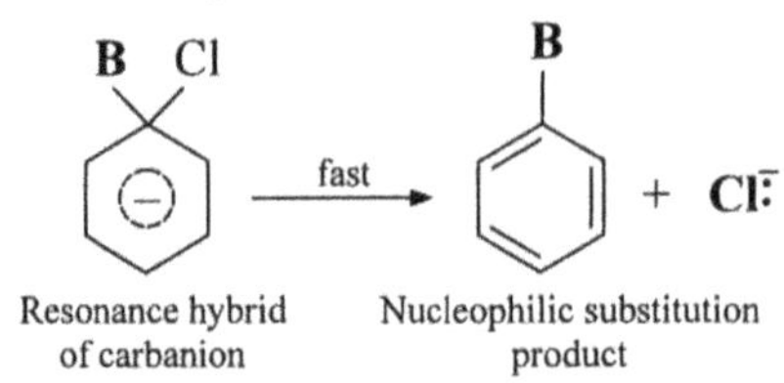

This mechanism is a bimolecular mechanism hence sometimes called S_N2 mechanism. This is also called addition–elimination mechanism.

(ii) *Benzyne mechanism* Benzyne is a highly reactive intermediate species, which contains an additional bond between two ortho carbons of benzene ring. Although benzynes are formally depicted as containing an alkyne, the linear geometry of such a unit means that two *sp*-hybridised carbon atoms cannot be incorporated into a 6-membered ring. Alternative ways of considering the structure are a singlet di-radical (electrons spin paired), a triplet di-radical (parallel spin) or a charge separated species. The true nature of benzyne is presumably a hybrid of all these possibilities resulting in a highly reactive, electrophilic species. There is a little interaction between the electron cloud of the new bond and the electron cloud lying above and below the ring.

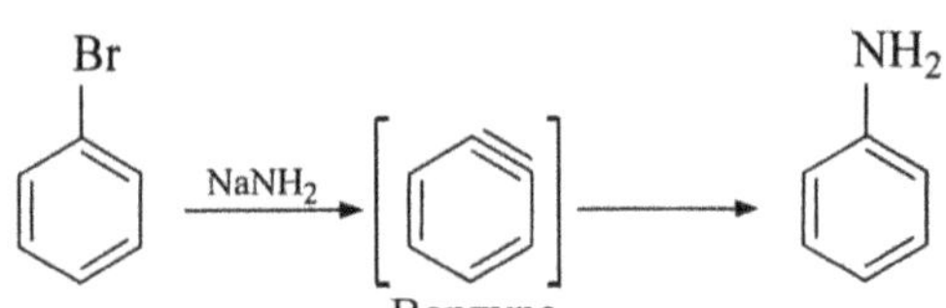

This mechanism requires a strong base (for example $NaNH_2$, BuLi) and is commonly used with haloaromatic substrates, which involves the following steps:

(a) *Elimination* The amide ion (nucleophile) removes hydrogen in the form of proton from one of the ortho positions with respect to halogen. The resulting carbanion loses a halide to form benzyne.

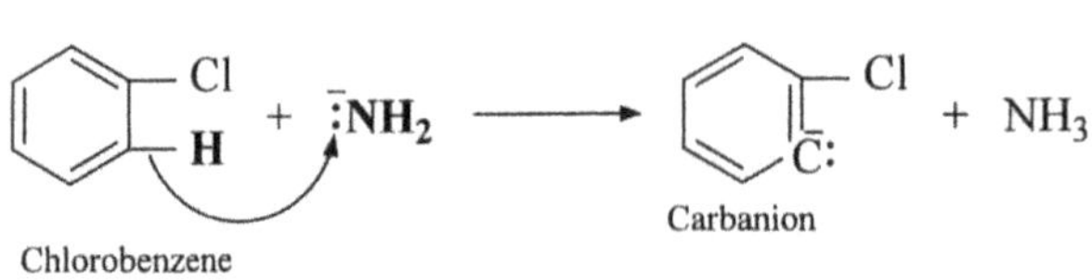

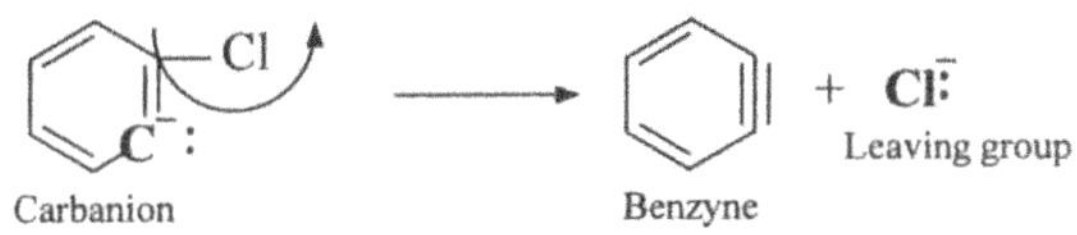

(b) *Addition* In this step, the amide ion gets attached to the benzyne to form the final product.

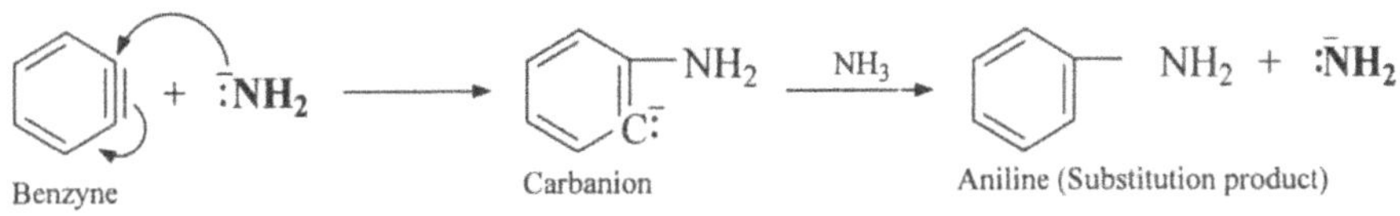

4. ***Electrophilic Aromatic Substitution*** Aryl halides undergo electrophilic aromatic substitution reactions. The halogens have deactivating influence on the aromatic ring and are ortho-, para-directing groups.

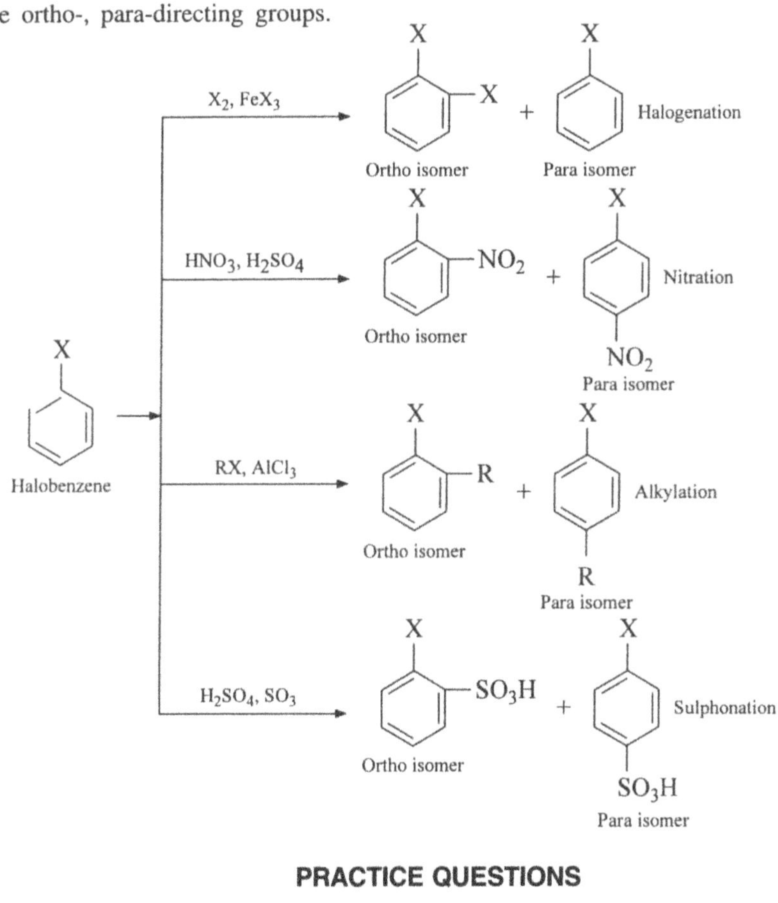

PRACTICE QUESTIONS

1. The reactions of aryl and alkyl halides are different in many ways. Give a pair of reactions that clearly illustrate this fact.
2. Provide a detailed curved-arrow mechanism.

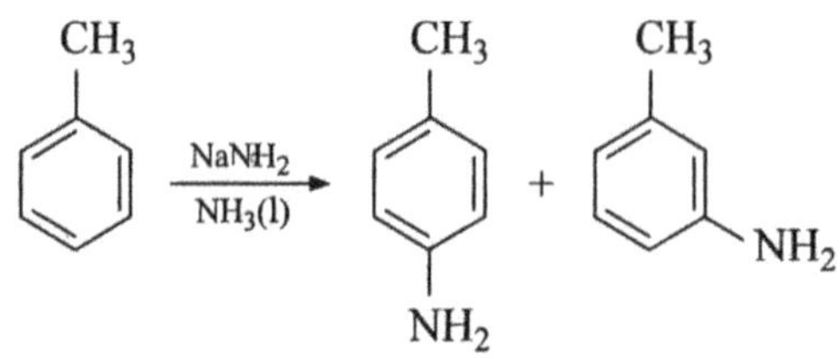

3. Suggest the two most important requirements for the addition–elimination aromatic substitution mechanism.
4. Suggest the three most important requirements for the elimination–addition substitution mechanism.

18

AROMATIC SULPHONIC ACIDS

18.1 INTRODUCTION

Aromatic sulphonic acids are the derivatives of aromatic hydrocarbons. These are obtained from aromatic hydrocarbons by the replacement of one or more hydrogen atom by sulphonic acid (—SO_3H) functional group and are generally named by adding 'suffix sulphonic acid' to the name of parent hydrocarbon.

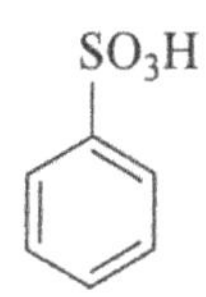

Benzenesulphonic acid

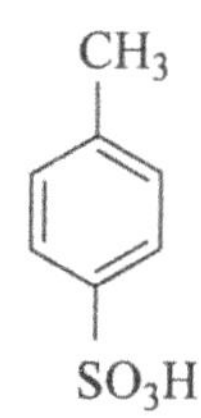

p-Toluenesulphonic acid

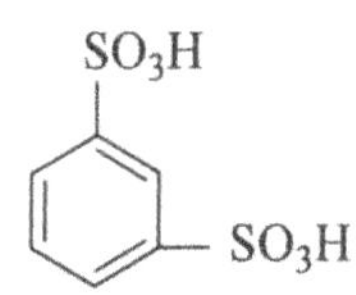

Benzene-1,3-sulphonic acid

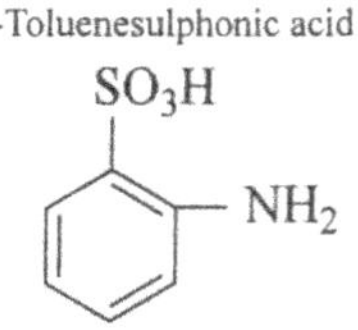

o-Aminobenzene sulphonic acid

18.2 SYNTHESIS OF AROMATIC SULPHONIC ACIDS

1. ***Sulphonation of Aromatic Hydrocarbons*** Aromatic hydrocarbons by direct sulphonation with sulphonic acid give aromatic sulphonic acids. Mono-, di- and tri-sulphonic acids can be prepared. Mono-sulphonic acids are prepared with concentrated sulphuric acid at room temperature, but di- and tri-sulphonic acids are prepared using fuming sulphuric acid ($H_2S_2O_7$) at high temperature. The activating groups and halogens orient the sulphonic acid group to *o*- and *p*-positions.

2. ***From Aromatic Hydrocarbons by the Action of Chlorosulphonic Acids*** Aromatic hydrocarbons on treatment with chlorosulphonic acid yield arylsulphonylchlorides, which on hydrolysis give arylsulphonic acids.

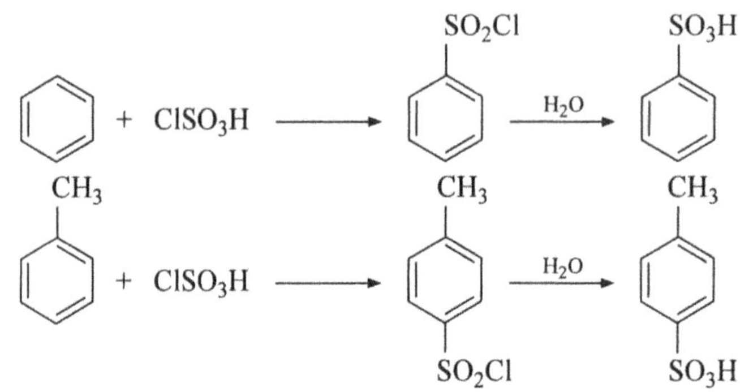

3. ***From Thiophenols by Oxidation*** Thiophenols on oxidation give aryl sulphonic acids.

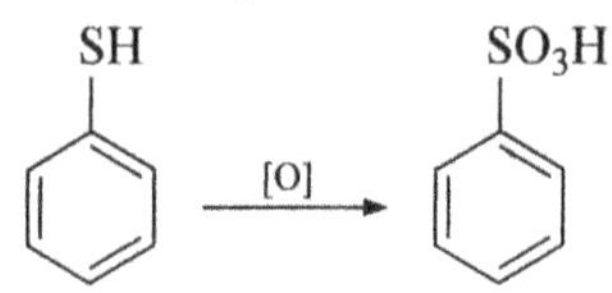

18.3 PHYSICAL PROPERTIES

1. Aromatic sulphonic acids are non-volatile, colourless, crystalline compounds.
2. They are hygroscopic in nature.
3. They have sour taste.
4. Aromatic sulphonic acids are freely soluble in water.
5. They have strong acidic properties.

18.4 CHEMICAL PROPERTIES

Aromatic sulphonic acids possess an aromatic nucleus and a sulphonic acid functional group. They exhibit the following general chemical reactions.

1. ***Acidity of Aromatic Sulphonic Acids*** Arylsulphonic acids are strongly acidic in nature. Hence, they form salts with bases. The acidity of aromatic sulphonic acids is equal to that of sulphuric acid.

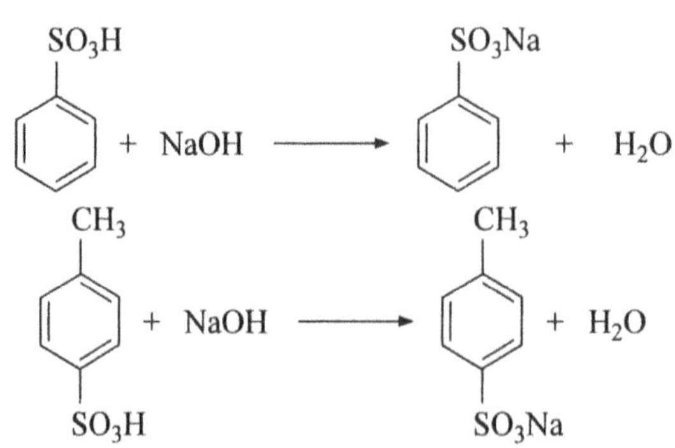

2. ***Conversion of Arylsulphonic Acid to Arylsulphonic Chloride*** Arylsulphonic acids can be converted to their respective arylsulphonic chlorides, on treatment with thionyl chloride or phosphorous pentachloride.

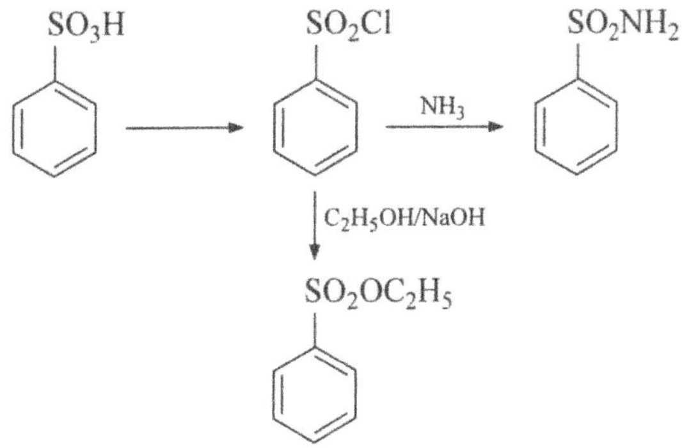

3. ***Formation of Sulphones*** Aromatic sulphonic acids give sulphones on reaction with aromatic hydrocarbons.

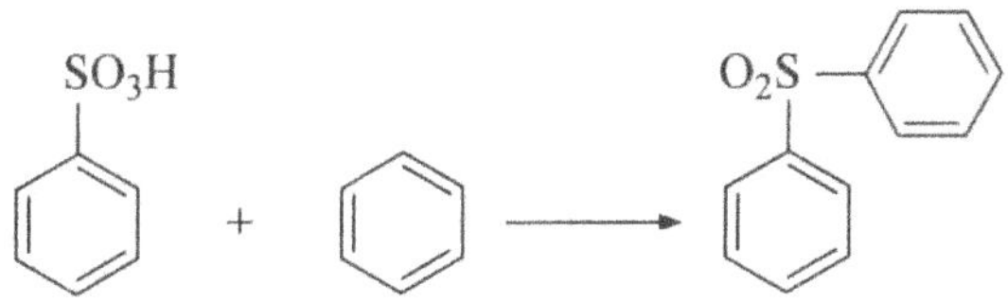

4. ***Desulphonation*** Aromatic sulphonic acids are converted to aromatic hydrocarbons on heating with aqueous acid.

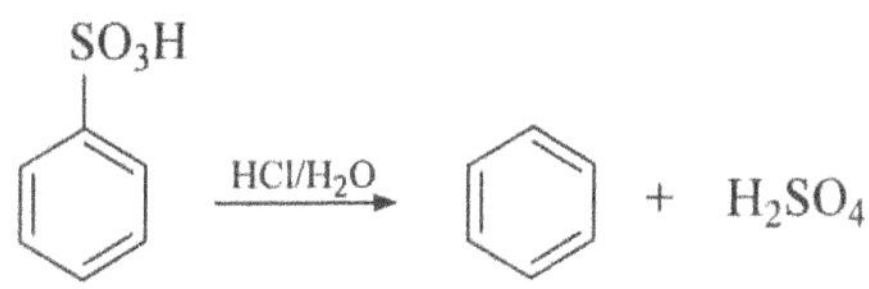

5. ***Conversion to Phenols*** Arylsulphonic acids give phenols on heating with solid sodium hydroxide.

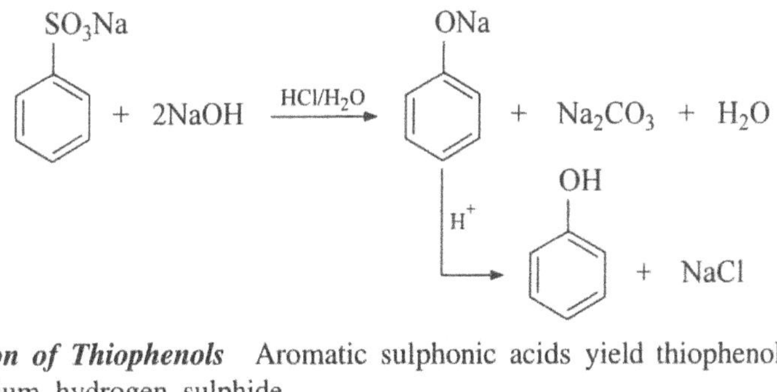

6. ***Formation of Thiophenols*** Aromatic sulphonic acids yield thiophenols on heating with potassium hydrogen sulphide.

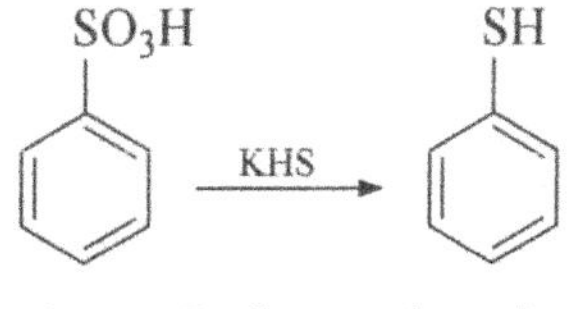

7. ***Formation of Aromatic Amines*** Sodium salts of aromatic sulphonic acids yield aromatic amines on treatment with sodamide.

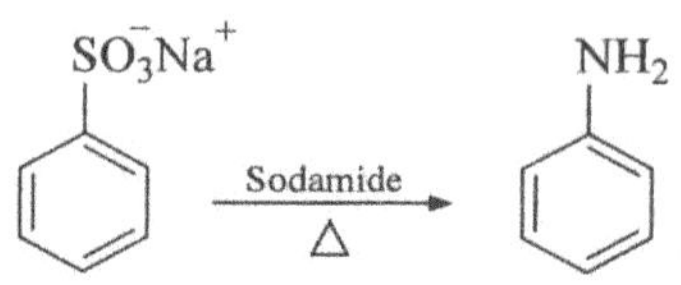

8. ***Electrophilic Aromatic Substitution*** Aromatic sulphonic acids undergo nitration, sulphonation and halogenation. The sulphonic acid group is meta-directing group.

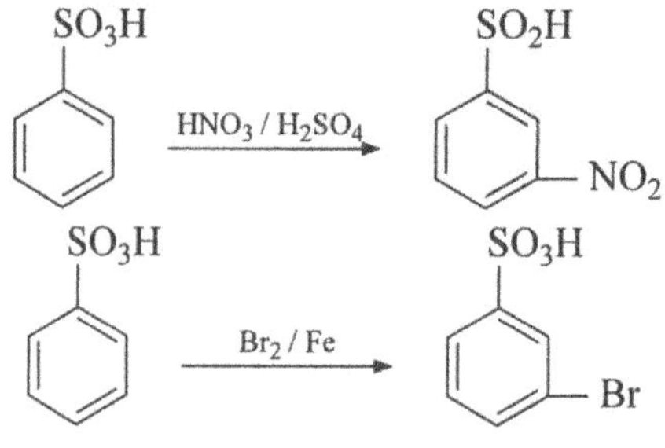

18.5 USES OF ARYLSULPHONIC ACIDS

1. Arylsulphonic acids have strong acidic and mild oxidising properties. Hence, they are used as catalysts.
2. Arylsulphonic acids are valuable synthetic compounds as a number of organic compounds can be synthesized from them.
3. Barium and calcium salts of sulphonic acids are used as lubricating oils for internal combustion engines.
4. Some arylsulphonic acids have detergent properties, e.g. *p*-dodecylbenzene sulphonate.

18.6 PHARMACEUTICAL COMPOUNDS

1. ***Saccharin*** Saccharin is a synthetic, white, crystalline powder with a chemical formula $C_6H_4CONHSO_2$, which in its pure state is 550 times as sweet as sugar cane. In its commercial form, saccharin is estimated to have a sweetening power 375 times that of sugar. The sweet taste of the substance was discovered accidentally in the late ninetheenth century in the course of investigations of toluene derivatives. When moderately large amounts of saccharin are dissolved in water, the solution has a bitter taste, the sweetness being evident only in dilute solutions. Saccharin is not digested by the body and has no food value. Persons suffering from diabetes (Diabetes Mellitus) and persons on weight-reducing diets consume it in place of sugar, for the psychological purpose of satisfying a taste for sweetness. Some evidence indicates, however, that saccharin can itself stimulate the appetite and the production of insulin by the body.

Saccharin is synthesised from toluene-*o*-sulphonic acid by the following steps:

(a) Toluene-*o*-sulphonic acid is converted into toluene-*o*-sulphonyl chloride on treatment with thionylchloride

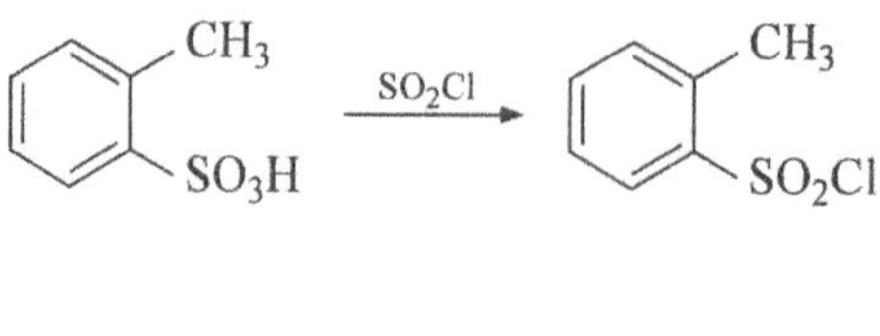

(b) Toluene-*o*-sulphonamide is obtained by adding ammonia to toluene-*o*-sulphonylchloride.

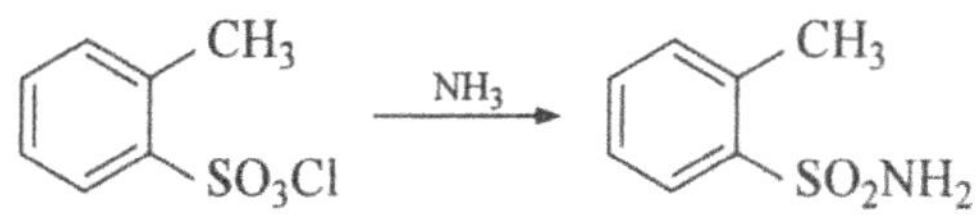

(c) Toluene-*o*-sulphonamide is oxidised to *o*-sulphamoyl benzoic acid by oxidation.

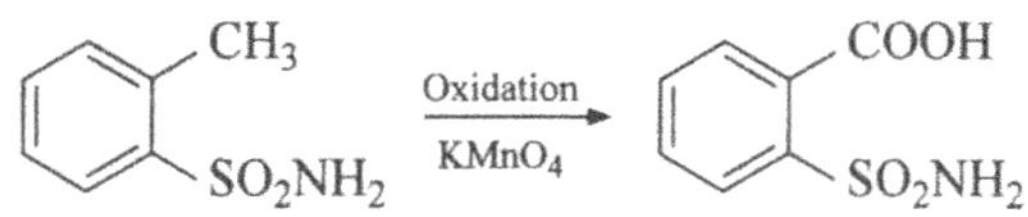

(d) Acidification of *o*-sulphamoyl benzoic acid yields saccharin.

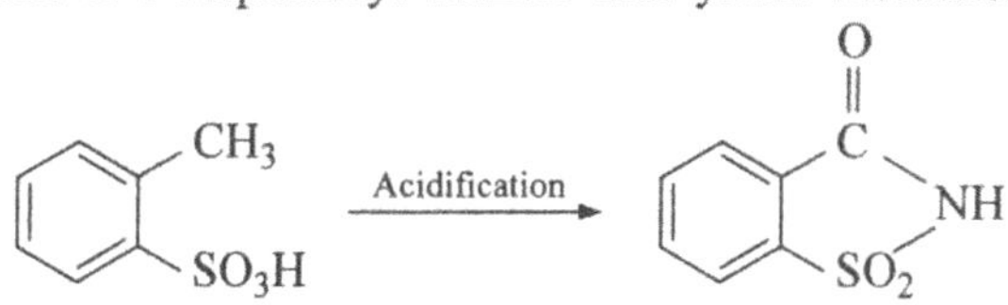

Saccharin is a colourless, crystalline, water insoluble powder. It is having an intensely sweet taste.

Use Saccharin is an intensely sweet substance. Hence, it is used as a sweetening agent in vehicles, canned foods, beverages and diets. It is sweeter than sucrose.

2. ***Sodium Lauryl Sulphate*** Sodium lauryl sulphate is a sodium salt of laurylsulphuric acid. The preparation of sodium laurylsulphate involves two steps.

(a) In the first step, lauryl alcohol is allowed to react with chlorosulphonic acid to give the lauryl ester of sulphuric acid.

$$\underset{\text{Laurylalcohol}}{CH_3(CH_2)_{10}CH_2OH} + \underset{\text{Chlorosulphonic acid}}{Cl-\overset{\overset{O}{\|}}{\underset{\underset{O}{\|}}{S}}-C} \longrightarrow \underset{\text{Lauyl ester of sulphuric acid}}{CH_3(CH_2)_{10}CH_2-O-\overset{\overset{O}{\|}}{\underset{\underset{O}{\|}}{C}}-OH}$$

(b) In the second step, aqueous sodium carbonate is added to produce sodium laurylsulphate.

$$\underset{\text{Lauryl ester of sulphuric acid}}{CH_3(CH_2)_{10}CH_2-O-\overset{\overset{O}{\|}}{\underset{\underset{O}{\|}}{S}}-OH} + Na_2CO_3$$

$$\downarrow$$

$$\underset{\text{Sodiumlaurylsulphate}}{CH_3(CH_2)_{10}CH_2-O-\overset{\overset{O}{\|}}{\underset{\underset{O}{\|}}{S}}-O^-Na^+} + H_2O + CO_2$$

PRACTICE QUESTIONS

1. What are aryl sulphonic acid derivatives? Enumerate their important derivatives and uses.
2. Write various chemical reactions of aryl sulphonic acids.
3. Write synthesis, properties and uses of:
   (a) Saccharin
   (b) Sodiumlaurylsulphate

19

CHEMISTRY OF ALDEHYDES AND KETONES

The compounds possessing of carbonyl group ($-\overset{|}{C}=O$) are called carbonyl compounds. In aldehydes, the carbonyl carbon is linked to one hydrogen atom and one alkyl or aryl group while in ketones it is linked to two alkyl or aryl groups.

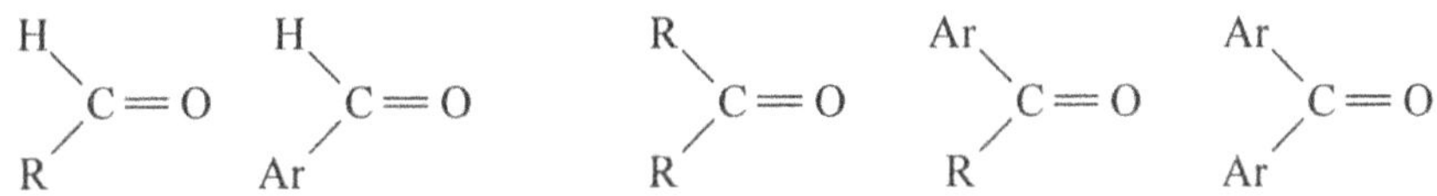

Aldehyde　　　　Ketone

A large number of aldehydes and ketones can be found in nature as highly fragrant substances. Many of these compounds are commercially important as fragrance additives to a wide variety of consumer products.

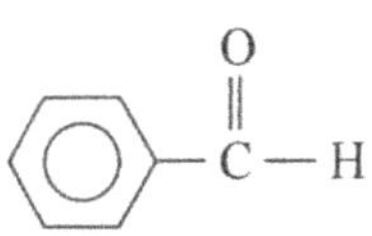

Benzaldehyde
(Oil of almonds)

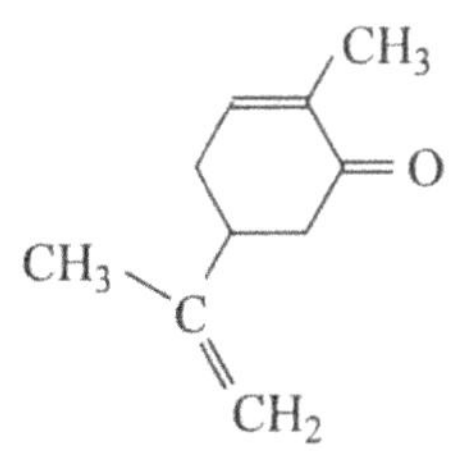

Carvone
(Spearmint oil)

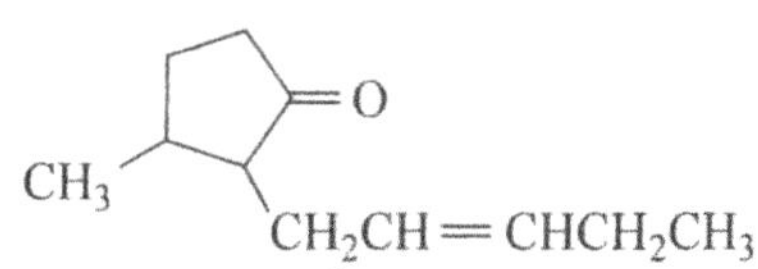

Jasmone
(Oil of jasmine)

19.1 NOMENCLATURE

Aldehyde nomenclature is governed by the following rules:

(i) Identify the longest continuous chain of carbons with the carbonyl carbon as part of the chain.

(ii) Number the carbon chain so that the carbonyl carbon is always at position 1.

(iii) Locate and identify alphabetically the branched groups by prefixing the carbon number attached to it.

(iv) After identifying the name, number and location of each branched group, use the alkane name corresponding to the number of carbons in the continuous chain.

(v) According to IUPAC system, aldehydes are named by replacing the 'e' of the corresponding alkane by '-al'. Hence, the general name for aldehydes is alkanals.

Formula	*Common Name*	*IUPAC Name*
HCHO	Formaldehyde	Methanal
CH_3CHO	Acetaldehyde	Ethanal
$CH_3.CH_2.CHO$	Propionaldehyde	Propanal
$CH_3.CH_2.CH_2CHO$	Butyraldehyde	Butanal

Nomenclature of ketones Ketones' nomenclature is based on the following rules:

(i) Identify the longest continuous chain of carbons with the carbonyl carbon as on the carbons in the chain.
(ii) Number the carbons so that the carbonyl carbon has the lowest possible number.
(iii) Identify the branched groups by naming them in alphabetical order and prefixing the carbon number they are attached to onto the name. If more than one of the same group is present use the Greek prefixes (di for 2, tri for 3, etc.).
(iv) Use the alkane name corresponding to the number of carbons in the chain.
(v) Drop the 'e' in the alkane name and add the characteristic IUPAC ending for ketones which is 'one'. Hence, the general name for ketones is alkanones.

Formula	*Common Name*	*IUPAC Name*
CH_3COCH_3	Acetone	Propanone
$CH_3CO.C_2H_5$	Ethylmethylketone	Butanone
$C_2H_5CO.C_3H_7$	Ethylpropylketone	3-Hexanone

19.2 ISOMERISM

Aldehydes and ketones exhibit the following types of isomerism:

1. ***Chain Isomerism*** Both aldehydes and ketones show chain isomerism, e.g. *n*-butyraldehyde ($CH_3CH_2CH_2CHO$) and isobutyraldehyde [$(CH_3)_2CHCHO$] are chain isomers. Similarly, methyl *n*-propyl ketone ($CH_3COCH_2CH_2CH_3$) and isopropyl methyl ketone [$CH_3COCH(CH_3)_2$] are also chain isomers.

2. ***Positional Isomerism*** Ketones exhibit positional isomerism. For example, 2-pentanone ($CH_3COCH_2CH_2CH_3$) and 3-pentanone ($CH_3CH_2COCH_2CH_3$) are positional isomers.

3. ***Functional Isomerism*** Ketones show functional isomerism with aldehydes and unsaturated alcohols. For example

CH_3COCH_2	CH_3CH_2CHO	$CH_2=CHCH_2OH$
Acetone	Propanal	2-Propen-1-ol

19.3 PREPARATION OF CARBONYL COMPOUNDS

The carbonyl compounds are prepared by the following methods.

19.3.1 Preparation of Aldehydes

1. ***Oxidation of Alcohols*** Primary alcohols are oxidised to aldehydes by using oxidising agents (acidic solutions of potassium permanganate, sodium dichromate, sodium chromate

or chromic acid). The reaction, however, does not stop at the aldehyde, which is further oxidised to a carboxylic acid. The oxidation of primary alcohol can be stopped at the aldehyde stage by using a milder oxidising agent (pyridinium chlorochromate, Tollens reagent, and Fehlings reagent) or by dehydrogenation with copper metal at high temperatures.

$$\underset{\text{Primary alcohol}}{RCH_2OH} \xrightarrow[\text{or Cu, Heating}]{\text{Pyridinium chlorochromate}} \underset{\text{Aldehyde}}{RCHO}$$

$$\underset{\text{Ethyl alcohol}}{CH_3CH_2OH} \xrightarrow[H_2SO_4]{Na_2Cr_2O_7} \underset{\text{Acetaldehyde}}{CH_3CHO} \xrightarrow{\text{Further oxidation}} \underset{\text{Acetic acid}}{CH_3COOH}$$

2. ***Reduction of Acid Chlorides*** Aldehydes are prepared by the reduction of acid chlorides with hydrogen gas in presence of palladium catalyst (poisoned with barium sulphate) or lithium aluminium hydride. This is known as *Rosenmund's reduction.*

$$\underset{\text{Acid chloride}}{RCOCl \text{ or } ArCOCl} \xrightarrow[\text{or } LiAlH_4]{\text{Hydrogen + Pd } (BaSO_4)} \underset{\text{Aldehyde}}{RCHO \text{ or } ArCHO}$$

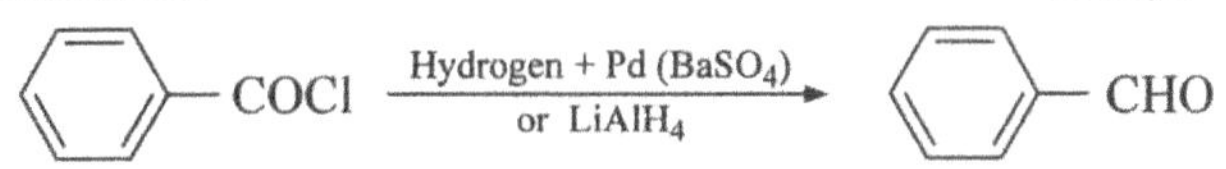

Benzoylchloride Benzaldehyde

3. ***Oxidation of Methylbenzenes*** Aldehydes are prepared by alkaline hydrolysis of gem dihalides or gem diacetates, which are prepared from methylbenzenes, by heating with chlorine or acetic anhydride respectively.

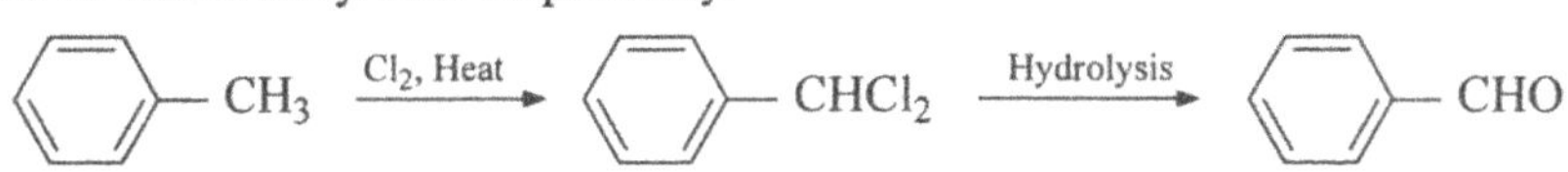

Methylbenzene Benzaldehyde

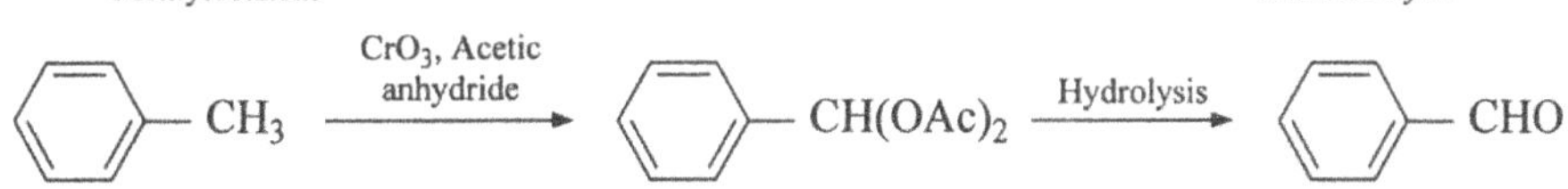

Methylbenzene (Toulene) Benzaldehyde

4. ***Reimer–Tiemann Reaction (Synthesis of Phenolic Aldehydes)*** When a phenol is treated with aqueous NaOH and $CHCl_3$ at 70°C, an aldehyde group (—CHO) is introduced at the ortho position of —OH group on to the aromatic ring. In this reaction, benzal chloride is initially formed which on alkaline hydrolysis converts to —CHO group. This reaction is known as Reimer–Tiemann reaction.

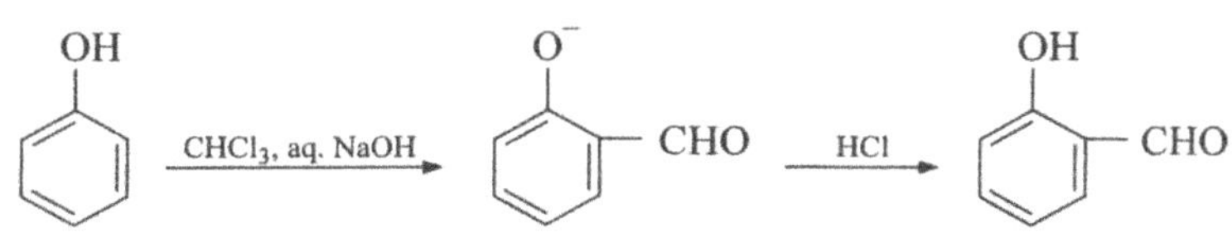

Phenol Salicylaldehyde

Mechanism Reimer–Tiemann reaction is an electrophilic substitution. This involves the following steps:

Substitution takes place on the highly reactive phenoxide ring. Although $:CCl_2$ is neutral, it is strongly electrophilic because the carbon atom is a sextet.

(a) The electrophilic reagent is dichlorocarbene ($:CCl_2$) which is generated from $CHCl_3$ by the action of a base. Although $:CCl_2$ is neutral, it is strongly electrophilic because the carbon atom is a sextet.

$$\underset{\text{Chloroform}}{CHCl_3} + \underset{\text{Base}}{^-{:}OH} \rightleftharpoons H_2O + \underset{\text{Trichlorocarbanion}}{Cl_3C{:}^-} \rightleftharpoons Cl^- + \underset{\text{Dichlorocarbene}}{Cl_2C{:}}$$

(b) Electrophile (dichlorocarbene $:CCl_2$) attacks on the highly reactive phenoxide ring.

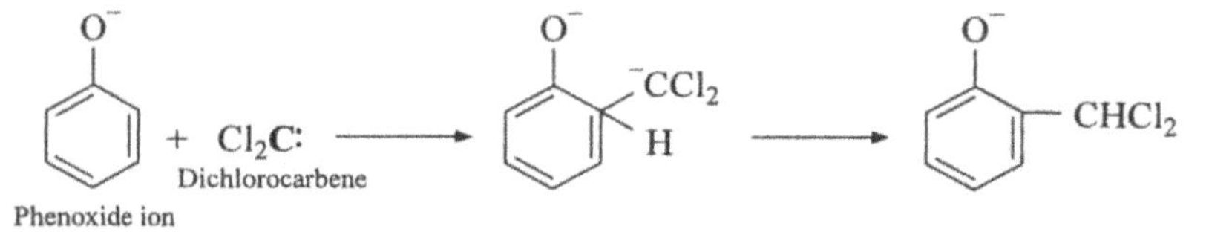

(c) Substitution product on alkaline hydrolysis yields an aromatic aldehyde.

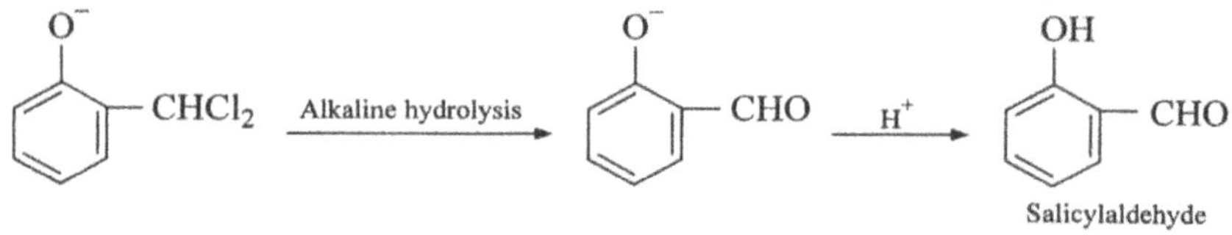

5. ***Ozonolysis of Alkenes*** Ozonolysis of alkenes is used as a synthetic tool for the preparation of aldehydes and ketones. This reaction involves addition of ozone to an alkene to form ozonide, which on hydrolysis in presence of zinc dust yields one or more aldehydes or ketones.

$$\underset{\text{Propene}}{H_3CCH{=}CH_2} \xrightarrow[\text{(ii) } H_2O/\text{Zinc}]{\text{(i) } O_3} \underset{\text{Acetaldehyde}}{CH_3CHO} + \underset{\text{Formaldehyde}}{HCHO}$$

19.3.2 Preparation of Ketones

1. ***Oxidation of Alcohols*** Secondary alcohols are oxidised to ketones by using oxidising agents or by heating with copper. This is similar to a dehydrogenation where hydrogen atoms are eliminated from the carbinol carbon and the hydroxylic oxygen to produce the π bond of the carbonyl carbon. The oxidising agent is chromic acid (H_2CrO_4), which can be prepared as needed by adding sulphuric acid to a potassium dichromate solution in which the alcohol has been added. Indeed, this reaction is usually carried out in acetone or acetic acid solutions.

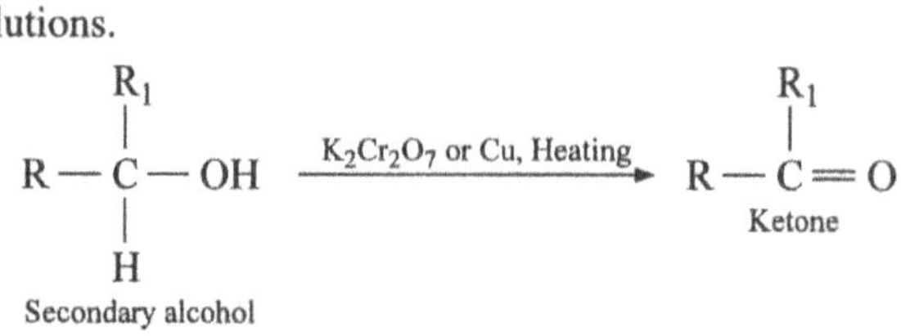

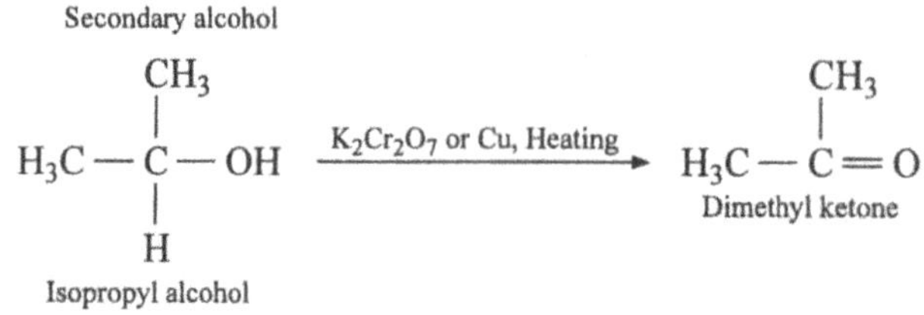

2. ***Reaction of Acid Chlorides with Organo Cadmium Compounds*** Acid chlorides on reaction with organo cadmium compounds yield ketones. The required organo cadmium compounds are prepared from corresponding organo magnesium compounds. The reason for using organo cadmium compounds is that, they are less reactive than organo magnesium compounds and do not react with the formed ketones.

$$\underset{\text{Grignard reagent}}{2R-MgX} + CdCl_2 \longrightarrow \underset{\text{Organo cadmium}}{R_2Cd} + 2Mg(X)Cl$$

$$\underset{\text{Acidchloride}}{2R_1-\overset{\overset{\displaystyle O}{\|}}{C}-Cl} + \underset{\text{Organo cadmium}}{R_2Cd} \longrightarrow \underset{\text{Ketone}}{2R_1-\overset{\overset{\displaystyle O}{\|}}{C}-R} + CdCl_2$$

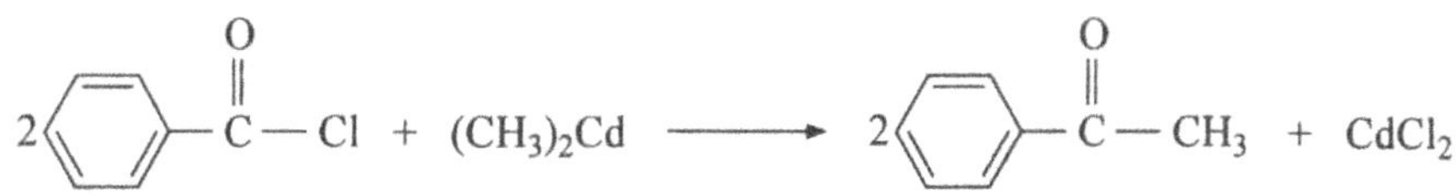

Benzoylchloride Acetophenone

3. ***Friedel–Crafts Acylation*** Friedel–Crafts acylation involves reaction between acyl halide and an aromatic compound to form ketones. This reaction is similar to the Friedel–Crafts alkylation reaction except that the electrophile is formed from an acid halide (acyl halide) instead of an alkyl halide.

$$\underset{\text{Aromatic hydrocarbon}}{ArH} + \underset{\text{Acyl chloride}}{R-\overset{\overset{\displaystyle Cl}{|}}{C}=O} \xrightarrow{AlCl_3} \underset{\text{Ketone}}{R-\overset{\overset{\displaystyle Ar}{|}}{C}=O} + HCl$$

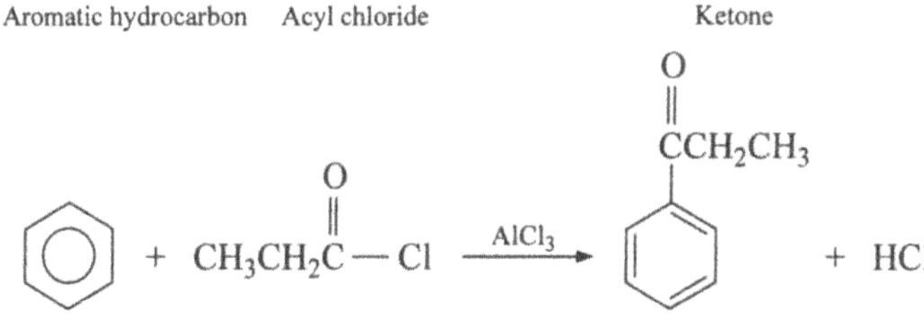

Mechanism Friedel–Crafts acylation reaction proceeds through the formation of acylium ion (electrophile) which undergoes electrophilic aromatic substitution in aromatic compound to form ketone.

(a) An electrophile is generated. The electrophile is an acyl cation (usually called an acylium ion). This acylium ion is relatively stable (all the atoms of acylium ion are in octet configuration).

$$\underset{\text{Acyl chloride}}{RCOCl} + AlCl_3 \longrightarrow \underset{\text{Acylium ion}}{R-\overset{\overset{\displaystyle O}{\|}}{C}\oplus} + \overline{AlCl_4}$$

(b) The electrophile (*acylium ion*) attacks benzene ring to form arenium ion.

$$\underset{\text{Aromatic hydrocarbon}}{ArH} + \underset{\text{Acylium ion}}{R-\overset{\overset{\displaystyle O}{\|}}{C}\oplus} \longrightarrow \underset{\text{Arenium ion}}{Ar^{+}\!\!<^{H}_{COR}}$$

(c) Arenium ion loses a proton to give acyl benzene.

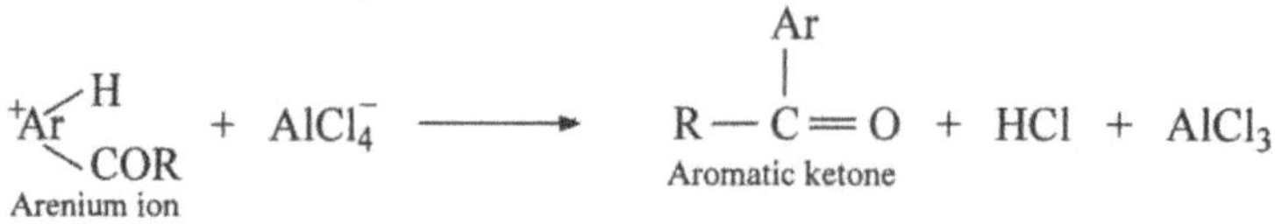

4. ***By Pinacol Rearrangement*** Pinacols can be converted into substituted ketones (pinacolones) in presence of mineral acids, acetyl chloride or acetic acid.

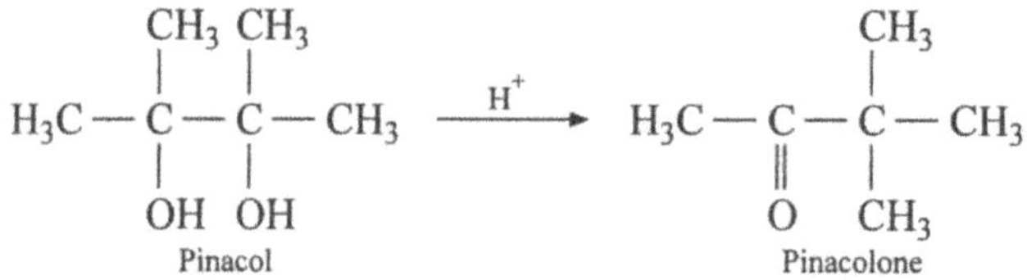

Mechanism Formation of substituted ketones from pinacol involves following steps through the intermediate formation of carbocation. In this rearrangement, the driving force for the migration of an alkyl group is the strong π-electrons release of a lone pair of electrons from the —OH group.

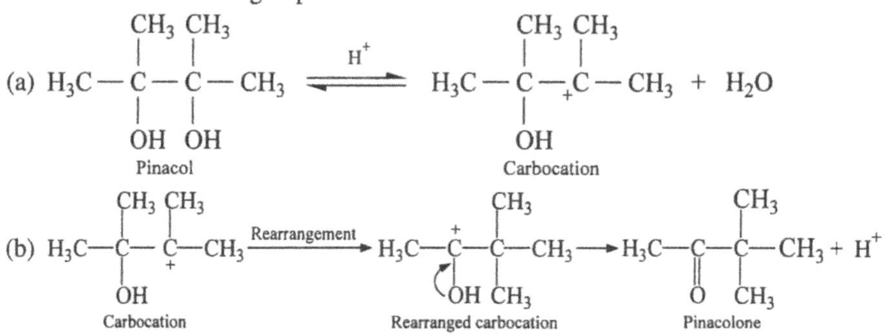

5. ***Ozonolysis of Alkenes*** Ozonolysis of alkenes reaction involves addition of ozone to an alkene to form ozonide, which on hydrolysis (in presence of zinc dust) yields one or more aldehydes or ketones.

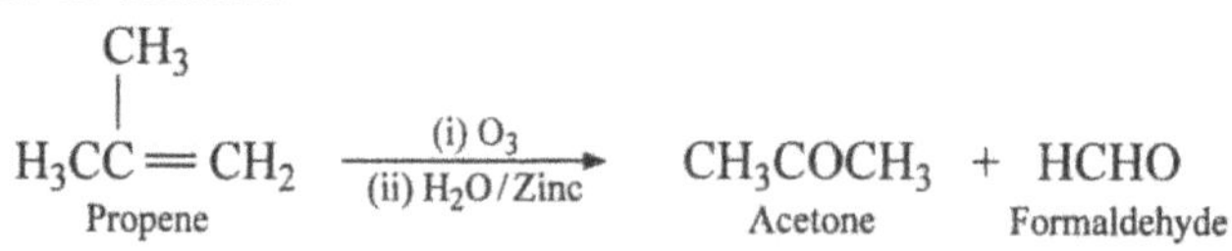

6. ***From Acetoacetic Ester*** Ketones can also be prepared from acetoacetic ester. In this method, the acetoacetic ester is converted into sodioacetoacetic ester which on reacting with alkyl halide forms alkylacetoacetic ester by nucleophilic substitution. The obtained alkylacetoacetic ester is hydrolysed to get β-keto acid, which is decarboxylated to give alkyl-substituted ketone.

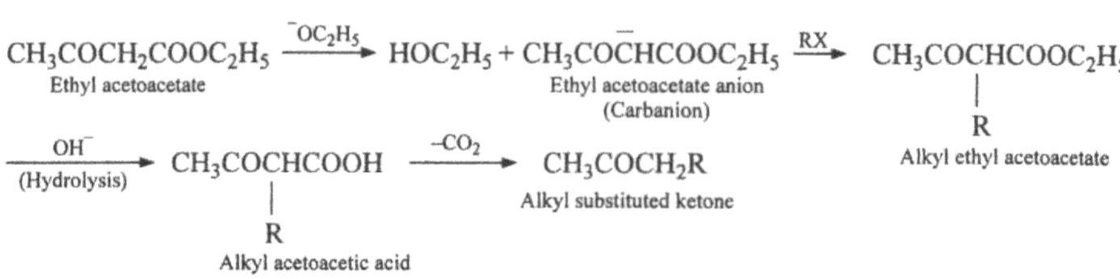

19.4 PHYSICAL PROPERTIES OF CARBONYL COMPOUNDS

1. The lower members up to C_{11} are colourless liquids (except formaldehyde which is a gas at room temperature) while the higher members are solids.
2. The lower members are soluble in water but the higher members are insoluble, as they are unable to develop intermolecular hydrogen bonding with water.
3. Aldehydes and ketones possess lower boiling and melting points than the corresponding alcohols and carboxylic acids due to the absence of intermolecular hydrogen bonding.
4. Aldehydes and ketones are capable of developing dipole–dipole intermolecular interactions, as they possess carbonyl group.

19.5 CHEMICAL PROPERTIES OF CARBONYL COMPOUNDS

The following chemical properties are exhibited by carbonyl compounds:

1. ***Reduction of Carbonyl Compounds*** Different reagents reduce carbonyl compounds as follows:

(i) *Reduction to alcohols* The carbonyl group of aldehydes and ketones can be reduced to primary and secondary alcohols respectively in presence of hydrogen gas and metal catalyst (Pt, Pd or Ni) or chemical reducing agents ($LiAlH_4$, or $NaBH_4$ or aluminium isopropoxide).

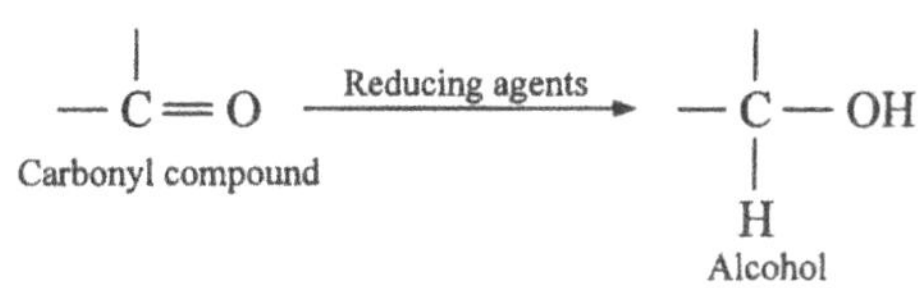

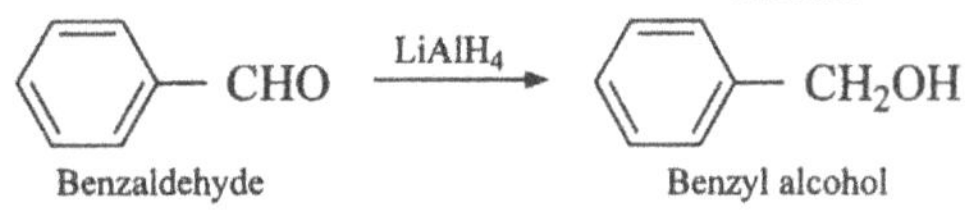

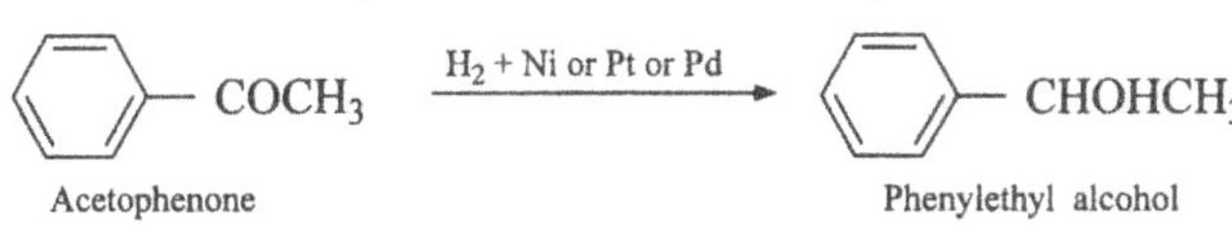

Metal hydride, such as $LiAlH_4$ or $NaBH_4$, reduces aldehydes and ketones to alcohols by the following reaction mechanism.

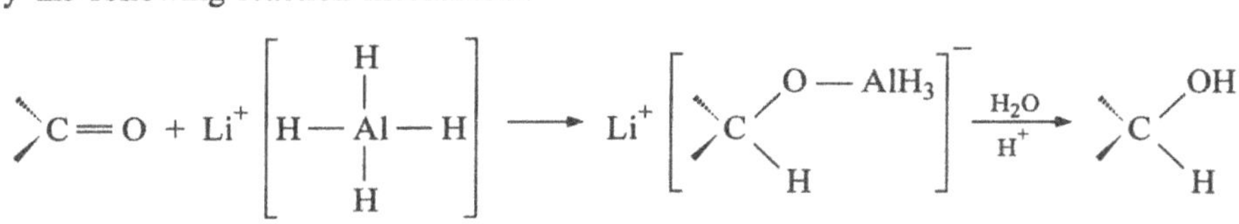

Reduction of aldehydes or ketones to the corresponding alcohols with aluminium alkoxides is known as Meerwein–Pondorf–Verley reduction (the reverse of the Oppenauer oxidation):

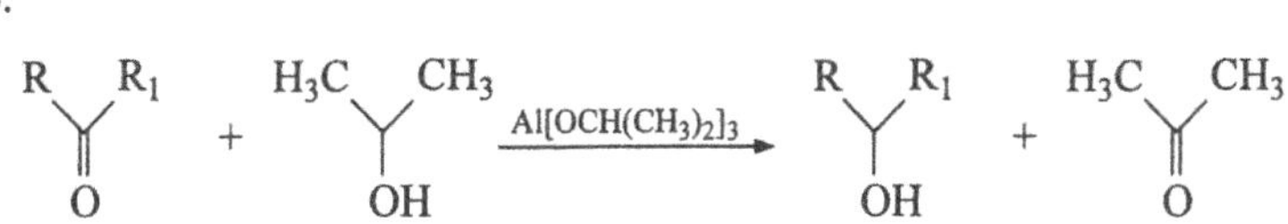

(ii) *Reduction to hydrocarbons* Aldehydes and ketones can also be reduced to hydrocarbons with zinc amalgam (Zn/Hg) in presence of HCl (Clemmensen reduction) or hydrazine ($NH_2 — NH_2$) in presence of sodium ethoxide (Wolf–Kishner reduction).

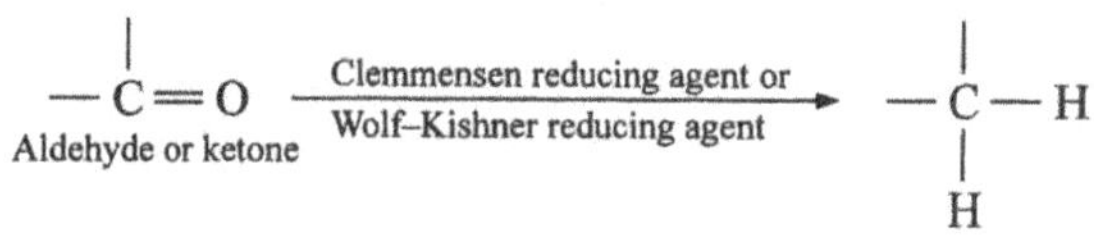

Aldehyde or ketone — Alkane

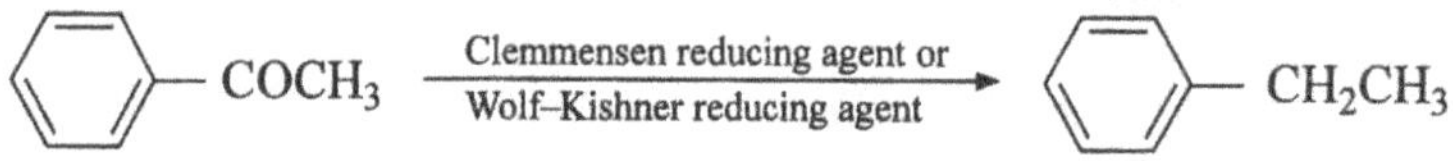

Acetophenone — Ethylbenzene

Mechanism The Clemmensen reduction proceeds through the intermediate formation of carbanion. It involves the following steps.

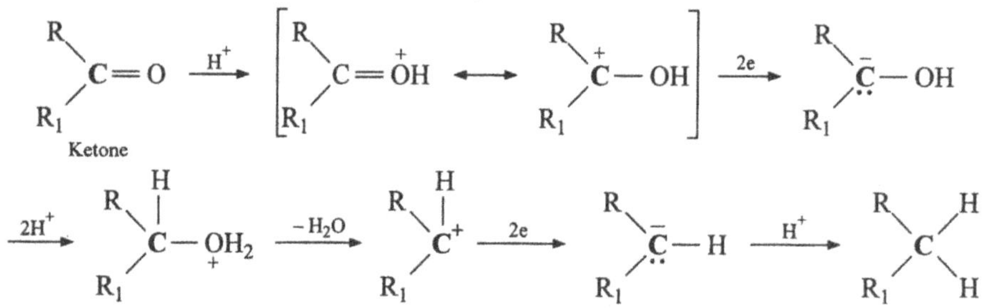

Mechanism Wolf–Kishner reduction is very useful synthetic tool for converting the carbonyl group (C=O) in an aldehyde or ketone to a $—CH_2—$ group. The reaction proceeds by the following steps.

(a) In the first step, hydrazine reacts with ketone to form hydrazone.

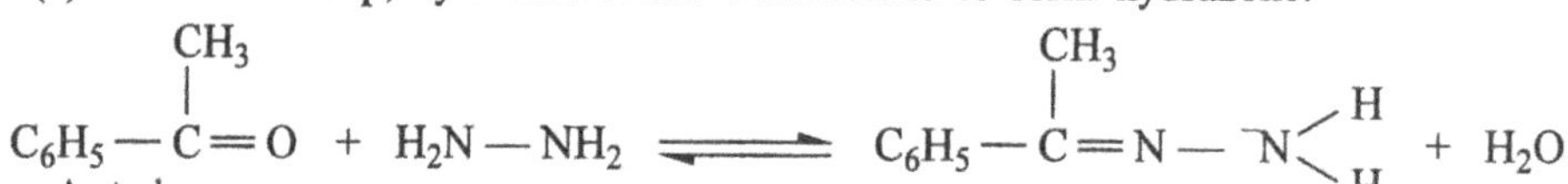

(b) The base removes proton from amino group of hydrazone to form carbanion.

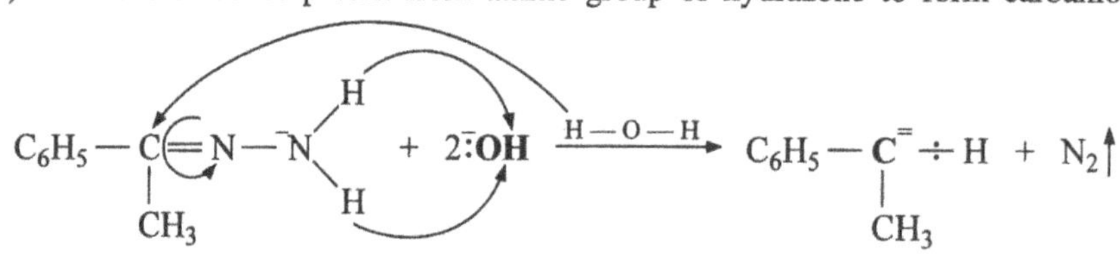

Acetophenone hydrazone

(c) The carbanion abstracts a proton from water molecule to an alkane.

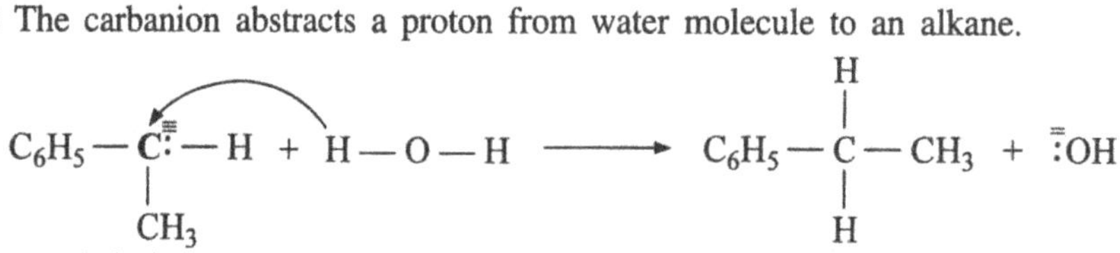

Carbanion — An alkane

(iii) *Reductive amination* Many aldehydes and ketones are converted into amines by catalytic reduction (H_2 + Ni or Pt or Pd) or chemical reduction ($NaBH_3CN$ or $LiBH_3CN$)

in presence of ammonia or an amine. This process is called reductive amination of aldehydes or ketones, which involves through the intermediate formation of imine (an organic compound containing carbon–nitrogen double bond). Primary, secondary and tertiary amines can be prepared by this reaction.

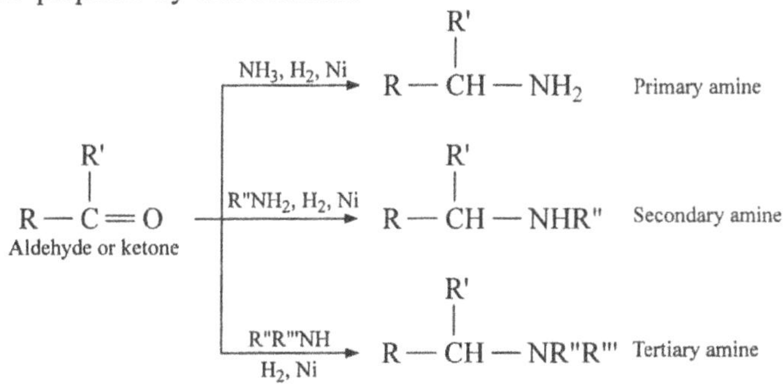

2. ***Oxidation of Aldehydes and Ketones*** Aldehydes are easily oxidised to carboxylic acids in presence of common oxidising agents ($KMnO_4$, $K_2Cr_2O_7$, etc.) or mild oxidising agents like Tollen's reagent [Ammoniacal solution of silver nitrate contains silver ammonia complex $[Ag(NH_3)_2^+]$, Fehling's reagent (solution of copper sulphate + solution of sodium hydroxide and sodium potassium tartarate), Benedict's reagent (copper sulphate + sodium citrate + sodium carbonate) due to the free hydrogen atom attached to the carbonyl carbon. During oxidation, this hydrogen is abstracted either as a proton or an atom. Ketones resist oxidation and get oxidised only under the influence of strong oxidising agents to form carboxylic acids with lesser number of carbon atoms. Hence, this test can be used to distinguish aldehydes from ketones.

$$RCHO \xrightarrow{\text{Oxidising agent}} RCOOH$$

$$CH_3CHO + \underset{\substack{\text{Fehling's}\\ \text{solution (blue)}}}{Cu^{2+}} \longrightarrow \underset{\text{(Brick red colour)}}{Cu_2O\downarrow} + CH_3COOH$$

$$CH_3CHO + \underset{\text{Tollen's reagent}}{2Ag(NH_3)_2^+} + 3OH^- \longrightarrow \underset{\text{Silver mirror}}{2Ag} + CH_3COO^- + 4NH_3 + 2H_2O$$

Tollen's reagent will oxidise only aldehydes to a salt of an acid with the result that the silver ion will be reduced to free silver. Depending on the concentration of Tollen's reagent and the surface of the reaction vessel, the free silver deposition will form a layer of silver atoms on the inside of the reaction vessel which is highly reflective.

Fehling's solution and Benedict's solution will also oxidise aldehydes to a salt of the acid. Both solutions have copper (II) ion which is reduced to copper (I). This ion reacts with the hydroxide present to produce a orange red coloured solid precipitate signalling the presence of an aldehyde.

3. ***The Baeyer–Villager Reaction of Ketones*** Ketones (RCOR) can be oxidised by peracids to esters (RCO_2R) by Baeyer–Villager reaction. This can be viewed as the insertion of oxygen into one of the carbon–carbon bonds adjacent to the carbonyl carbon.

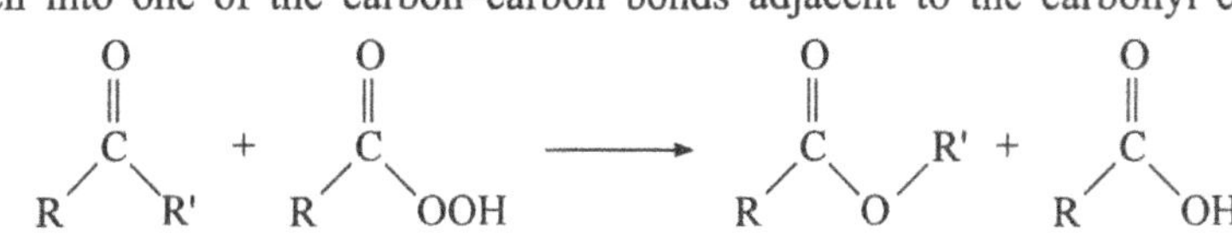

Cyclic ketones by Baeyer–Villager reaction give cyclic esters, which are also known as lactones.

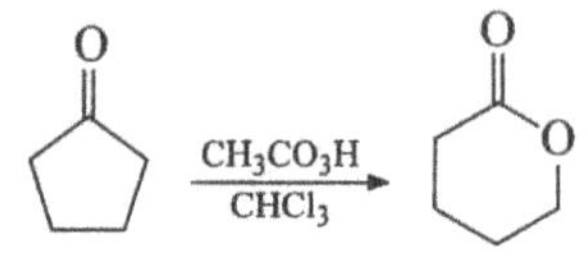

Mechanism of the Baeyer–Villager Reaction

Step 1 Protonation of the carbonyl carbon by peracid. It is an acid/base reaction.

Step 2 In the second step, the nucleophilic oxygen of percarboxylate ion attacks the carbonyl carbon (electrophilic).

Step 3 This step involves the migration of the C—C electrons to form a new C—O bond displacing the carboxylate as a leaving group.

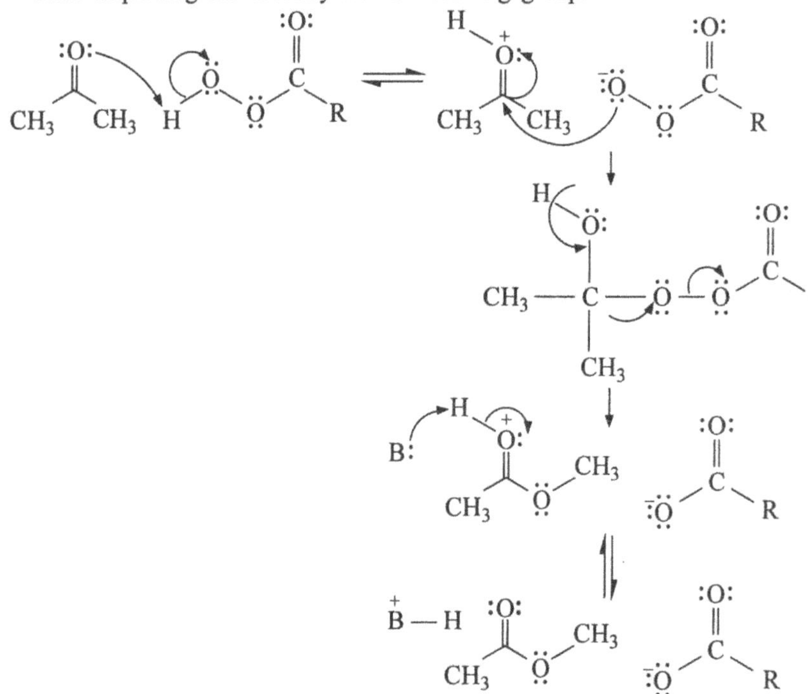

Step 4 Finally ester is produced.

4. ***Haloform Reaction*** When methyl ketones [$RCOCH_3$] react with halogens ($X_2 = Cl_2$, Br_2 or I_2) in aqueous sodium hydroxide solution, they get cleaved to yield a carboxylic acid and haloform (CHX_3). Hence, this reaction is known as haloform reaction. When halogen is iodine, iodoform is obtained. This reaction is also positive with a methyl carbinol group if one hydrogen atom is attached to the carbon bearing the hydroxyl group. The methyl carbinol first oxidised to methyl ketones, which further undergoes haloform reaction.

$$\underset{\text{Methyl ketone}}{R-\overset{\overset{\displaystyle O}{\|}}{C}-CH_3} + 3I_2 + 4NaOH \longrightarrow \underset{\text{Sodium carboxylate}}{RCOONa} + 3NaI + H_2O + \underset{\text{Haloform}}{CHI_3}$$

Mechanism The haloform reaction proceeds through the intermediate formation of carbanion. This involves following steps:

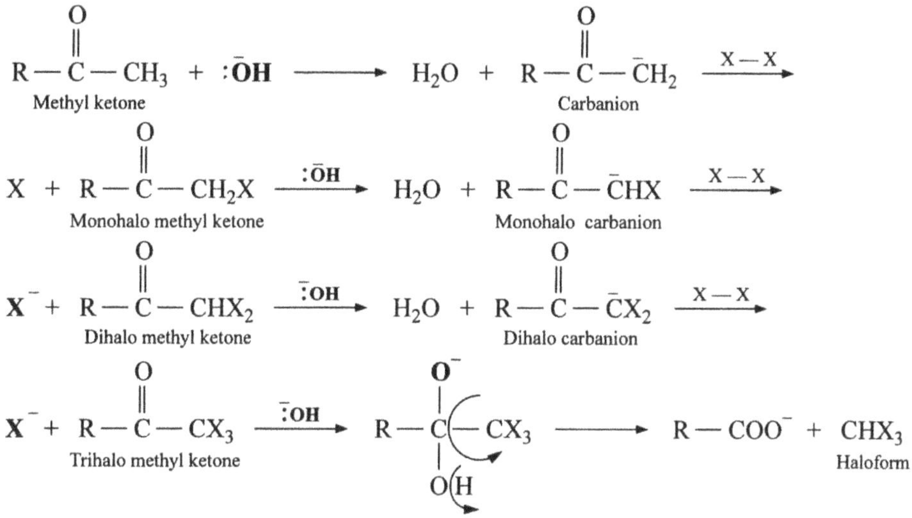

5. ***Nucleophilic Addition*** An addition reaction initiated by a nucleophile is called nucleophilic addition reaction. Nucleophilic addition is a characteristic reaction of carbonyl compounds due to the presence of carbonyl group.

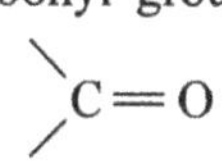

The carbonyl group contains a double bond between two heteroatoms, i.e. carbon and oxygen. The oxygen is more electronegative than carbon; the bonded π-electrons are withdrawn strongly towards oxygen. As a result, the carbonyl group is highly polar, the carbonyl carbon is electron deficient (electrophilic) and the carbonyl oxygen being electron rich (nucleophilic).

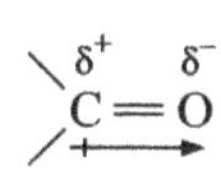

Consequently a nucleophile readily attacks the electrophilic carbon and forms a σ bond with carbonyl carbon with its electron pair. The ability of oxygen to acquire π-electrons or to accommodate negative charge is the real cause of the reactivity of carbonyl group with nucleophilic reagents. In general, the addition of a nucleophile to a carbonyl compound may be represented as below:

The carbonyl group is trigonal and the carbonyl carbon in the starting compound is sp^2 hybridised, whereas in the transition state started acquiring sp^3, which will be ultimately there in the product. The ability of oxygen to acquire electrons or to accommodate negative charge is the real cause of the reactivity of carbonyl group with nucleophilic reagents.

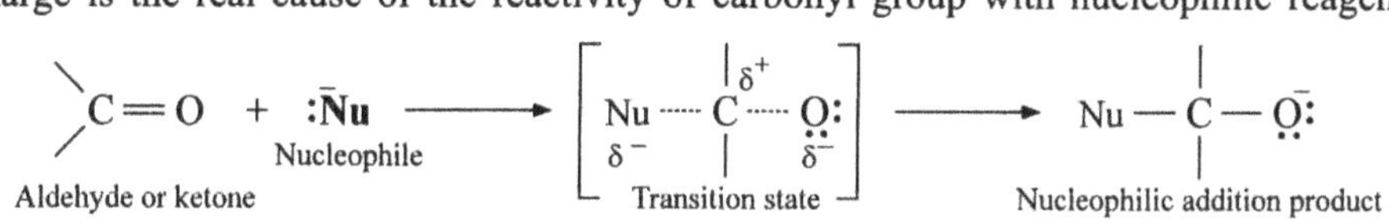

Catalysis of nucleophilic reactions The attack of nucleophile at carbonyl carbon can be catalysed under slight acidic conditions. The H^+ ion generated by the acid combines readily with electron rich oxygen. This oxygen acquires π-electrons without bearing negative charge. This leads to decrease in E_a and improves the rate of nucleophilic addition reaction.

It should be noted that, if the reaction is made too acidic, the H^+ ions would combine with nucleophilic reagents, thus decreases rate of reaction.

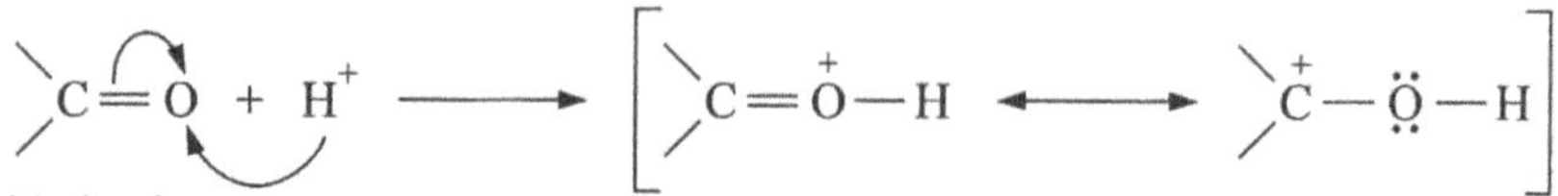

Aldehyde or ketone

Relative reactivities of aldehydes and ketones in nucleophilic reactions In nucleophilic reactions aldehydes are more reactive than ketones and aliphatic aldehydes or ketones are more reactive than the aromatic ones.

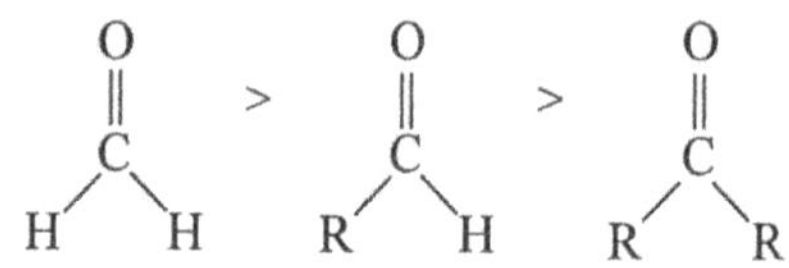

Ketones have one more alkyl or aryl group in place of hydrogen of aldehydes. The alkyl or aryl groups are bulkier than hydrogen. Therefore, in ketones there is steric hindrance and the molecule resists crowding. Moreover, the alkyl groups are electron-releasing groups and thus they decrease partial positive charge on carbonyl carbon and increase negative charge on oxygen atom thus makes the transition state less stable. Hence, aldehydes are more reactive due to less steric hindrance and more stability of transition state than ketones. The following are various nucleophilic addition reactions of aldehydes and ketones:

(i) *Addition of sodium bisulphite* The reaction is carried out by adding carbonyl compound to a concentrated aqueous solution of sodium bisulphite when the product separates as a crystalline solid.

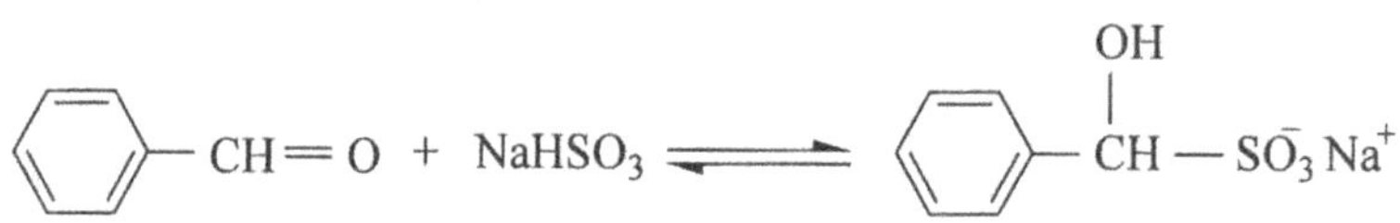

Benzaldehyde — Benzaldehyde sodiumbisulphite

This is a reversible reaction. Ketones containing bulky groups fail to react with $NaHSO_3$ due to steric hindrance. The reaction is often employed for the purification of aldehydes and ketones.

Mechanism The reaction involves initial nucleophilic attack of bisulphite ion on electrophilic carbon, followed by addition of a hydrogen ion to carbonyl oxygen.

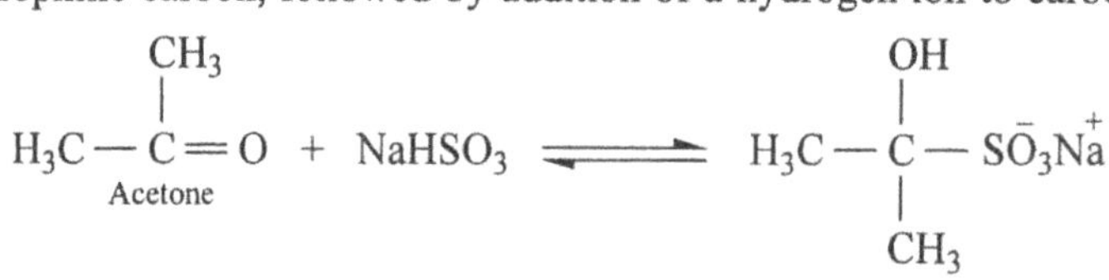

Acetone — Acetone sodiumbisulphite

(ii) *Addition of hydrogen cyanide* This reaction is an example of nucleophilic addition, often carried out in presence of mineral acid. Aldehydes and ketones on treatment with HCN, the elements of HCN add to the carbonyl group to yield cyanohydrins. The reaction is not normally done using hydrogen cyanide itself, because this is an extremely poisonous gas. Instead, the aldehyde or ketone is mixed with a solution of sodium or potassium cyanide in water to which a little sulphuric acid has been added. The *pH* of the solution is adjusted to about 4 to 5, because this gives the fastest reaction. The reaction is useful since the cyano group can be converted into other useful functional groups (—CO_2H or —CH_2NH_2). In this reaction the nucleophilic cyanide anion attacks electrophilic carbon.

For Example

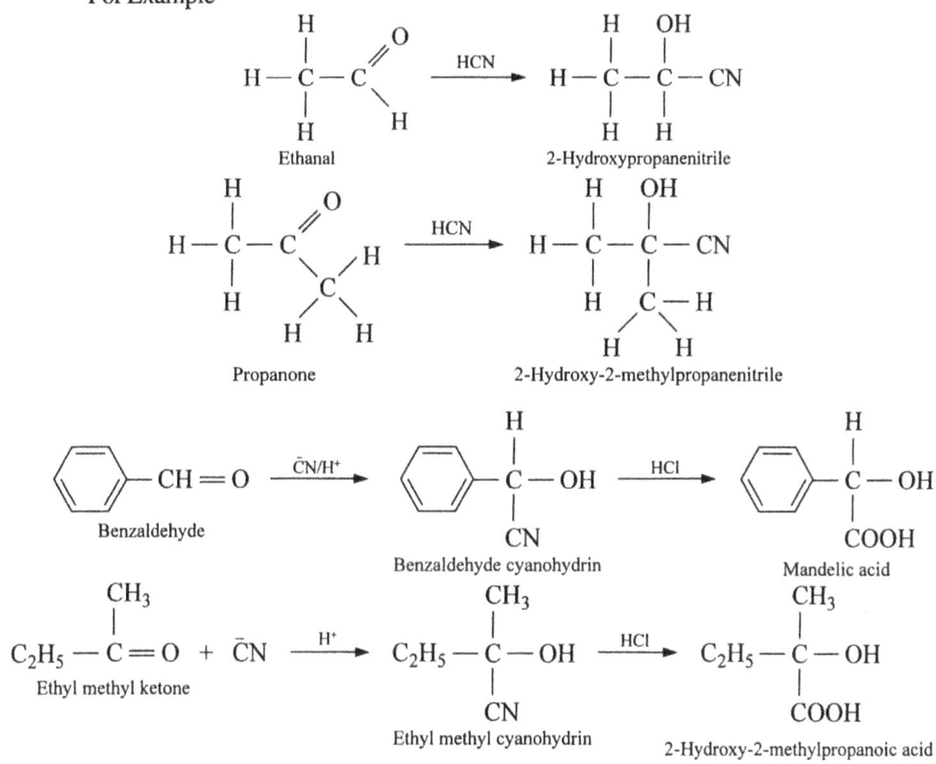

Mechanism of Addition Cyanide to an Aldehyde

Step 1 The nucleophilic carbon in the cyanide adds to the electrophilic carbon in the polar carbonyl group, electrons from the C=O move to the electronegative oxygen creating an intermediate alkoxide.

Step 2 It is an acid/base reaction. Protonation of the alkoxide oxygen creates the cyanohydrin product.

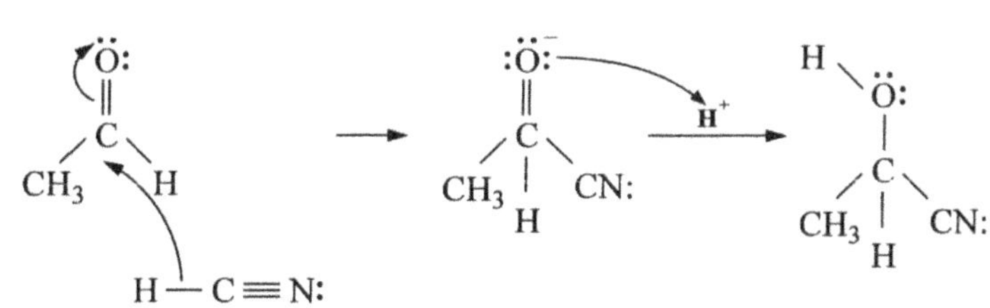

(iii) *Reformatsky reaction* Aldehydes or ketones on reaction with α-bromo ester and metallic zinc in presence of dry ether or benzene yield addition product. The addition product is decomposed to β-hydroxy esters with dilute mineral acids.

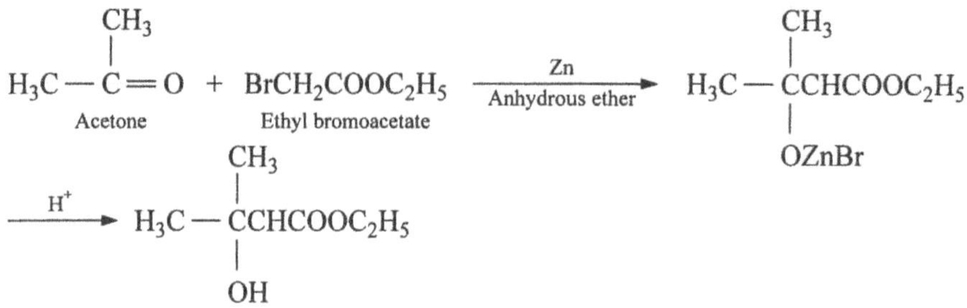

Ethyl-3-hydroxy-3-methylbutanoate

Mechanism The reaction involves formation of organo zinc compound by the reaction between α-bromo ester and zinc. The bond between carbon and zinc is polar hence organic group (nucleophile) of organo zinc compound attacks electrophilic carbonyl carbon to form addition product.

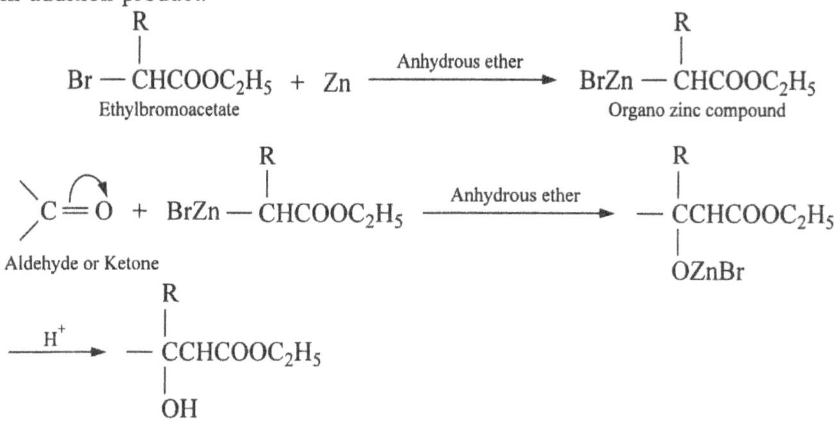

Addition compound

(iv) *Addition of alcohols* Under appropriate conditions aldehydes or ketones react with two molecules of alcohols in presence of anhydrous HCl and form ethereal compounds called acetals or ketals respectively.

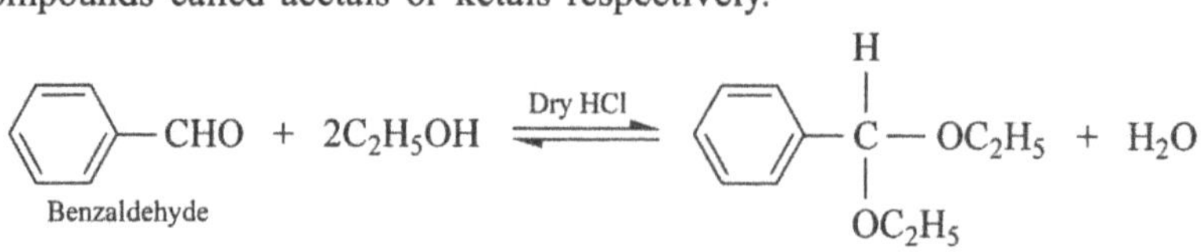

Diethyl acetal of benzaldehyde

Mechanism This reaction occurs in three reversible steps to form hemiacetals or hemiketals. The hemiacetals or hemiketals (the prefix hemi means half) are not normally isolable compounds. Hemiacetals or hemiketals can further react in the presence of excess alcohol to form acetals or ketals.

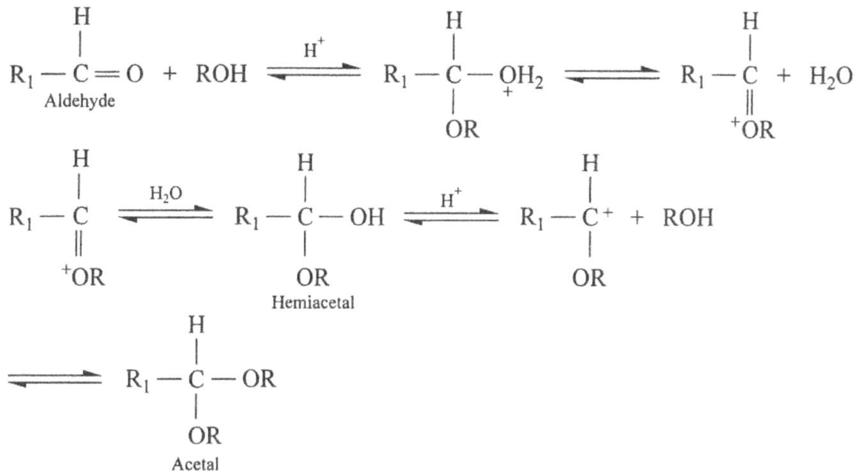

Importance Many important examples of hemiacetals, acetals, hemiketals and ketals may be found in sugars.

(v) *Addition of Grignard reagents* Grignard reagent react with aldehydes and ketones followed by acidification give alcohols. This reaction involves nucleophilic addition of organic group (alkyl or aryl) of Grignard reagent to electrophilic carbonyl carbon of aldehydes or ketones.

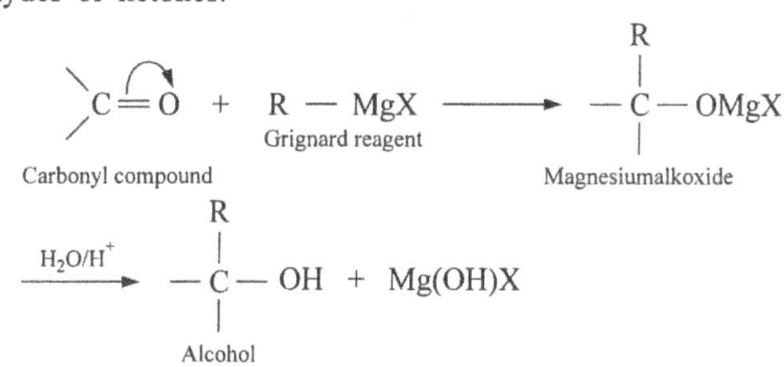

Formaldehyde gives 1° alcohol on reaction with Grignard reagent and followed by hydrolysis with acidified H_2O, whereas higher aldehydes give 2° alcohol. All ketones react with Grignard reagent and produces 3° alcohol.

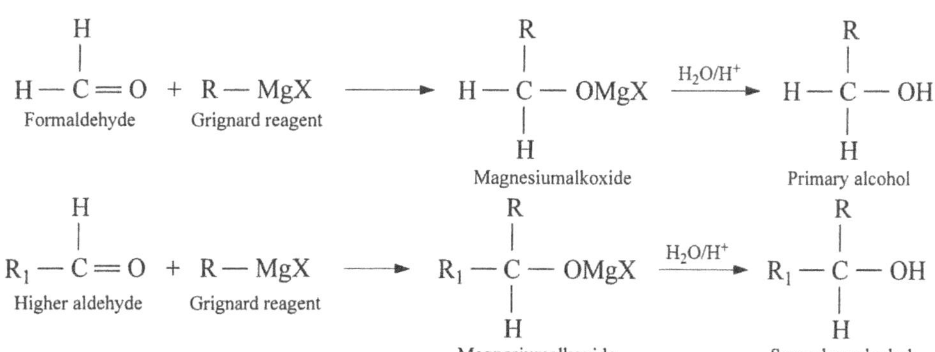

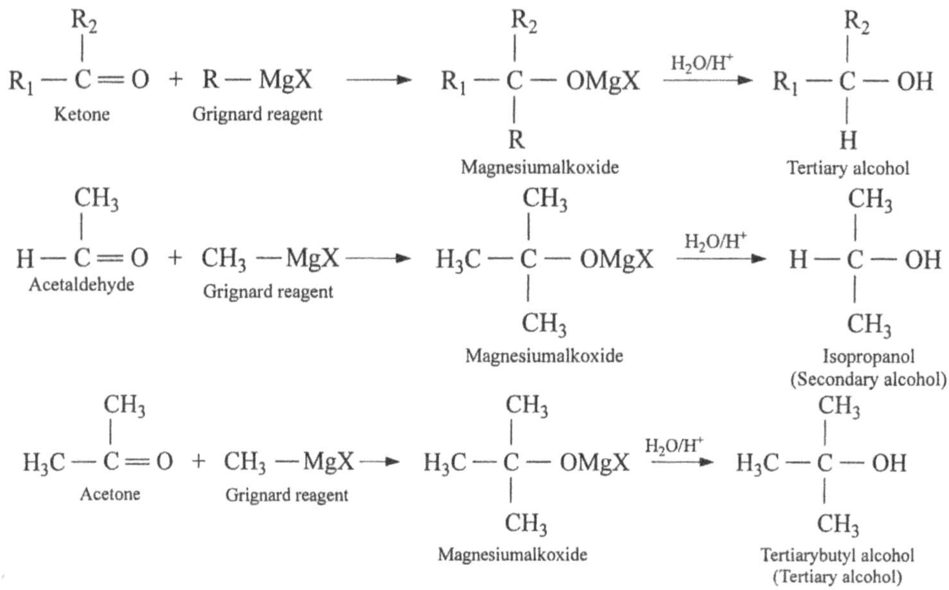

Importance This reaction is very useful for producing a wide variety of alcohols since depending on the number of alkyl groups attached to the carbonyl carbon, it is possible to produce primary, secondary, or tertiary alcohols.

(vi) *Addition of ammonia derivatives* Certain ammonia derivatives (hydroxylamine, hydrazine, phenyl hydrazine, 2,4-dinitrophenyl hydrazine, semicarbazide) add to the carbonyl group to form nucleophilic addition product. The product contains a carbon–nitrogen double bond resulting from the elimination of water from the initial addition product. These derivatives have very specific melting points and this fact can be used to determine the original aldehyde or ketone used to form the derivative.

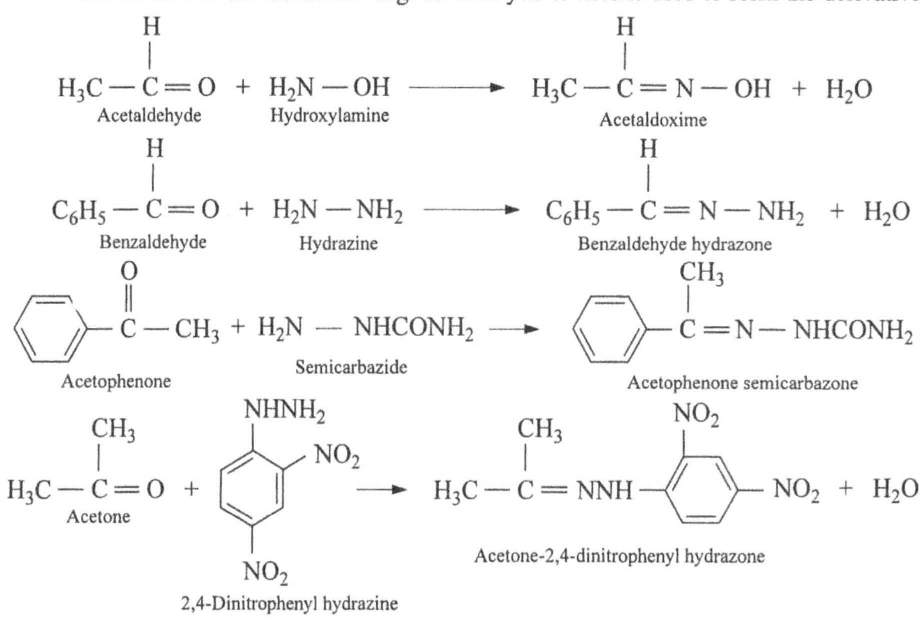

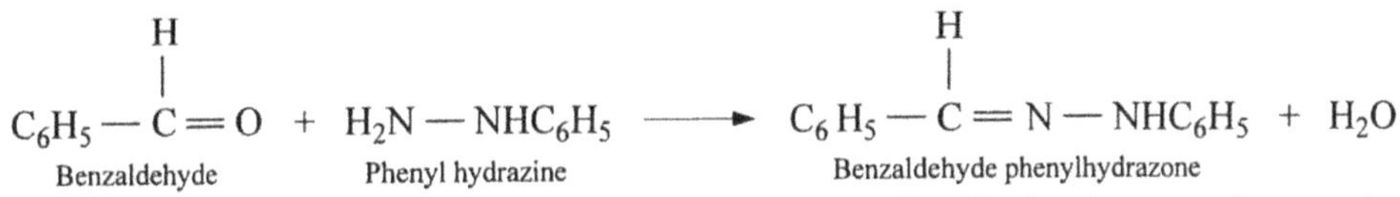

Mechanism This reaction involves nucleophilic attack of basic nitrogen of ammonia derivative on electrophilic carbon of carbonyl group. The overall reaction is an addition-elimination process, with water being the molecule removed from the reactants.

The reaction must be acidic enough for protonation of carbonyl compound, but not so acidic that the concentration of free nitrogen compound is too low.

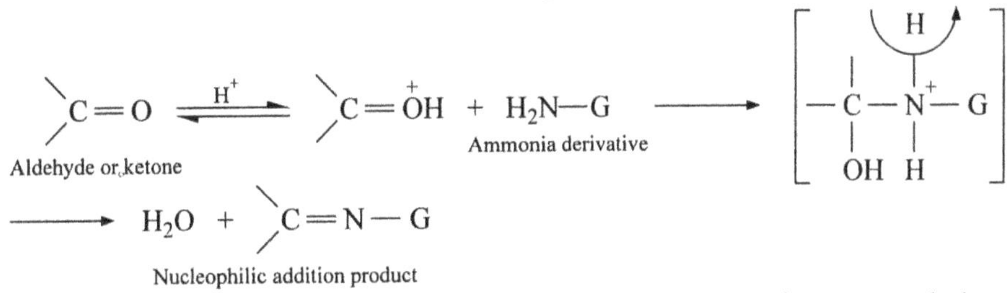

Importance These derivatives have very large molar masses and consequently have high melting points. They are also brightly coloured either orange or red. This fact can be used for identification of aldehydes and ketones.

(vii) *Aldol condensation* Two molecules of an aldehyde or a ketone having α-hydrogen atoms undergoes self-condensation in presence of dilute base or dilute acid at room temperature to form product called aldol (β-hydroxy aldehyde or ketone). Hence, this reaction is known as aldol condensation.

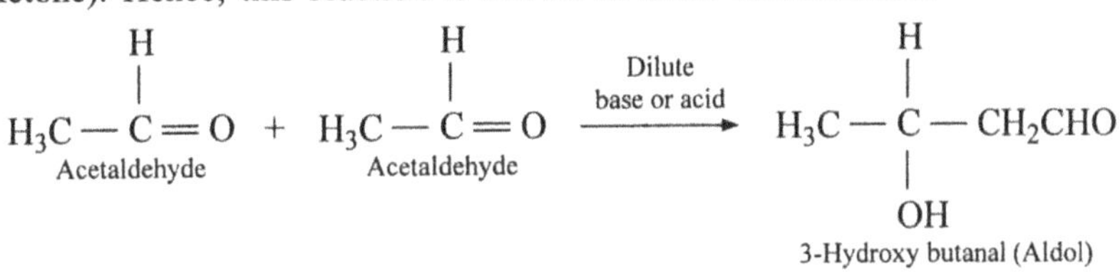

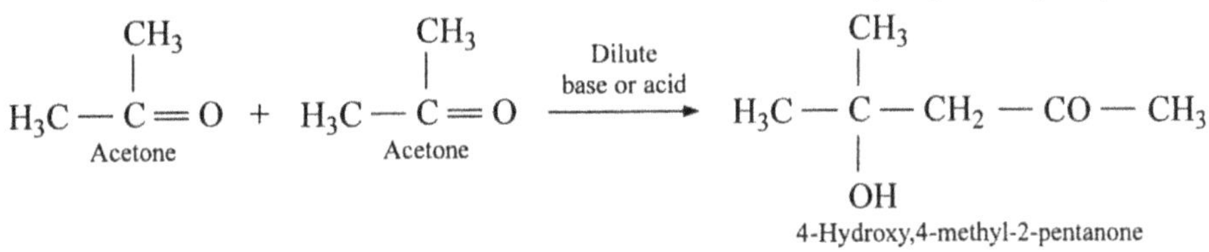

Mechanisms The following mechanisms were proposed for aldol condensation.

(a) *Base catalysed mechanism*

- The base (:OH⁻) abstracts hydrogen from β-carbon of carbonyl compound to form carbanion.

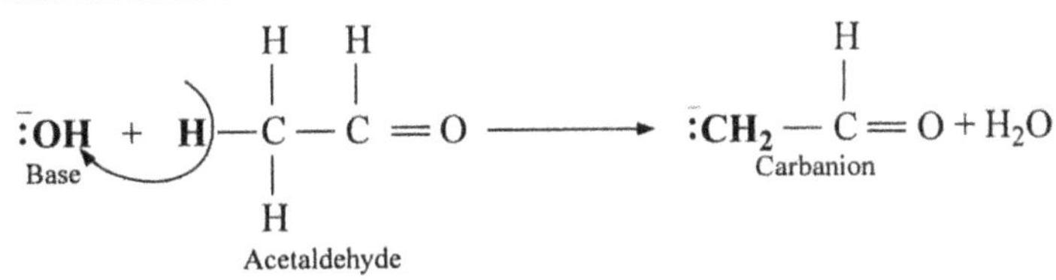

- The nucleophilic carbanion attack carbonyl carbon of second molecule to form an anion, which picks up a proton from water to form aldol.

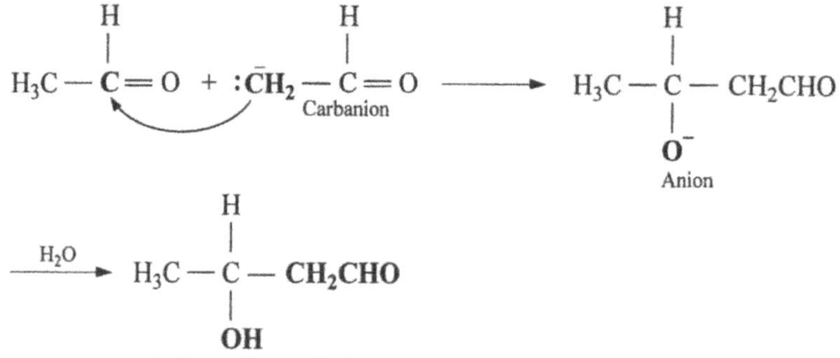

3-Hydroxy butanal (Aldol)

(b) *Acid catalysed mechanism* Acid catalysed mechanism proceeds through the intermediate formation of carbocation.

- Acid adds at the carbonyl oxygen and forms carbocation.

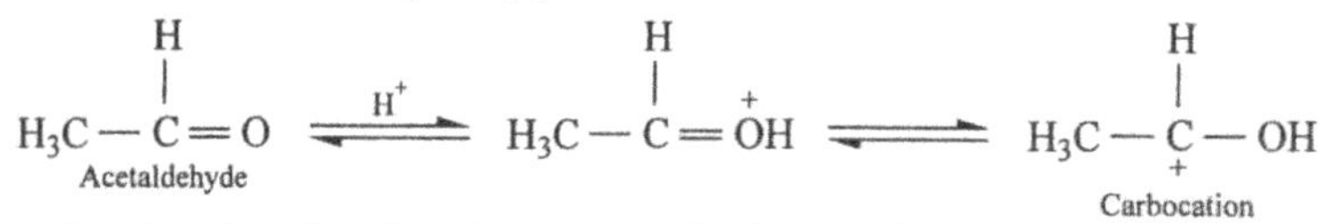

- Second molecule of carbonyl compound adds to electrophilic carbocation to form aldol.

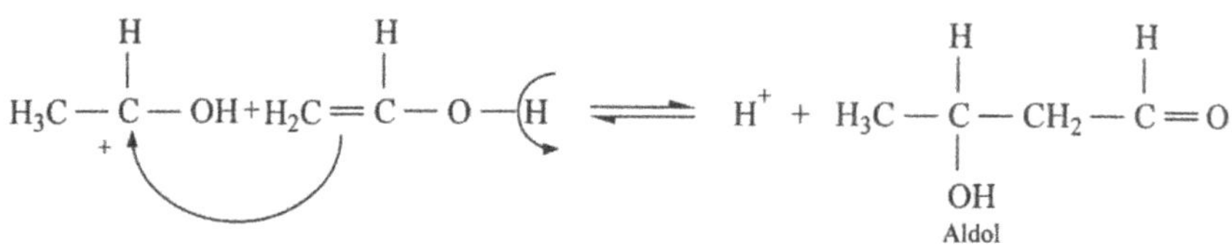

Crossed aldol condensation If aldol condensation takes place between two different carbonyl compounds a mixture of four different products may be formed. This condensation reaction is known as crossed aldol condensation.

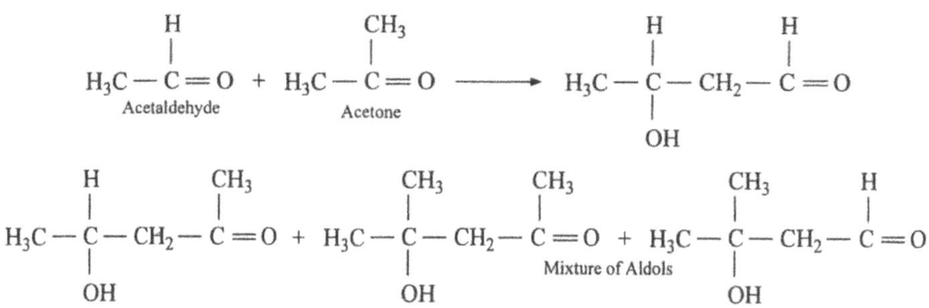

(viii) *Perkin reaction* Aromatic aldehydes on reaction with anhydride of aliphatic acid (containing α-hydrogens) in presence of its sodium salt yields β-aryl acrylic acid. The reaction is known as Perkin reaction. For example, benzaldehyde with acetic anhydride and sodium acetate, cinnamic acid is formed.

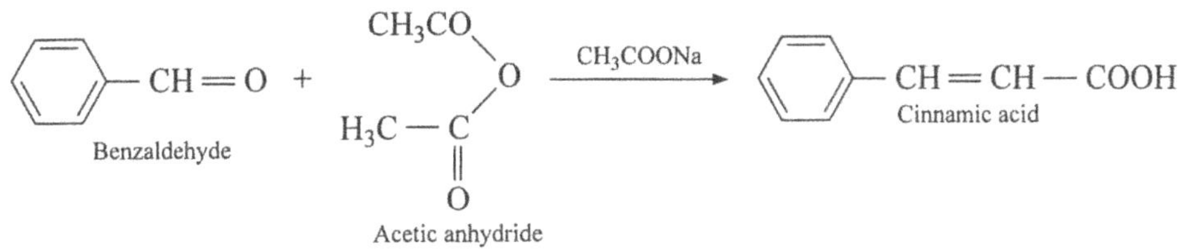

Mechanism (a)

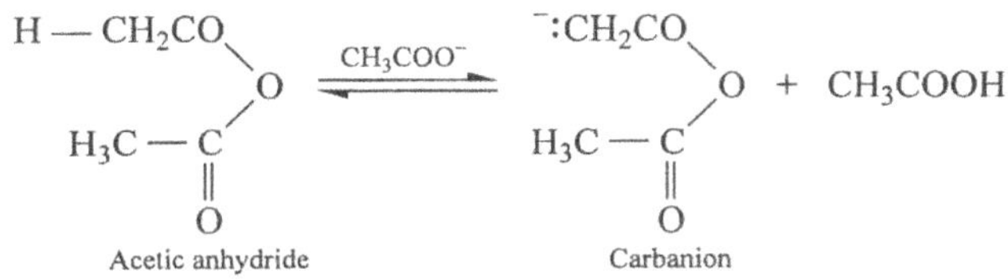

(b)

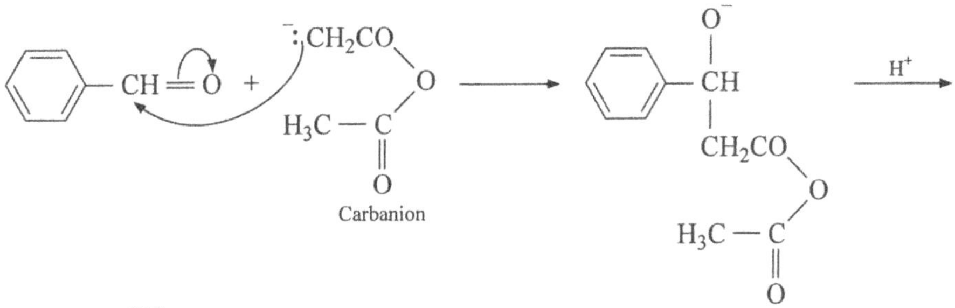

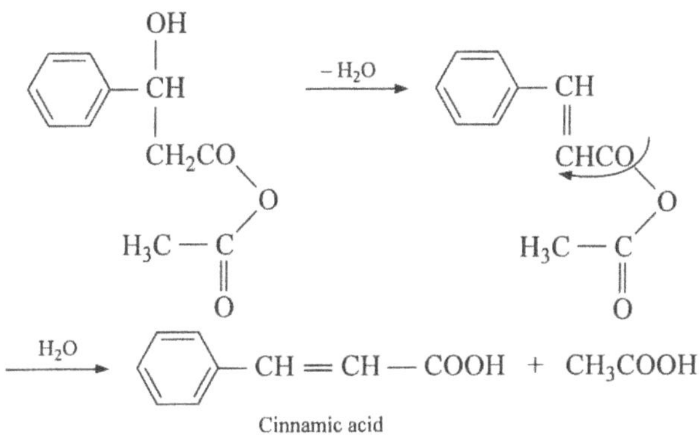

(ix) *Benzoin condensation* Aromatic aldehydes containing no α-hydrogen atoms undergo self-condensation in presence of KCN to form benzoins (ArCHOHCOAr). This reaction is known as benzoin condensation, which is also another example for nucleophilic addition.

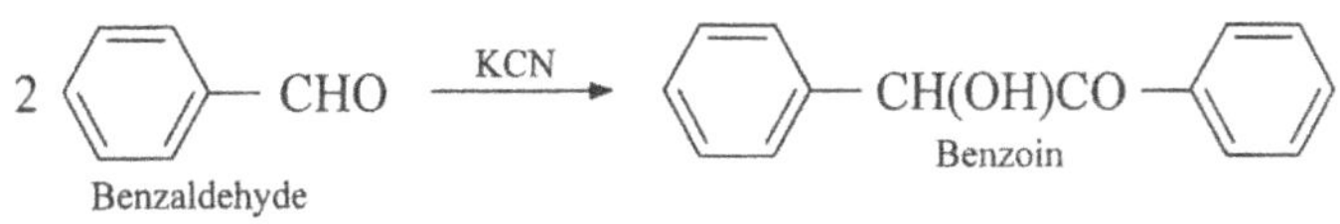

Mechanism The reaction proceeds by the following steps.

(a)

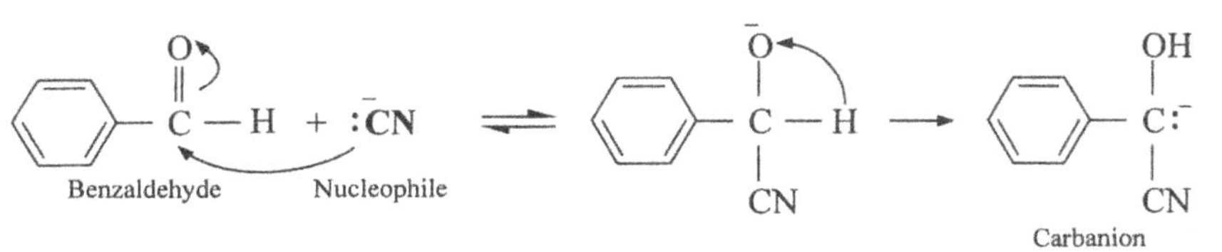

(b)

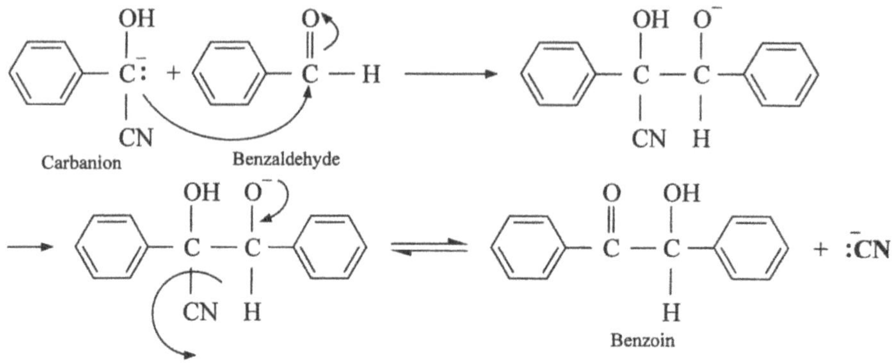

(x) *Cannizzaro reaction* Aldehydes containing no α-hydrogens undergo self-oxidation and reduction in presence of concentrated aqueous or alcoholic solution of sodium or potassium hydroxide to form a salt of carboxylic acid and an alcohol is known as Cannizzaro reaction.

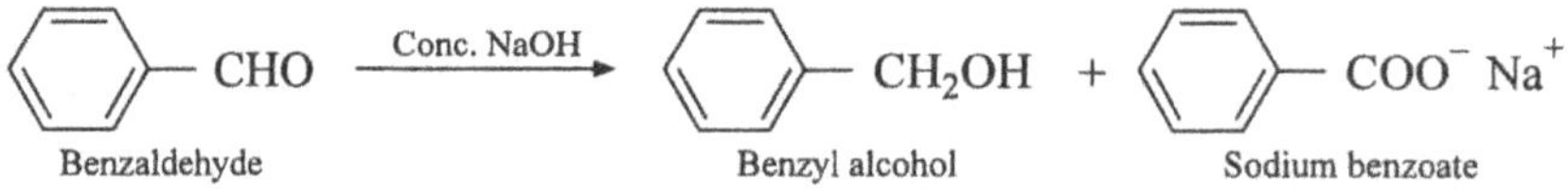

Mechanism Mechanism of Cannizzaro reaction involves the following steps.

(a) Hydroxide ion attacks carbonyl carbon to form an intermediate anion (I)

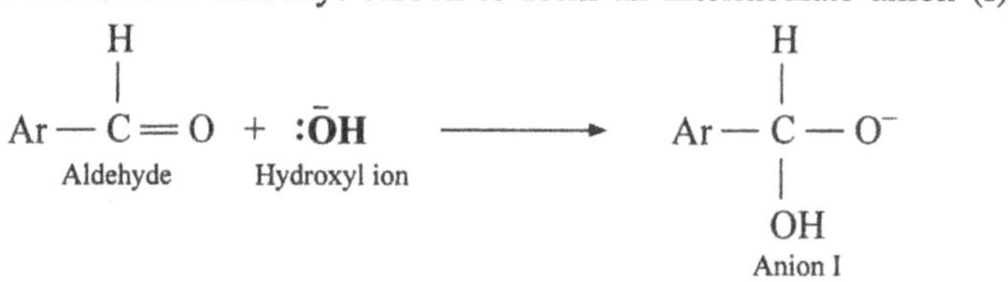

(b) Transfer of hydride ion from intermediate anion (I) to carbonyl carbon of second aldehyde molecule.

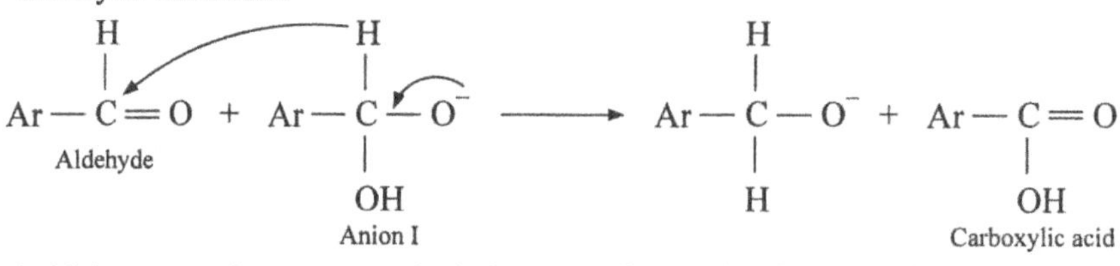

(c) Acid–base reactions to get alcohol and sodium salt of carboxylic acid.

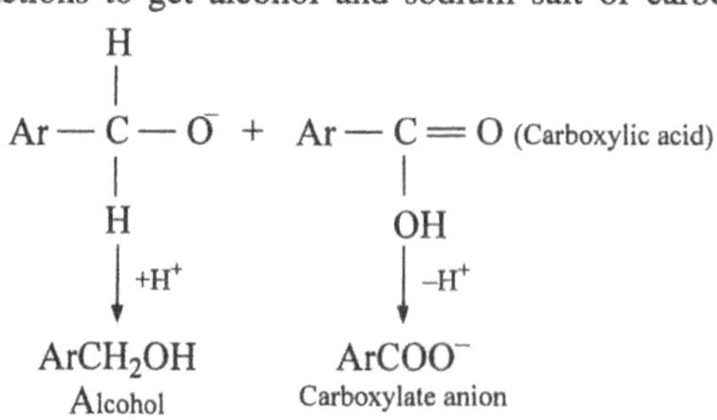

Crossed Cannizzaro reaction Cannizzaro reaction between two different aldehydes is known as crossed Cannizzaro reaction. When a mixture of formaldehyde and benzaldehyde is treated with caustic soda solution, a crossed Cannizzaro reaction takes place and benzyl alcohol forms along with sodium formate.

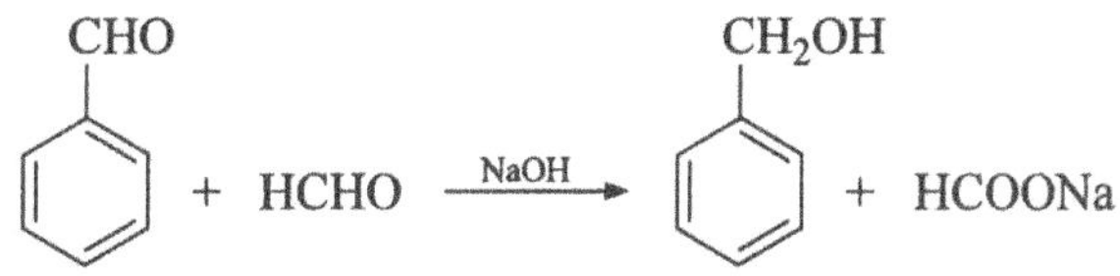

During this reaction formaldehyde gets oxidised to formate and benzaldehyde gets reduced to benzyl alcohol. This is because the carbonyl carbon of formaldehyde is more electrophilic and less stearically crowded than benzyl alcohol hence ^{-}OH attacks the carbonyl carbon of formaldehyde to form an anion which transfers H^+ directly.

p-Methoxybenzyl alcohol may be prepared form *p*-methoxy benzaldehyde by the crossed Cannizzaro reaction.

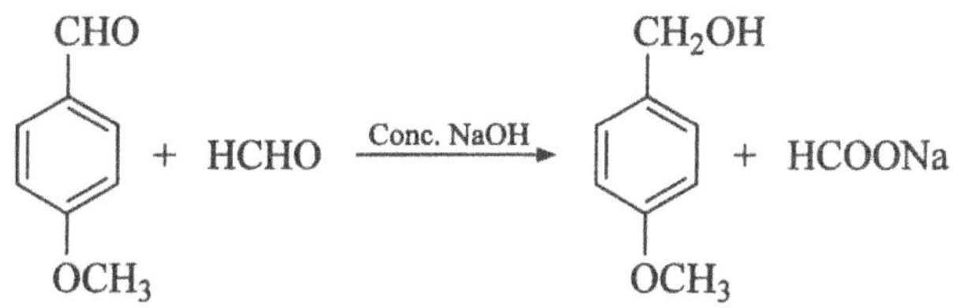

(xi) *Wittig reaction* This reaction involves between aldehydes or ketones and phosphorus ylides to form substituted alkenes. Ylides are neutral molecules but have +ve and –ve centres on adjacent atoms that are connected by a σ bond. The ylide is prepared by an S_N2 reaction between triphenyl phosphine and an alkyl halide followed by treatment with a strong base such as an organolithium reagent:

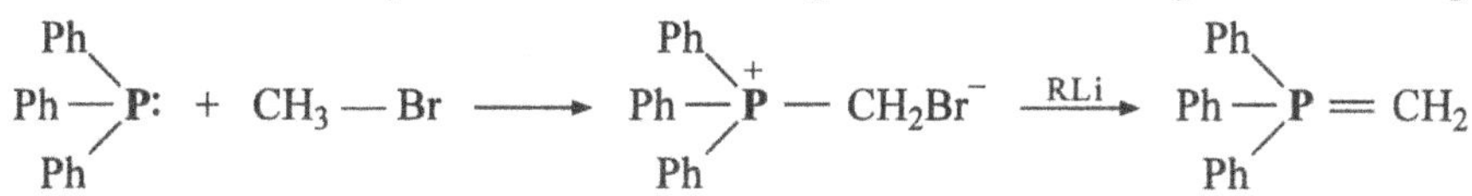

The Wittig reaction is an important method for the formation of alkenes. This is also an example for nucleophilic addition of organic group of ylide to carbonyl carbon.

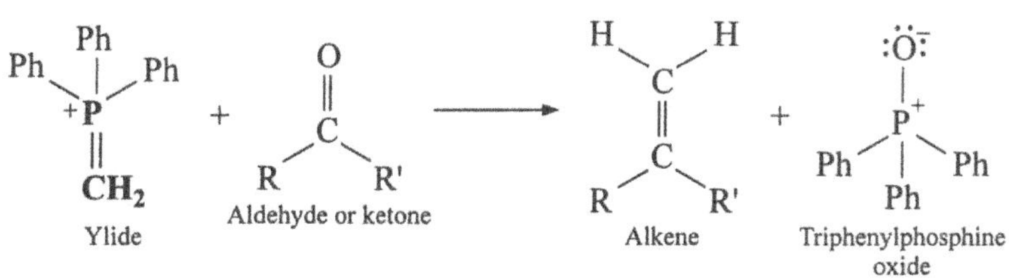

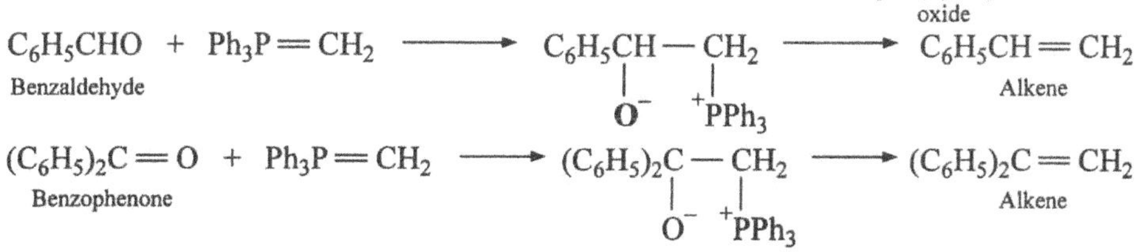

19.6 PHARMACEUTICAL COMPOUNDS

1. ***Chloral (Trichloroacetaldehyde)*** Chloral is a colourless oily liquid. This is prepared by the action of chlorine on ethyl alcohol. Chloral is used as hypnotic and to prepare DDT.

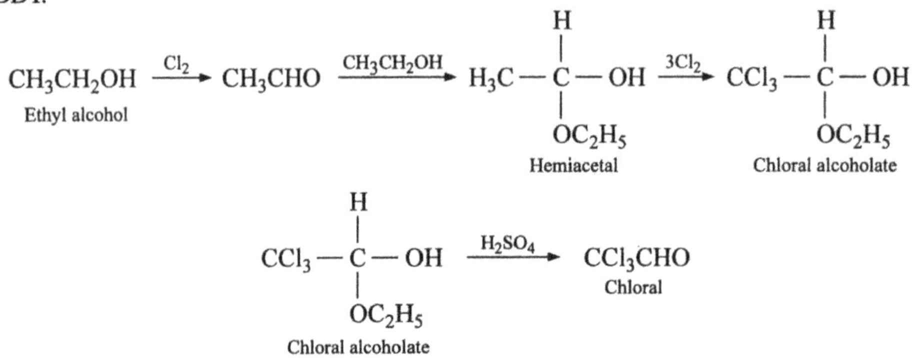

2. ***Paraldehyde*** Paraldehyde is a cyclic trimer of acetaldehyde. It is a colourless liquid having strong characteristic odour. It is prepared by adding a drop of concentrated sulphuric acid to acetaldehyde. It is used as a hypnotic and sedative.

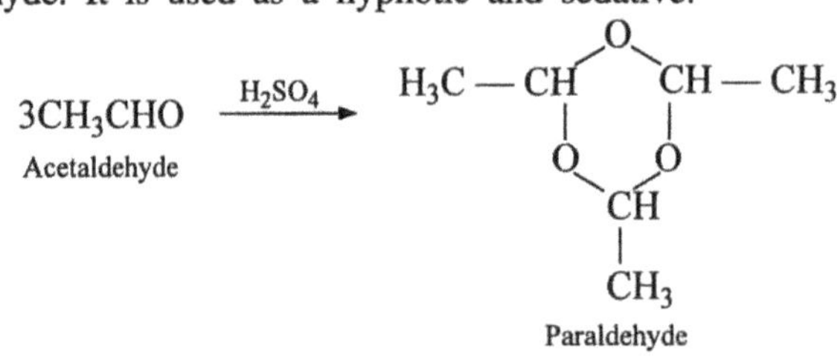

3. ***Hexamine*** Hexamine is a complex derivative of formaldehyde. It is prepared by mixing aqueous solutions of formaldehyde and ammonia and evaporating the liquid to dryness on a water bath. This is used as an urinary antiseptic.

$$6HCHO + 4NH_3 \longrightarrow C_6H_{12}N_4 + 6H_2O$$

4. ***Formaldehyde*** Formaldehyde (or methanal) is the simplest aldehyde and can be prepared by a decomposition reaction of methanol, catalysed by silver.

$$CH_3OH \xrightarrow[600°–700°C]{\text{Ag catalyst}} H_2C{=}O + H_2$$

Formaldehyde is an unstable gas in its pure state. It is normally produced as a 37% aqueous solution called formalin. Formaldehyde is a colour liquid having pungent, irritating odour. It is miscible with water and alcohol. Usually 10 to 15% methanol is added to formaldehyde solution to prevent polymerisation of gas to solid paraformaldehyde.

Uses

1. Formaldehyde is used as a disinfectant for surgical instruments, storage house, utensils, clothes, dwellings, etc.
2. It is used as a germicide and fungicide for plants and vegetables.
3. Phenolic resins, artificial silk and cellulose esters, dyes, organic chemicals, glass mirror and explosives are manufactured from formaldehyde.

4. Formaldehyde is used for tanning and preserving hides, in photography for hardening gelatin plates and also in chemical analysis.
5. Formaldehyde has local anaesthetic effect. It has been used in tymphony, diarrhoea, mastitis, pneumonia and internal bleeding.
6. Formalin is well known as a preservative used for biological samples, but most is used as one of the components of certain two part glues.

5. ***Vanillin*** Vanillin is 4-hydroxy-3-methoxy benzaldehyde. It is the active constituent of *Vanilla Planifolia* or other species of *Vanilla*. Vanillin can be synthesised from guaiacol by Reimer-Tiemann reaction.

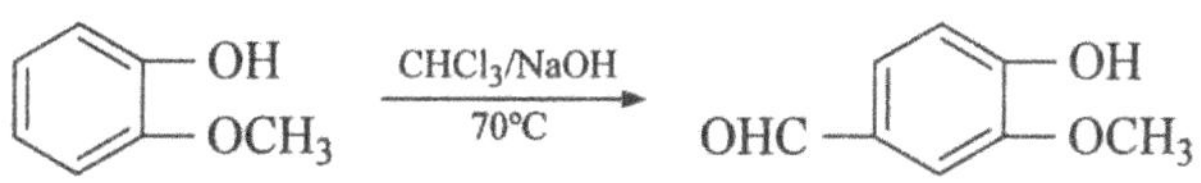

Vanillin is available as colourless or cream-coloured needle like crystals or powder. It melts at 81°C. The odour and taste of Vanillin are characteristic of Vanilla. It is soluble in 100 parts of water, freely soluble in alcohol, fixed oils and volatile oils.

Use Vanillin is used as a flavouring agent.

6. ***Ketamine*** Ketamine is a cyclohexanol derivative. Chemically ketanine is 2-(*o*-chlorophenyl)-2-(methylamino)-cyclohexanone. Ketamine is prepared by Grignard reaction of *o*-chlorobenzonitrile with bromocyclopentane in presence of strong alkali to form an expoxy compound which converts to an imine by the action of methylamine. The imine rearranges to ketamine on heating with HCl.

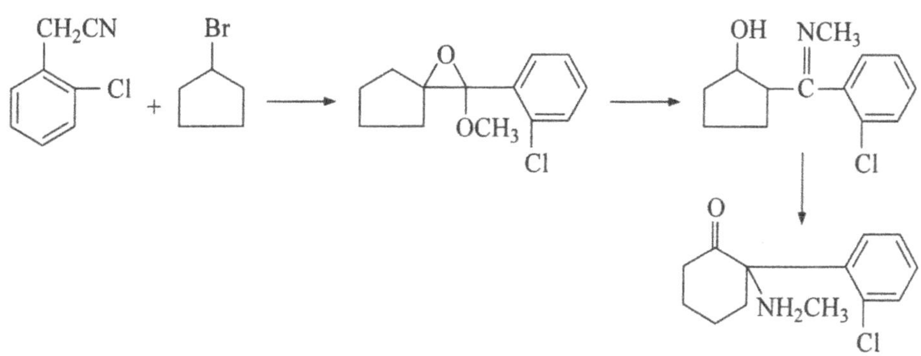

Ketamine is available as colourless crystalline compound having characteristic odour. It melts at 258°C.

Uses

1. Ketamine is used as a general anaesthetic.
2. It also has analgestic effect.
3. Ketamine relaxes skeletal muscles.

7. ***Ketoprofen*** Ketoprofen is an arylpropionic acid derivative. Chemically ketoprofen is 2-(3-benzoyl phenyl)-propionic acid. Ketoprofen is a colourless crystalline powder. It is practically insoluble in water.

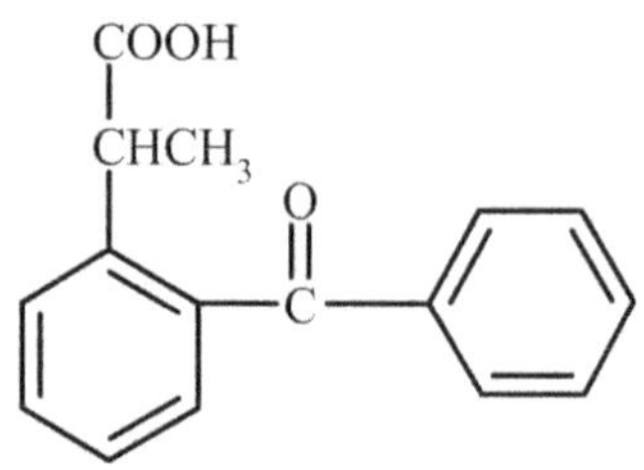

Uses

1. Ketoprofen is a non-stereoidal anti-inflammatory agent. It is used for the relief of mild to moderate pain.
2. It is used to treat various rheumatic disorders and in other non-rheumatid musculoskeletal and joint disorders.

8. *Phenindione* Phenindione is an indan derivative. Chemically phenindione is 2-phenyl-1,3-indanedione.

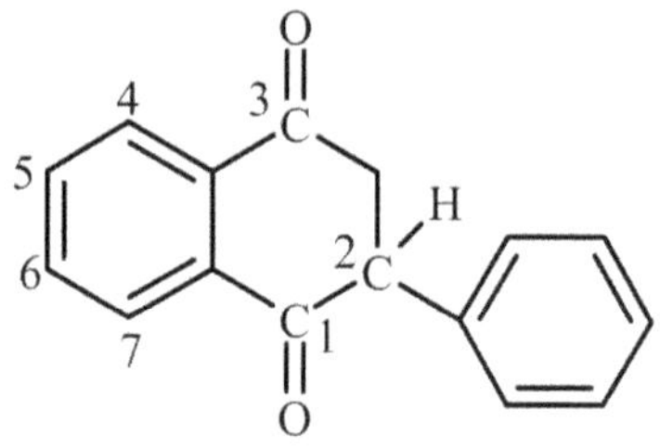

Phenindione is used as a blood anti-coagulant.

9. *Benzaldehyde* Benzaldehyde is an aromatic aldehyde bearing a single formyl group. Benzaldehyde is a clear colorless to yellow liquid with a bitter almond odor. It is denser than water and insoluble in water.

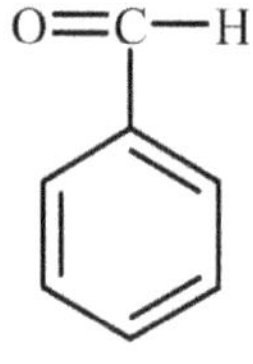

Uses

1. Benzaldehyde used in the preparation of various aniline dyes, perfumes, flavorings and pharmaceuticals.
2. Benzaldehyde is commonly employed to confer almond flavor to foods and scented products.
3. Benzaldehyde sometimes used in cosmetics products.
4. Benzaldehyde used as a bee repellant.

10. *Cinnamaldehyde* Cinnamaldehyde occurs naturally in the bark of cinnamon trees and other species of the genus Cinnamomum. Cinnamaldehyde yellow oily liquid with a cinnamon odor and sweet taste.

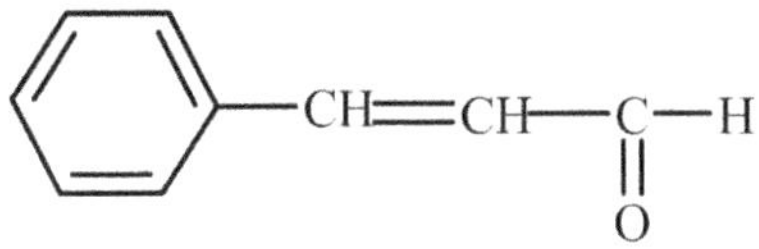

Uses

1. Cinnamaldehyde is also used as a fungicide.
2. Cinnamaldehyde helps to reduce infections of antifungal and antibacterial property.
3. Cinnamaldehyde exhibit anti-microbial activity.

11. *Acetone* Acetone occurs naturally in plants, trees and forest fires. Acetone is a colorless, volatile, flammable organic solvent.

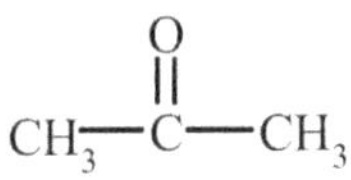

Uses

1. Acetone used as a solvent and an antiseptic.
2. Acetone used as adhesives and sealant chemicals.
3. Acetone used as viscosity adjustors.
4. Acetone is an irritant and inhalation may lead to hepatotoxic effects (causing liver damage).

PRACTICE QUESTIONS

1. (a) Mention different classes of carbonyl compounds giving the structure of one compound from each group.
   (b) Explain the similarities and differences between aldehydes and ketones.
   (c) Formulate the reactions of benzaldehyde with the following compounds, giving the conditions. Indicate the names and structures of expected products.
      (i) Potassium cyanide
      (ii) Conc. sodium hydroxide
      (iii) 2,4-Dinitrophenyl hydrazine
      (iv) Sodium bisulphate.
2. An organic compound A with molecular formula C_3H_6O is not really oxidised. It gives on reduction C_3H_6O (B) which reacts with HBr to give a bromide C. Grignard reagent obtained from C reacts with A to give $C_6H_{14}O$(D). Identify the compounds from A to D.

3. Write short notes on the following:
   (a) Clemmensen reduction with suitable examples
   (b) Wittig reaction
   (c) Reimer-Tiemann reaction
   (d) Benzoin condensation
   (e) Perkin condensation
4. Write short notes on:
   (a) Addition reactions of acetaldehyde
   (b) The importance of following reagents in the laboratory:
      (i) Tollen's reagent
      (ii) Fehling's solution
      (iii) Benedict's reagent
5. How do you convert
   (i) Acetic acid into methyl cyanide
   (ii) Acetaldehyde into acetone
6. (a) How will you distinguish between the following pairs of compounds in the laboratory?
      (i) Acetaldehyde and Acetone
      (ii) 2-Pentanone and 3-Pentanone
   (b) Write the mechanism of Aldol condensation and Cannizzaro reactions
7. Outline and discuss the evidence for the proposition that 'reagents which attack carbon-carbon double bonds do not attack carbon-oxygen double bonds and vice versa.
8. Complete the following reaction schemes stating the products and any essential conditions.

$$CH_3\,CHO + HSO_3 \longrightarrow$$

9. How do you prepare the following?
   (a) Acetaldehyde from acetylene
   (b) Acetaldehyde from acetone
10. What is Clemenson reduction? Give its mechanism with suitable example. Mention its application in the synthesis of two medicinally important compounds.
11. Give the chemical structure and uses of:
    (a) Ketamine
    (b) Ketoprofen
    (c) Chloral hydrate
    (d) Phenindione
    (e) Formaldehyde
    (f) Paraldehyde
    (g) Hexamine
    (h) Vanillin

20

CARBOXYLIC ACIDS

20.1 INTRODUCTION

Organic compounds containing a carbonyl group $(-\overset{|}{C}=O)$ and a hydroxyl (—OH) group on the same carbon atom are called carboxylic acids. The functional group of carboxylic acids is —COOH. They are acidic in nature. This class of compounds has the general formula of R—COOH, where R may be hydrogen, alkyl, substituted alkyl, aryl or substituted aryl group.

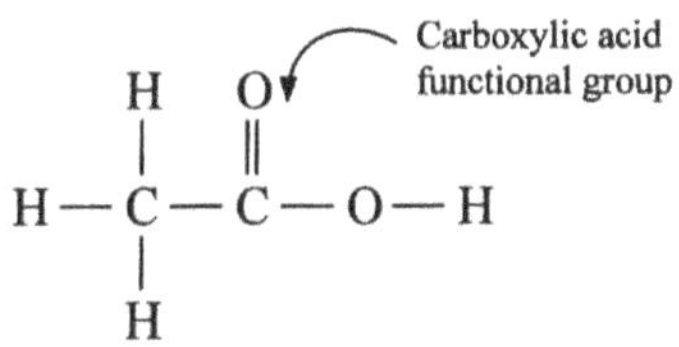

Acetic acid

20.2 CLASSIFICATION

The carboxylic acids are classified according to the number of carboxylic groups present in the molecule. These may be:

1. ***Monocarboxylic Acids*** Table 20.1 lists the important monocarboxylic acids.

Table 20.1 Names of the Simplest Carboxylic Acids

Compound	*Systematic Name*	*Trivial Name*
HCOOH	Methanoic acid	Formic acid
CH_3COOH	Ethanoic acid	Acetic acid
C_2H_5COOH	Propanoic acid	Propionic acid
C_3H_7COOH	Butanoic acid	Butyric acid
C_4H_9COOH	Pentanoic acid	Valeric acid
$C_5H_{11}COOH$	Hexanoic acid	Caproic acid
$C_6H_{13}COOH$	Heptanoic acid	Enanthic acid

Carboxylic acids containing long unbranched carbon chains are called *fatty acids.* Fatty acids are major components of the fats or lipids found in living organisms. Although over 70 different fatty acids are known, most have an even number of carbon atoms between 12 and 24. Of these, the most common and most important have either 16 or 18 carbon atoms and may contain a few double bonds. Fatty acids are usually known by their trivial names, which are given in Table 20.2.

Table 20.2 Systematic and Trivial Names of Simple Fatty Acids

Systematic Name	*Trivial Name*	*Carbon Atoms*
n-Dodecanoic acid	Lauric acid	12
n-Tetradecanoic acid	Myristic acid	14
n-Hexadecanoic acid	Palmitic acid	16
n-Hexadecan-9-enoic acid	Palmitoleic acid	16
n-Octadecanoic acid	Stearic acid	18
n-Octadecan-9-enoic acid	Oleic acid	18
n-Octadecan-9,12-dienoic acid	Linoleic acid	18
n-Octadecan-9,12,15-trienoic acid	Linolenic acid	18
n-Eicosanoic acid	Arachidic acid	20
n-Eicosan-5,8,11,14-tetraenoic acid	Arachidonic acid	20
n-Tetracosanoic acid	Lignoceric acid	22

2. ***Dicarboxylic Acids*** Organic compounds consisting of two carboxylic acids are known as dicarboxylic acids.

Chemical Structure	*Trivial (Common) Name*
HO_2CCO_2H	Oxalic acid
$HO_2CCH_2CO_2H$	Malonic acid
$HO_2CCH_2CH_2CO_2H$	Succinic acid
cis-$HO_2CCH{=}CHCO_2H$	Maleic acid
trans-$HO_2CCH{=}CHCO_2H$	Fumaric acid
$HO_2C(CH_2)_3CO_2H$	Glutaric acid
$HO_2C(CH_2)_4CO_2H$	Adipic acid
$HO_2C(CH_2)_5CO_2H$	Pimelic acid
$HO_2C(CH_2)_6CO_2H$	Suberic acid
$HO_2C(CH_2)_7CO_2H$	Azelaic acid
$HO_2C(CH_2)_8CO_2H$	Sebacic acid

20.3 IUPAC NOMENCLATURE

The sequence of steps taken for naming the carboxylic acids is as follows:

1. ***Identify the Parent Hydrocarbon*** Find the longest continuous chain of carbon atoms containing the carboxyl group. Change the -ane ending of the parent alkane to -oic acid.

Compound	*Common Name*	*IUPAC Name*
HCOOH	Formic acid	Methanoic acid
CH_3COOH	Acetic acid	Ethanoic acid
$CH_3CH_2CH_2COOH$	Butyric acid	Butanoic acid
C_6H_5COOH	Benzoic acid	Benzoic acid
$CH_3CH{=}CHCOOH$	Crotonic acid	2-Butenoic acid

2. ***Number the Parent Chain and Name each Substituent*** Number the parent chain starting from the carboxyl carbon. Number 1 is understood and is not used as part of the name. Name and number any other substituents and attach them as a prefix to the parent name.

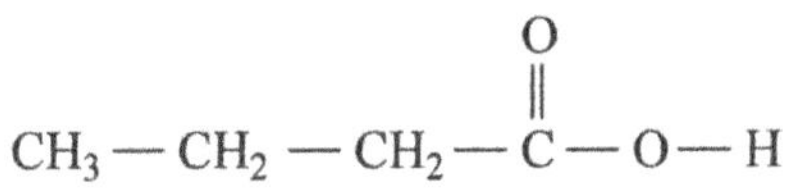

Butanoic acid

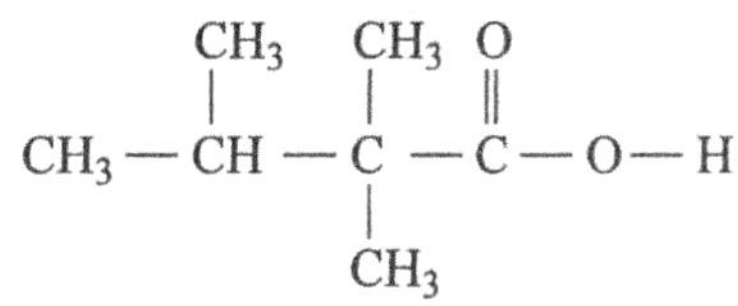

2,2′,3-Trimethyl butanoic acid

3. ***If other Functional Groups are Present*** The carboxylic acid group has priority over alkyl, halo, hydroxy, alkoxy, aldehyde and ketone groups. Name and number these substituents and attach them as prefixes to the parent name.

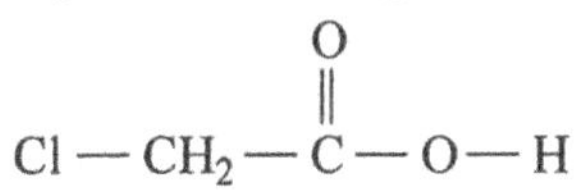

2-Chloroethanoic acid

The carboxylic acid group has priority over carbon–carbon double and triple bonds. If these groups are present, name the parent hydrocarbon as an alkene or alkyne and change the -e ending to -oic acid.

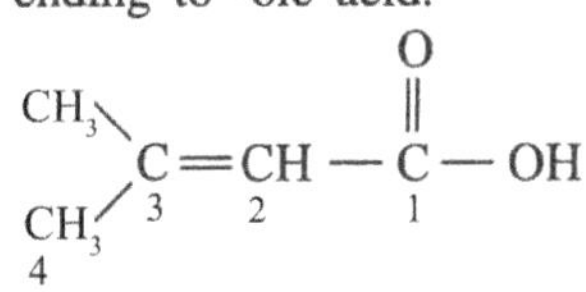

3-Methyl-2-butenoic acid

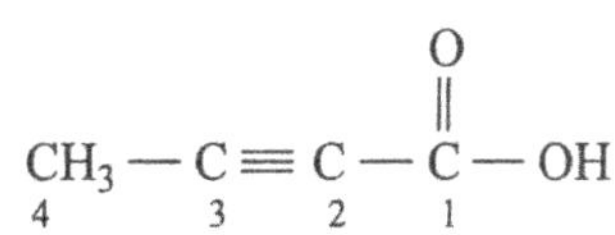

2-Butynoic acid

The carboxylic acid group has priority over aldehydes and ketones. If these groups are present give the carbonyl group the prefix oxo- and indicate its position.

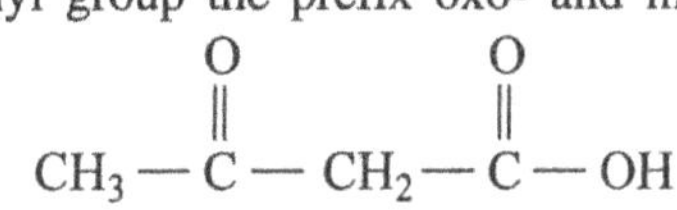

Acetoxy-ethanoic acid

4. ***If the Carboxylic Acid is attached to a Ring*** If the carboxylic acid is attached to a ring, give the —COOH group the suffix -carboxylic acid and begin numbering the ring from this group. Do not use this number as part of the name.

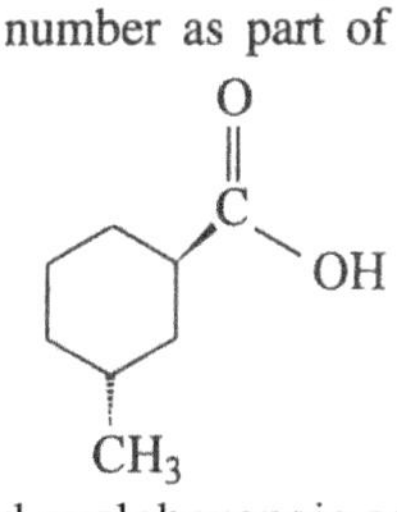

3-Methyl cyclohexanoic acid

5. ***If two Carboxylic Acid Groups are Present*** If two carboxylic acid groups are present, use the suffix -dioic acid. The parent hydrocarbon contains both carboxyl groups.

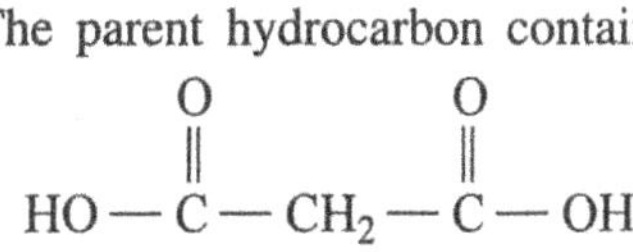

Propanedioic acid

20.4 SYNTHESIS OF CARBOXYLIC ACIDS

The important methods to prepare carboxylic acids are as follows:

1. ***Oxidation of Primary Alcohols or Aldehydes*** Carboxylic acids are readily obtained by the oxidation of primary alcohols or aldehydes using oxidising agents like $KMnO_4$ or HNO_3 or acidified $K_2Cr_2O_7$.

(a) $$\underset{\text{Alcohol or aldehyde}}{RCH_2OH \text{ or } RCHO} \xrightarrow{[O]} \underset{\text{Carboxylic acid}}{RCOOH}$$

(b) $$\underset{\text{Ethyl alcohol}}{H_3CCH_2OH} \xrightarrow[KMnO_4 \text{ or } K_2Cr_2O_7]{\text{Oxidation}} \underset{\text{Ethanal}}{H_3CCHO} \xrightarrow[KMnO_4 \text{ or } K_2Cr_2O_7]{\text{Oxidation}} \underset{\text{Ethanoic acid}}{H_3CCOOH}$$

(c) $$\underset{\text{Isobutyl alcohol}}{H_3C\overset{\overset{CH_3}{|}}{C}HCH_2OH} \xrightarrow{KMnO_4} \underset{\text{Isobutyric acid}}{H_3C\overset{\overset{CH_3}{|}}{C}HCOOH}$$

2. ***Oxidation of Alkylbenzenes*** On heating alkyl benzenes with acidified $K_2Cr_2O_7$ or $KMnO_4$, the alkyl sidechain gets oxidised to carboxyl group.

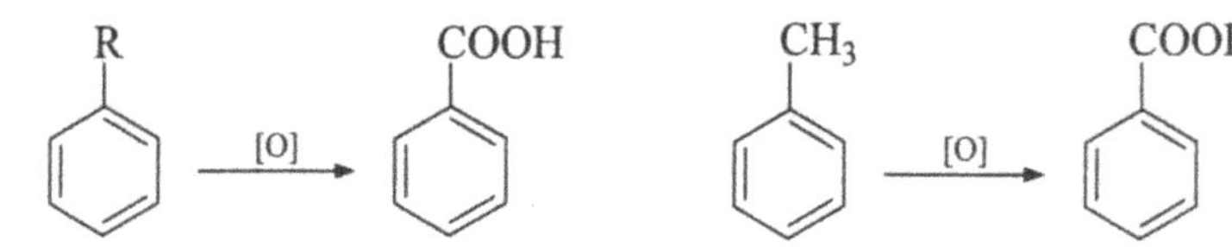

Alkylbenzene Benzoic acid Methylbenzene Benzoic acid

3. ***Hydrolysis of Nitriles*** Aliphatic and aromatic nitriles (Nitriles may be prepared by S_N2 displacement of halides by the cyanide ion) give the corresponding carboxylic acids on hydrolysis in either acidic or alkaline solution.

$$\underset{\text{Nitrile}}{R-CN} \xrightarrow[\Delta]{H_3O^+} \underset{\text{Carboxylic acid}}{R-\overset{\overset{O}{\|}}{C}-OH} + \overset{+}{N}H_4$$

$$\underset{\text{Methyl cyanide}}{H_3CCN} \xrightarrow{\text{Acidic hydrolysis}} \underset{\text{Ethanoic acid}}{H_3CCOOH}$$

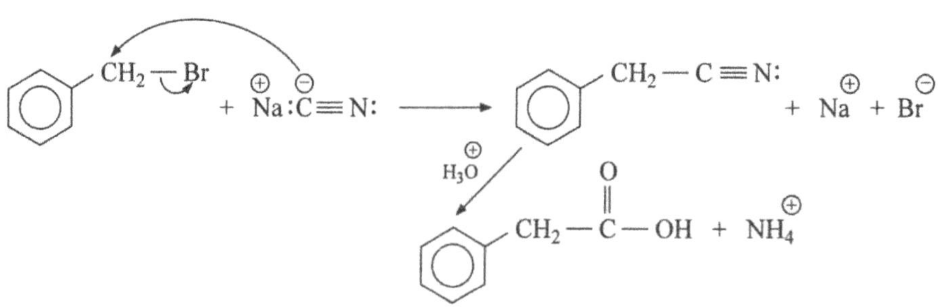

4. ***Hydrolysis of Acid Chlorides, Anhydrides, Esters or Amides*** The acid derivatives (acid chlorides, anhydrides, esters or amides) can be hydrolysed to produce carboxylic acids with varying difficulty. The acid chlorides and anhydrides react with water as such whereas hydrolysis of esters and amides is carried out in the presence of mineral acids or alkalis.

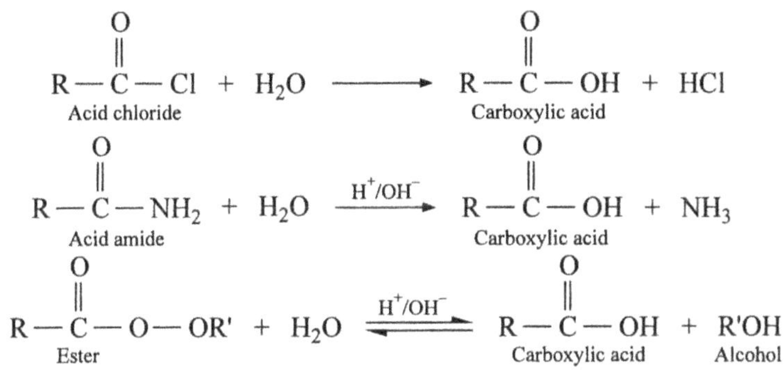

5. ***Kolbe–Schmidt Synthesis*** Phenolic carboxylic acids can be synthesised by this reaction. Kolbe's reaction is an electrophilic aromatic substitution, which involves heating the nucleophilic phenolate salt with carbon dioxide under high pressure/temperature. This results in regioselective ortho-substitution. *o*-hydroxybenzoic acid is more commonly known as salicylic acid.

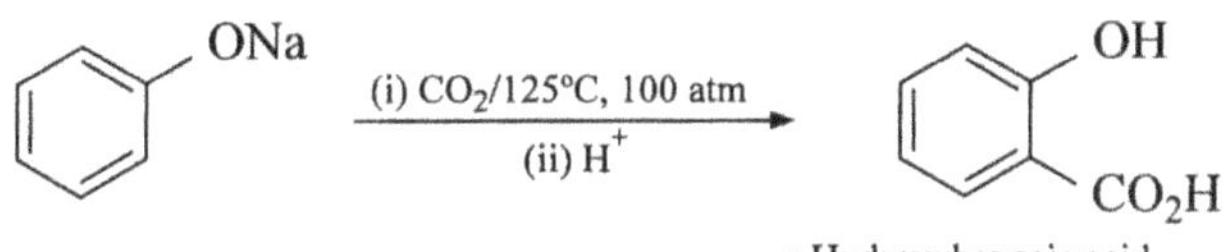

o-Hydroxybenzoic acid
(Salicylic acid)

6. ***Carbonation of Grignard Reagent*** Grignard reagents can react with carbon dioxide to form a carboxylate anion having one more carbon atom than the reactant. Experimentally, this reaction is usually accomplished by pouring the Grignard reagent onto dry ice (solid CO_2). The resulting anion is treated with dilute aqueous acids, such as hydrochloric acid, to generate the carboxylic acid.

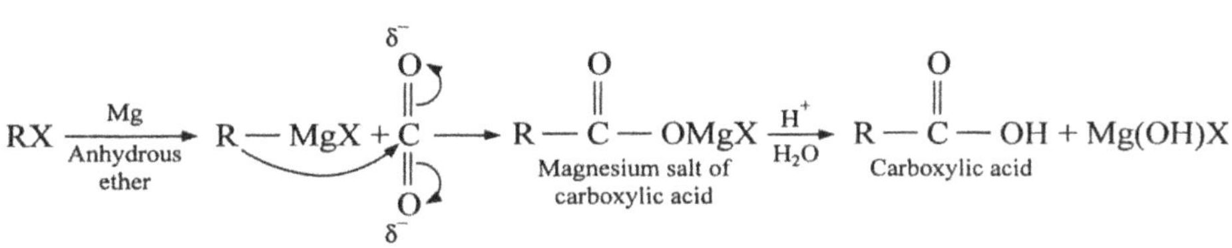

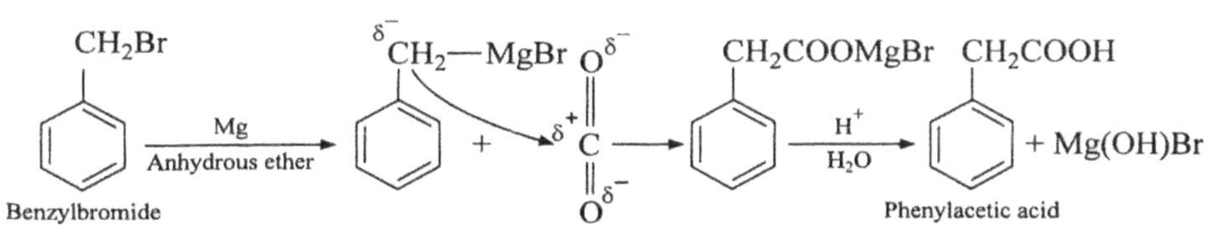

7. ***From Malonic Ester (Diethylmalonate)*** The mono or dialkyl derivative of malonic ester is hydrolysed to form mono or dialkyl malonic acid. These acids in turn can be decarboxylated by heating to get mono- or di-alkyl derivative of acetic acid.

Mono- or di-alkyl derivative of malonic ester is formed on treatment of sodium salt of malonic ester (malonic ester forms its sodium salt on reaction with metallic sodium or sodium ethoxide) with alkyl halide. Following chemical reactions are involved in the synthesis of carboxylic acids from malonic ester:

$$\underset{\text{Malonic ester}}{H_2C(COOC_2H_5)_2} \xrightarrow[-\,2C_2H_5OH]{C_2H_5ONa} \underset{\text{Sidiomalonic ester}}{Na^+\,\overset{-}{H}C(COOC_2H_5)_2} \xrightarrow{RX} \underset{\text{Alkyl malonic ester}}{RCH(COOC_2H_5)_2}$$

$$\xrightarrow[-\,2C_2H_5OH]{NaOH} RCH(COONa)_2 \xrightarrow[-\,2NaCl]{HCl} RCH(COOH)_2 \xrightarrow[\Delta]{\text{Decarboxylation}} \underset{\text{Alkyl acetic acid}}{RCH_2COOH} + CO_2$$

20.5 PHYSICAL PROPERTIES OF CARBOXYLIC ACIDS

1. First nine-monocarboxylic acids are colourless liquids, while the higher ones are colourless wax-like solids.
2. First three members possess pungent odour, while the higher ones have goat-like odour.
3. Lower members (up to C_4) are completely soluble in water due to the formation of intermolecular hydrogen bonds between the hydroxyl group of acid and oxygen of water and oxygen of acid and hydrogen of water.

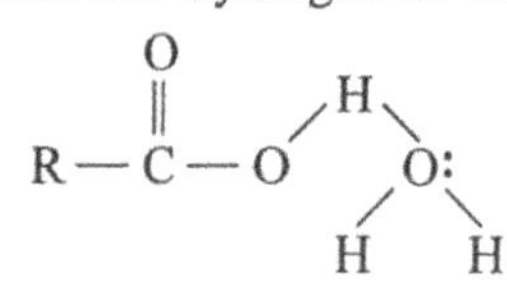

The higher members are insoluble in water. All the acids are soluble in organic solvents (alcohol, benzene, ether, etc.).

4. The carboxylic acids have higher boiling points, than alkenes, ketones, and alcohols because of greater strengths of the intermolecular hydrogen bonds, e.g. propanoic acid (mol. wt. 74) boils at 141°C while *n*-butanol (mol. wt. 74) boils at 118°C.

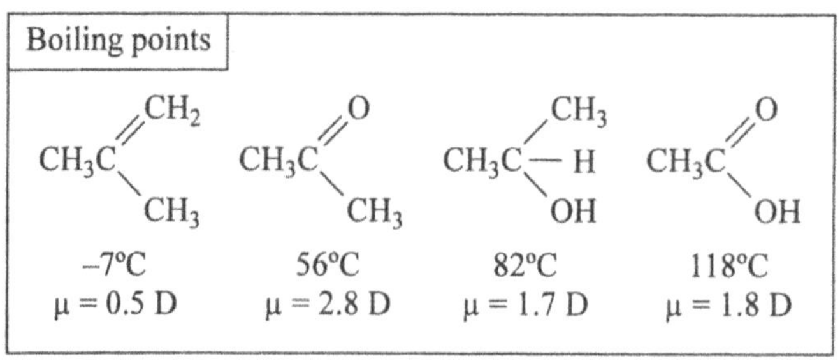

20.6 CHEMICAL PROPERTIES OF CARBOXYLIC ACIDS

1. ***Acidity of Carboxylic Acids*** Carboxylic acids are considerably acidic in nature and are the acids of organic chemistry. In aqueous solution, molecules of carboxylic acid interact with water molecules and form carboxylate ions and hydronium ions.

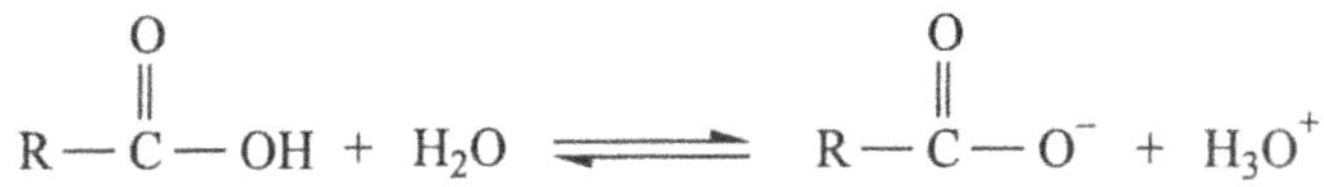

Carboxylic acid Carboxylate ion

Carboxylic acids are weak acids and the extent of ionisation is described by acidity constant (K_a).

$$K_a = [RCOO^-][H_3O^+] / [RCOOH]$$

The value of K_a is directly proportional to the concentration of hydrogen ions. The larger the value of K_a the stronger the acid and smaller the value of K_a weaker the acid. If K_a is greater than 10, the given acid will be completely dissociated in water. For convenience pK_a is introduced.

$$pK_a = -\log K_a$$

Higher the value of K_a lower will be the value of pK_a. Hence, lower pK_a value indicates a higher strength of the acid.

The cause of acidity may be explained on the basis of the following considerations:

(i) *Resonance effect* The reasons for the acidity of carboxylic acids is that they lose a proton readily because the carboxylate ion formed is stabilised by resonance. In case of a carboxylic acid both the acid and the carboxylate ion exist in two canonical forms.

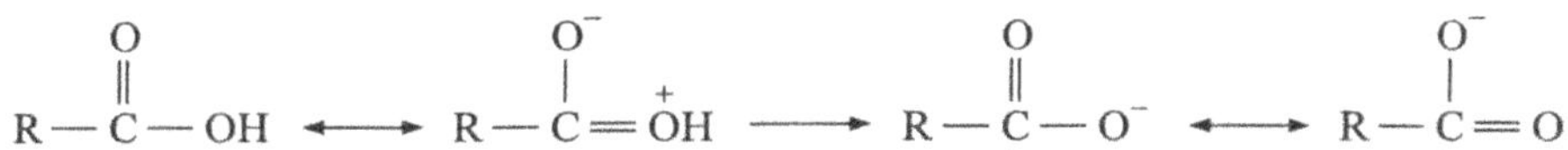

A B C D

Carboxylic acid Carboxylate ion

In canonical form B, there is charge separation, therefore, it would contain more energy and hence less stable than form A. On the other hand, in the canonical forms C and D, carboxylate ions have equivalent structures and are equally stable. Thus, both acid and carboxylate ions are resonance stabilised but stabilisation is greater for the carboxylate ion than for acid. The driving force for ionisation of carboxylic acids moves from acid to carboxylate ion.

According to the resonance theory, a carboxylate ion is a hybrid of two canonical forms. These forms are equally stable, hence the hybrid is more stable, the carbon is joined to each oxygen by equivalent one-and-a-half bond. The negative charge is evenly distributed over both oxygen atoms.

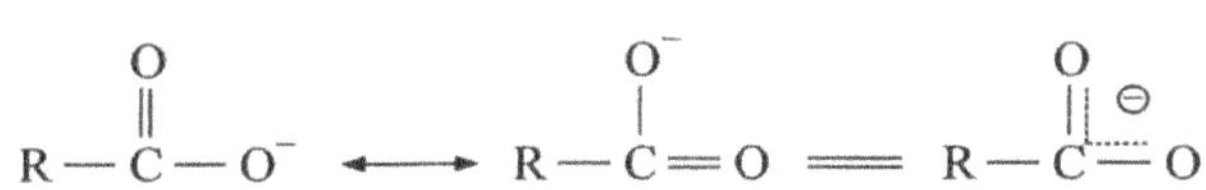

C D Resonance hybrid of carboxylate ion

Contributors of carboxylate ion

For example, formic acid contains one carbon–oxygen bond of 1.36 Å (single bond) and another 1.23 Å (double bond) whereas sodium formate contains two equal carbon–oxygen bonds each 1.27 Å long. These results were confirmed by X-ray and electron diffraction studies.

Formic acid Sodium formate

(ii) *Molecular orbital structure* The stability of carboxylate ion can be explained on the basis of molecular orbital theory. Carbon atom of carboxylate ion is sp^2 hybridised. Two of the sp^2 orbital of this carbon atom form σ-bonds with the *p* orbitals of oxygen atoms, the third sp^2 orbital of the carbon forms σ-bond with the carbon of the alkyl group or hydrogen atom in the case of formic acid. The unhybridised *p* orbital of carbon and *p* orbitals of both the oxygen atoms form a stable delocalised molecular orbital. Thus, the π-electrons are delocalised and hence the carboxylate ion is more stable.

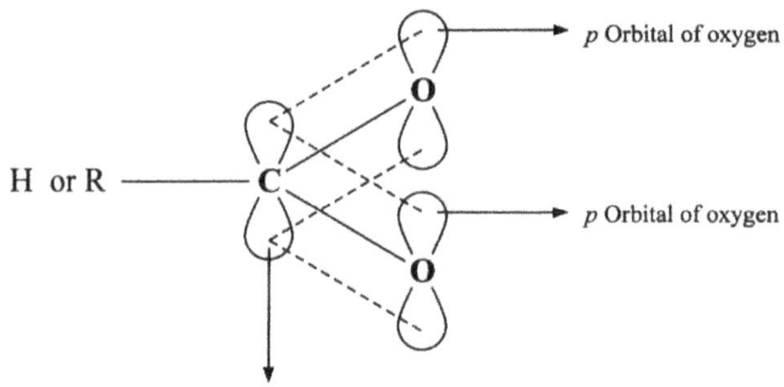

Molecular orbital diagram of carboxylate anion

(iii) *Effect of substituents on acidity* The carboxylic acids are acidic in nature because of the stabilisation of carboxylate ion. Any factor that stabilises the carboxylate ion should increase the acidity and any factor that makes carboxylate ion less-stable should decrease acidity. Electron-withdrawing substituents should disperse the negative charge, stabilise the carboxylate ion and thus increase acidity. Electron-releasing substituents should intensify the negative charge there by destabilise the carboxylate ion and thus lead to decrease in acidity, e.g. chloroacetic acid is about 100 times stronger than acetic acid, dichloroacetic acid is still stronger than chloroacetic acid.

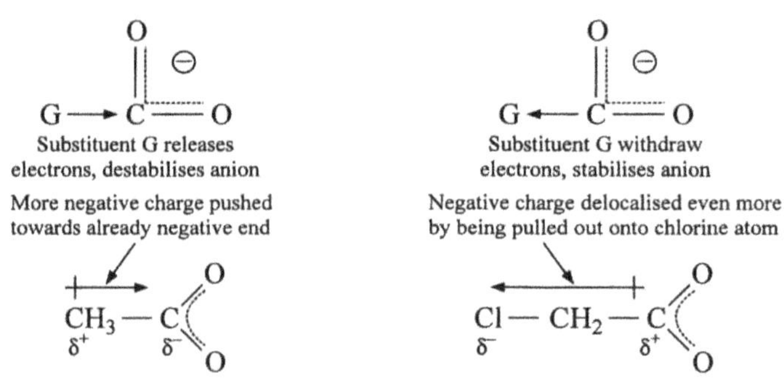

Carboxylic Acid	pK_a	*Carboxylic Acid*	pK_a
CH_3COOH	4.76	FCH_2COOH	2.66
$ClCH_2COOH$	2.86	$BrCH_2COOH$	2.90
$Cl_2CHCOOH$	1.29	ICH_2COOH	3.17
Cl_3CCOOH	0.65	NO_2CH_2COOH	1.7

2. ***Salt Formation*** Carboxylic acids are attacked by strongly electropositive metals (sodium, potassium and zinc) to form their salts and liberate hydrogen. They also react with hydroxides, metallic oxides and bicarbonates to form salts.

$$\underset{\text{Carboxylic acid}}{R-\overset{\overset{\displaystyle O}{\|}}{C}-OH} + NaOH \longrightarrow \underset{\text{Sodium carboxylate}}{R-\overset{\overset{\displaystyle O}{\|}}{C}-O^-Na^+} + H_2O$$

$$\underset{\text{Acetic acid}}{CH_3-\overset{\overset{\displaystyle O}{\|}}{C}-OH} + NaOH \longrightarrow \underset{\text{Sodium acetate}}{CH_3-\overset{\overset{\displaystyle O}{\|}}{C}-O^-Na^+} + H_2O$$

$$\underset{\text{Benzoic acid}}{C_6H_5-\overset{\overset{\displaystyle O}{\|}}{C}-OH} + NaHCO_3 \longrightarrow \underset{\text{Sodium benzoate}}{C_6H_5-\overset{\overset{\displaystyle O}{\|}}{C}-O^-Na^+} + CO_2 + H_2O$$

$$\underset{\text{Acetic acid}}{CH_3-\overset{\overset{\displaystyle O}{\|}}{C}-OH} + NH_3 \longrightarrow \underset{\text{Ammonium acetate}}{CH_3-\overset{\overset{\displaystyle O}{\|}}{C}-O^-\overset{+}{N}H_4}$$

$$\underset{\text{Benzoic acid}}{2C_6H_5-\overset{\overset{\displaystyle O}{\|}}{C}-OH} + Na_2CO_3 \longrightarrow \underset{\text{Sodium benzoate}}{2C_6H_5-\overset{\overset{\displaystyle O}{\|}}{C}-O^-Na^+} + CO_2\uparrow + H_2O$$

3. ***Nucleophilic Acyl Substitution*** Acyl compounds (carboxylic acids and their derivatives) undergo nucleophilic substitution, in which —OH, —Cl, —OOCR, —NH_2 or —OR is replaced by some other basic group.

$$\underset{\text{Carboxylic acid}}{R-\overset{\overset{\displaystyle C}{\|}}{C}-OH} + \underset{\text{Nucleophile}}{\mathbf{Z}\colon} \longrightarrow \underset{\text{Substitution product}}{R-\overset{\overset{\displaystyle O}{\|}}{C}-Z} \qquad (Z = -Cl, -OR', -NH_2)$$

Nucleophilic acyl substitution proceeds by the following steps:

(a) Nucleophile attacks at electrophilic carbon of acyl compound to form a tetrahedral intermediate.

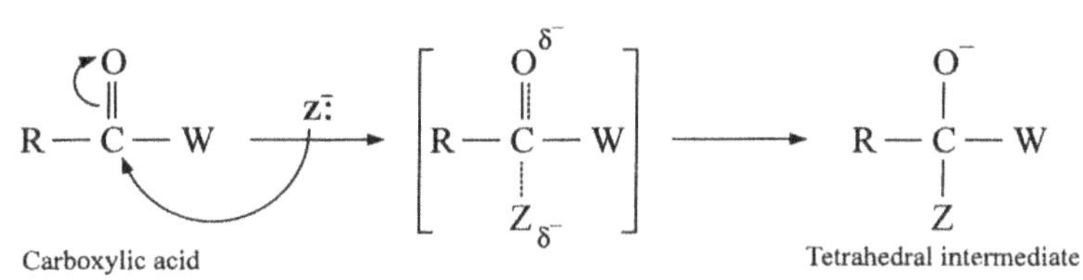

(b) The tetrahedral intermediate ejects (:w = —OH, —Cl, —NH_2, —OR) group and changes to trigonal compound results in substitution. The second step depends on the nucleophilicity of the leaving group (w:).

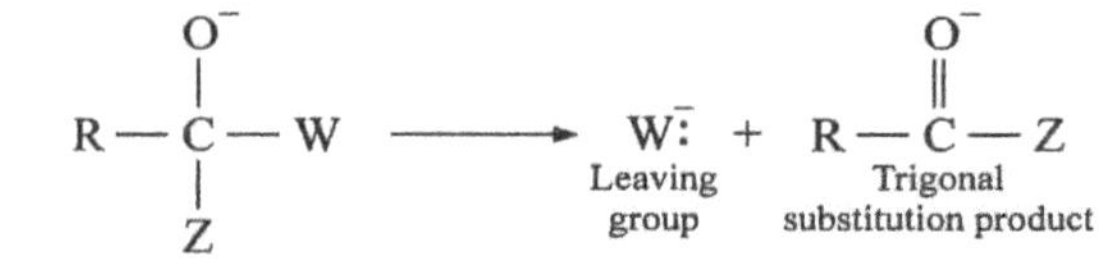

Tetrahedral intermediate

Kinetics The overall rate of nucleophilic acyl substitution reaction is affected by the rate of both steps, but the first step is more important hence it is the rate-detrmining step.

Relative Reactivities of Carboxylic Acids and their Derivatives

(i) *Electronic factors* The nucleophilic acyl substitution reactions are favoured by electron-withdrawing groups, which stabilise the negative charge of the oxygen in the itermediate.

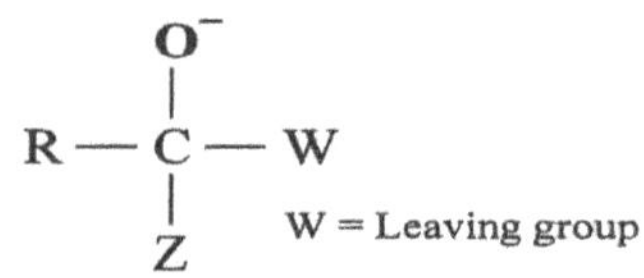

Tetrahedral intermediate

The reactivity of a carboxylic acid derivative depends on the nucleophilicity of the leaving group attached to the acyl carbon. Lesser the nucleophilicity of leaving group more the reactivity of carboxylic acid derivative because a weaker nucleophile has greater resonance stabilisation. Relative basicities of the leaving groups is $Cl^- < {}^-OCOR < {}^-OR < {}^-OH < {}^-NH_2$. Hence, the relative reactivities of carboxylic acid derivatives is $Cl^- > {}^-OCOR > {}^-OR > {}^-OH > {}^-NH_2$. Therefore, the more electrophilic this carbon (acyl carbon) is, the more reactive it will be.

(ii) *Stearic factors* Bulky groups attached to the carbonyl group can hinder the approach of nucleophiles and result in lowered reactivity. Bulky nucleophiles will also react more slowly.

(i) *Esterification* Carboxylic acids react with alcohols in the presence of mineral acid catalyst (HCl or H_2SO_4) to form esters. This reaction is reversible, the forward reaction is esterification and the backward reaction is known as hydrolysis.

$$\underset{\text{Carboxylic acid}}{RCOOH} + \underset{\text{Alcohol}}{R'OH} \overset{H^+}{\rightleftharpoons} \underset{\text{Ester}}{RCOOR'} + H_2O$$

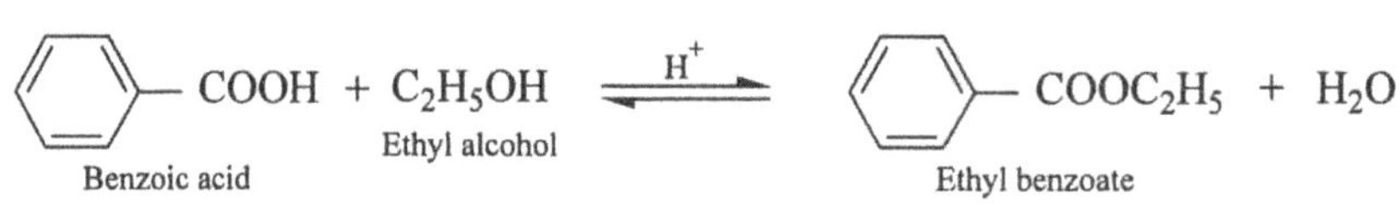

Mechanism The mechanism of esterification is an example of nucleophilic acyl substitution, which involves the following steps:

- Protonation of the carboxylic group by H^+ of the acid catalyst.
- This makes the carbonyl carbon more strongly electropositive which is attacked by the nucleophile, the alcohol molecule.
- The transfer of proton to one of the —OH groups takes place.
- The —OH group leaves as water molecule giving protonated ester.
- The resonance stabilised protonated ester loses a proton to form ester.

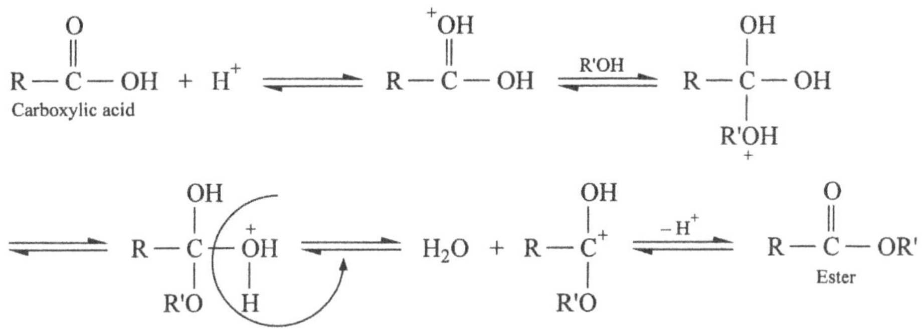

(ii) *Formation of acid halides* Carboxylic acids can be converted into corresponding acid halides by reaction with PCl_5, PCl_3, PBr_3, or $SOCl_2$. Of all these reagents, thionyl chloride is the best and the mildest reagent for the preparation of acid halides. This is because the products (SO_2 and HCl) being gaseous can be easily removed from acid halide.

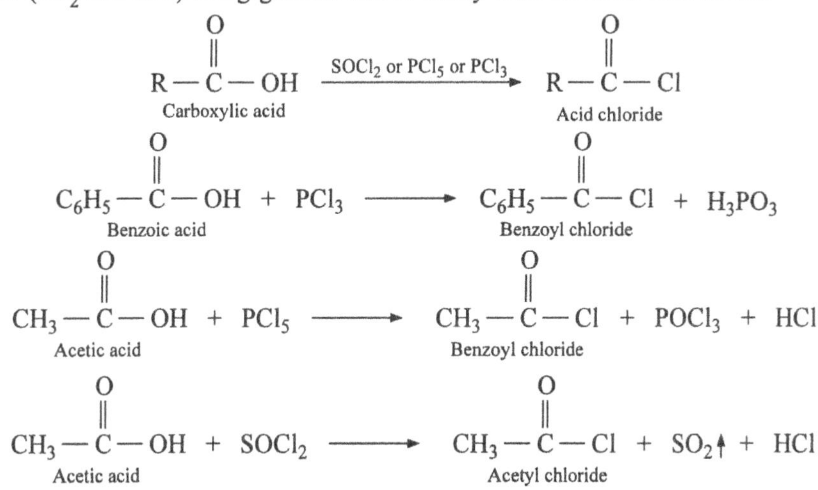

Mechanism

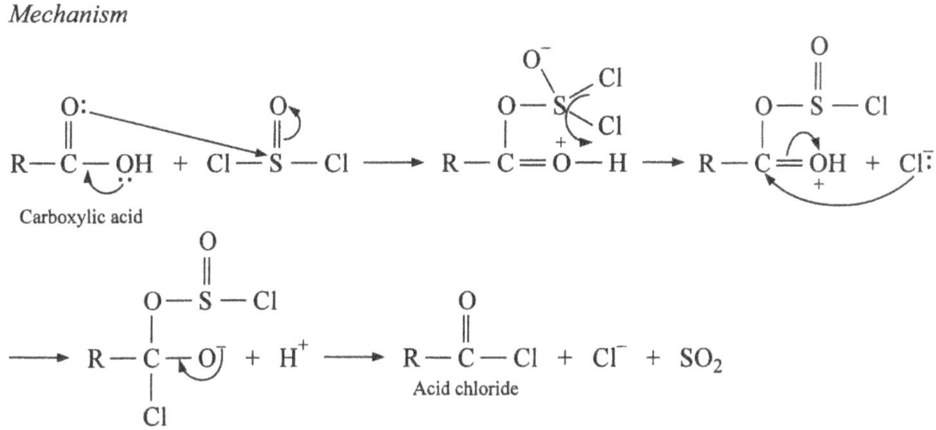

(iii) *Formation of acid anhydrides* Carboxylic acids undergo intermolecular anhydride formation in the presence of a strong dehydrating agent like phosphorous pentoxide.

$$\underset{\text{Carboxylic acid}}{2R-\overset{\overset{\displaystyle O}{\|}}{C}-OH} \xrightarrow{P_2O_5} \underset{\text{Acid anhydride}}{R-\overset{\overset{\displaystyle O}{\|}}{C}-O-\overset{\overset{\displaystyle O}{\|}}{C}-R}$$

$$\underset{\text{Acetic acid}}{2CH_3-\overset{\overset{\displaystyle O}{\|}}{C}-OH} \xrightarrow{P_2O_5} \underset{\text{Acetic anhydride}}{CH_3-\overset{\overset{\displaystyle O}{\|}}{C}-O-\overset{\overset{\displaystyle O}{\|}}{C}-CH_3}$$

(iv) *Formation of acid amides* Carboxylic acids give amides on treating acid chloride of carboxylic acid with ammonia. This reaction follows nucleophilic acyl substitution.

$$\underset{\text{Carboxylic acid}}{R-\overset{\overset{\displaystyle O}{\|}}{C}-OH} \xrightarrow{SOCl_2 \text{ or } PCl_5 \text{ or } PCl_3} \underset{\text{Acid chloride}}{R-\overset{\overset{\displaystyle O}{\|}}{C}-Cl} \xrightarrow{NH_3} \underset{\text{Acid amide}}{R-\overset{\overset{\displaystyle O}{\|}}{C}-NH_2}$$

$$\underset{\text{Benzoic acid}}{C_6H_5-\overset{\overset{\displaystyle O}{\|}}{C}-OH} \xrightarrow{SOCl_2 \text{ or } PCl_5 \text{ or } PCl_3} \underset{\text{Benzoyl chloride}}{C_6H_5-\overset{\overset{\displaystyle O}{\|}}{C}-Cl} \xrightarrow{NH_3} \underset{\text{Benzamide}}{C_6H_5-\overset{\overset{\displaystyle O}{\|}}{C}-NH_2}$$

4. ***Reduction of Carboxylic Acids*** Carboxylic acids are resistant to catalytic hydrogenation. However, they can be reduced by $LiAlH_4$ to form primary alcohol.

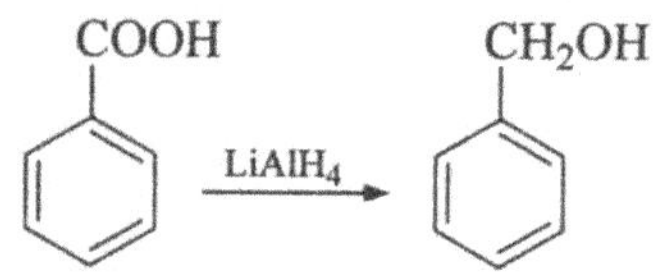

Benzoic acid Benzylalcohol

5. ***Decarboxylation of Carboxylic Acid*** When the sodium salt of a carboxylic acid is heated strongly with sodalime (NaOH + CaO), an alkane is formed. The alkane, so obtained, contains one carbon less than original acid. This reaction is known as *decarboxylation.*

$$\underset{\text{Sodium carboxylate}}{RCOONa} + \underset{\text{Sodalime}}{NaOH/CaO} \rightarrow \underset{\text{Alkane}}{RH} + Na_2CO_3$$

$$\underset{\text{Sodium acetate}}{CH_3COONa} + NaOH/CaO \rightarrow \underset{\text{Methane}}{CH_4} + Na_2CO_3$$

6. ***Kolbe's Electrolytic Reaction*** When a concentrated solution of sodium or potassium salt of a monocarboxylic acid is electrolysed, a symmetrical alkane is obtained at the anode. This reaction takes place through the intermediate formation of free radicals.

$$2RCOONa + 2H_2O \rightarrow R-R + 2CO_2 + 2NaOH + H_2$$

$$\underset{\text{Sodium acetate}}{2CH_3COONa} + 2H_2O \rightarrow \underset{\text{Ethane}}{C_2H_6} + 2CO_2 + 2NaOH + H_2$$

7. ***Electrophilic Aromatic Substitution*** Aromatic carboxylic acids undergo electrophilic aromatic substitution reactions (halogenation, nitration and sulphonation) on benzene ring. Carboxyl group is a meta-directing and deactivating.

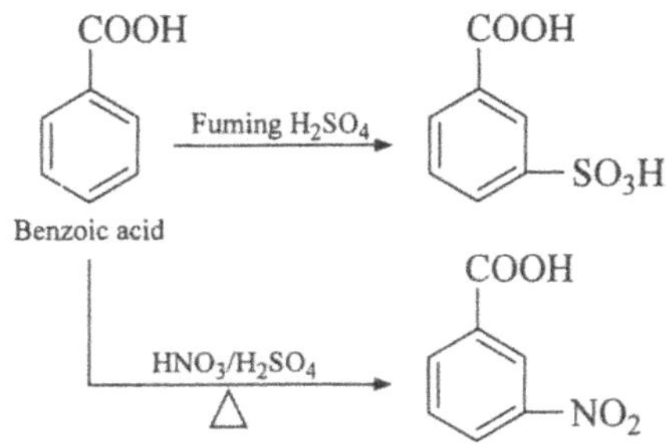

8. ***Halogenation (Hell–Volhard–Zelinsky Reaction)*** If a carboxylic acid is treated with halogens (Cl_2 or Br_2) and red phosphorus, the latter reacts with Br_2 or Cl_2 to form phosphorous trihalide (PBr_3 or PCl_3). The halogenation occurs at α-carbon. This reaction is known as Hell–Volhard–Zelinsky reaction (HVZ reaction).

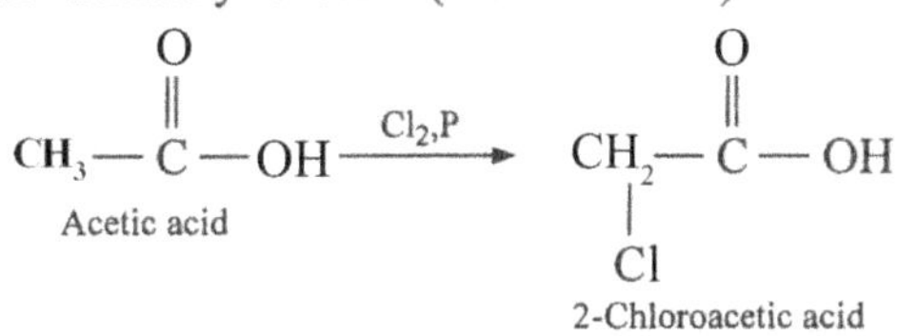

Mechanism This reaction involves conversion of a carboxylic acid into an acyl chloride. The acyl chloride is in equilibrium with its enol. Chlorination of enol followed by loss of a proton gives α-chlorinated acyl chloride, which is hydrolysed to α-chlorinated carboxylic acid.

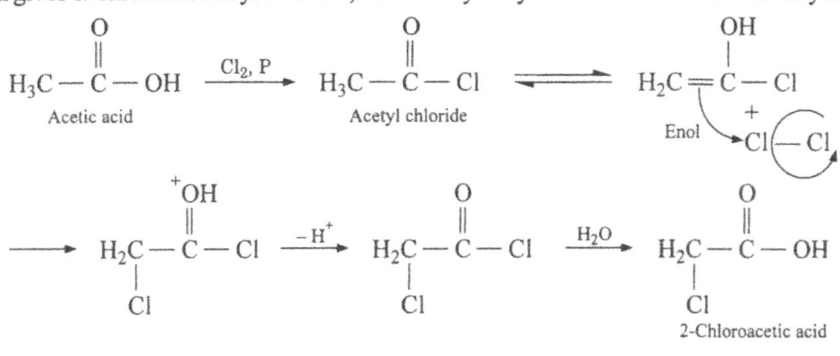

20.7 DICARBOXYLIC ACIDS

Organic compounds consisting of two carboxylic acids are known as dicarboxylic acids. According to IUPAC nomenclature, the suffix '*dioic* acid' is added after the name of the parent alkane. The dicarboxylic acids may be saturated or unsaturated. The names of some important saturated dicarboxylic acids are:

Common Name	*IUPAC Name*	*Formula*
Oxalic acid	Ethane*dioic* acid	$(COOH)_2$
Malonic Acid	Propane*dioic* acid	$CH_2(COOH)_2$
Succinic acid	Butane*dioic* acid	$HOOC - CH_2 - COOH$
Glutaric acid	Hexane*dioic*	$HO_2C(CH_2)_3CO_2H$
Adipic acid	Heptane*dioic* acid	$HO_2C(CH_2)_4CO_2H$

20.7.1 Methods of Preparation

Dicarboxylic acids can be prepared by the following methods:

1. ***From Glycols by Oxidation*** Glycols on oxidation give dicarboxylic acids.

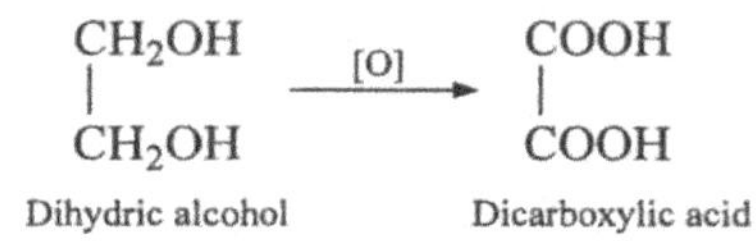

2. ***From Dinitriles by Hydrolysis*** Dinitriles on acidic hydrolysis yield dicarboxylic acids.

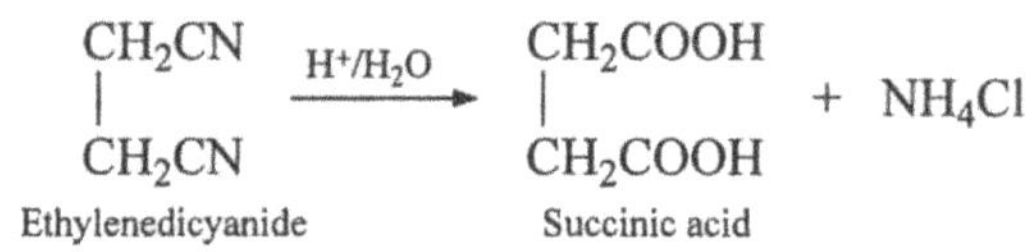

3. ***From Malonic Ester*** Dicarboxylic acids and its derivatives can be prepared by heating monosodiomalonic ester with iodine, followed by hydrolysis and decarboxylation.

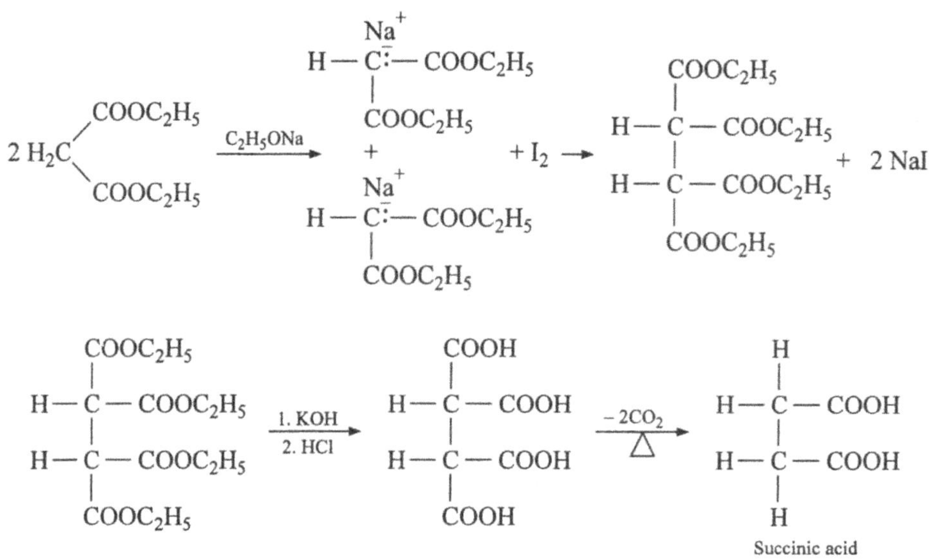

20.7.2 General Properties

1. All dicarboxylic acids are crystalline solids.
2. They are more soluble in water than the monocarboxylic acids containing the same number of carbon atoms. This is due to the formation of more number of hydrogen bonds with water.
3. The dicarboxylic acids have two pK_a values due to the presence of two ionisable carboxylic groups.

20.7.3 Chemical Properties

1. ***Formation of Esters and Amides*** Generally dicarboxylic acids undergo similar chemical reactions as that of monocarboxylic acids like formation of esters, amides:

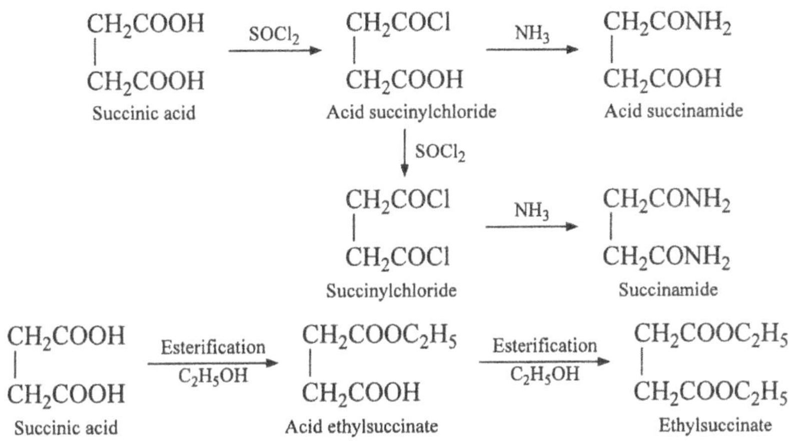

2. ***Acidity*** Dicarboxylic acids are acidic in nature. They give two series of derivatives and dissociate in two steps. The first dissociation constant of dicarboxylic acids is greater than the second one due to electron withdrawal inductive effect of carboxylic acid group.

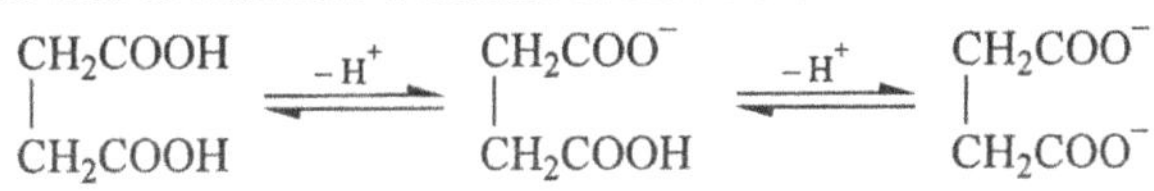

The acidity decreases by increasing the molecular weight.

3. ***Action of Heat*** Dicarboxylic acids behave differently on heating.

(a) Dicarboxylic acids containing two carboxyl groups attached to the same carbon atom like oxalic acid, malonic acid eliminate a molecule of carbon dioxide on heating.

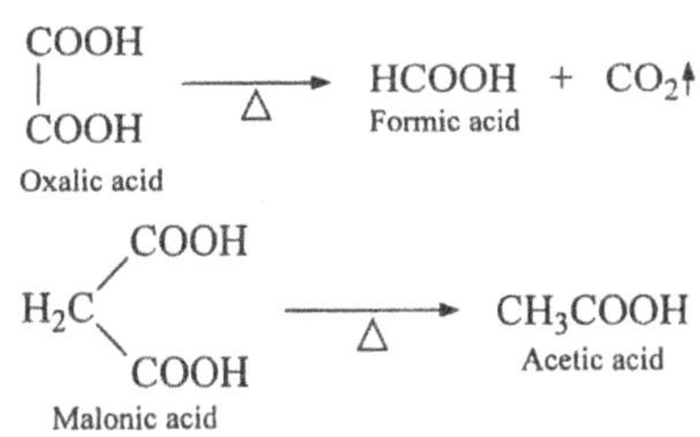

(b) The dicarboxylic acids (1,5) form cyclic anhydrides on heating with acetic anhydride.

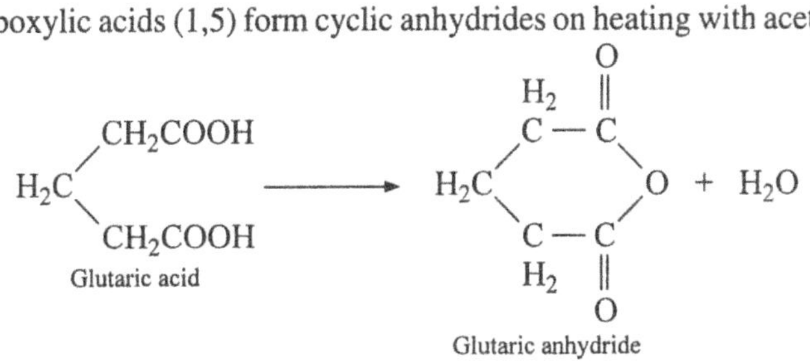

(c) Some dicarboxylic acids (1,6 or 1,7) like adipic acid and higher members (the two carboxylic acid groups are separated by four or more carbon atoms) yield cyclic ketones on heating.

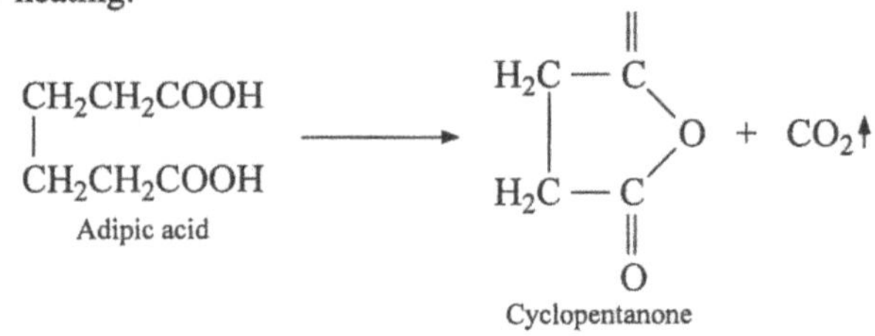

20.8 ALDEHYDIC AND KETO ACIDS

20.8.1 Introduction

The carboxylic acids consisting of an aldehyde or keto group along the carboxylic acid functional group are called aldehydic or keto acids. They are classified as α, β, γ, δ on the basis of relative positions of aldehyde (or keto) group and carboxylic acid group. Some examples of aldehydic or keto acids with trivial names are:

$CH_3C(=O)CO_2H$	Pyruvic acid
$CH_3C(=O)CH_2CH_2CO_2H$	Levulinic acid
$HO_2CCH_2C(=O)CH_2CO_2H$	Acetonedicarboxylic acid
$CH_3C(=O)CH_2CO_2H$	Acetoacetic acid

20.8.2 Methods to Prepare

Aldehydic and keto acids can be prepared by the following methods:

1. ***Glyoxalic Acid (α-aldehydic acid)*** It can be prepared by the oxidation of 1,2-ethanediol with nitric acid.

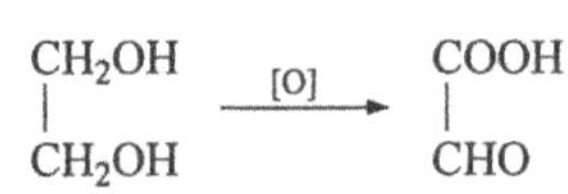

2. ***Preparation of α-Keto Acid (pyruvic acid)*** Pyruvic acid is prepared by heating tartaric acid with potassium hydrogen sulphate.

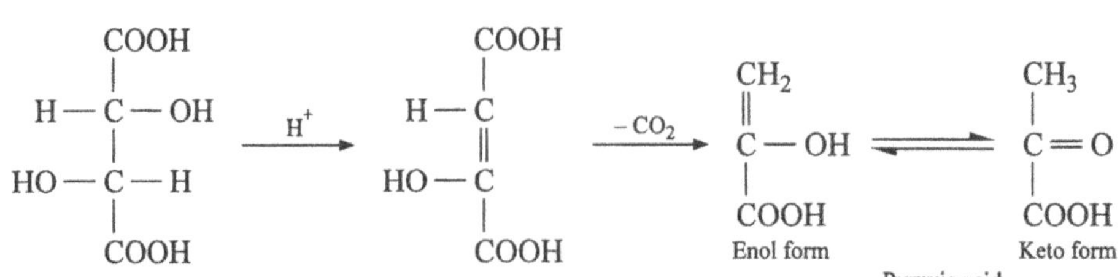

3. ***Preparation of β-Acids*** β-keto acid is prepared by crossed Claisen condensation of ethyl acetate and ethyl formate.

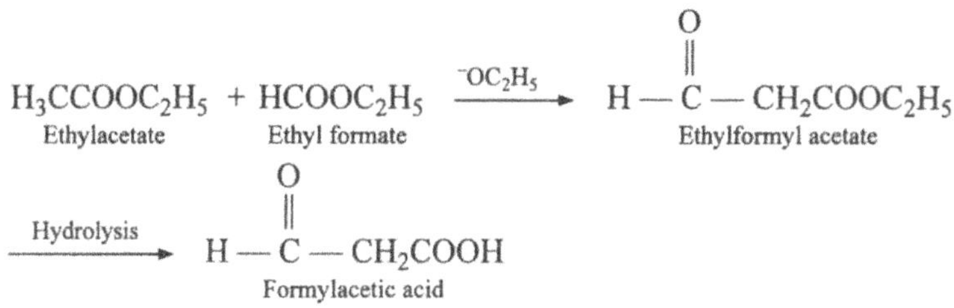

20.9 HYDROXY ACIDS

20.9.1 Introduction

Hydroxy acids are the substituted derivatives of monocarboxylic acids. They are obtained from monocarboxylic acids by replacing a hydrogen atom of hydrocarbon by hydroxyl group.

Examples of hydroxy acids are

$HOCO_2H$	Carbonic acid
$HOCH_2CO_2H$	Glycolic acid
$CH_3CH(OH)CO_2H$	Lactic acid
$HO_2CCH(OH)CH_2CO_2H$	Malic acid
$HO_2CCH(OH)CH(OH)CO_2H$	Tartaric acid
$HO_2CCH_2C(OH)(CO_2H)CH_2CO_2H$	Citric acid

20.9.2 Methods of Preparation

Hydroxy acids can be prepared by the following methods:

1. ***Hydrolysis of Cyanohydrins*** Cyanohydrins of aldehydes or ketones give α-hydroxy acids on hydrolysis.

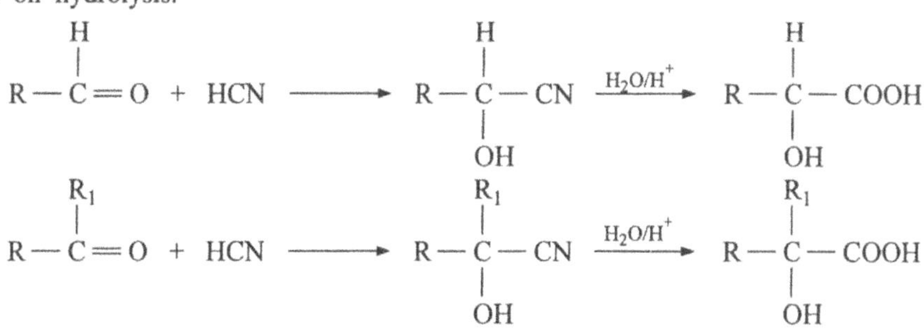

2. ***Hydrolysis of α-Halogen Acids*** α-Halogen carboxylic acids on hydrolysis yield α-hydroxy acids. The required α-halogen acids can be prepared from the respective carboxylic acids by Hell–Volhard–Zelinsky reaction.

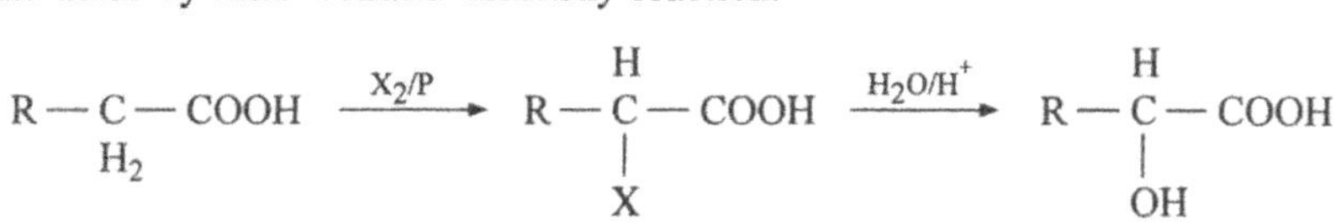

3. ***From α-Amino Acids*** α-Amino acids on treatment with nitrous acid yield α-hydroxy acids.

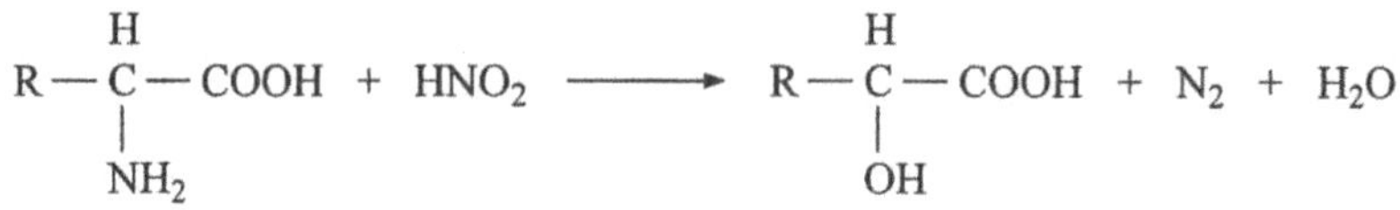

4. ***Reformatsky Reaction*** β-Hydroxy acids can be prepared by treating aldehyde or ketone with α-bromoester and metallic zinc in presence of dry ether or benzene.

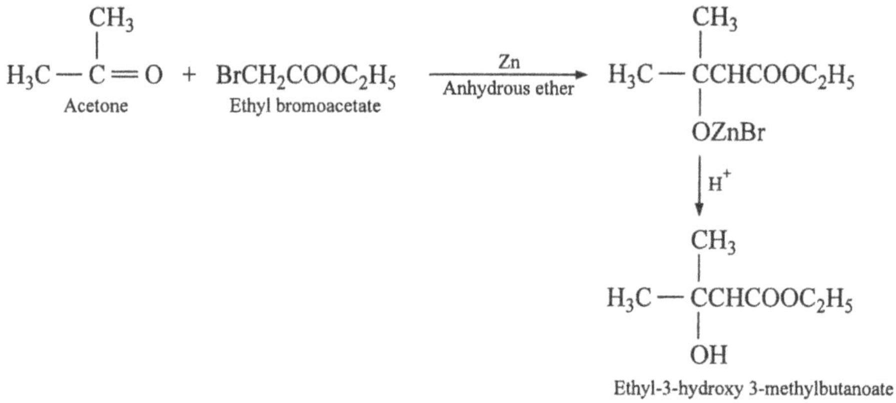

5. ***By Oxidation of Aldol with Tollen's Reagent*** α-Hydroxy acids are prepared by oxidation of aldol with mild-oxidising agents.

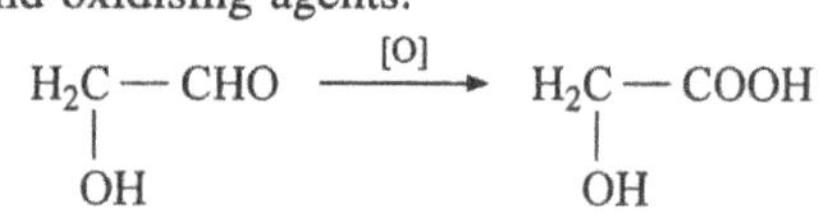

6. β-Hydroxy acids can also be prepared by catalytic reduction of the keto esters followed by acidic or alkaline hydrolysis.

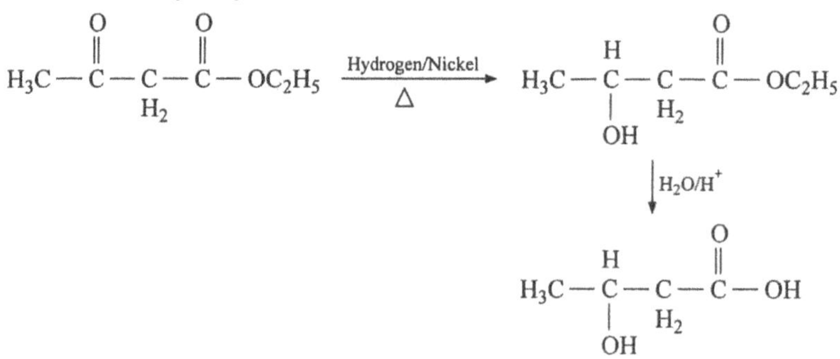

20.9.3 Properties

Hydroxy acids possess two functional groups, namely, the alcoholic hydroxyl group and carboxyl groups. Therefore, hydroxy acids exhibit the following chemical reactions:

1. ***Reactions of Carboxyl Group*** Hydroxy acids undergo the characteristic reactions of carboxyl group due to the presence of free carboxyl group.

(i) *Reaction with bases*

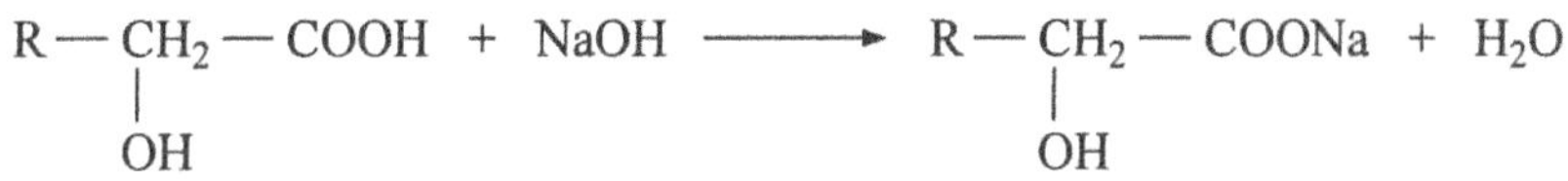

(ii) *Reaction with alcohols (Esterification)*

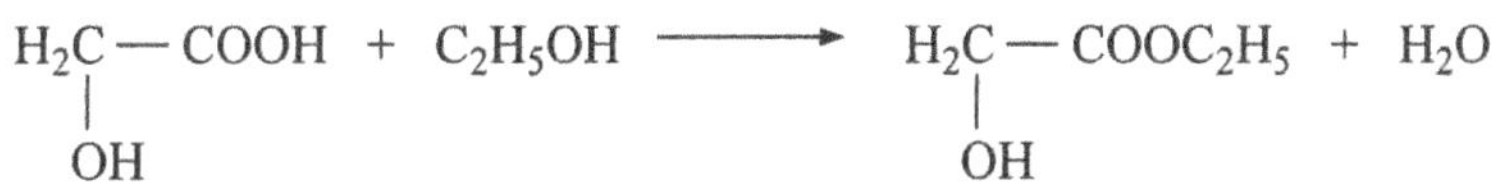

(iii) *Reaction with phosphorous halides or thionyl chloride*

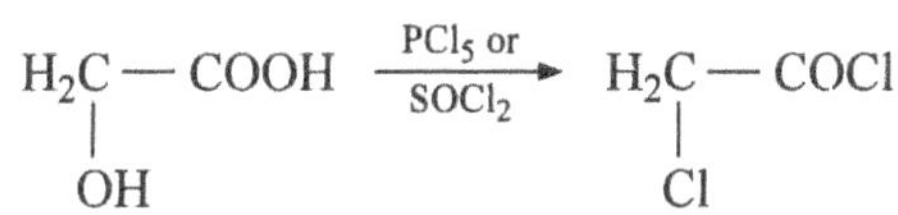

2. ***Reactions of Hydroxyl Group*** Hydroxy acids undergo the characteristic reactions of hydroxyl group.

(i) *Oxidation*

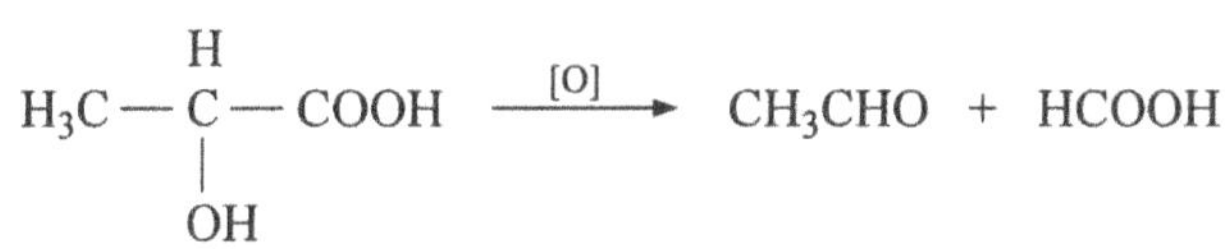

(ii) *Reaction with halogen acids*

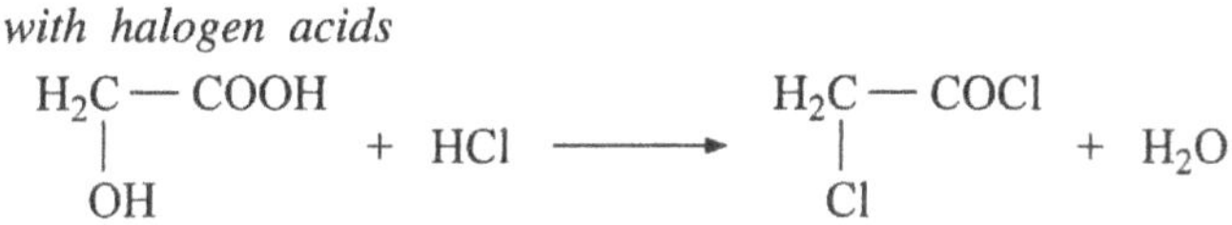

3. ***Special Reactions***

(i) α-Hydroxy acids form cyclic esters on heating due to the reaction of hydroxyl and carboxyl groups.

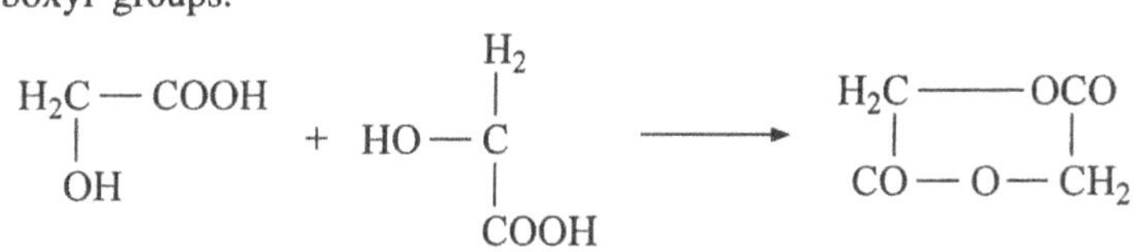

(ii) β-Hydroxy acids yield α,β-unsaturated acids on heating by dehydration

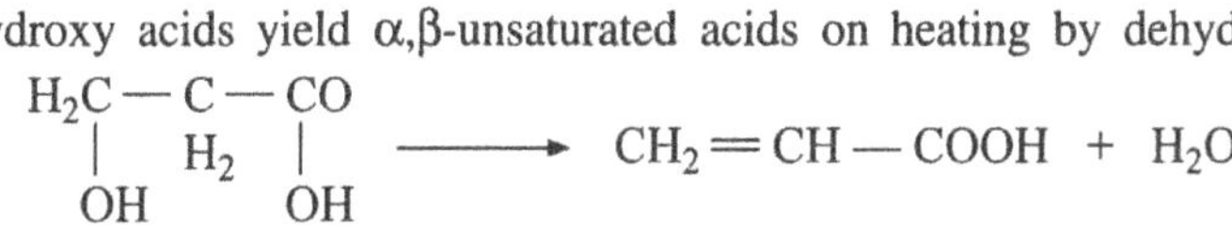

(iii) γ-Hydroxy acids form lactones on heating.

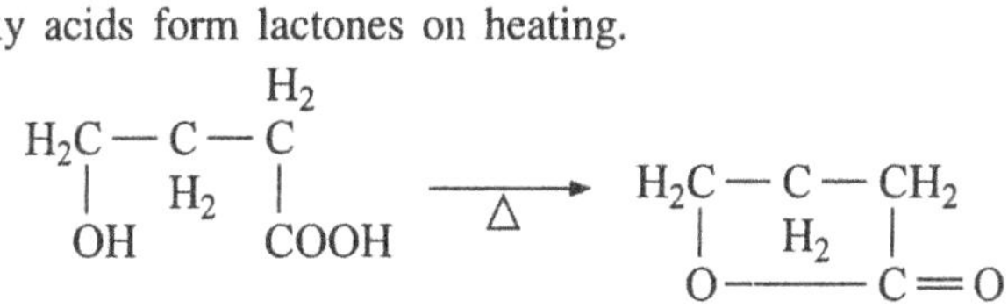

20.10 PHARMACEUTICAL COMPOUNDS

20.10.1 Formic Acid

Preparation Formic acid is prepared industrially by heating NaOH with carbon monoxide at 150ºC under 8 atmospheric pressure. Then dilute H_2SO_4 is added to the slurry of sodium formate and the mixture is distilled to get formic acid.

$$NaOH + CO \xrightarrow[\text{Pressure (8 atms)}]{150^\circ C} HCOO^- Na^+$$

$$HCOO^- Na^+ + H_2SO_4 \longrightarrow HCOOH + NaHSO_4$$

Properties

(i) Formic acid is the strongest of all other carboxylic acids of the homologous series (It is 13 times stronger than acetic acid).
(ii) It is corrosive and it exposed develops blisters on the skin.
(iii) Formic acid exists as dimer in aqueous solution.
(iv) Formic acid is unique among simple carboxylic acids because it contains an H atom instead of alkyl group. Thus, formic acid has the structure of both carboxylic acid and aldehyde. Hence, formic acid undergoes carboxylic acid reactions (like salt formation with bases, reaction with PCl_5, formation of esters) and aldehyde type reactions (reduction of Fehling's reagent, Tollens reagent).

Uses

1. Formic acid is used as an antiseptic and as a food preservative.
2. It is used to treat gout.
3. Formic acid is used as a growth stimulant of yeast.
4. Formic acid is also used in textile industries, plastic industries and in hydrogenation of oils.

20.10.2 Acetic Acid

Pure acetic acid was first isolated in 1700 AD by the distillation of vinegar. Acetic acid is the chemical compound responsible for the characteristic odour and sour taste of vinegar. Typically, vinegar is about 4 to 8% acetic acid. As the defining ingredient of vinegar, acetic acid has been produced and used by humans even before the dawn of recorded history. In fact, its name comes from the Latin for vinegar, *acetum*. Vinegar is formed from dilute solutions of alcohol, such as wine, by the action of certain bacteria in the presence of oxygen. These bacteria require oxygen, and the overall chemical change is the reaction of ethanol with oxygen to form acetic acid and water.

$$CH_3CH_2OH + O_2 \longrightarrow CH_3\overset{\overset{\displaystyle O}{\|}}{C}OH + H_2O$$

For many years, the bulk of commercial acetic acid was produced by the oxidation of ethanol. Today, most industrial production of acetic acid is by the Monsanto process, in which carbon monoxide reacts with methanol under the influence of a rhodium complex catalyst at 180°C and pressures of 30–40 atm.

$$CO + CH_3OH \xrightarrow{[Rh(CO)_2I_2]} CH_3\overset{\overset{\displaystyle O}{\|}}{C}OH$$

Properties

(i) Acetic acid is a clear, colourless liquid with a sharp, irritating odour of vinegar. The term glacial (ice-like) came to be applied to the pure acid in either its solid or liquid state.

(ii) Glacial acetic acid boils at 118°C, and has a density of 1.049 g/ml at 25°C.

(iii) It is flammable with a flash point of 39°C.

(iv) Through hydrogen-bonding interactions, acetic acid is miscible (mixable) in all proportions with water, ethyl alcohol, and diethyl ether.

(v) Pure or concentrated solutions of acetic acid are very corrosive and can cause painful burns.

(vi) Aqueous solutions of acetic acid freeze at temperatures below the freezing point of water.

(vii) Acetic acid is classified as a weak acid, because it does not completely dissociate into its component ions when dissolved in aqueous solution; at a concentration of 0.1 M, only about 1% of the molecules are ionised.

(viii) In solution, there is a dynamic equilibrium between the neutral molecules and the acetate and hydronium ions.

$$CH_3\overset{\overset{\displaystyle O}{\|}}{C}OH + H_2O \rightleftharpoons CH_3\overset{\overset{\displaystyle O}{\|}}{C}O^- + H_3O^+$$

(ix) The acid dissociation constant (K_a value) for acetic acid is 1.8×10^{-5} at 25°C.

Uses

1. Acetic acid is an important industrial chemical.
2. The primary use of acetic acid is in the manufacture of assorted acetate esters. These are substances formed by reacting acetic acid with a substance containing a hydroxyl (—OH) group. Cellulose, found in cotton and wood, is a polymeric material containing multiple hydroxyl groups. It reacts with acetic acid to yield cellulose acetate, which is used to make films and textiles. Some photographic films are made of cellulose acetate, and rayon is made from cellulose acetate fibres.
3. Vinyl acetate, another ester of acetic acid, polymerises to form poly(vinyl acetate), which is used in water-based latex paints and in glues for paper and wood.

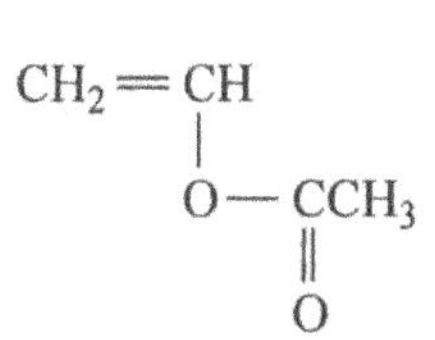

Vinyl acctate

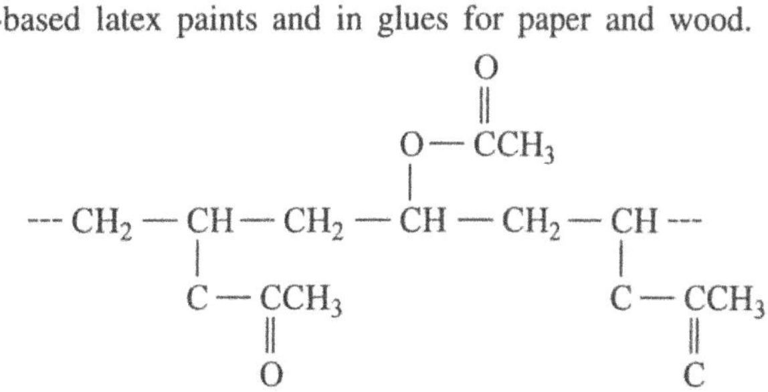

Pol y(vinyl acetate)

4. Acetic acid is also used as a fungicide and as a solvent for many organic compounds.
5. Acetic acid is also used in the preparation of pharmaceuticals. Aspirin (acetylsalicylic acid) is formed by the reaction between acetic acid and salicylic acid.

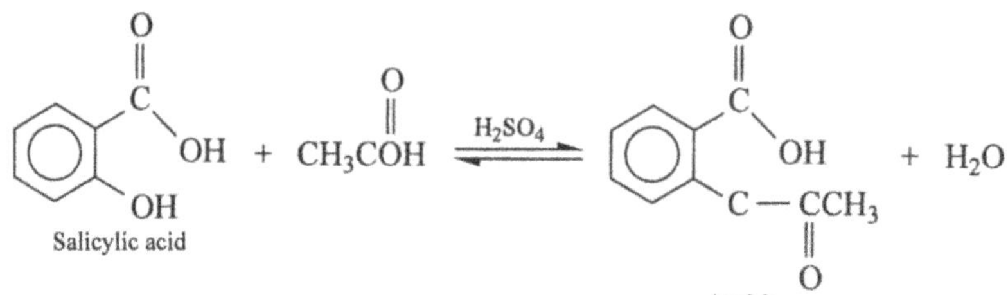

Salicylic acid

Aspirin

20.10.3 Propionic Acid

Preparation Propionic acid can be obtained from wood pulp waste liquor by bacterial fermentation process using bacteria *Propioni bacterium*. It can also be synthesised by oxidising *n*-propyl alcohol or propanal with an oxidising agent ($KMnO_4$ or $K_2Cr_2O_7$).

$$\underset{\text{Propanol}}{CH_3CH_2CH_2OH} \xrightarrow{[O]} \underset{\text{Propanal}}{CH_3CH_2CHO} \xrightarrow{[O]} \underset{\text{Propionic acid}}{CH_3CH_2CHO}$$

Properties Propionic acid is a water-soluble, colourless liquid having pungent odour. It boils at 122°C and is soluble in water, alcohol, ether and chloroform.

Use Propionic acid and its salts are used to treat fungal infection.

20.10.4 Ibuprofen

Ibuprofen is an arylacetic acid derivative. Chemically, ibuprofen is 2-4-(isobutylphenyl) propionic acid. It is available as colourless, crystalline powder and is insoluble in water.

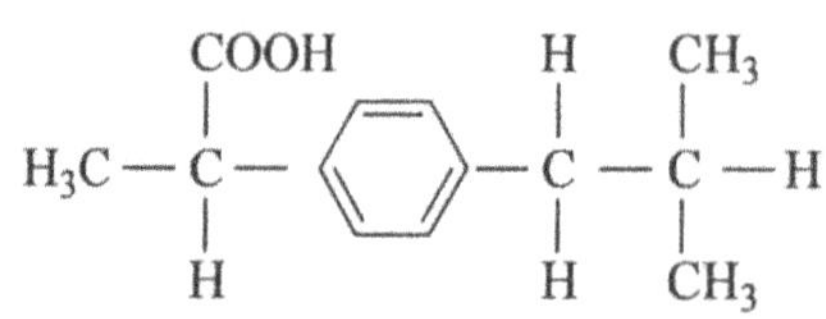

Ibuprofen is available as R and S isomers, but the activity resides in the S-(+)-isomer. There have been many commercial and laboratory methods available for the synthesis of Ibuprofen. Two of the most popular ways to obtain Ibuprofen are the Boot process and the Hoechst process. The Boot process is an older commercial process developed by the Boot Pure Drug Company, and the Hoechst process is a newer process developed by the Hoechst Company. Most of these routes to Ibuprofen begin with isobutylbenzene and use Friedel–Crafts acylation. The Boot process requires six steps, while the Hoechst process, with the assistance of catalysts, is completed in only three steps.

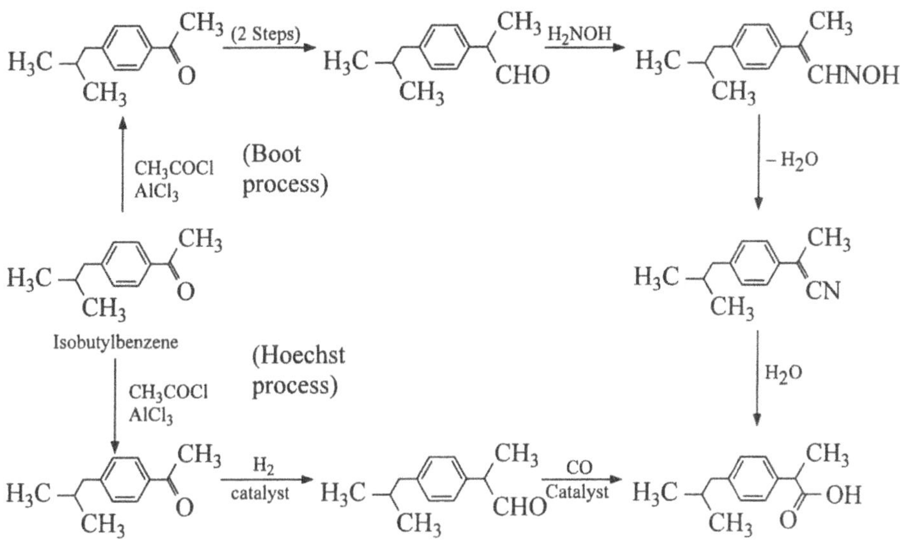

Uses

1. Ibuprofen is used for primary dysmenorrhea.
2. Ibuprofen is an important anti-inflammatory and analgesic drug. It is also used in the treatment of rheumatoid arthritis.

20.10.5 Acetylsalicylic Acid

Acetylsalicylic acid is an acetyl derivative of salicylic acid. It was introduced into medicine by dreser in 1899. Acetyl salicylic acid (aspirin) can be prepared by the reaction between salicylic acid and acetic anhydride.

In this reaction, the hydroxyl group on the benzene ring in salicylic acid reacts with acetic anhydride to form an ester functional group. Thus, the formation of acetyl salicylic acid is referred to as an esterification reaction. This reaction requires the presence of an acid catalyst.

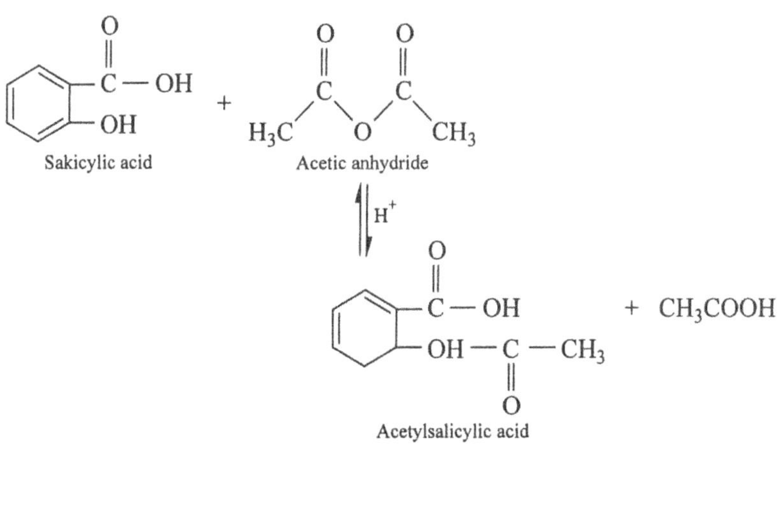

Properties

(i) Aspirin occurs as colourless crystals or crystalline powder.
(ii) It is slightly soluble in water and soluble in alcohol, chloroform, ether and glycerin.
(iii) Aspirin is stable in dry air but in presence of moisture, it hydrolyses slowly into salicylic acid and acetic acid.
(iv) Aspirin is acidic and produces effervescence with carbonates and bicarbonates.

Use Aspirin is used as an antipyretic, analgesic and antirheumatic.

20.10.6 Probenecid

Probenecid is a sulphonamide derivative. Probenecid is a colourless crystalline solid. It is insoluble in water.

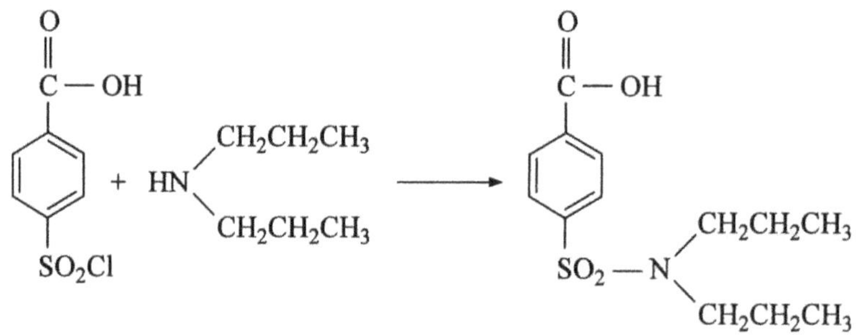

Probenecid is used to control gout.

20.10.7 Oleic Acid

Oleic acid is a long-chain monocarboxylic acid. Chemically, it is *cis*-octadec-9-enoic acid.

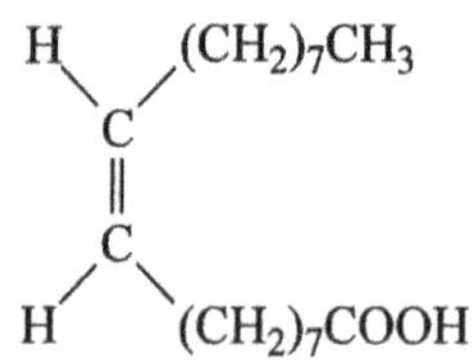

Oleic acid occurs as glyceryl esters in oils and fats (olive oil, cottonseed oil). It is prepared by alkaline hydrolysis of fat or oil followed by acidification. The oleic acid is separated from stearic acid and palmitic acid by cooling.

$$\begin{array}{l} CH_2OCOC_{15}H_{31} \\ | \\ CHOCOC_{17}H_{35} \\ | \\ CH_2OCOC_{17}H_{35} \end{array} + 3NaOH \longrightarrow \begin{array}{l} CH_2OH \\ | \\ CHOH \\ | \\ CH_2OH \end{array} + C_{17}H_{35}COONa + C_{17}H_{35}COONa + C_{15}H_{31}COONa$$

Oleic acid is available as colourless to pale yellow oil. It boils at 286°C. Oleic acid is immiscible in water but miscible in ether and alcohol and fixed oils.

Uses

1. Oleic acid is used to prepare various pharmaceutical preparations like benzylbenzoate lotion and green soap. In these preparations oleic acid reacts with alkalis to form sodium or potassium oleate which acts as an emulsifying agent.
2. Oleic acid is also used to prepare oleate salts of bases.

20.10.8 Oxalic Acid

Oxalic acid is one of the most important dicarboxylic acids. Chemically, oxalic acid is ethanedioic acid. It occurs in rhubarb, sorrel and other plants of oxalis group as potassium hydrogen oxalate and calcium oxalate. Oxalic acid is prepared from sodium formate, which is prepared by passing carbon monoxide into sodium hydroxide. Sodium formate on heating at 360°C forms sodium oxalate, which on treatment with calcium hydroxide solution forms calcium oxalate. Calcium oxalate on acidification with dilute sulphuric acid produces oxalic acid.

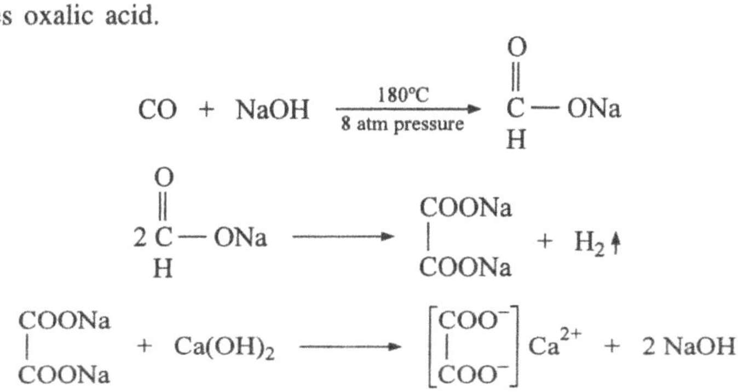

Oxalic acid is available as colourless, crystalline solid. It melts at 102°C. Oxalic acid is soluble in water, alcohol but insoluble in ether. It has an acidic taste.

Uses

1. Oxalic acid is used for the manufacture of inks, dyes and bleaching straw.
2. Antimony oxalates prepared from oxalic acid is used as mordant in printing and dyeing.
3. It is used as a primary standard in quantitative analysis.

20.10.9 Lactic Acid

Chemically, lactic acid is 2-hydroxy propionic acid. Lactic acid exhibit optical isomerism. It has been prepared from propionic acid by halogenation (Hell–Velhard–Zelinsky reaction) and hydrolysing the α-halo propionic acid with dilute alkali to form sodium lactate.

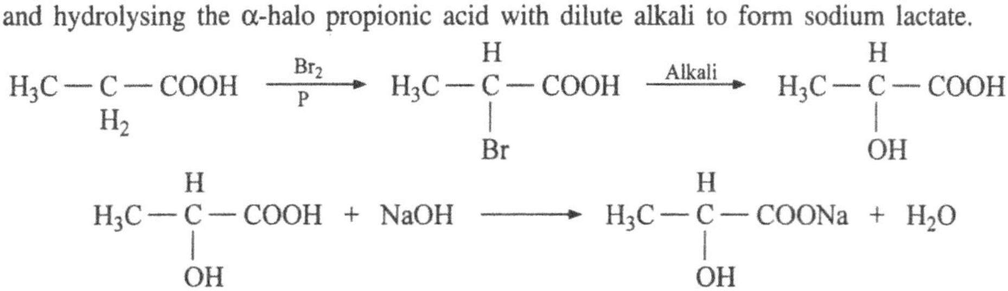

Uses

1. Lactic acid is used in dying and tanning industries.
2. Derivatives of lactic acids are used as medicinal agents (calcium and iron) and as pharmaceutical excipient (ethyllactate).
3. Lactic acid is used to prepare sodium lactate injection.

20.10.10 Citric Acid

Citric acid is 2-hydroxy-1,2,3-propanetricarboxylic acid. It is an example of substituted tricarboxylic acid.

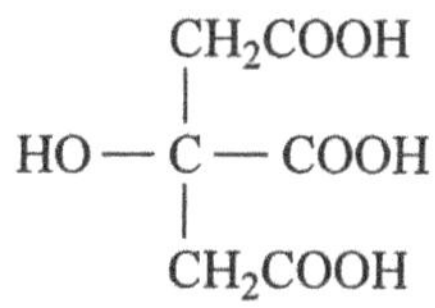

Citric acid

Citric acid is found in many fruits (orange, lemon, tomato, etc.) especially in citrus family. Citric acid is prepared largely by fermentation of sucrose solution with fungi (*Aspergillus niger*).

$$C_{12}H_{22}O_{11} + 3O_2 \rightarrow 2C_6H_8O_7 + 3H_2O$$

However, it may be prepared from glycerin by the following chemical reactions:

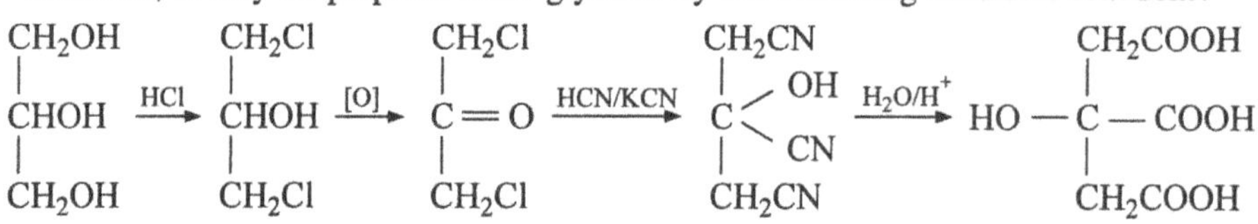

Citric acid

Citric acid is available as colourless crystals or crystalline powder. It melts at 130°C. It is freely soluble in water, alcohol, methanol and slightly soluble in ether.

Uses

1. Citric acid is used to prepare anticoagulant citrate dextrose solution, citric acid syrup and effervescent salts.
2. It is used to dissolve urinary bladder calculi and as an astringent.
3. Citric acid esters are used to prepare plasticisers for varnishes and lacquers.
4. It is used as a mordant in print and dyeing.
5. Citric acid salts like sodium citrate, potassium citrate, ferric citrate are used as medicines.

20.10.11 Tartaric Acid

Tartaric acid is a dicarboxylic acid. It is a dihydroxy succinic acid. Tartaric acid is an important plant acid and occurs in the juice of many fruits and tamarinds either in free state or as potassium salt.

The acid was first isolated in 1769 by the Swedish chemist Carl Wilhelm Scheele, who boiled tartar with chalk and decomposed the product with sulphuric acid. Tartaric acid has been synthesised from succinic acid by bromination and followed by hydrolysis with silver oxide and water.

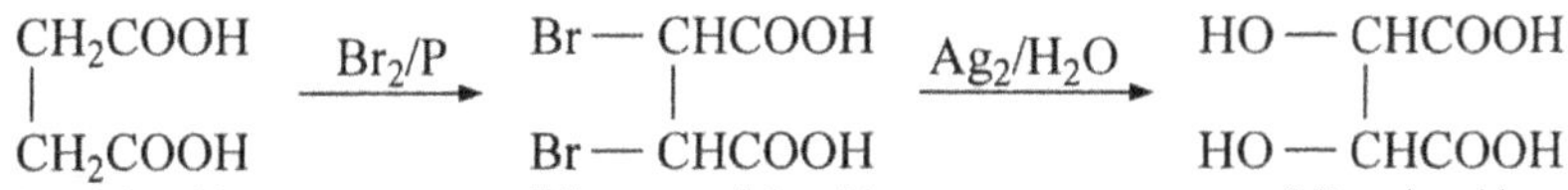

Succinic acid — Dibromosuccinic acid — *dl*-Tartaric acid

Tartaric acid is available as large, colourless crystals or crystalline powder. It is odourless and has an acidic taste. It is freely soluble in water, alcohol and insoluble in ether. Tartaric acid possesses two identical asymmetric carbon atoms. Hence, it exists in four stereoisomeric forms. The various stereoisomeric forms are dextro, laevo, meso and racemic. The naturally occurring tartaric acid is dextrorotatory.

Uses

1. Tartaric acid is an important ingredient of effervescent salts.
2. It is used as a buffering agent.
3. Tartaric acid is used in printing and dyeing.
4. Sodium potassium tartarate is used to prepare Fehling's solution B.
5. Some tartaric acid derivatives (e.g. potassium antimony tartarate) are used in medicine.

20.10.12 Salicylic Acid

Salicylic acid is ortho hydroxy benzoic acid. It is prepared from methyl salicylate (oil of wintergreen) by hydrolysis with an aqueous base followed by acidification. The overall organic products of the reaction are salicylic acid and methanol. The salicylic acid is a solid, which can be isolated and purified by crystallisation.

Properties Salicylic acid occurs as colourless needle-like crystals or as a fluffy, crystalline powder. It is slightly soluble in water but freely soluble in organic solvents. It has strong acidic character (pK_a: 2.5). The strong acidic properties and minimum solubility of salicylic acid in water is due to intermolecular hydrogen bonding.

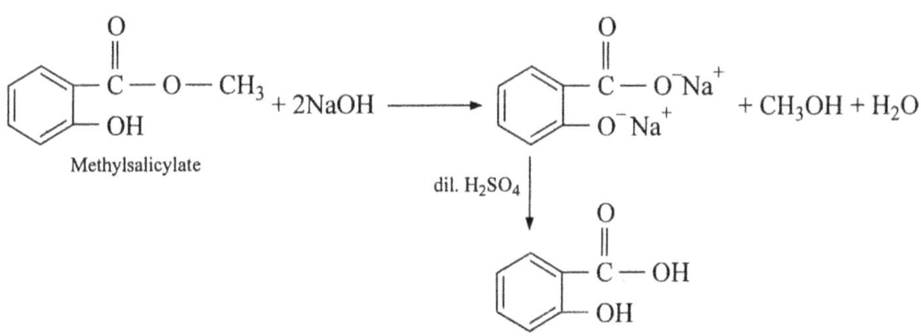

Uses

1. Salicylic acid has antiseptic and keratolytic properties. It is used externally in the form of ointments and solutions.
2. It is used for the treatment of athlete's foot and corns.

20.10.13 Carbidopa

Levodopa is required by the brain to produce dopamine, an important neurotransmitter. People with Parkinson's disease have depleted levels of dopamine, leading to debilitating symptoms. Levodopa is given to increase production of dopamine, which in turn reduces the symptoms of Parkinson's disease. When taken by mouth, the body breaks down most levodopa before it reaches the brain. Therefore, levodopa is combined with carbidopa, a drug that prevents the breakdown, allowing levodopa to reach the brain to increase dopamine levels. Carbidopa is available as colourless or yellowish white powder. It is insoluble in water and decomposes on exposure to daylight.

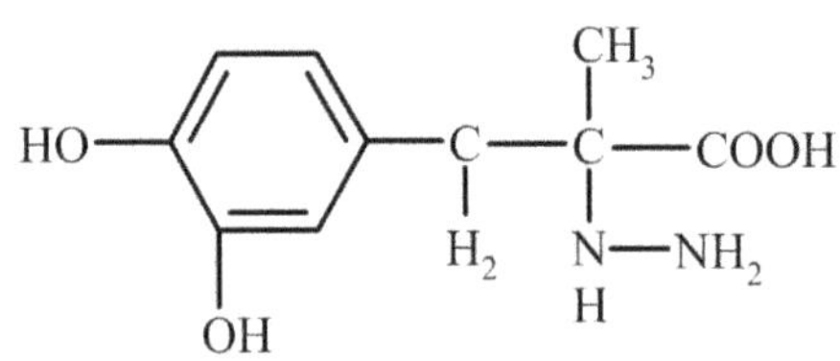

Uses

1. Carbidopa is administered in combination with levodopa in the treatment of Parkinson's disease.
2. Carbidopa inhibits decarboxylation of peripheral levodopa in extra-cerebral tissues.

20.10.14 Succinic Acid

Succinic acid is a dicarboxylic acid with molecular formula $C_4H_6O_4$. It is also called as butanedioic acid which is water soluble, colorless crystal with an acid taste. Succinic acid is synthesized by hydrogenation of maleic acid, maleic anhydride, or fumaric acid

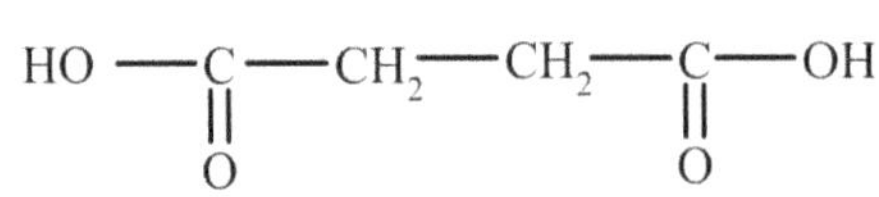

Uses

1. Succinic acid is a precursor to some polyesters, organic solvent like tetrahydrafuran and also a precursor to polybutylene terephthalate.
2. Succinic acid is used primarily as an acidity regulator in the food and beverage industry.
3. It is used as a flavoring agent and also dietary supplement.

20.10.15 Benzoic Acid

Benzoic acid is a simple aromatic carboxylic acid. It occurs naturally in many plants. It is also called as dracylic acid. Benzoic acid is a colorless crystalline solid, pleasant odor with melting point of 122.41 °C.

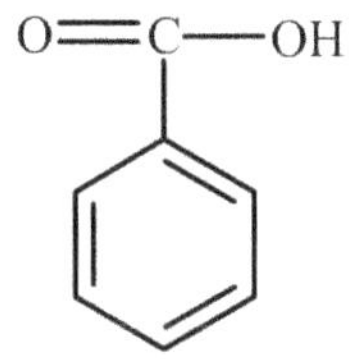

Uses

1. Benzoic acid is a fungistatic compound that is widely used as a food preservative.
2. It is used as precursor for many plasticizers such as the glycol esters, diethyleneglycol esters, and triethyleneglycol esters.
3. Benzoic acid was used as an expectorant, analgesic and antiseptic.

PRACTICE QUESTIONS

1. Describe the general methods for the preparation of carboxylic acids. Explain why carboxylic acids are more acidic than alcohols. Write a note on the preparation and properties of hydroxy monocarboxylic acids.
2. (a) How do you say carboxylic acids are more acidic than alcohols?

   (b) Suggest suitable methods to prepare the following:

   (i) Chloroaceticacid from acetic acid

   (ii) Lactic acid from acetaldehyde

   (c) Chloroacetic acid is more acidic than acetic acid. Explain.
3. (a) How will you distinguish the following pairs of compounds in the laboratory:

   (i) Acetic acid and formic acid

   (ii) Benzoic acid from salicylic acid

   (b) How do you convert:

   (i) Acetic acid into methyl cyanide

   (ii) Propionic acid from acetic acid
4. Write the reactions of carboxylic acids.
5. Formic acid differs chemically from acetic acid because it contains a hydrogen group but not an alkyl group. Give example to justify this statement.

6. Name the reagents and explain the chemistry involved in the following conversions.
   (a) Phenol to salicylic acid
   (b) Acetic acid to propionic acid
   (c) Acetylene to lactic acid
7. (a) Explain the acidity of carboxylic acid group.
   (b) Explain the effect of substituents on the acidity of carboxylic acids.
   (c) Give the names and structures of various carboxylic acid derivatives.
8. Write preparation and uses of the following:
   (a) Formic acid
   (b) Ibuprofen
   (c) Citric acid
   (d) Tartaric acid
   (e) Lactic acid
   (f) Probenecid
   (g) Oleic acid

21

CHEMISTRY OF CARBOXYLIC ACID DERIVATIVES

The derivatives of carboxylic acids are compounds in which the —OH of a carboxyl group has been replaced by —Cl (acid chlorides), —OOCR (acid anhydrides), —NH_2 (amides) and —OR (esters). These functional derivatives contain acyl group and are closely related to carboxylic acids and to each other.

21.1 ACID CHLORIDES

21.1.1 Preparation

Acid chlorides are prepared by the reaction of carboxylic acids with thionyl chloride, phosphorous pentachloride or phosphorous trichloride. Thionyl chloride is particularly convenient, since the products formed besides the acid chlorides are gases and thus easily separated from the acid chloride.

$$\underset{\text{Carboxylic acid}}{RCOOH} + \underset{\text{Thionyl chloride}}{SO_2Cl} \longrightarrow \underset{\text{Acid chloride}}{RCOCl} + \underset{\text{Sulphur dioxide}}{SO_2} + \underset{\text{Hydrogen chloride}}{HCl}$$

Mechanism This reaction takes place through formation of intermediate tetravalent sulphur by attacking sulphur of thionyl chloride at carbonyl oxygen and involves following steps:

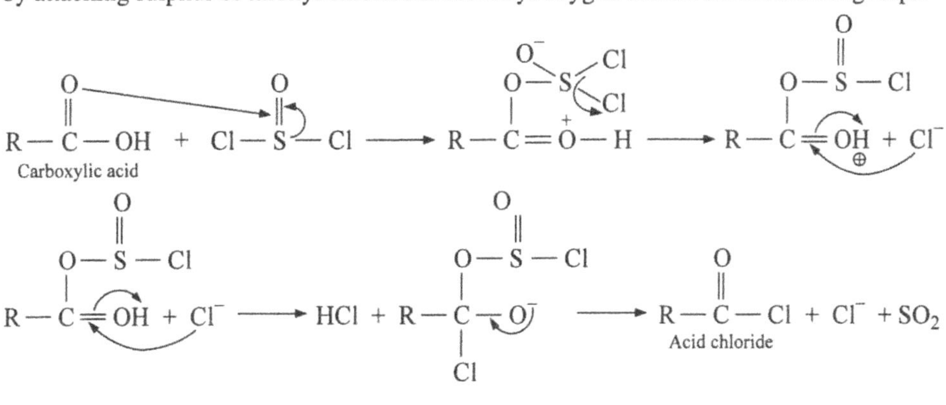

21.1.2 Physical Properties

1. Acid chlorides are colourless liquids or low melting solids.
2. They are soluble in organic solvents (ether, alcohol).

3. They have lower boiling points than their parent acids as acid chlorides do not contain acidic hydrogen and they do not form hydrogen bond.
4. They have an irritating odour.

21.1.3 Chemical Reactions

Acid chlorides undergo nucleophilic substitution. Nucleophile easily attacks at acyl carbon because of electron withdrawal effect of both chlorine and oxygen. The nucleophilic acyl substitution of acid chloride involves two steps:

(a) *Addition of nucleophile at acyl carbon*

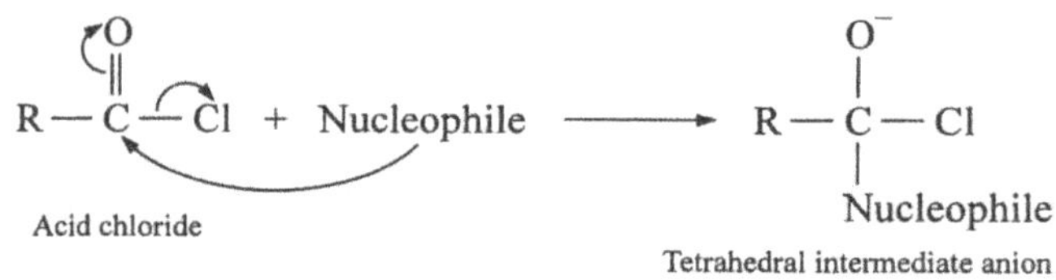

(b) *Elimination of chlorine as a nucleophile*

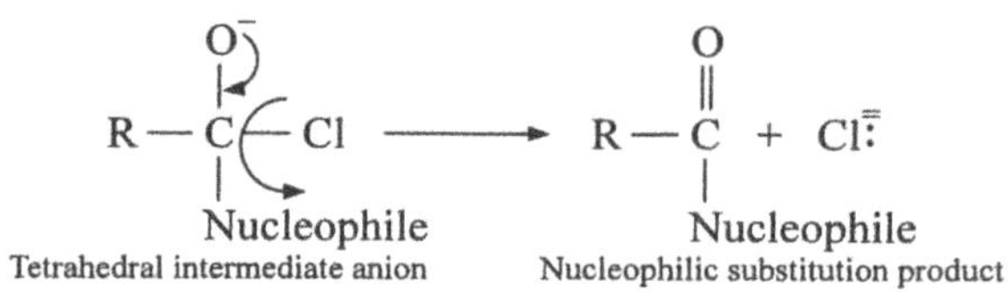

Of all carboxylic acid derivatives, acid chlorides are highly reactive towards nucleophilic substitution due to the presence of weakly basic leaving group. The following are important reactions of acid chlorides:

1. ***Hydrolysis of Acid Chlorides (Conversion into Acids)*** Acid chlorides are highly reactive and do not require catalysts for hydrolysis. The hydrolysis reaction is often an unwanted side reaction and requires anhydrous solvents and exclusion of water from a reaction.

Acid chloride + H_2O ⟶ Acid + HCl

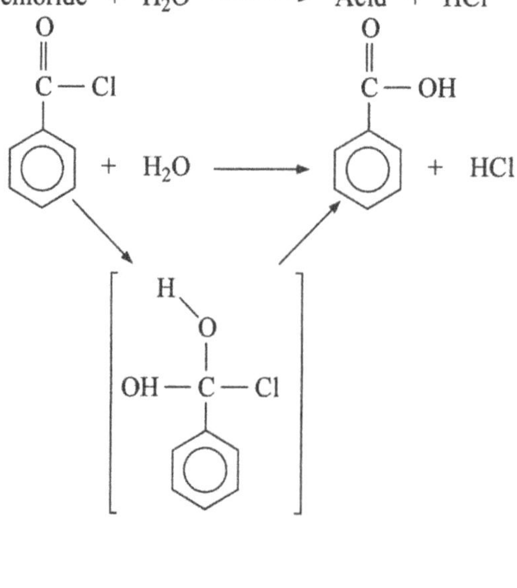

$$\underset{\text{Acetyl chloride}}{CH_3COCl} + H_2O \longrightarrow \underset{\text{Acetic acid}}{CH_3COOH} + HCl$$

2. ***Alcoholysis (Conversion into Esters)*** Primary and secondary alcohols and phenols readily react with acid chlorides to yield esters. The reaction, known as alcoholysis, constitutes a very good method for preparing esters.

$$\underset{\text{Acid chloride}}{RCOCl} + R'OH \longrightarrow \underset{\text{Ester}}{RCOOR'} + HCl$$

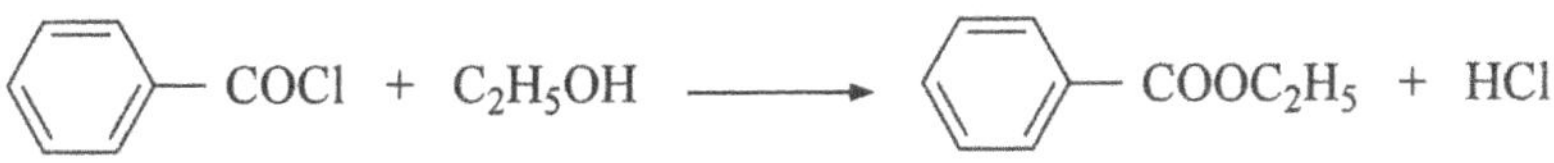

Benzoyl chloride Ethyl benzoate

3. ***Ammonolysis (Conversion into Amides)*** Acid chlorides react with ammonia and primary and secondary amines to yield amides.

$$\underset{\text{Acetyl chloride}}{CH_3COCl} + 2HN_3 \longrightarrow \underset{\text{Acetamide}}{CH_3CONH_2} + NH_4Cl$$

4. ***Reaction with Carboxylic Acids (Conversion into Anhydrides)*** Acid chloride reacts with carboxylic acids in the presence of pyridine to yield anhydrides.

$$\underset{\text{Acetyl chloride}}{CH_3COCl} + \underset{\text{Acetic acid}}{CH_3COOH} \longrightarrow \underset{\text{Acetic anhydride}}{CH_3COOCOCH_3} + HCl$$

5. ***Reduction*** When reduced with $LiAlH_4$ acid chlorides are conveniently changed into primary alcohols.

$$\underset{\text{Acid chloride}}{RCOCl} \xrightarrow{LiAlH_4,\ H^+} \underset{\text{Alcohol}}{RCH_2OH}$$

6. ***Rosenmunds Reduction*** Acid chlorides with hydrogen in the presence of partially poisoned palladium catalyst undergo partial reduction to form aldehydes.

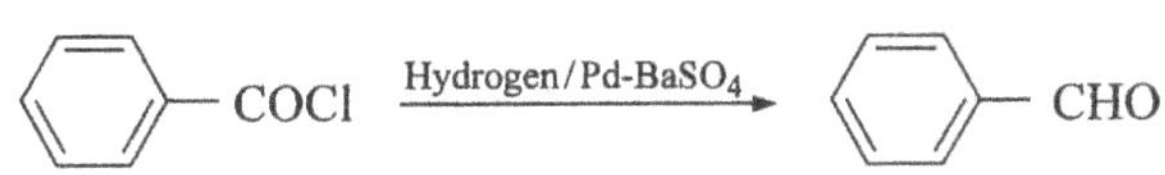

Benzoyl chloride Benzaldehyde

7. ***Friedel–Crafts Acylation*** Acid chlorides react with aromatic compounds in the presence of lewis acids, such as anhydrous aluminium chloride, to form aromatic ketones.

$$\underset{\text{Acid chloride}}{RCOCl} + ArH \xrightarrow{\text{Anhyd. } AlCl_3} \underset{\text{Ketone}}{ArCOR} + HCl$$

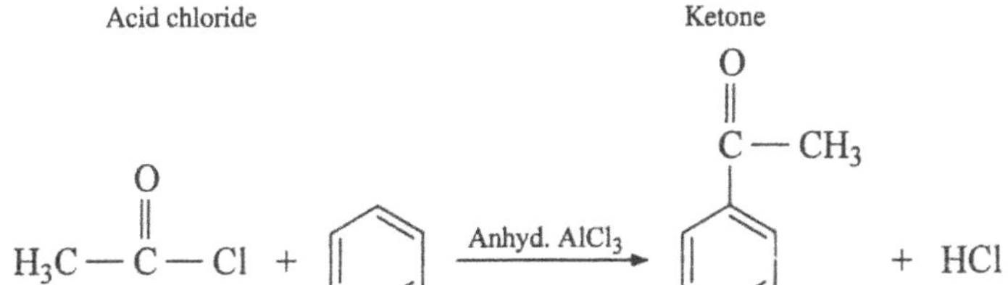

Acetyl chloride Benzene Acetophenone

8. ***Aromatic Substitution*** Aromatic acid chlorides can also undergo the usual electrophilic substitution reaction of the benzene ring. However, —COCl group has a deactivating influence on benzene ring and directs the entering group to meta-position.

21.2 ACID ANHYDRIDES

Acid anhydrides are named by changing the name of the parent acid from -oic acid to -ic anhydride.

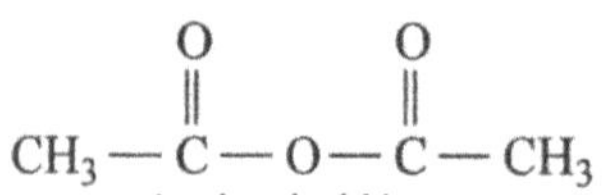

Acetic anhydride

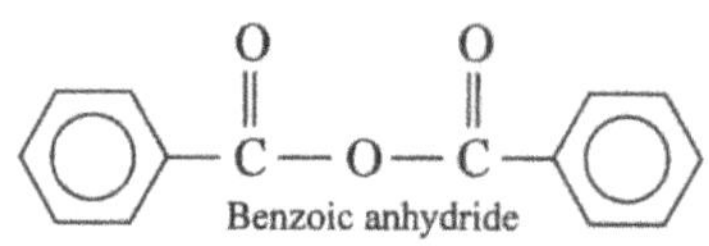

Benzoic anhydride

21.2.1 Preparation

By the Reaction between Acid Chlorides and Carboxylic Acids Acid anhydrides are obtained by the reaction of acid chlorides with carboxylic acids in the presence of pyridine.

$$\underset{\text{Acetyl chloride}}{CH_3COCl} + \underset{\text{Acetic acid}}{CH_3COOH} \longrightarrow \underset{\text{Acetic anhydride}}{CH_3COOCOCH_3} + HCl$$

21.2.2 Physical Properties

1. Acid anhydrides are colourless, sharp smelling liquids while aromatic anhydrides are colourless solids.
2. The boiling points of acid anhydrides are higher than those of the acids formed by their hydrolysis. Acid anhydrides do not form intermolecular hydrogen bonds. The size of anhydride molecules is much larger in comparison to the acid molecules. This leads to larger van der Walls forces of attraction, which is responsible for higher boiling points.

21.2.3 Chemical Properties

Acid anhydrides undergo nucleophilic substitution reactions typical of acid derivatives. The important reactions of acid anhydrides are described below.

1. ***Hydrolysis (Conversion into Acids)*** Acid anhydrides are hydrolysed by water to form carboxylic acids. Acids or bases can accelerate this reaction.

$$\underset{\text{Acetic anhydride}}{CH_3COOCOCH_3} + H_2O \longrightarrow \underset{\text{Acetic acid}}{2CH_3COOH}$$

2. ***Alcoholysis*** Acid anhydrides form esters on reacting with alcohols.

$$\underset{\text{Acetic anhydride}}{CH_3COOCOCH_3} + C_2H_5OH \longrightarrow \underset{\text{Ethyl acetate}}{CH_3COOC_2H_5} + \underset{\text{Acetic acid}}{CH_3COOH}$$

21.2.4 Acetic Anhydride

Acetic anhydride is a clear, colourless, mobile (free-flowing) liquid with a sharp odour similar to that of acetic acid. It hydrolyses in water to yield acetic acid. In its liquid or vapour state, acetic anhydride can irritate body tissues, possibly leading to the death of such tissue. Acetic anhydride melts at – 73°C, boils at 139°C and has a density of 1.080 g/ml at 15°C. It is inflammable with a flash point of 54°C. This compound is readily combustible and represents a fire hazard.

Acetic anhydride can by prepared by the dehydration of acetic acid at 800°C.

$$\underset{\text{Acetic acid}}{2CH_3\overset{\overset{O}{\|}}{C}OH} \longrightarrow \underset{\text{Acetic anhydride}}{CH_3\overset{\overset{O}{\|}}{C}-O-\overset{\overset{O}{\|}}{C}CH_3} + H_2O$$

Alternatively, the reaction between the acetyl chloride and a salt of acetic acid (e.g. sodium acetate) yields acetic anhydride and a salt.

$$\underset{\text{Acetyl chloride}}{CH_3\overset{\overset{O}{\|}}{C}Cl} + \underset{\text{Sodium acetate}}{NaO\overset{\overset{O}{\|}}{C}CH_3} \longrightarrow \underset{\text{Acetic anhydride}}{CH_3\overset{\overset{O}{\|}}{C}-O-\overset{\overset{O}{\|}}{C}CH_3} + NaCl$$

Acetic anhydride is primarily used in the manufacture of cellulose acetate for films and plastic goods. It is used in the synthesis of aspirin. Other uses include the manufacture of industrial chemicals, pharmaceuticals, perfumes, plastics, synthetic fibres, explosives, and weed killers. Acetic anhydride reacts with water hence it is sometimes used as a dehydrating agent in reaction mixtures where removal of water is necessary.

21.3 ACID AMIDES

21.3.1 Introduction

Acid amides are the derivatives of carboxylic acids. They are obtained from carboxylic acids by the replacement of —OH group of —COOH by amino (—NH_2) group. Acid amides have the general formula of $RCONH_2$. Amides are named by changing the name of the parent acid from -oic acid to -amide. If alkyl groups are attached to the nitrogen, the prefix N- is used to show attachment to the amine group. An N- is needed for each alkyl group.

$$\underset{\text{Propanamide}}{CH_3CH_2-\overset{\overset{O}{\|}}{C}-NH_2} \qquad \underset{N\text{-Ethylpropanamide}}{CH_3CH_2-\overset{\overset{O}{\|}}{C}-\underset{H}{N}-CH_2CH_3}$$

$$\underset{N,N'\text{-Diethyl propanamide}}{CH_3CH_2-\overset{\overset{O}{\|}}{C}-\overset{\overset{CH_3}{|}}{\overset{CH_2}{\overset{|}{N}}}-CH_2CH_3}$$

If the amide is attached to a ring, the suffix -carboxamide is used.

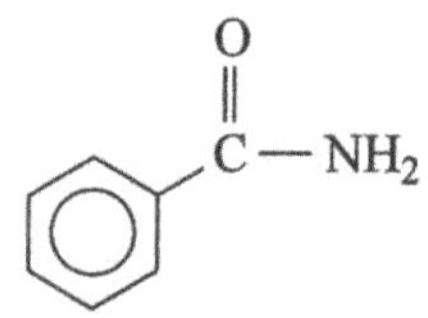

Amide	*Common Name*	*IUPAC Name*
$HCONH_2$	Formamide	Methanamide
CH_3CONH_2	Acetamide	Ethanamide
$C_6H_5CONH_2$	Benzamide	Benzamide

21.3.2 Preparation of Amides

Amides are frequently prepared by the following methods:

1. ***Preparation of Amides by Ammonolysis of Carboxylic Acids and its Derivatives*** Amides can be prepared from carboxylic acid and its derivatives (acid chlorides, acid anhydrides or esters) by nucleophilic acyl substitution reaction with ammonia or an amine (primary or secondary amine). This reaction is known as ammonolysis of acid derivatives.

$$\underset{\text{Acid chloride}}{RCOCl} + 2NH_3 \longrightarrow \underset{\text{Acid amide}}{RCONH_2} + NH_4Cl$$

$$\underset{\text{Benzoyl chloride}}{C_6H_5COC} + 2NH_3 \longrightarrow \underset{\text{Benzamide}}{C_6H_5\,CONH_2} + NH_4Cl$$

An example of this reaction can be found in the preparation of N,N-diethyl-*m*-toluamide, commonly known as DEET, an ingredient in many insect repellants.

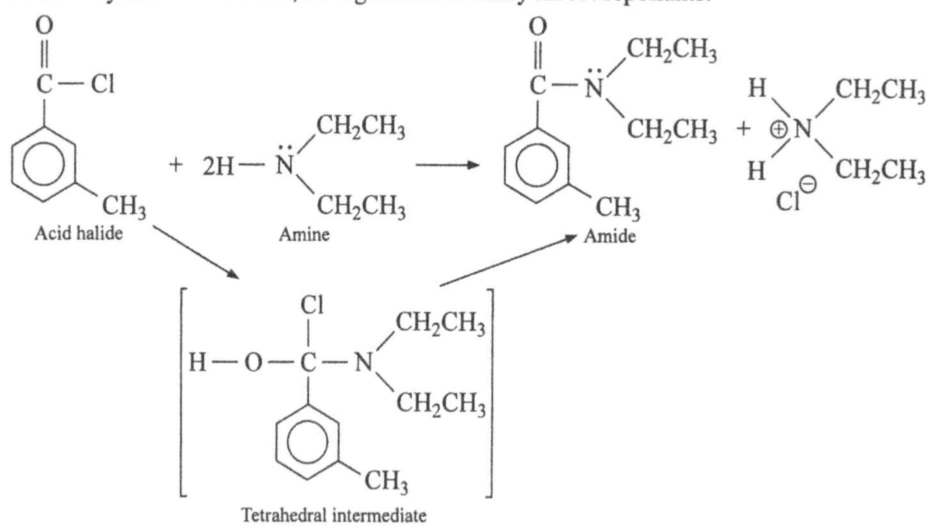

2. ***Preparation of Amides from Carboxylic Acid Anhydrides*** Acetic anhydride is commonly used to prepare acetamides. The acetic acid produced in the reaction undergoes an acid-base reaction with an amine to produce a salt. To complete the reaction, it is necessary to use two equivalents of amine. The product of this reaction, acetanilide, is an analgesic.

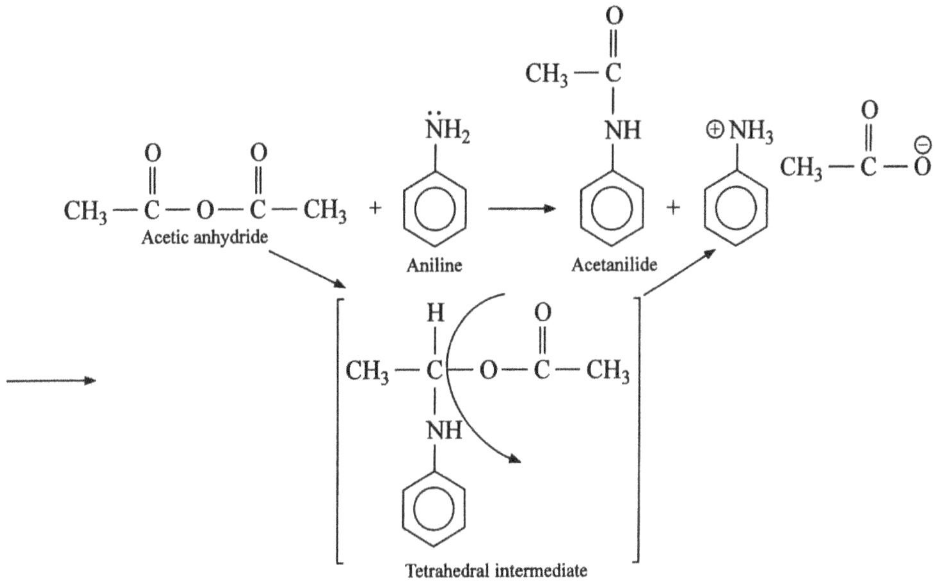

Mechanism The nucleophilic acyl substitution of acid chloride proceeds by initial nucleophilic attack at acyl carbon followed by an elimination of chloride anion.

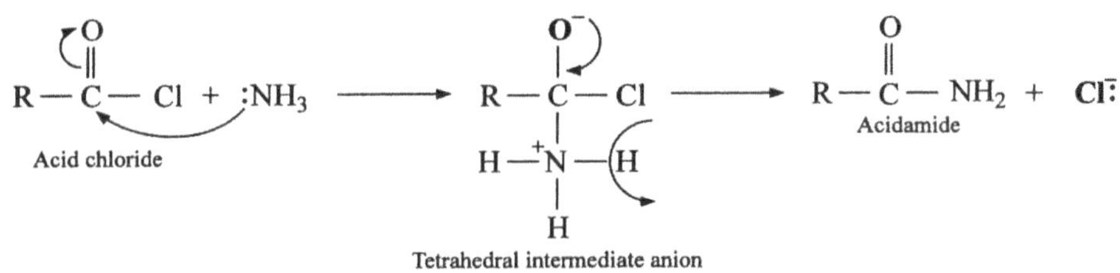

3. ***Preparation of Amides from Esters*** Amides can be prepared from esters by the exchange reaction with amines or ammonia. Esters are less reactive toward amines than either acid chlorides or anhydrides.

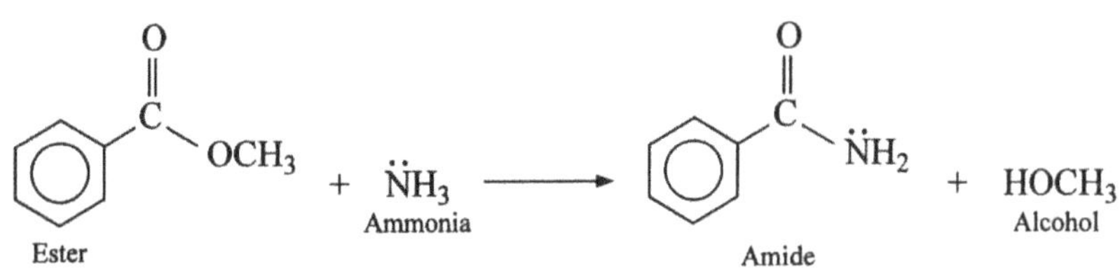

21.3.3 Physical Properties

1. All amides are colourless crystalline solids at room temperature (except formamide).
2. The lower members (up to about C_6) are soluble in water.
3. Amides have quite high boiling points (due to strong intermolecular hydrogen bonding).
4. Unlike amines, amides are not bases (proton acceptors).

21.3.4 Chemical Properties

1. ***Amides are Neutral*** Amides are practically neutral in character. These are expected to be basic in nature (like amines) due to the presence of a lone pair of electrons on nitrogen.

2. ***Hydrolysis of Amides*** Amides are the least reactive of the acid derivatives and hydrolysis requires acids or bases and vigorous reaction conditions. Acids activate the carbonyl group for nucleophilic addition of water. With amides, the acid does not act as a catalyst because the amine product of the reaction undergoes an acid-base reaction with the acid.

$$\underset{\text{Acid amide}}{RCONH_2} + NaOH \longrightarrow \underset{\text{Sodium carboxylate}}{RCOO^- Na^+} + NH_3$$

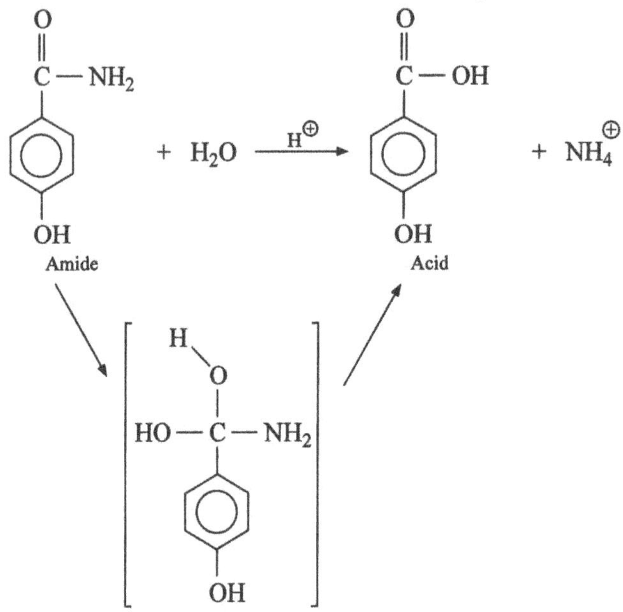

As with esters, the strong hydroxyl nucleophile attacks the carbonyl group and yields the carboxylate anion and the amine.

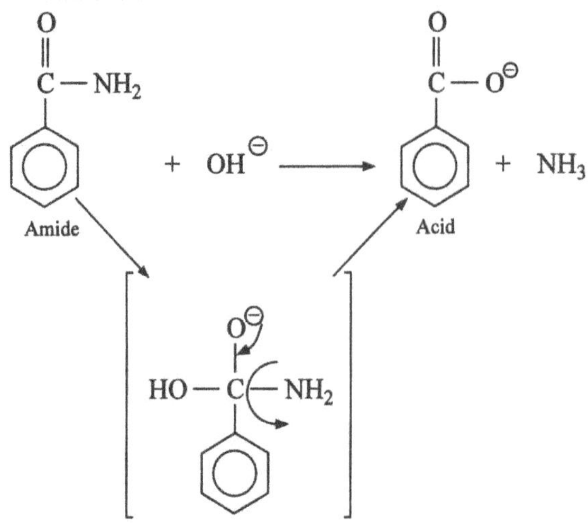

3. ***Dehydration*** Amides get dehydrated on heating with dehydrating agents (phosphorous pentoxide) to form nitriles.

$$\underset{\text{Acid amide}}{RCONH_2} + P_2O_5 \longrightarrow \underset{\text{Nitrile}}{RC{\equiv}N} + 2H_3PO_4$$

4. ***Hofmann Degradation of Amides*** Amides give amines containing one carbon less than starting amide, on treatment with bromine or chlorine in presence of alkaline solution.

$$R-\overset{\overset{\large O}{\|}}{C}-NH_2 + X_2 + 4NaOH \longrightarrow R-NH_2 + 2NaX + Na_2CO_3 + 2H_2O$$

$$(X_2 = Cl_2 \text{ or } Br_2)$$

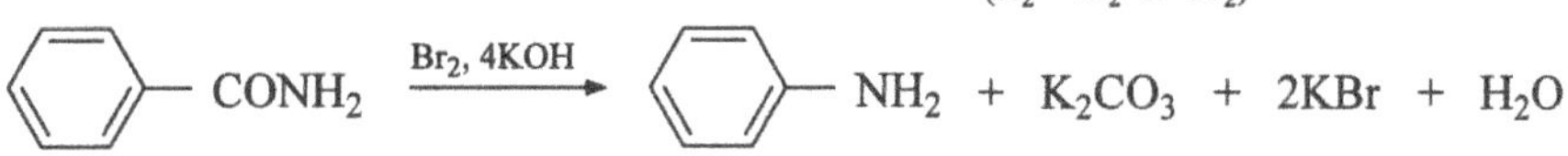

Benzamide Aniline

5. ***Reduction of Amides*** Amides are reduced to amines in presence of lithium aluminium hydride.

$$\underset{\text{Amide}}{RCONH_2} \xrightarrow{LiAlH_4} \underset{\text{Amine}}{RCH_2NH_2}$$

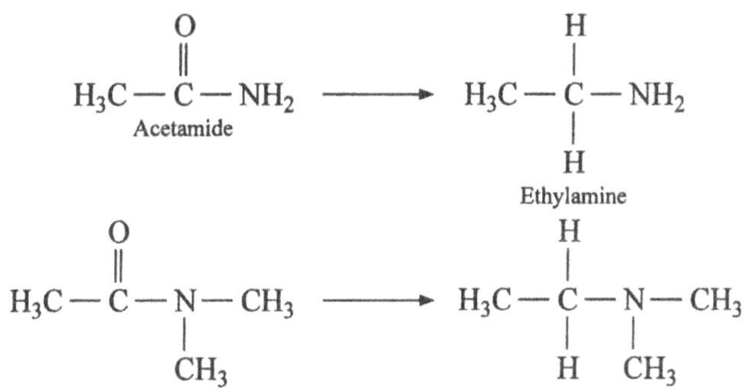

Acetamide Ethylamine

N,N-Dimethylacetamide N,N-Dimethylethylamine

21.4 ESTERS

21.4.1 Introduction

Esters are widely distributed in nature. The simplest esters have pleasant odours. In many cases, the characteristic flavours and fragrances of flowers and fruits are due to esters. Esters are the derivatives of carboxylic acids having the general formula RCOOR. They are obtained from carboxylic acids by the replacement of —OH group of — COOH by alkoxy group (— OR).

Ester	*Common Name*	*IUPAC Name*
$HCOOCH_3$	Methyl formate	Methyl methanoate
$CH_3COOC_2H_5$	Ethyl acetate	Ethyl ethanoate
$C_6H_5COOC_2H_5$	Ethyl benzoate	Ethyl benzoate

Esters are named by combining the name of the alkyl group attached to the oxygen atom with the name of the carboxylate group.

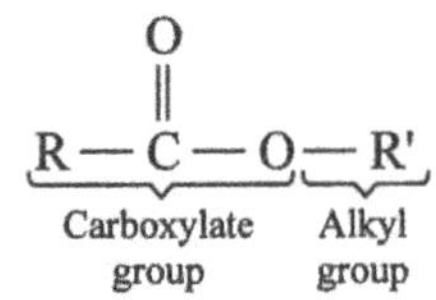

The carboxylate group is named by changing the *-ic* acid ending of the parent acid to *-ate*.

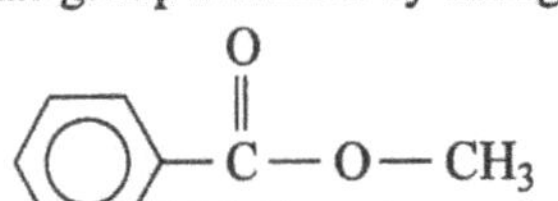

Methylbenzoate

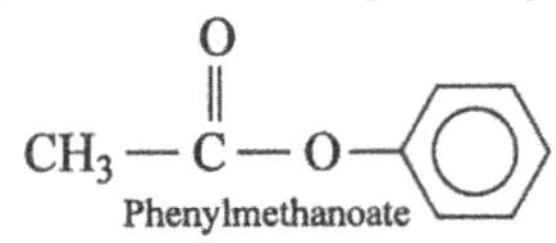

Phenylmethanoate

Esters are very important compounds. Low molecular weight esters often have pleasant 'fruity' odours and, in fact, are responsible for the odour of fruits. Table 21.1 gives several examples of esters and the typical flavours associated.

Table 21.1 Some Naturally Occurring Esters Useful as Flavours and Fragrances

Ester	*Structure*	*Odour*
3-Methyl-1-butyl acetate (isoamyl acetate)	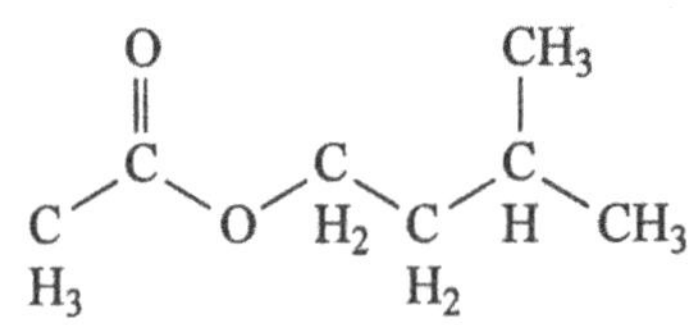	Banana
Ethyl butyrate	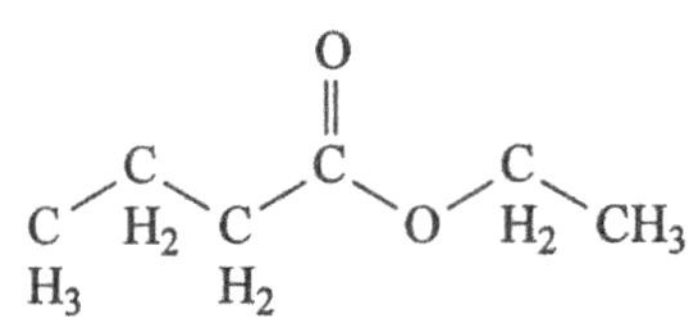	Pineapple
Methyl butyrate	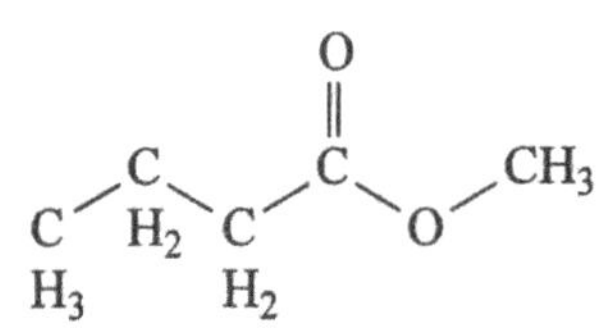	Apple
Methyl salicylate	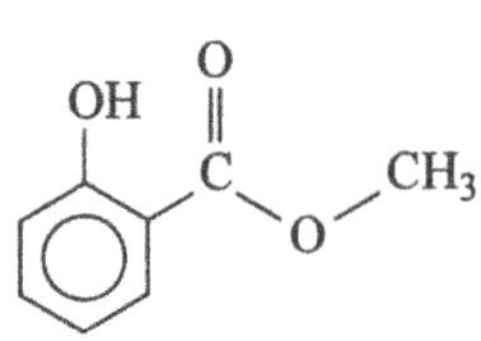	Wintergreen
Methyl anthranilate	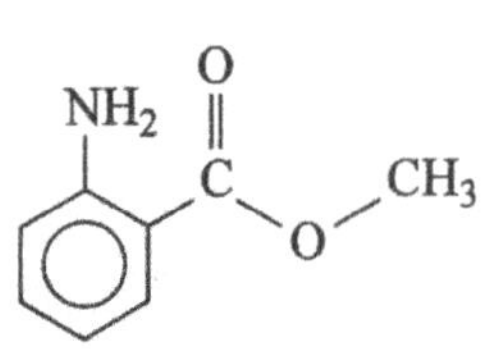	Grape

Esters of long-chain carboxylic acids (fatty acids) and long-chain alcohols are waxes. These compounds are produced by birds to serve as water repellants for their feathers. Other esters make orderly arrays and form the liquid crystals that we use as the displays in calculators and laptop computers.

21.4.2 Preparation

1. ***By the Reaction between a Carboxylic Acid and Alcohol*** Esters are generally prepared by direct esterification of carboxylic acids with alcohols in the presence of a strong mineral acid or a Lewis acid (such as BF_3). The reaction is reversible in nature and is known as Fisher's esterfication.

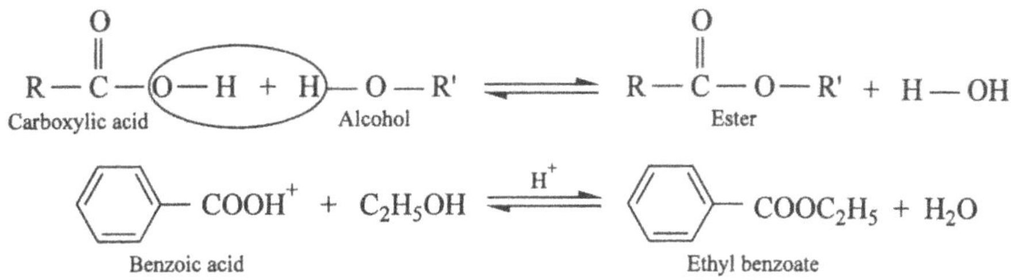

2. ***Reaction between an Acid Chloride or an Anhydride and an Alcohol*** Esters can also be prepared by the reaction of acid chloride with alcohol.

$$\underset{\text{Acid chloride}}{RCOCl} + \underset{\text{Ethyl alcohol}}{R'OH} \longrightarrow \underset{\text{Ester}}{RCOOR'}$$

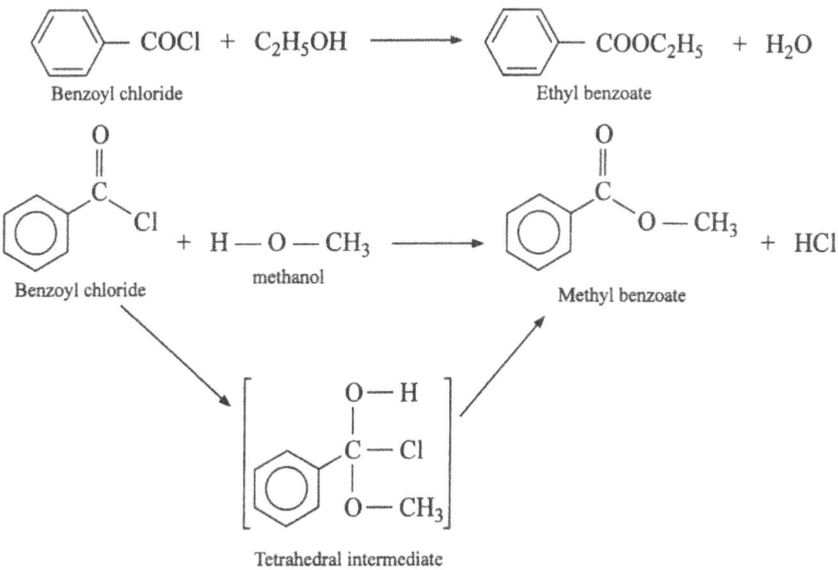

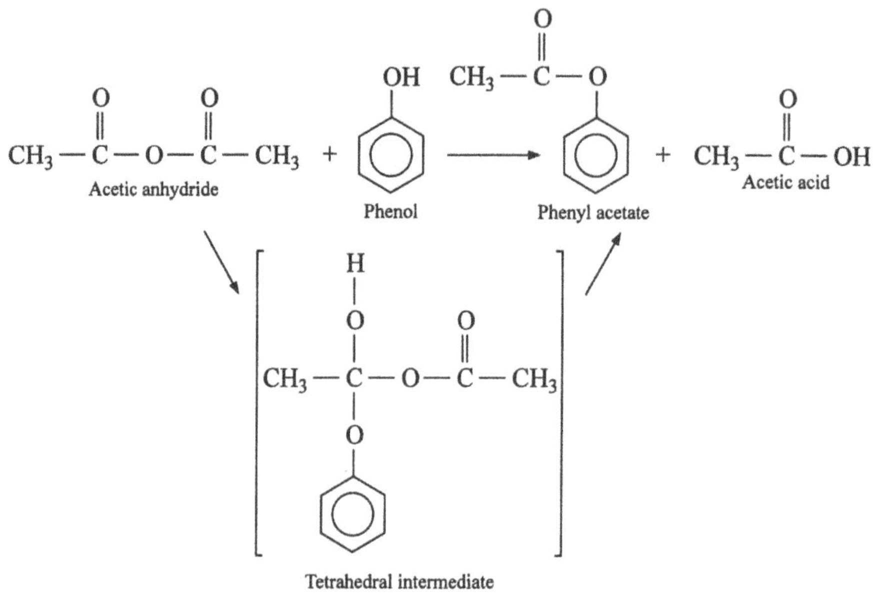

3. ***Trans-esterification Reaction*** This reaction is alcoholysis of an ester in presence of an acid or a base, when the alkoxy part of alcohol displaces the alkoxy part of ester. Thus, one ester may be obtained from another ester.

$$RCOOR' + R''OH \xrightleftharpoons{H^+ \text{ or } OR^{-''}} RCOOR'' + R'OH$$

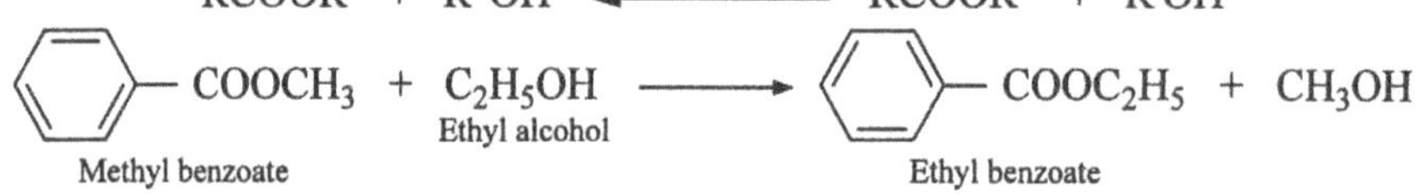

21.4.3 Physical Properties

1. Esters are colourless, pleasant-smelling liquids or solids. They are in general, insoluble in water but soluble in most organic solvents.
2. The boiling points of the methyl, ethyl and propyl esters are lower than those of the corresponding free acids. This is probably due to lack of hydrogen bond formation amongst esters.

21.4.4 Chemical Properties

Like other acid derivatives, esters undergo nucleophilic acyl substitution.

1. ***Hydrolysis*** Esters are hydrolysed very slowly in neutral medium. However, the hydrolysis takes place much more rapidly in acidic or alkaline solution. Acidic hydrolysis of esters yields a carboxylic acid and an alcohol whereas basic hydrolysis gives an alcohol and the salt of carboxylic acid.

$$RCOOR' + H_2O \xrightleftharpoons{H^+} RCOOH + R'OH$$

$$RCOOR' + H_2O \xrightleftharpoons{OH^-} RCOO^- + R'OH$$

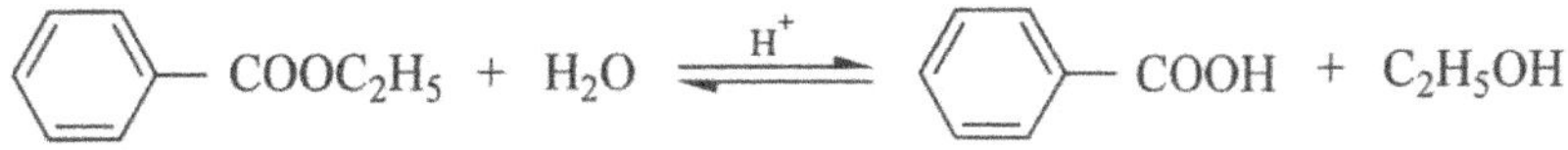

Ethyl benzoate Benzoic acid

(i) *Alkaline hydrolysis of esters* Alkaline hydrolysis of ester is a nucleophilic acyl substitution reaction in which nucleophile is a hydroxide anion. The mechanism of alkaline hydrolysis of esters involves the following steps:

(a) Addition of nucleophile at acyl carbon to form tetrahedral intermediate anion.

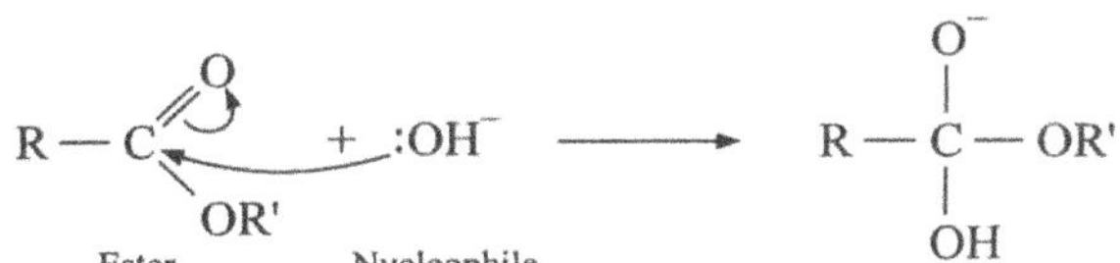

Ester Nucleophile Tetrahedral intermediate anion

(b) Tetrahedral intermediate anion eliminates alkoxide anion to form carboxylic acid.

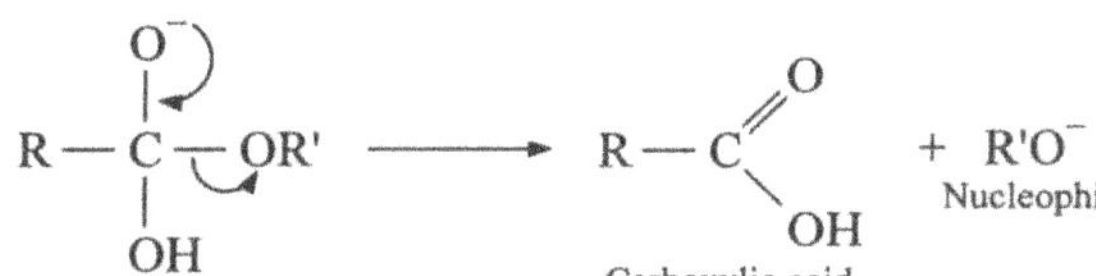

Tetrahedral intermediate anion Carboxylic acid Nucleophile

Free carboxylic acid reacts with a base to form a sodium salt of carboxylic acid (soap).

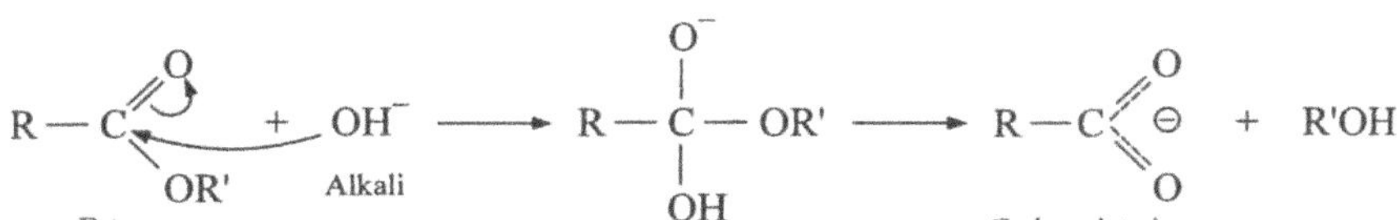

Ester Alkali Carboxylate ion

Kinetics Alkaline hydrolysis of ester involves nucleophilc attack on the ester by hydroxide ion. The rate of reaction should depend upon the concentration of both the ester and the hydroxide ion hence it follows second-order kinetics. This process is known as saponification.

$$\text{Rate of reaction} \propto \text{(ester) (nucleophile)}$$

(ii) *Acidic hydrolysis of esters* The mechanism of acidic hydrolysis is the same as that described for acid-catalysed Fischer esterification, because all the steps in acidic hydrolysis as well as esterification are reversible. This equilibrium process is driven to favour the acid and alcohol by using excess water, usually as the solvent.

The mechanism may be depicted as follows:

1. Protonation of the carboxylic group by H^+ of the acid catalyst.
2. This makes the carbonyl carbon more strongly electropositive that is attacked by the nucleophile, the alcohol molecule.
3. The transfer of proton to one of the —OH groups takes place.
4. The —OH group leaves as water molecule giving protonated ester.
5. The resonance-stabilised protonated ester losses a proton to form ester.

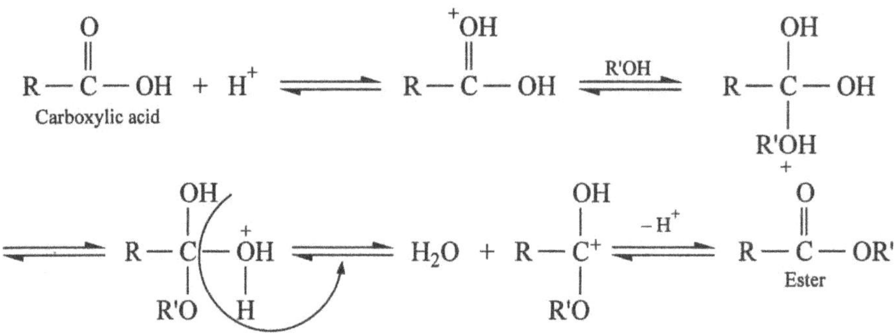

2. ***Ammonolysis (Conversion into Amides)*** Esters react slowly with ammonia to yield amides and alcohols.

$$\underset{\text{Ester}}{RCOOR'} + NH_3 \longrightarrow \underset{\text{Amide}}{RCONH_2} + R'OH$$

3. ***Reaction with Grignard Reagents*** Esters, other than those of formic acid, react with Grignard reagents to form tertiary alcohols.

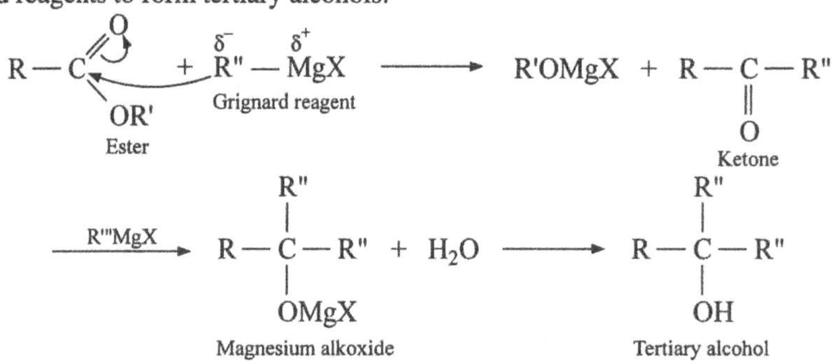

4. ***Reduction of Esters*** Esters can be reduced into alcohols by the catalytic hydrogenation or metallic hydrides or Bouveault-Blanc reducing agent (sodium and ethanol or *n*-butanol).

$$\underset{\text{Ester}}{RCOOC_2H_5} \xrightarrow{\text{Reducing agent}} \underset{\text{Alcohol}}{RCH_2OH + C_2H_5OH}$$

5. ***Reaction with Ammonia Derivatives*** Esters react with hydroxylamine and hydrazine to form hydroxamic acid and hydrazide respectively.

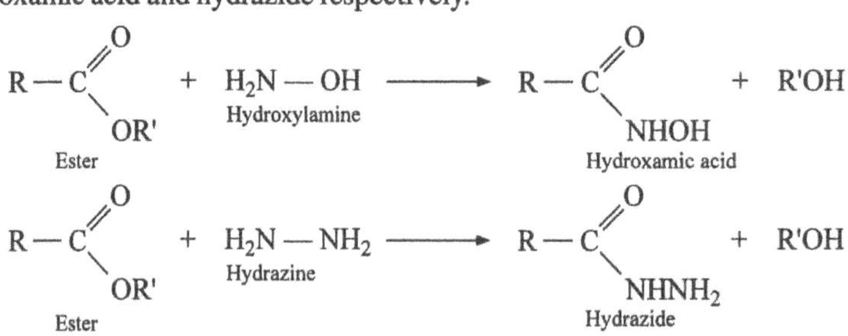

6. ***Claisen Condensation Reaction*** Ethyl acetate reacts with sodium ethoxide gives a condensation product (sodioacetoacetic ester) which on acidification gives a β-ketoester (ethyl acetoacetate or acetoacetic ester). These types of condensations are generally known as Claisen condensations.

$$\underset{\text{Ethylacetate}}{2CH_3COOC_2H_5} \xrightarrow{C_2H_5ONa} C_2H_5OH + \underset{\text{Sodioacetoacetic ester}}{CH_3CO\overset{-}{C}H\overset{Na^+}{C}OOC_2H_5} \xrightarrow{HCl} \underset{\text{Ethylacetoacetate}}{CH_3COCH_2COOC_2H_5}$$

Mechanism This reaction proceeds through carbanion mechanism.

(i) An ethoxide ion abstracts a proton from ester (ethylacetate) to form a carbanion.

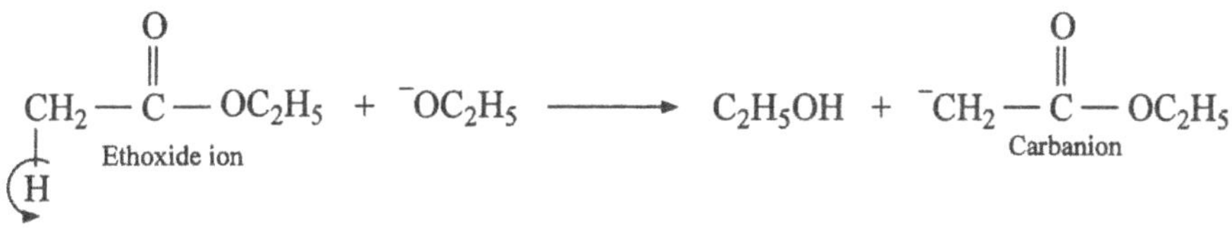

(ii) The carbanion formed in the first step attacks the electrophilic carbonyl carbon of second ester molecule to form substitution product.

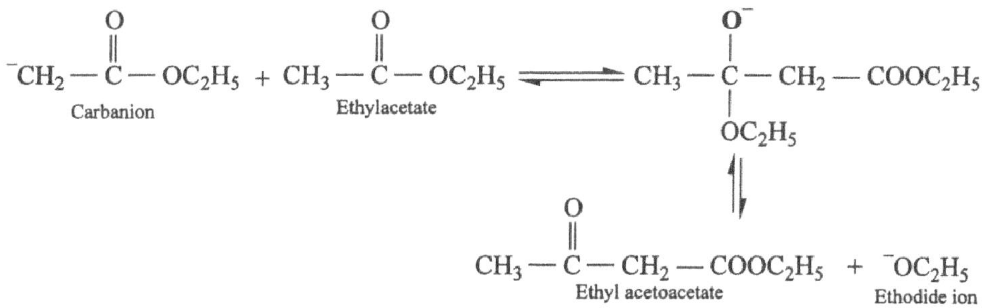

21.5 RELATIVE REACTIVITY OF ACID DERIVATIVES

The relative reactivity of acid derivatives is summarised in the chart given below.

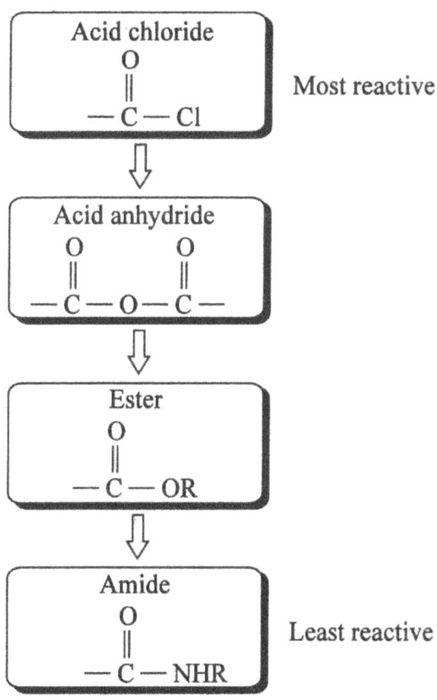

This order is important in planning organic syntheses. In general, an acid derivative can be prepared from another derivative that is more reactive. Esters can be prepared by reacting alcohols with acid chlorides or anhydrides. Amides are the least reactive and can be prepared from any other acid derivative.

21.6 ACETOACETIC ESTER

Acetoacetic ester is the ethyl ester of acetoacetic acid (β-ketobutyric acid). The structure of acetoacetic ester possesses two carbonyl groups flanked through a methylene group. The structure of acetoacetic ester is represented as:

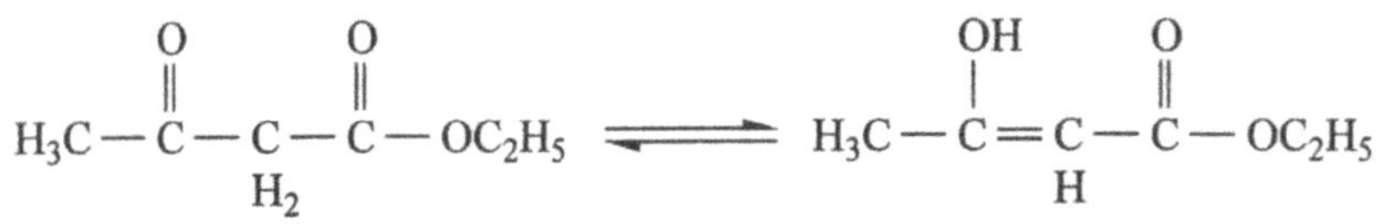

A B

Acetoacetic ester

Structures A (keto form) and B (enol form) are isomers of ethyl acetoacetate which are in dynamic equilibrium. The two isomers are called tautomers and the isomerism is keto-enol tautomerism. Tautomerism is rare in solid state but the two forms exist in dynamic equilibrium in presence of a solvent.

21.6.1 Preparation

Ethyl acetoacetate is prepared by Claisen condensation reaction. In this reaction, two molecules of ethyl acetate are condensed in presence of sodium ethoxide.

$$\underset{\text{Ethyl acetate}}{2CH_3COOC_2H_5} \xrightarrow{C_2H_5ONa} C_2H_5OH + \underset{\text{Sodioacetoacetic ester}}{CH_3CO\bar{C}HCOOC_2H_5} \xrightarrow{HCl} \underset{\text{Ethyl acetoacetate}}{CH_3COCH_2COOC_2H_5}$$

21.6.2 Properties

1. Acetoacetic ester is a colourless, pleasant smelling liquid. It boils at 181°C. It is sparingly soluble in water but freely soluble in organic solvents (alcohol, ether, etc.).
2. Ethyl acetoacetate possesses a keto group, enol group and methylene group. Hence, it shows the characteristic reactions of keto compounds, alcohol and methylene group.

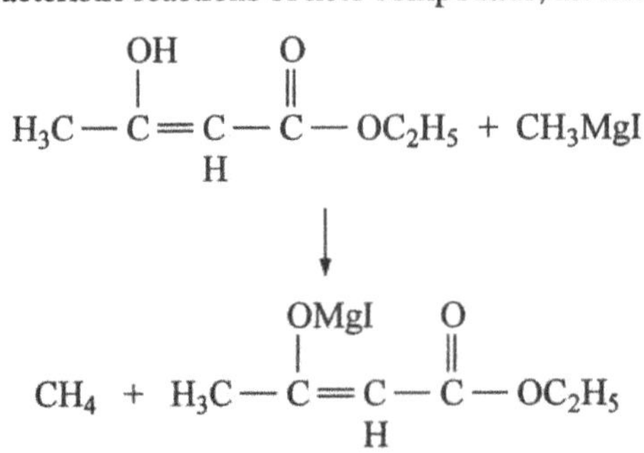

21.6.3 Uses

Acetoacetic ester is an extremely useful synthetic reagent. It is used to prepare the following organic compounds.

1. ***Synthesis of Mono- or Di-alkyl Derivatives of Acetoacetic Ester*** Acetoacetic ester is treated with a base to form an anion. The anion is allowed to react with an alkyl halide to form mono- or di-alkyl acetoacetic ester by nucleophilic substitution.

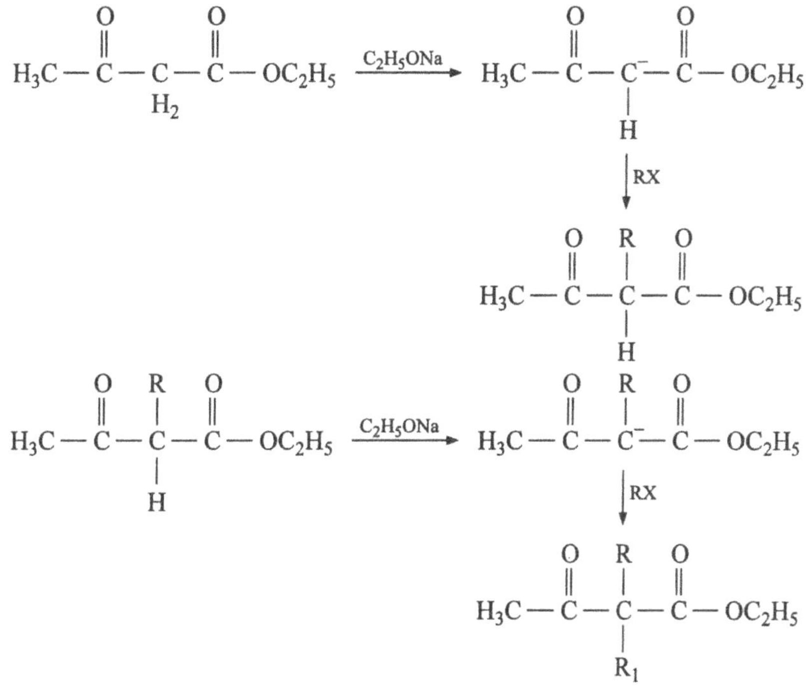

2. ***Synthesis of Fatty Acids*** Fatty acids can be prepared from mono- or di-alkyl derivatives of acetoacetic ester by acidic hydrolysis.

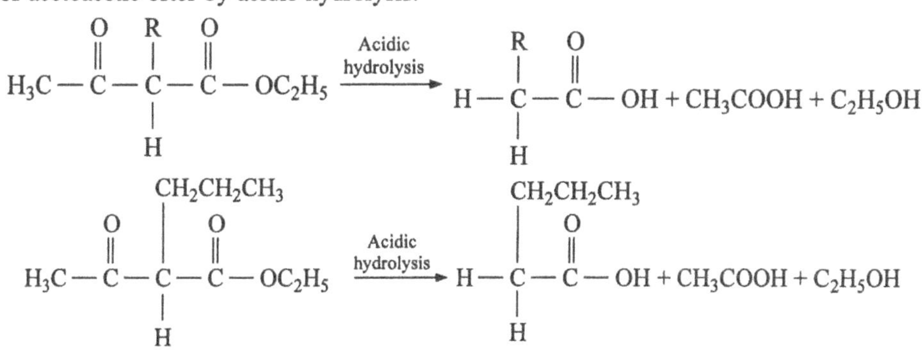

3. ***Synthesis of Dicarboxylic Acids*** Dicarboxylic acids are prepared by acid hydrolysis of sodium salt of ethyl acetoacetate.

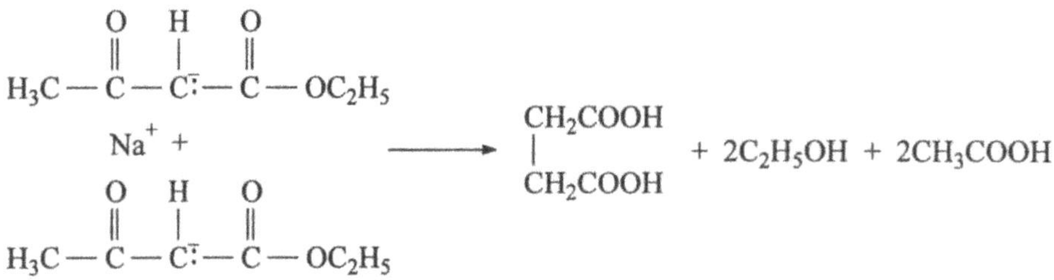

4. ***Synthesis of Unsaturated Acids*** Ethyl acetoacetate is allowed to react with an aldehyde or ketone to form condensed product in presence of base. The condensed product on hydrolysis yields α,β-unsaturated acids.

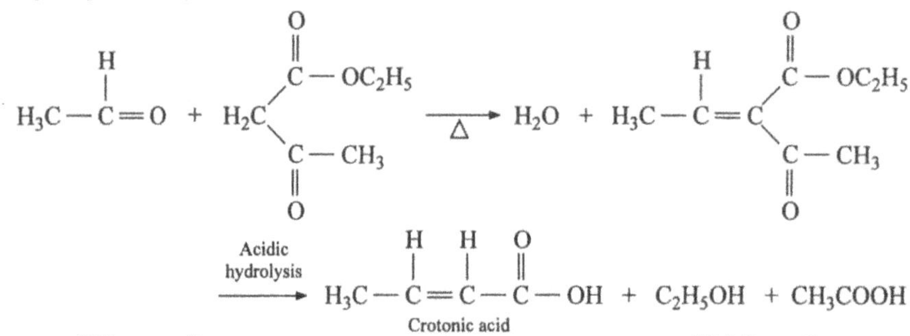

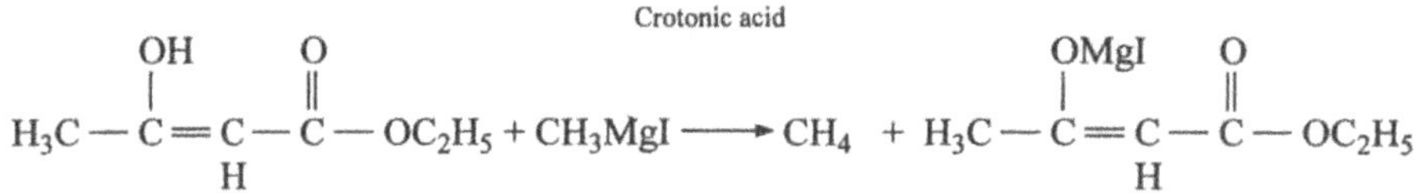

5. ***Synthesis of Keto Acids*** Keto acids are prepared by treating sodio derivative of acetoacetic ester with α-haloester to get acetosuccinic ester, which on ketonic hydrolysis form γ-keto acids.

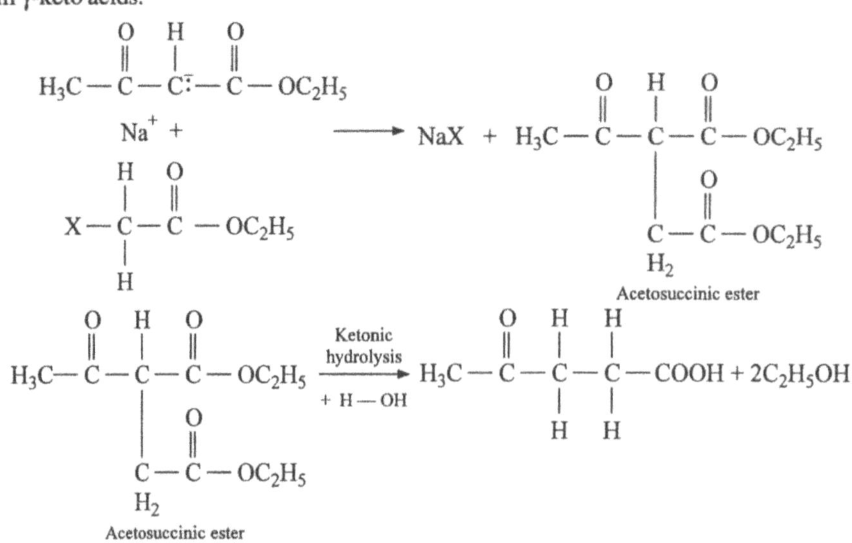

6. ***Synthesis of Ketones*** Mono- or di-alkyl acetoacetic ester on keto hydrolysis yields ketones.

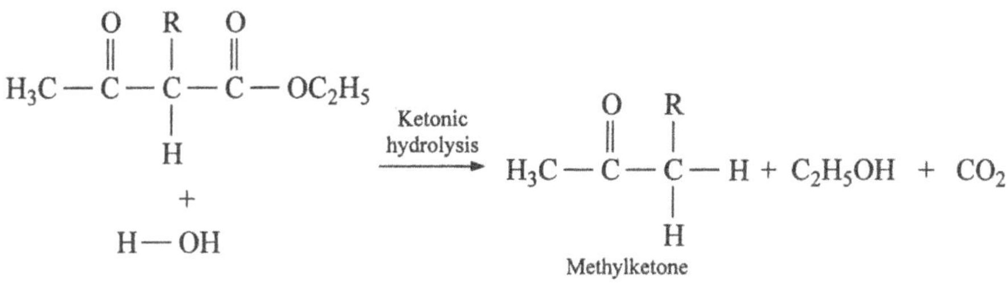

7. ***Synthesis of Cyclic Compounds*** Ethyl acetoacetate condenses with urea to form a cyclic compound (4-methyl uracil).

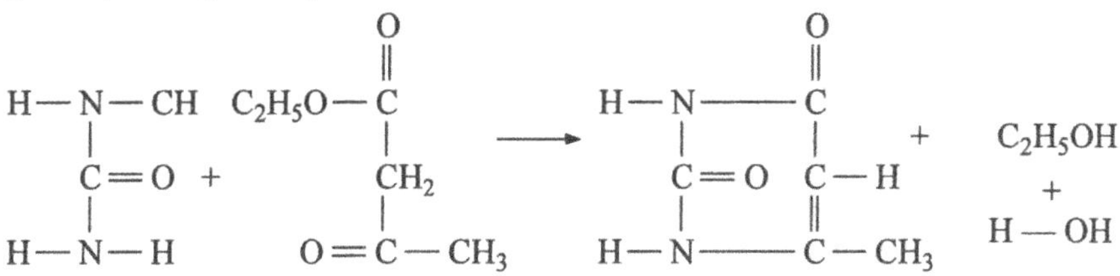

21.7 MALONIC ESTER

Malonic ester is a diethyl ester of malonic acid. Malonic ester contains a methylene group flanked between two carbonyl groups.

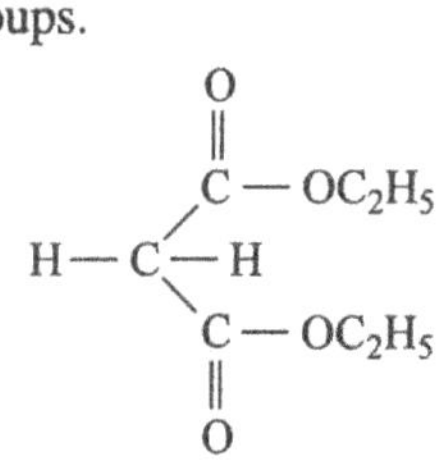

21.7.1 Preparation

Malonic ester is synthesised from chloroacetic acid on reaction with potassium cyanide (KCN) followed by boiling with ethanolic hydrochloric acid.

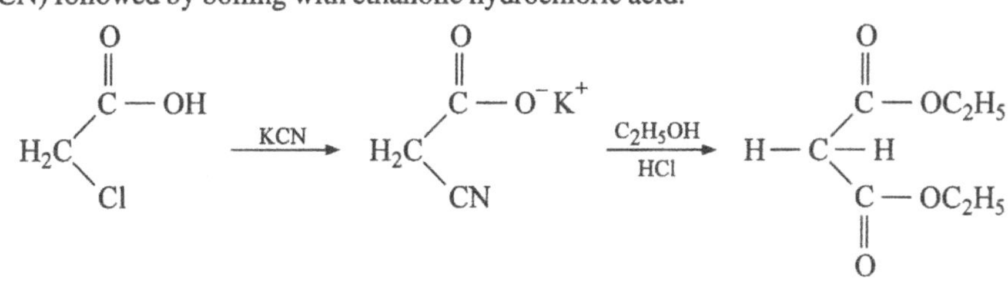

21.7.2 Properties

Malonic ester is a colourless, pleasant-smelling liquid. It boils at 199°C. It is sparingly soluble in water but freely soluble in organic solvents (alcohol, ether, benzene, etc.). Malonic ester exhibits keto-enol tautomerism.

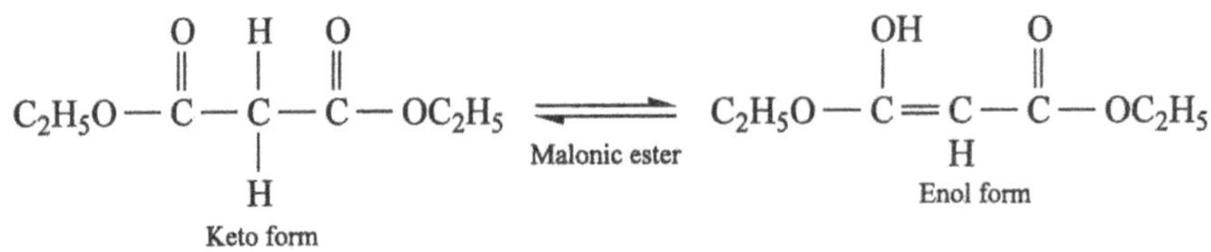

21.7.3 Uses

Malonic ester is a valuable synthetic organic reagent. The synthetic uses of malonic ester are as follows:

1. ***Synthesis of Fatty Acids*** Malonic ester is an acidic compounds (pK_a =13). Malonic ester on treatment with a strong base sodium salt of malonic ester is formed. Sodio malonic ester readily undergoes nucleophilic substitution with primary/secondary alkyl halides to form alkyl (mono- or di-) malonic ester.

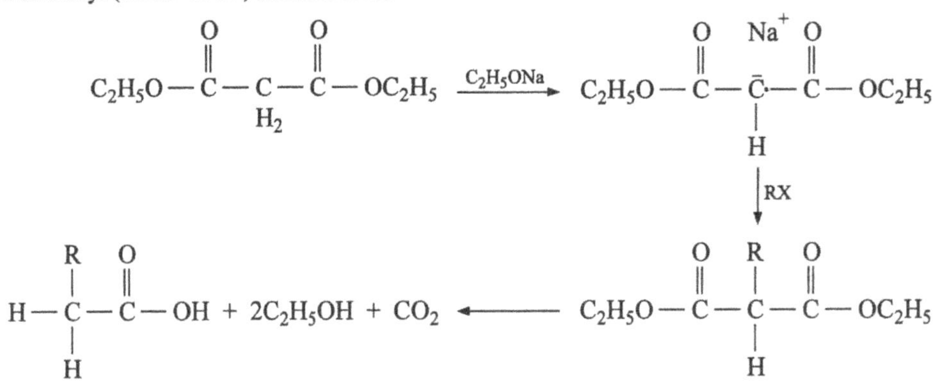

The mono- or di-alkyl malonic ester on hydrolysis yields substituted malonic acid which on heating (above its melting point) forms fatty acids.

2. ***Synthesis of Dicarboxylic Acids*** Dicarboxylic acids can be synthesised on treatment of sodium salt of diethyl malonate with ethylene di-iodide followed by hydrolysis and decarboxylation.

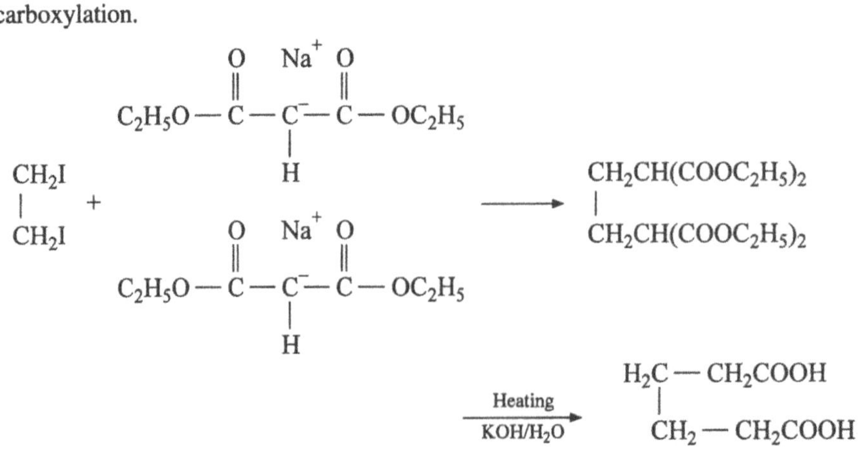

3. ***Synthesis of Unsaturated Acids*** Diethyl malonate condenses with an aldehyde or ketone in presence of base (pyridine or piperdine) to form a condensed product (alkylidene diethyl malonate) which on hydrolysis and heating forms an unsaturated acid.

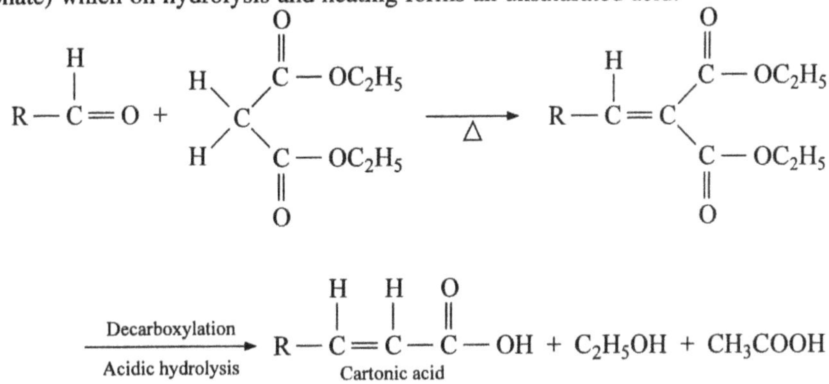

4. ***Synthesis of Keto Acids*** Diethyl malonate reacts with an acid chloride to form acetyl derivative of malonic ester which on hydrolysis and heating gives a keto acid.

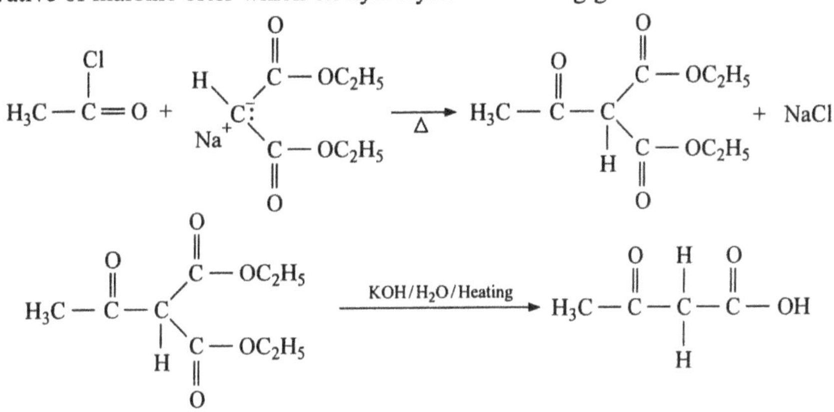

5. ***Synthesis of Ketones*** Ketones can be synthesised from diethyl malonate by the following procedure.

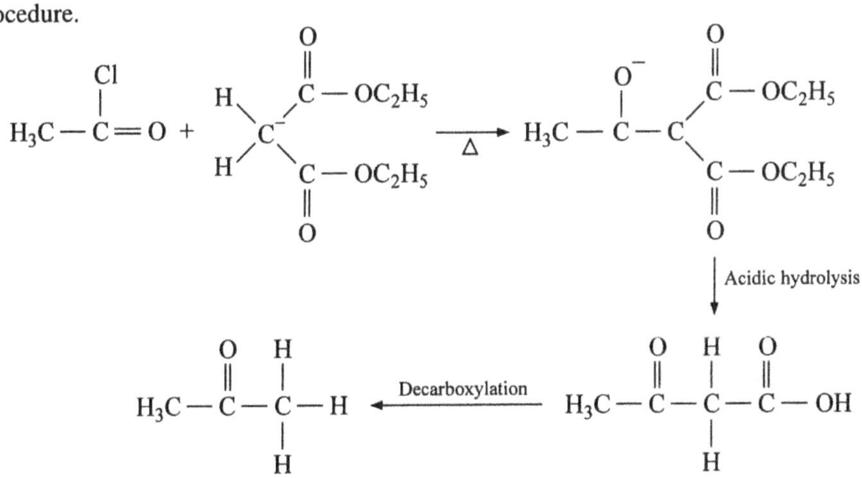

6. ***Synthesis of Amino Acids*** Diethyl malonate reacts with nitrous acid to form diethyl oxinomalonate which on reduction and hydrolysis yield amino acid.

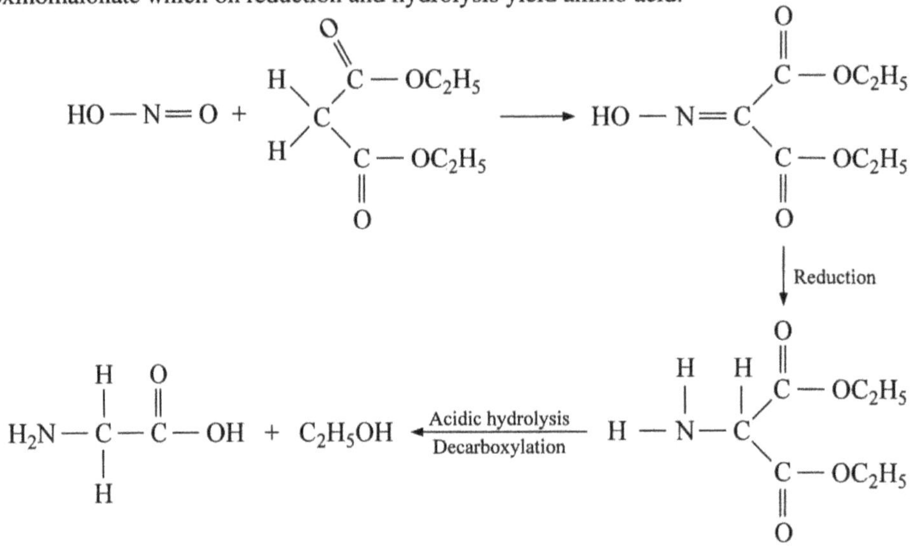

7. ***Synthesis of Cyclic Compounds*** Malonic ester condenses with urea in presence of phosphorous oxychloride to form barbituric acid.

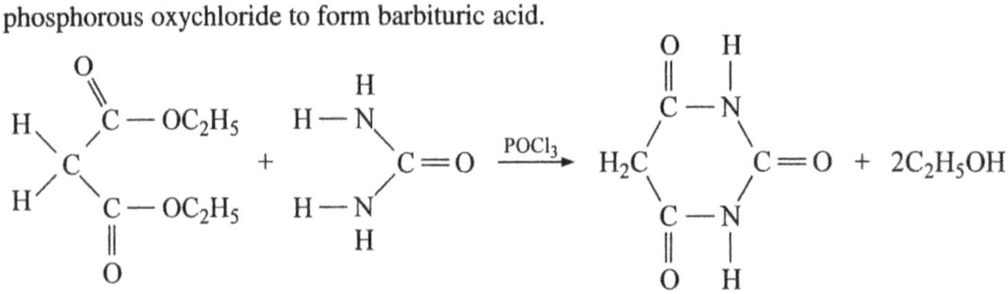

Barbituric acid

21.8 PHARMACEUTICAL COMPOUNDS

1. ***Ethyl Benzoate*** Ethyl benzoate is an ester. Ethyl benzoate is prepared by treating benzoyl chloride with ethyl alcohol by esterifcation reaction.

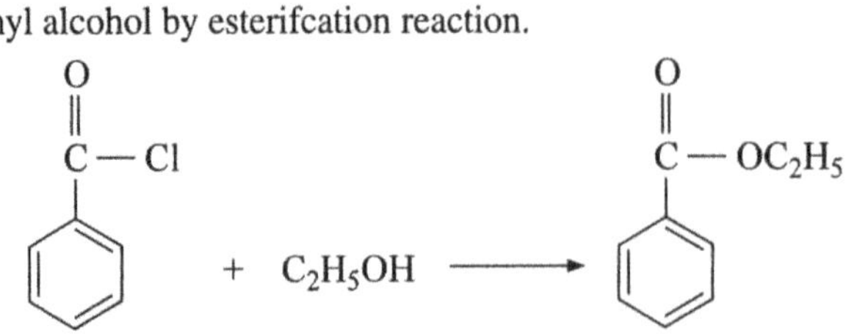

Ethylbenzoate is a colourless liquid. It boils at 213°C. It has a characteristic aromatic odour. Chemically, ethylbenzoate exhibits all chemical reactions of esters (hydrolysis, alcoholysis, ammonolysis, reduction, etc.).

2. ***Dimethyl Phthalate*** Dimethyl phthalate is dimethyl benzene 1,2-dicarboxylate. It is available as a colourless liquid with faint pleasant odour. It is slightly soluble in water.

Dimethyl phthalate is prepared by esterification of phthalic acid with two moles of methanol in acidic medium.

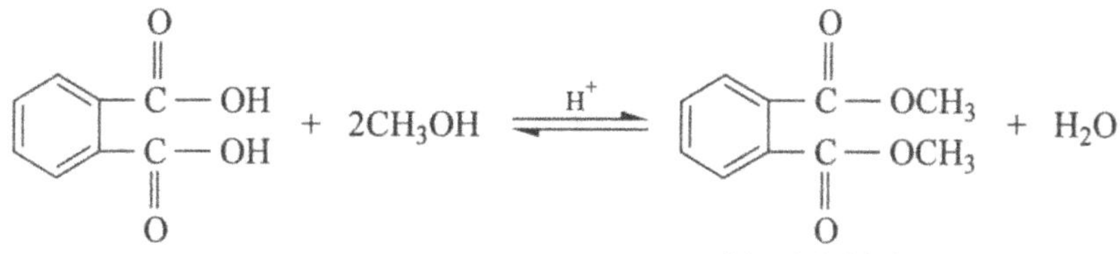

Phthalic acid   Dimethyl phthalate

Dimethyl phthalate is an insect repellant against mosquitoes, midges, mites, ticks and fleas.

3. ***Methyl Salicylate*** Methyl salicylate was first detected in 1843 by extraction from the wintergreen plant (*Gaultheria*). Methyl salicylate is an ester. It is prepared by esterification of salicylic acid by boiling with methyl alcohol in presence of a small amount of concentrated sulphuric acid.

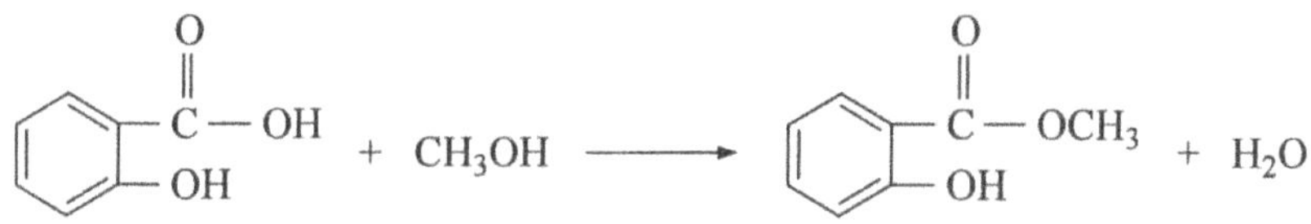

Salicylic acid   Methyl salicylate

Methyl salicylate is a colourless or pale yellow coloured oily liquid. It has a characteristic aroma and is sweet to taste. Methyl salicylate is slightly miscible with water but completely miscible with alcohol. It boils at 220°C.

Uses

1. Methyl salicylate is used as a flavouring agent.
2. It is used for the treatment of rheumatic pain.

4. ***Niclosamide*** Niclosamide is a substituted amide derivative. Chemically, niclosamide is 5-chloro-N-(2-chloro-4-nitrophenyl)–2-hydroxybenzamide.

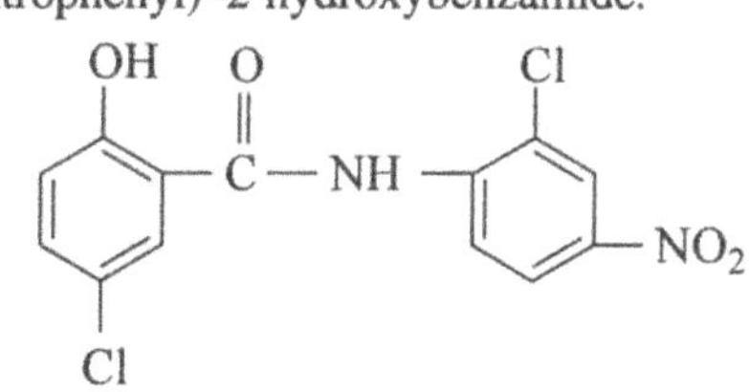

Niclosamide

Niclosamide may be prepared by heating 5-cholorsalicylic acid and 3-chloro-4-amino nitrobenzene in presence of thionyl chloride and chlorobenzene.

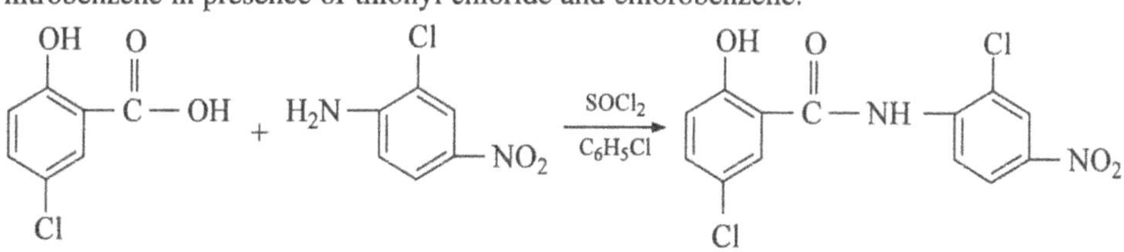

Niclosamide

Niclosamide is available as yellowish-white, water-insoluble powder.

Uses Niclosamide belongs to the family of medicines called anthelmintics, used in treatment of worm infections, and is potent taeniacide. It disintegrates the scolex and worm segments rapidly.

5. ***Benzyl Benzoate*** Benzyl benzoate can be prepared by esterification of benzyl alcohol with benzoic acid in presence of a catalyst.

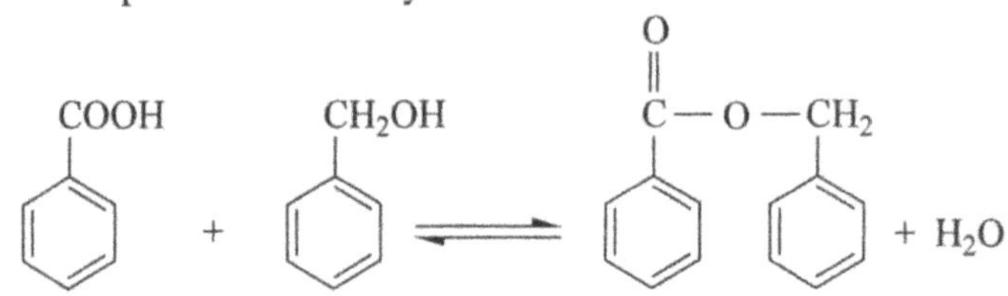

Benzoic acid Benzyl alcohol Benzyl benzoate

Benzyl benzoate is a colourless, crystalline solid.

Use

1. Benzyl benzoate is applied externally as scabicide for the treatment of scabies.
2. It is also useful for the treatment of pediculosis.

6. ***Urea*** Urea is a product of protein metabolism. It is present in human urine in about 3%. In the laboratory, urea is prepared by evaporating a solution of ammonium cyanate.

$$\underset{\text{Ammonium cyanate}}{NH_4OCN} \rightleftharpoons \underset{\text{Urea}}{H_2N-\overset{\overset{\displaystyle O}{\|}}{C}-NH_2}$$

Urea is available as colourless, hygroscopic crystalline powder. It is soluble in water, alcohol but insoluble in chloroform and ether.

Uses Urea is used as a diuretic and antiseptic.

7. ***Triclofos Sodium*** Triclofos is 2,2,2- trichloroethanol dihydrogen phosphate. Triclofos sodium is prepared by esterification of trichloroethanol with orthophosphoric acid and by heating at 100°C for 6 hours. Triclofos is first extracted with an organic solvent followed by extraction with sodium hydroxide solution form triclofos sodium.

$$CCl_3-CH_2OH + HO-\underset{\underset{\displaystyle O}{\|}}{\overset{\overset{\displaystyle OH}{|}}{P}}-OH \longrightarrow CCl_3CH_2O-\underset{\underset{\displaystyle O}{\|}}{\overset{\overset{\displaystyle OH}{|}}{P}}-ONa$$

Triclofos sodium is a colourless, odourless, water soluble, hygroscopic powder. It is insoluble in ether.

Use Triclofos sodium is used as hypnotic and sedative.

PRACTICE QUESTIONS

1. How will you distinguish between the following pairs of compounds in the laboratory?
   (a) Acetic acid and ethylacetate
   (b) Benzoic acid and benzamide

(c) Benzoic acid and benzyl benzoate
(d) Benzamide and acetamide
(e) Acetyl chloride and Aceticanhydride
(f) Urea and acetamide
(g) Ethanamide and ethylamine

2. Complete the following reaction schemes stating the products and any essential conditions.

$$C_2H_5 - COOCH_3 + OH^- \longrightarrow$$

3. Give the mechanisms of:
   (a) Esterification
   (b) Hydrolysis of amide
   (c) Acidic hydrolysis of ester
4. What are esters? Write about various uses of malonic ester with examples.
5. Give various functional derivatives of carboxylic acids. Discuss the chemistry of acid chlorides.
6. How do you account for:
   (a) Acetyl chloride has lower boiling point than acetic acid
   (b) Acetyl chloride is more reactive than acetic anhydride
   (c) Acetamide does not exhibit the characteristic reactions of amines
7. Give the chemical structure, synthesis and uses of:
   (a) Aspirin
   (b) Dimethyl phthalate
   (c) Benzyl benzoate
   (d) Ethyl benzoate
   (e) Urea
   (f) Niclosamide
   (g) Methylsalicylate

22

CHEMISTRY OF α,β-UNSATURATED CARBONYL COMPOUNDS

22.1 INTRODUCTION

Compounds that contain both a carbon–carbon double bond and a carbon–oxygen double bond are called α,β-unsaturated carbonyl compounds. In unsaturated carbonyl compounds, the carbon–carbon double bond and the carbon–oxygen double bond are separated by just one carbon–carbon single bond, i.e. the double bonds are conjugated. The table given here is self-explanatory.

Name	*Formula*
Acrolein	$CH_2{=}CHCHO$
Crotonaldehyde	$CH_3CH{=}CHCHO$
Cinnamaldehyde	$C_6H_5CH{=}CHCHO$
Benzal acetone	$C_6H_5CH{=}CHCOCH_3$
Dibenzal acetone	$C_6H_5CH{=}CHCOCH{=}CHC_6H_5$
Acrylic acid	$CH_2{=}CHCOOH$
Crotonic acid	$CH_3CH{=}CHCOOH$
Methylacrylate	$CH_2{=}CHCOOCH_3$
Acrylonitrile	$CH_2{=}CH{-}CN$

22.2 PREPARATION

The following methods are used to prepare α,β-unsaturated carbonyl compounds:

1. ***Aldol Condensation*** Two molecules of an aldehyde or a ketone having α-hydrogen atoms undergoes self-condensation in presence of dilute base or dilute acid at room temperature to form a product called aldol (β-hydroxy aldehyde or ketone). Hence, this reaction is known as aldol condensation.

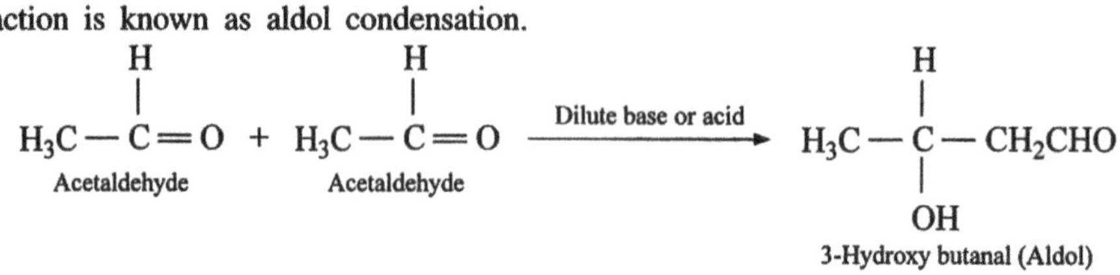

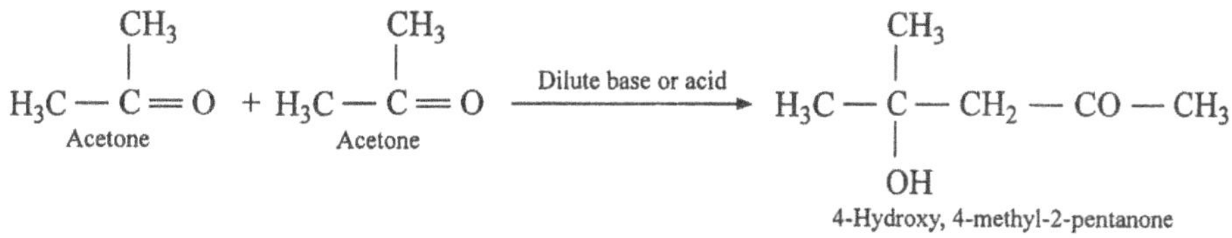

2. ***Perkin reaction*** Aromatic aldehydes on reaction with anhydride of aliphatic acid (containing α-hydrogens) in presence its sodium salt yields β-aryl acrylic acid. The reaction is known as Perkin reaction, e.g. benzaldehyde on reacting with acetic anhydride and sodium acetate forms cinnamic acid.

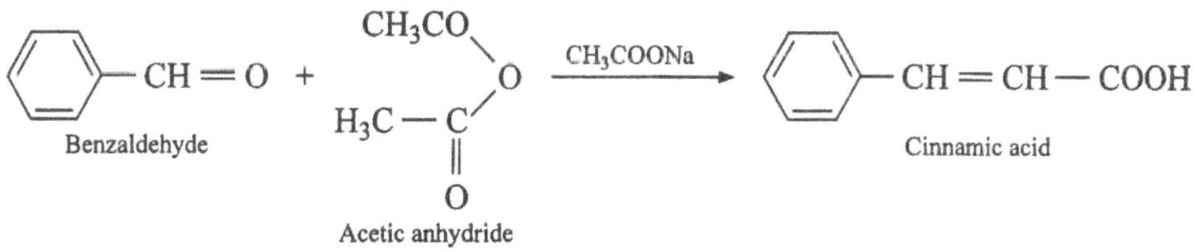

22.3 CHEMICAL REACTIONS

α, β-unsaturated carbonyl compounds undergo the following classes of chemical reactions:

1. Electrophilic addition
2. Nucleophilic addition

1. ***Electrophilic Addition*** The carbon–carbon double bond serves as a source of electrons for the electrophilic reagent. The presence of electron-withdrawing groups (—C=O, —COOR and —CN) at carbon atom not only lowers the reactivity of carbon–carbon double bond towards electrophilic addition but also controls the orientation of addition. The electron-releasing substituent stabilises the carbocation and transition state by dispersing the positive charge.

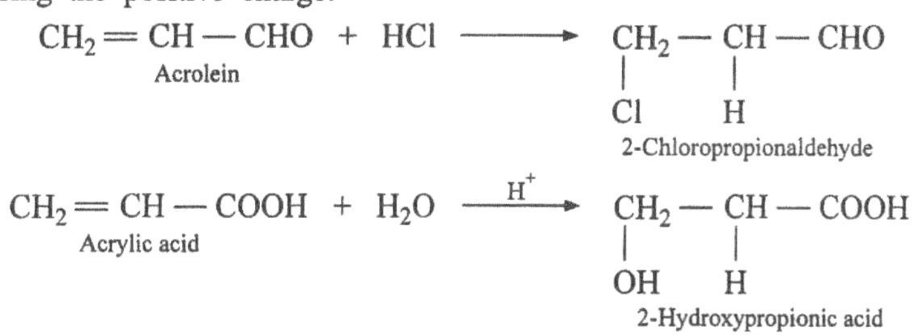

Mechanism Electrophilic addition to α,β-unsaturated carbonyl compounds proceeds through the intermediate formation of *resonance-stabilised carbocation.* This involves following steps:

(i) In the *first step,* electrophile is added to the carbonyl oxygen to yield carbocation I.

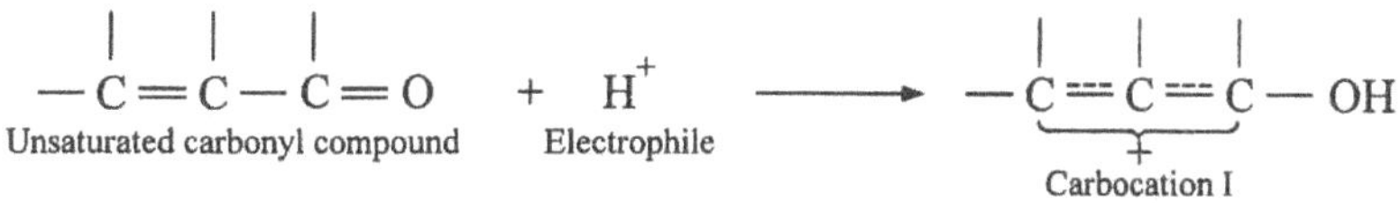

(ii) In the *second step*, a negative ion or basic molecule attaches to the β-carbon of carbocation I and yields a stable product.

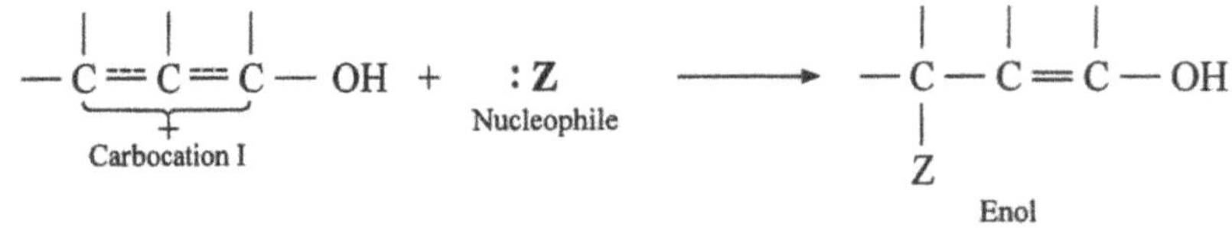

(iii) The enol formed in the above step undergoes tautomerisation to form ketone.

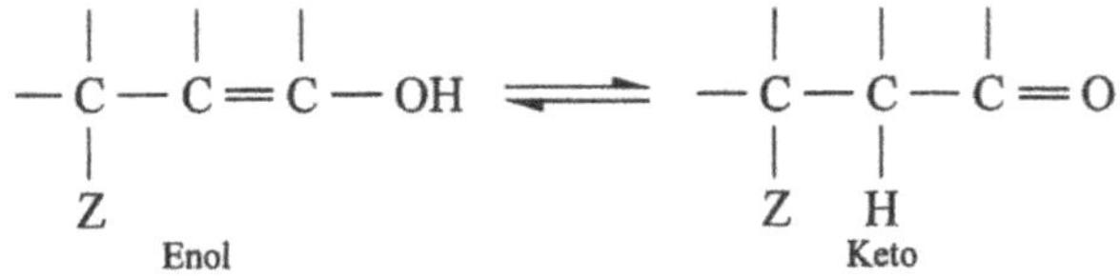

2. ***Nucleophilic Addition*** The electron-withdrawal groups deactivate carbon–carbon double bond towards electrophilic reagents and at the same time activates towards nucleophilic reagents. As a result the carbon–carbon double bond of an unsaturated ketone or acid or ester or nitrile is susceptible to nucleophilic (cyanide anion or ammonia and its derivatives) attack and undergoes nucleophilic addition, that is uncommon for simple alkenes.

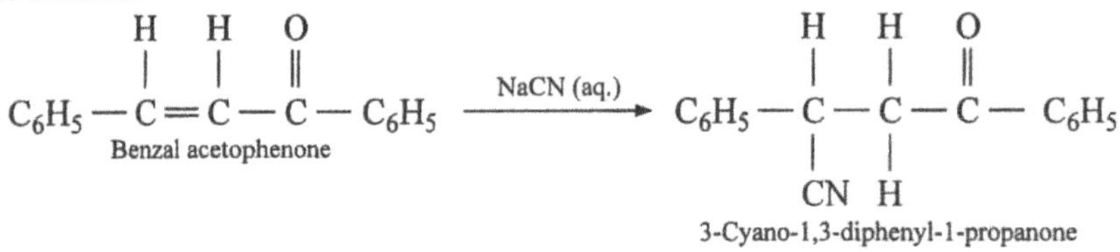

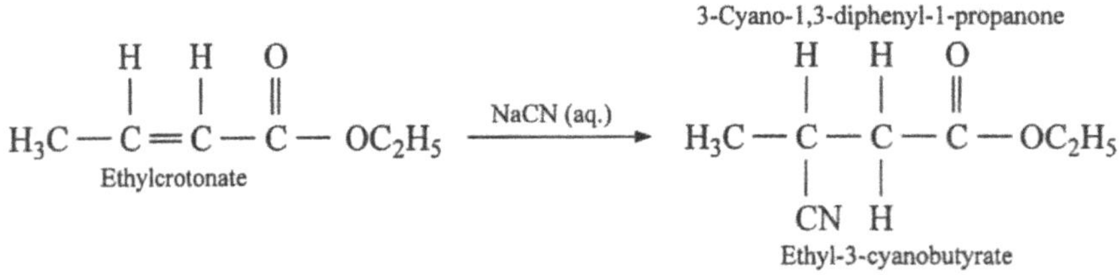

Mechanism (i) Nucleophile adds to the carbon–carbon double bond to get *hybrid anion I.*

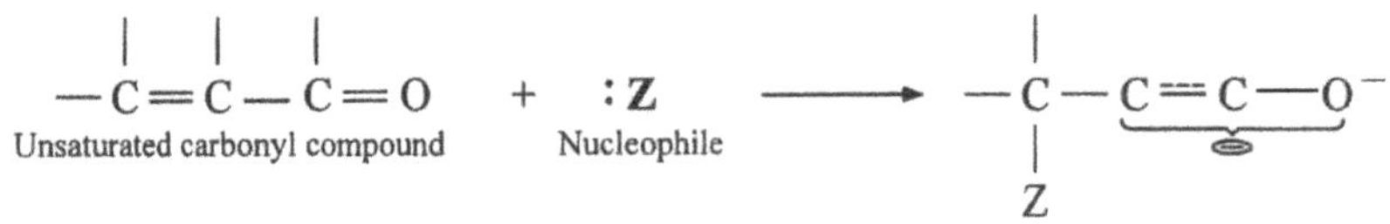

(ii) The hybrid anion I, accepts a proton from the solvent to form final product, i.e. keto compound.

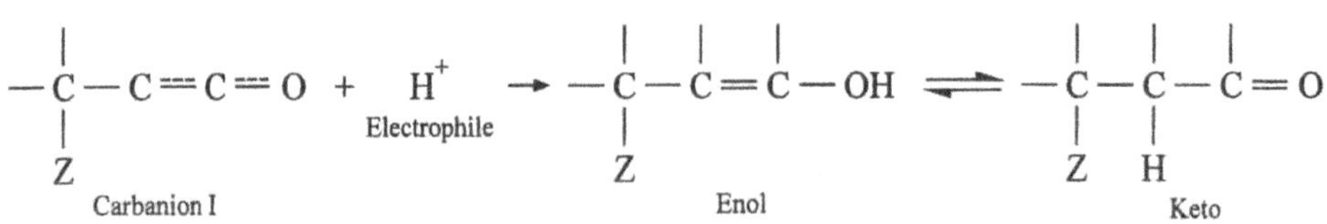

3. ***The Michael Addition*** Nucleophilic addition of carbanions to unsaturated carbonyl compounds is known as Michael addition.

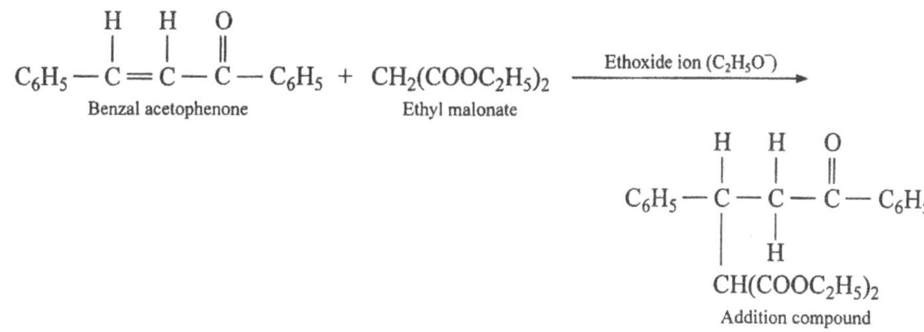

Mechanism This reaction proceeds by the following mechanism.

(i) The base (ethoxide ion) abstracts a hydrogen ion from malonic ester to form a carbanion I (nucleophile).

$$\underset{\text{Ethyl malonate}}{CH_2(COOC_2H_5)_2} + \textbf{Ethoxide ion } (\mathbf{C_2H_5O^-}) \longrightarrow \underset{\substack{\text{Ethyl malonate anion}\\ \text{[Carbanion I]}}}{\bar{C}H(COOC_2H_5)_2} + C_2H_5OH$$

(ii) The carbanion I (nucleophile) attacks the carbon of conjugated system to form a resonance-stabilised anion II (carbanion II).

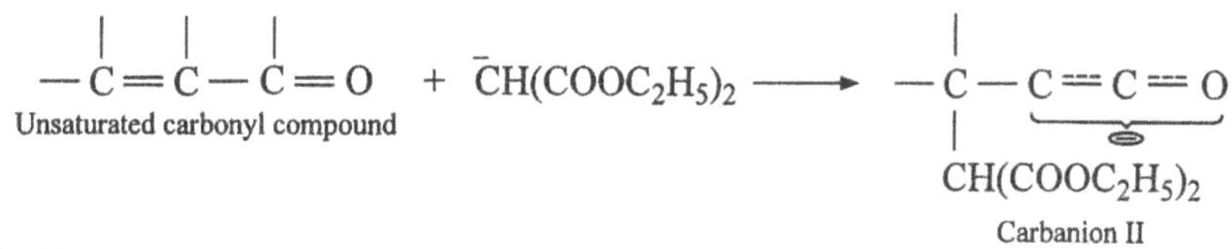

(iii) The carbanion II abstracts a proton from solvent to form product.

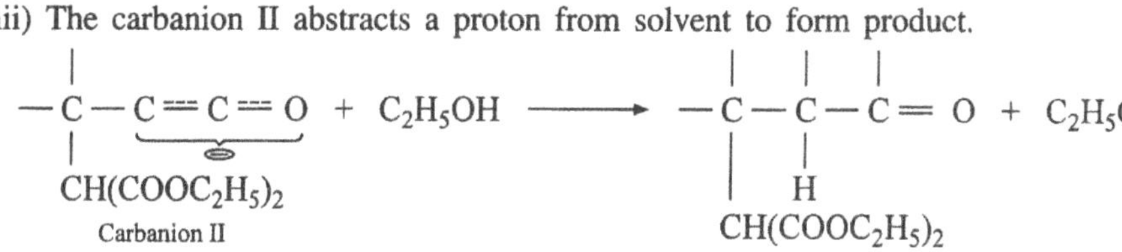

4. ***The Diels–Alder Reaction*** The Diels–Alder reaction is an important reaction because it creates two new carbon–carbon bonds in the formation of a cyclic molecule. Hence, this reaction is also known as *cycloaddition reaction.*

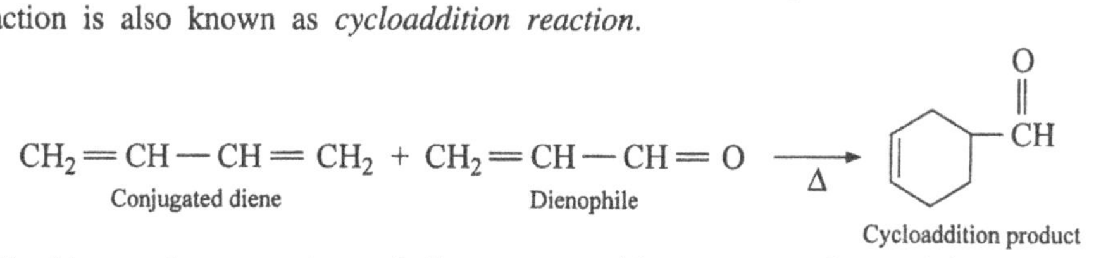

In this reaction, a conjugated diene reacts with a compound containing a carbon–carbon double bond (dienophile). Dienophiles with electron-withdrawing groups bonded to one of the sp^2 hybridised carbons are more reactive. The electron-withdrawing group polarises the double bond, making the reaction easier to initiate. This reaction is more precisely called as (4+2)-cycloaddition reaction because the 6π electrons involved in the cyclic transition state, 4 come from the conjugated diene and 2 come from the dienophile.

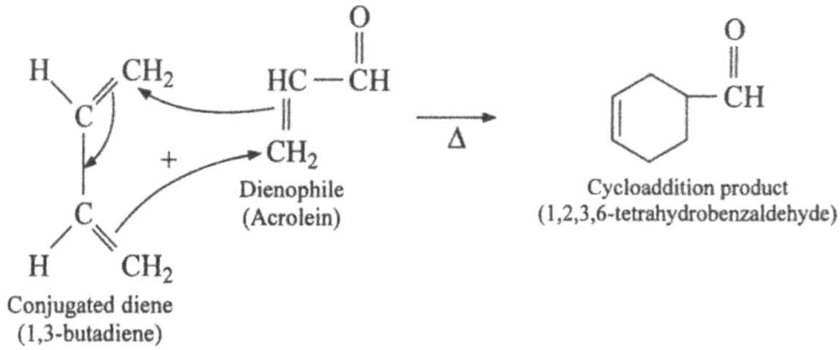

PRACTICE QUESTIONS

1. What are α,β-unsaturated carbonyl compounds? Write various methods to prepare α,β-unsaturated carbonyl compounds.
2. Write about electrophilic and nucleophilic addition reactions of α,β-unsaturated carbonyl compounds.
3. Explain why α,β-unsaturated carbonyl compounds react with both nucleophiles and electrophiles.
4. Write notes on:
   (a) Perkin reaction
   (b) Conjugate addition
   (c) Michael addition
   (d) Aldol condensation

23

CHEMISTRY OF PHENOLS

23.1 INTRODUCTION

Phenols are aromatic compounds in which the hydroxyl group is directly attached to the carbon atom of an aromatic ring. They may be represented by the general formula ArOH where Ar represents a phenyl, a substituted phenyl or some other aryl group such as naphthyl. Depending upon the number of hydroxyl groups attached to the aromatic ring, the phenols may be classified as monohydric, dihydric or trihydric phenols.

Monohydric phenols

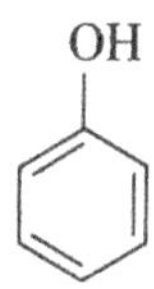
Phenol

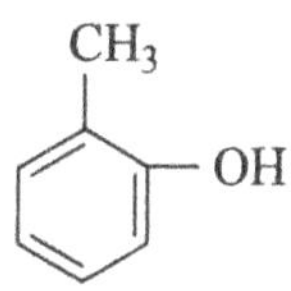
o-Cresol

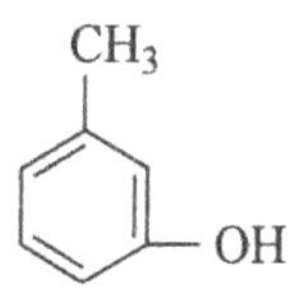
m-Cresol

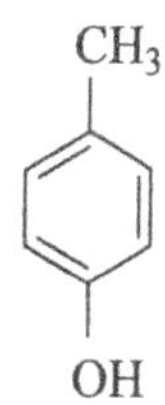
p-Cresol

Dihydric phenols

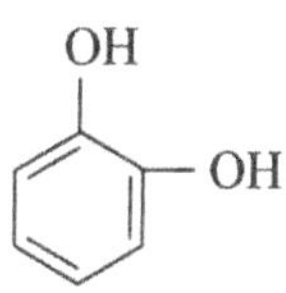
Catechol

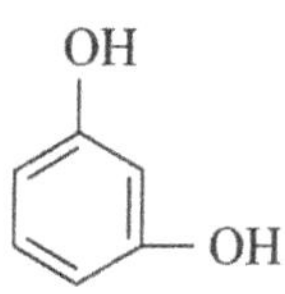
Resorcinol

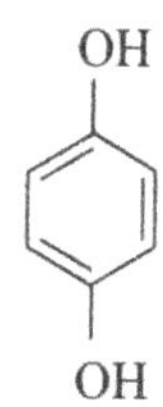
Quinol

Trihydric phenols

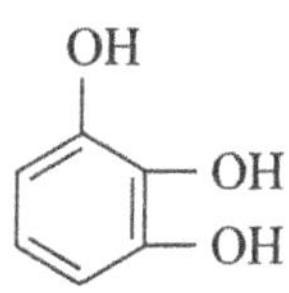
Pyrogallol

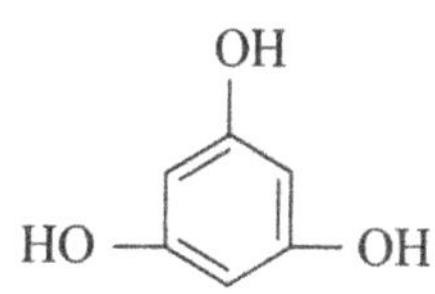
Phloroglucinol

23.2 GENERAL METHODS OF PREPARATION

The following methods are used to prepare phenols: (1) laboratory methods and (2) industrial methods.

1. ***Laboratory Method*** In the laboratory, phenols are generally prepared from aromatic diazonium salts. The procedure involves treatment of an aromatic amine at 0°– 5°C with

dilute HCl and $NaNO_2$ followed by warming up of the reaction mixture with water to get phenol.

$$\underset{\text{Amine}}{ArNH_2} \xrightarrow{NaNO_2/HCl} \underset{\text{Diazonium salt}}{Ar-\overset{+}{N_2}Cl^-} \xrightarrow[\Delta]{} \underset{\text{Phenol}}{Ar-OH} + N_2 + HCl$$

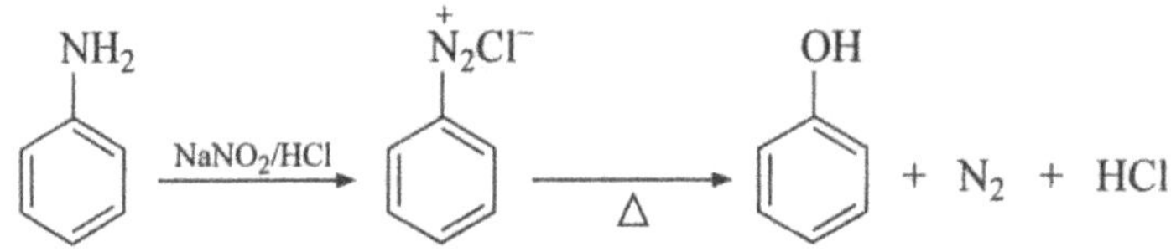

Aniline Benzenediazonium chloride Phenol

Alternatively, phenols may also be prepared by the fusion of aromatic sulphonic acids with alkali.

$$\underset{\text{Aromatic sulphonic acid}}{ArSO_3H} \xrightarrow[\text{Fuse}]{NaOH} \underset{\text{Sodium phenoxide}}{Ar-ONa} \xrightarrow{HCl} \underset{\text{Phenol}}{Ar-OH} + NaCl$$

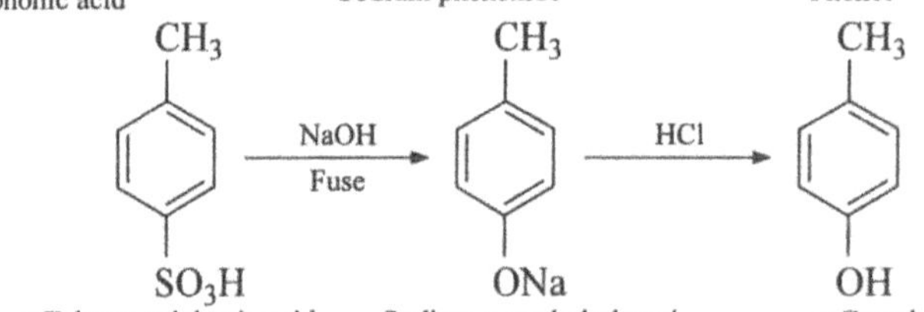

p-Toluene sulphonic acid Sodium *p*-methyl phenol *p*-Cresol

2. ***Industrial Methods*** A few phenols (the parent phenol and cresols) are generally obtained during fractionation of coal tar. The phenols occur in the middle-oil fraction of coaltar distillation, which are isolated by treatment with alkali followed by separation and acid hydrolysis.

Synthetically, phenols are obtained on a commercial scale by either of the following two processes:

(i) *From cumene* This method involves oxidation of cumene (isopropyl benzene) with oxygen/air to yield cumene hydroperoxide followed by acid hydrolysis resulting in phenol. The mechanism of this reaction involves a simple free-radical mediated oxidation of cumene to yield cumene hydroperoxide. The latter on acid hydrolysis undergoes ionic transformation to phenol and acetone.

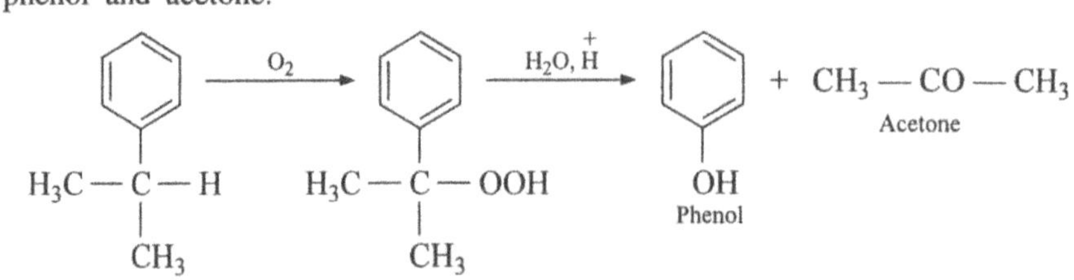

Cumene Cumene hydroperoxide

(ii) *Dow process* Aryl halides on alkali hydrolysis under drastic conditions yield phenols by nucleophilic substitution.

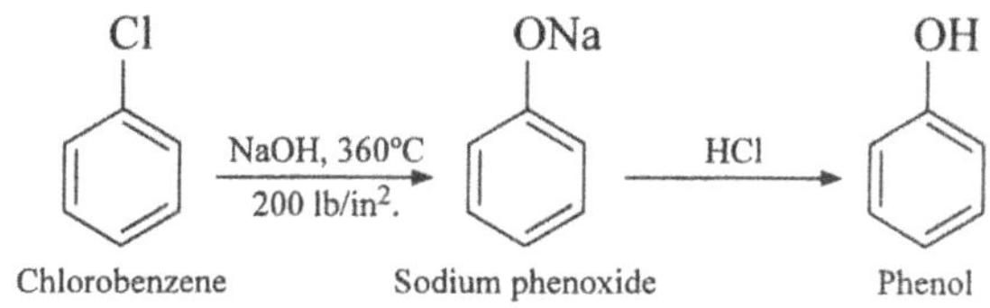

23.3 PHYSICAL PROPERTIES

1. Pure phenols are generally colourless liquids or solids. But they usually appear slightly coloured as they readily get oxidised even in air and the oxidation products are coloured (Substituents like NO_2 group also impart colour to phenols.)
2. Phenols boil at considerably higher temperatures than corresponding hydrocarbons and aryl halides due to intermolecular hydrogen bonding.

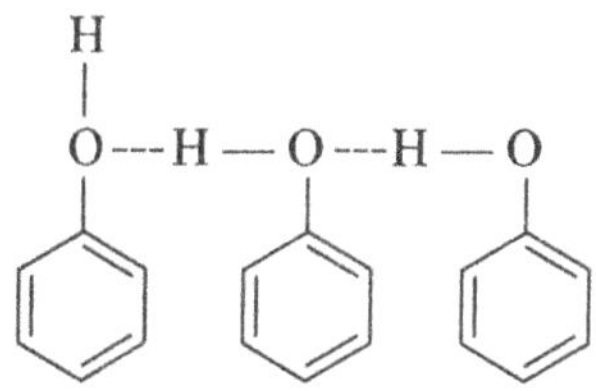

3. Phenols are generally insoluble in water although phenol itself and some di- and tri-hydrophenols are fairly soluble due to formation of intermolecular hydrogen bond with water, e.g. resorcinol.

23.4 CHEMICAL PROPERTIES

The chemical behaviour of phenols is different in some respects from that of the alcohols, so it is sensible to treat them as a similar but characteristically distinct group.

1. ***Acidity of Phenols*** Phenols are appreciably acidic compounds. They react with aqueous alkali metal hydroxides to form phenoxides. However, phenols do not react with aqueous carbonates or bicarbonates.

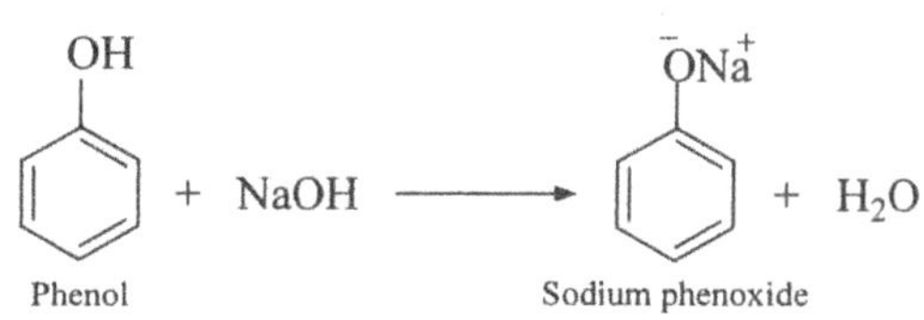

Phenol and phenoxide ion exhibit resonance and both of them are a resonance hybrid of various contributing structures:

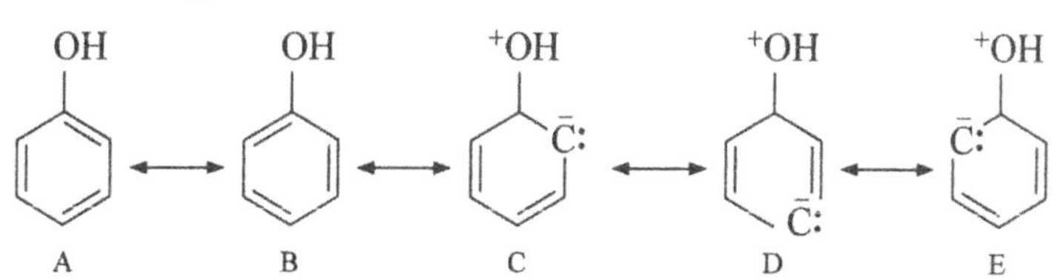

Contributors of phenol

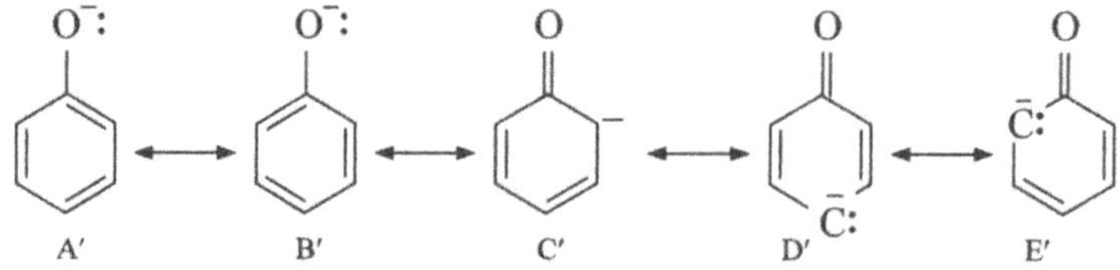

Contributors of phenoxide ion

Structures C, D, E involve charge separation hence less stable. The charge separation diminishes the importance of canonical contributors to the resonance hybrid and reduces the overall stabilisation. On the other hand, the phenoxide anion is already charged, and the canonical contributors act to disperse the charge, resulting in a substantial stabilisation of this species. So phenoxide ion is more stable than phenol, hence phenol gets ionised to phenoxide ion.

Why is phenol a much stronger acid than alcohol? The conjugate bases of simple alcohols are not stabilised by charge delocalisation, so the acidity of these compounds is similar to that of water.

$$\underset{\text{Alcohol}}{R-OH} \rightleftharpoons \underset{\text{Alkoxide anion}}{R-O^-} + H^+$$

An energy diagram showing the effect of resonance on cyclohexanol and phenol acidities is given here:

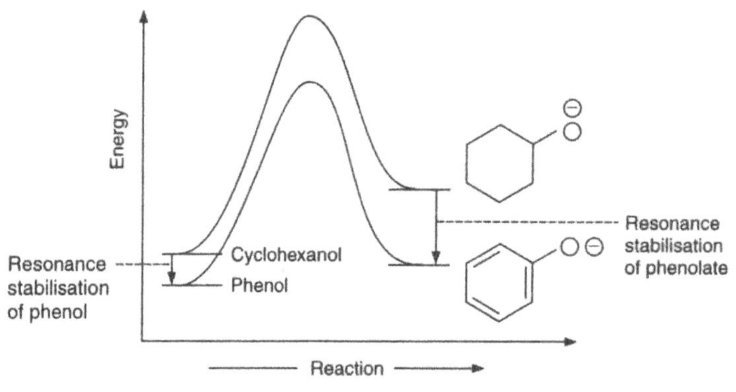

Since the resonance stabilisation of the phenoxide conjugate base is much greater than the stabilisation of phenol itself, the acidity of phenol relative to cyclohexanol is increased. Hence, phenols are more acidic than alcohols.

Effect of substituents on acidity of phenols The electron-withdrawing substituents increase the acidic strength because they stabilise the phenoxide ion greatly by dispersing the negative charge of this ion. This phenolic acidity is further enhanced by electron-withdrawing substituents ortho and para to the hydroxyl group. On the other hand, electron-releasing substituents destabilise the phenoxide ion by intensifying its negative charge. It is noteworthy that if the electron-withdrawing substituent is present at para-location rather than at meta then the phenol is more stronger, e.g. picric acid is a very strong acid.

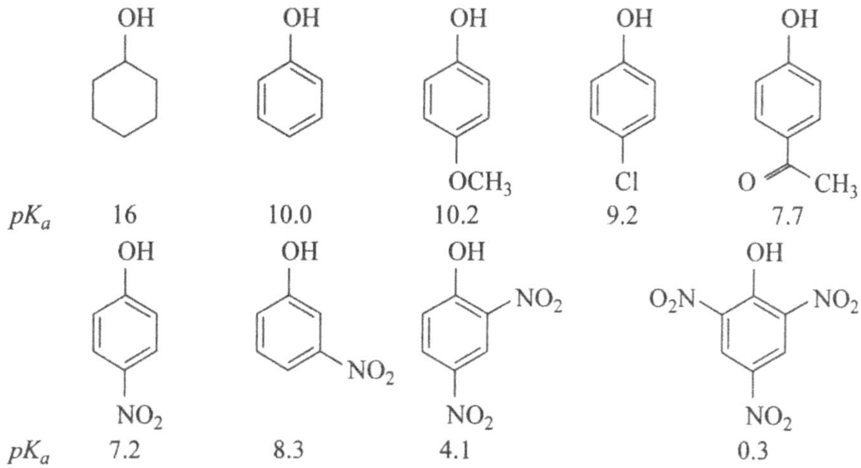

2. ***Ether Formation*** When phenols react with alkyl halides in alkaline medium, ethers are produced. This reaction is known as *Williamson's synthesis*. The alkyl halide (methyl or primary alkyl) undergoes nucleophilic substitution by phenoxide ion.

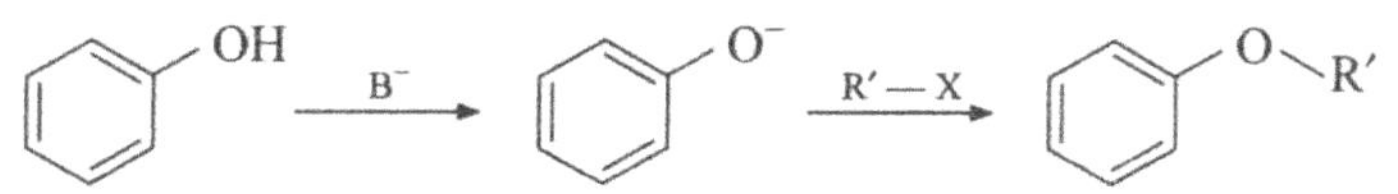

$$C_2H_5ONa + C_2H_5I \longrightarrow C_2H_5-O-C_2H_5 + NaI$$

Sodium ethoxide, Ethyl iodide, Diethyl ether

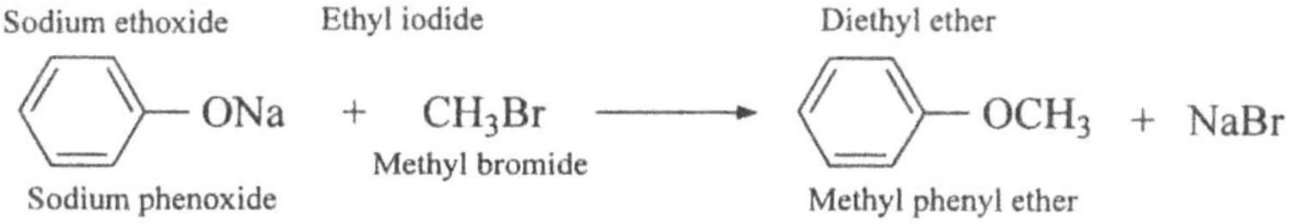

3. ***Oxidation of Phenols*** Phenols are rather easily oxidised despite the absence of a hydrogen atom on the hydroxyl-bearing carbon. In general, phenols are more easily oxidised than simple alcohols. Oxidation can be achieved by reaction with silver oxide (Ag_2O) or chromic acid ($Na_2Cr_2O_7$), or other oxidising agents. The coloured product obtained from phenol by oxidation with chromic acid is para-benzoquinone (also known as 1,4-benzoquinone or simply quinone). These compounds are easily reduced to their dihydroxybenzene analogs, and it is from these compounds that quinones are best prepared.

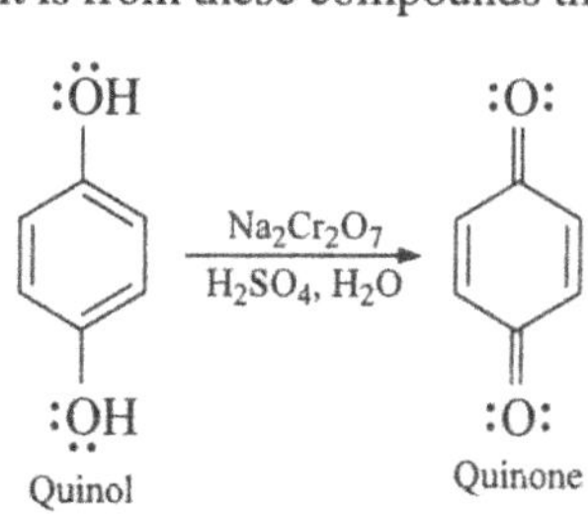

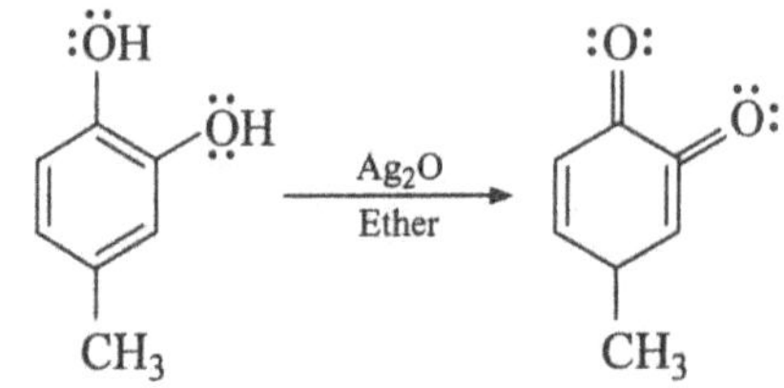

4. ***Ester Formation*** Phenols react with carboxylic acids, acid chlorides or anhydrides to form esters. The reaction is catalysed by both acids and bases. As with the alcohols, the phenolic hydroxyl hydrogen is rather easily replaced by other substituents. For example, phenol reacts easily with acetic anhydride to give phenyl acetate. Likewise, the phenoxide anion is an effective nucleophile in S_N2 reactions, as in the second example below.

$$C_6H_5\text{—}OH + (CH_3CO)_2O \longrightarrow C_6H_5\text{—}O\text{—}COCH_3 + CH_3CO_2H$$

$$C_6H_5\text{—}O^{(-)}Na^{(+)} + CH_3CH_2CH_3\text{—}Br \longrightarrow C_6H_5\text{—}O\text{—}CH_2CH_2CH_3 + NaBr$$

Fries Rearrangement When phenol ester is heated with $AlCl_3$, the acyl group migrates from phenolic oxygen to the ortho or para position of the ring. This is called Fries rearrangement.

$$ArOH + RCOCl \longrightarrow ArOCOR + HCl$$

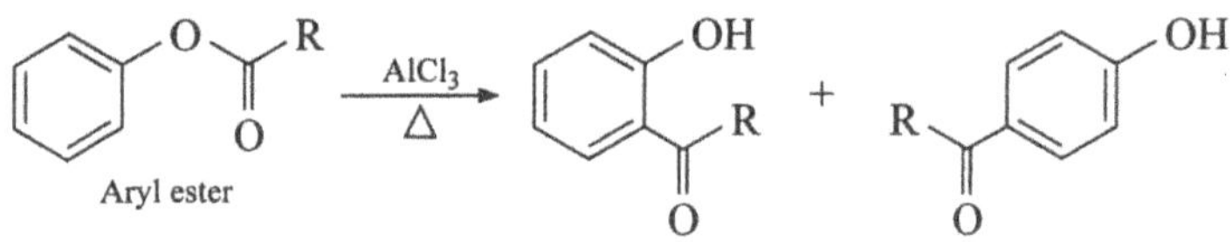

Aryl ester

o- and *p*-Aryl ketones

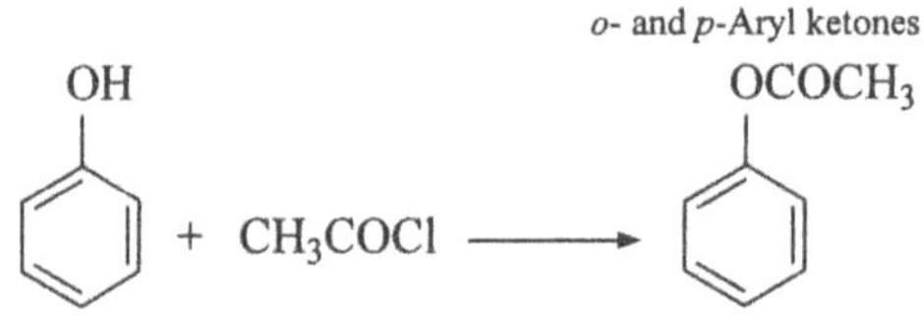

Phenol

Phenyl acetate

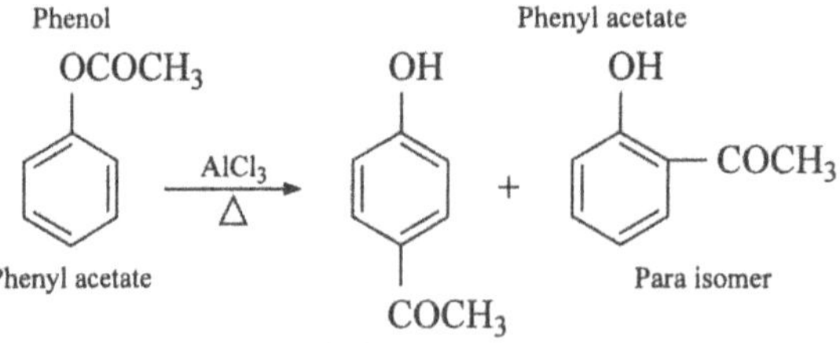

Phenyl acetate

Para isomer

Ortho isomer

Mechanism Fries rearrangement involves the following steps:

Step 1

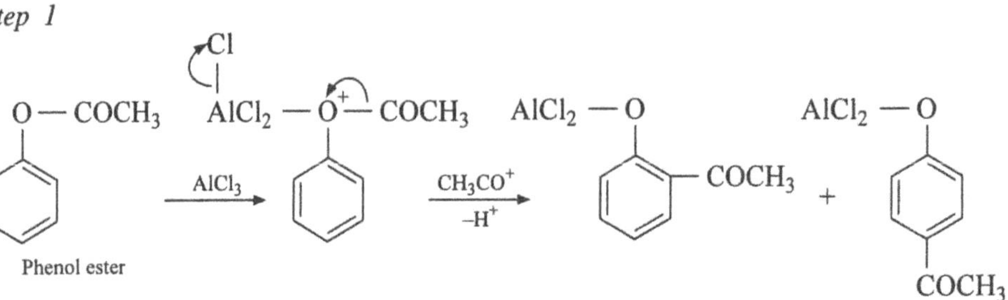

Phenol ester

Step 2

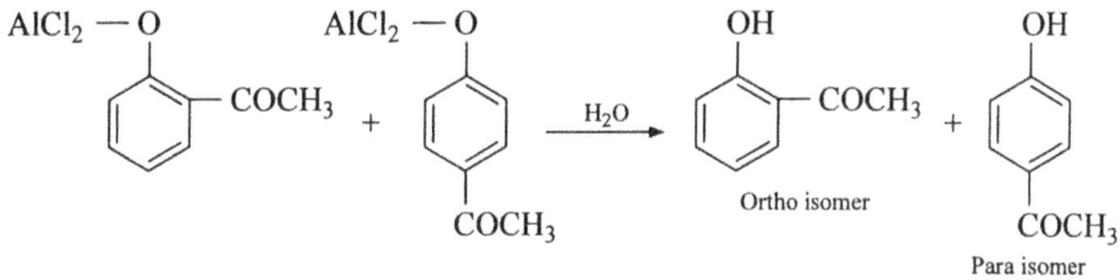

5. ***Reaction with Zinc Dust*** When phenol is distilled with zinc dust, we get corresponding hydrocarbon.

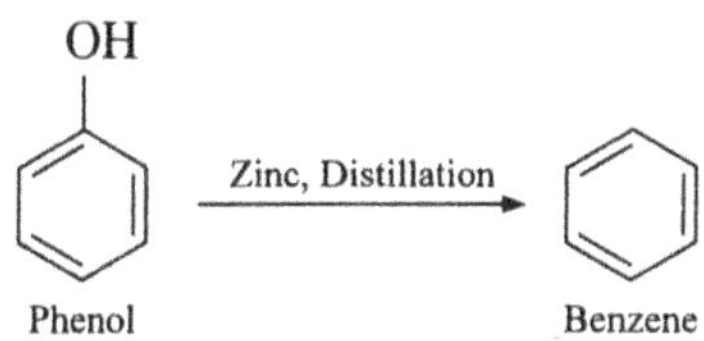

6. ***Reaction with Ferric Ions*** Phenols react with ferric ions in neutral solution to form greenish to blue–violet coloured solutions due to the formation of ferric phenoxide complex.

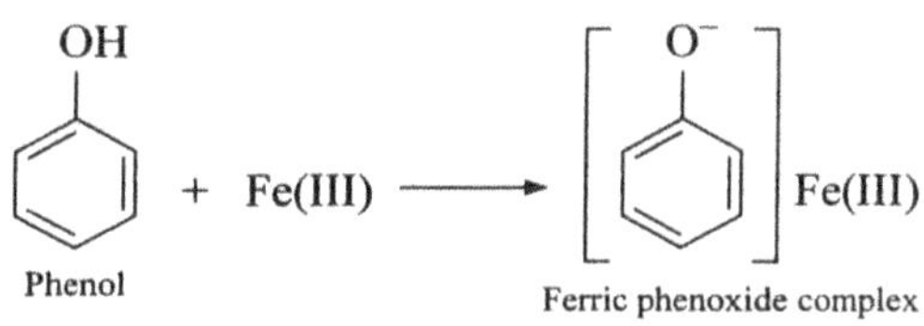

7. ***Electrophilic Aromatic Substitution*** Phenols are potentially very reactive towards electrophilic aromatic substitution. This is because the hydroxy group, (**—OH**), is a strongly activating, *ortho-* or *para*-directing substituent. Substitution typically occurs *para* to the hydroxyl group unless the *para* position is blocked, in which case *ortho* substitution occurs.

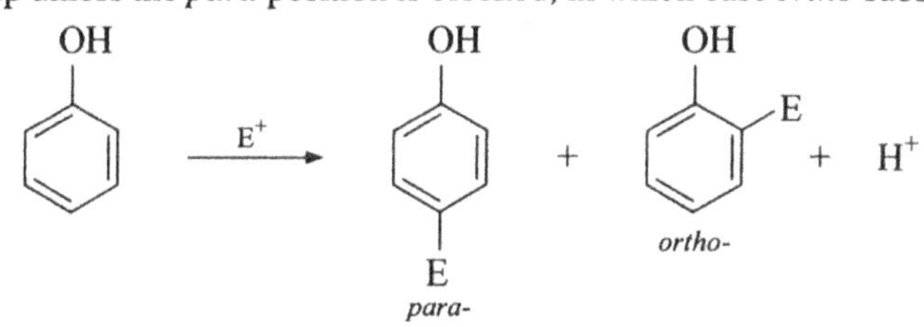

The strong activation of hydroxyl group often means that milder reaction conditions are sufficient for electrophilic substitution of phenols than those used for benzene itself:

Reaction	*Phenol*	*Benzene*
Nitration	Dil. HNO_3 in H_2O or CH_3CO_2H	HNO_3/H_2SO_4
Sulphonation	Conc. H_2SO_4	H_2SO_4 or SO_3/H_2SO_4
Halogenation	X_2	X_2/Fe or FeX_3
Alkylation	ROH/H^+ or $RCl/AlCl_3$	$RCl/AlCl_3$
Acylation	$RCOCl/AlCl_3$	$RCOCl/AlCl_3$
Nitrosation	Aq. $NaNO_2/H^+$	

(i) *Nitration* Nitration of a phenol with nitrating mixture at room temperature gives a mixture of products, picric acid being one of them.

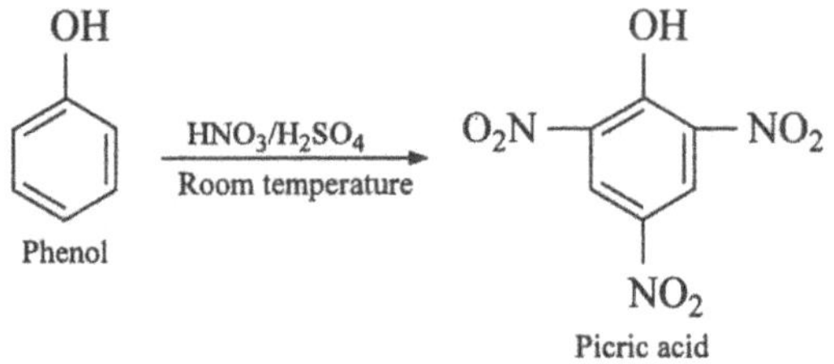

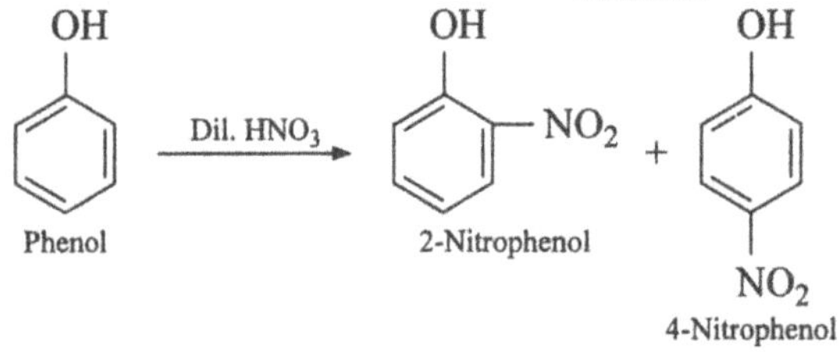

(ii) *Halogenation* Phenols on treatment with halogens give polyhalogenated derivative.

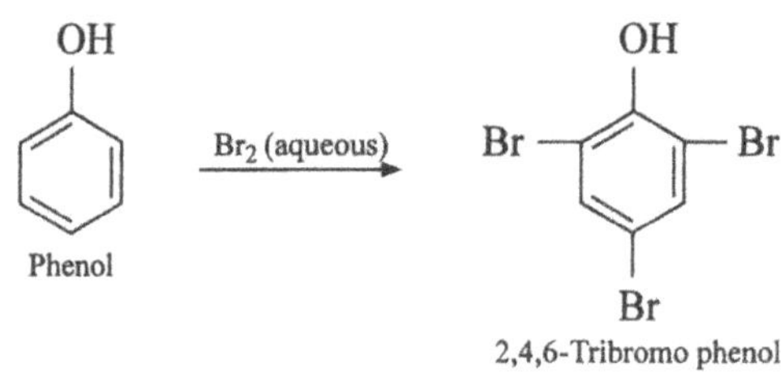

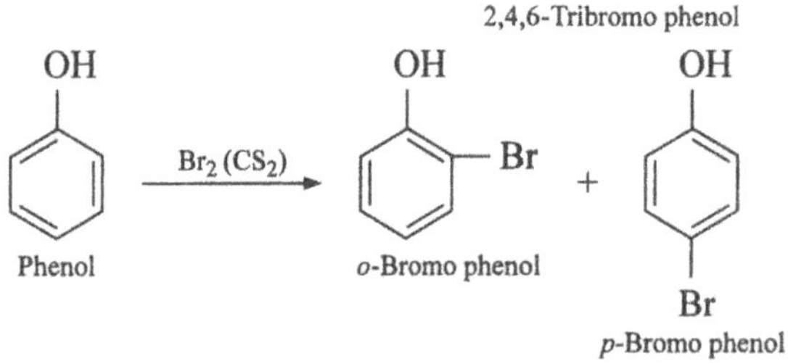

(iii) *Sulphonation* Phenols undergo sulphonation with concentrated sulphuric acid at room temperature and yield a mixture of ortho and para sulphonated phenols.

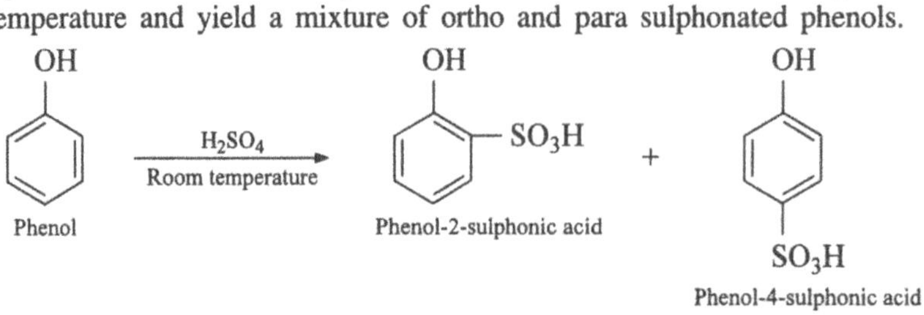

(iv) *The diazocoupling reaction* Phenoxide ion couples with benzenediazonium chloride to give a dye (*p*-hydroxyazobenzene). The diazonium ions are weak electrophiles and react with highly reactive aromatic compounds like phenols to give azo compounds.

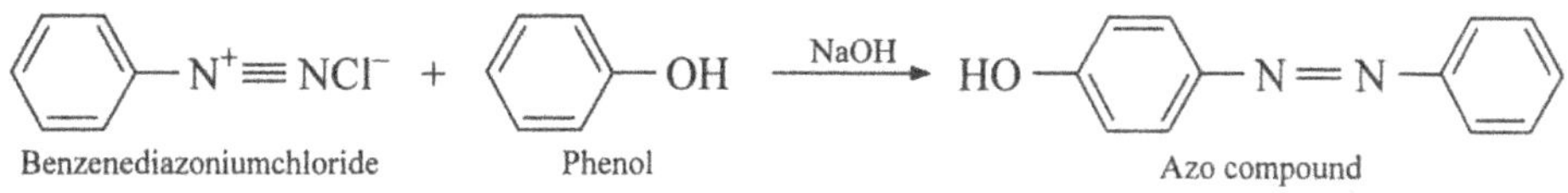

(v) *Kolbe's reaction (Electrophilic Aromatic Substitution)* Heating the nucleophilic phenoxide salt with carbon dioxide under high pressure/temperature results in regio-selective *ortho*-substitution. This process is also known as the *Kolbe–Schmidt synthesis*. *o*-Hydroxybenzoic acid is more commonly known as *salicylic acid* and is prepared by this reaction from sodiumphenoxide.

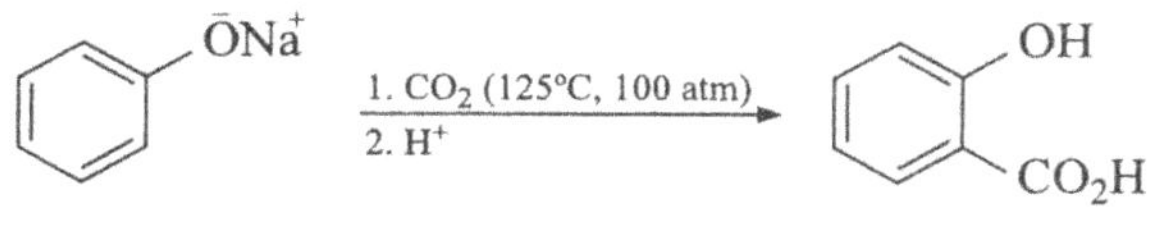

Mechanism for Carboxylation of Phenols

Step 1 The nucleophilic phenolate reacts with the electrophilic carbon of carbon dioxide in the *ortho* position (compare this with an Aldol reaction).

Step 2 The non-aromatic cyclohexadienonecarboxylate intermediate *tautomerises* to the more stable aromatic enol, which is further stabilised by an intramolecular hydrogen bond. An acidic work-up will generate the carboxylic acid.

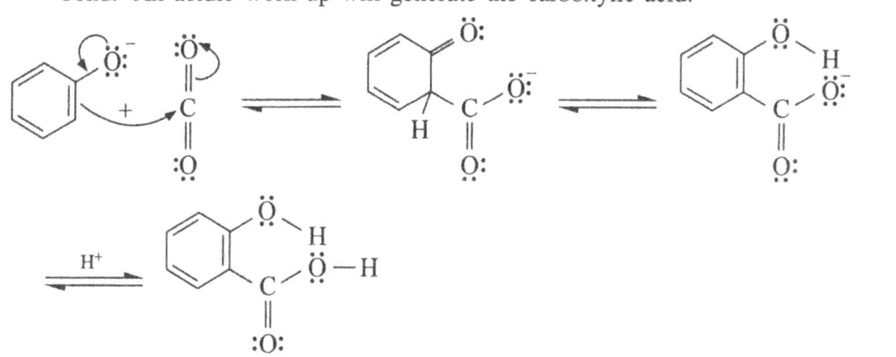

(vi) *Reimer–Tiemann reaction (Synthesis of Phenolic Aldehydes)* In a phenol, on treatment with NaOH and $CHCl_3$, an aldehyde group (—CHO) is introduced at the ortho position of —OH group on to the aromatic ring. This reaction is known as Reimer–Tiemann reaction. In this reaction, benzal chloride is initially formed which on alkaline hydrolysis gets converted to —CHO.

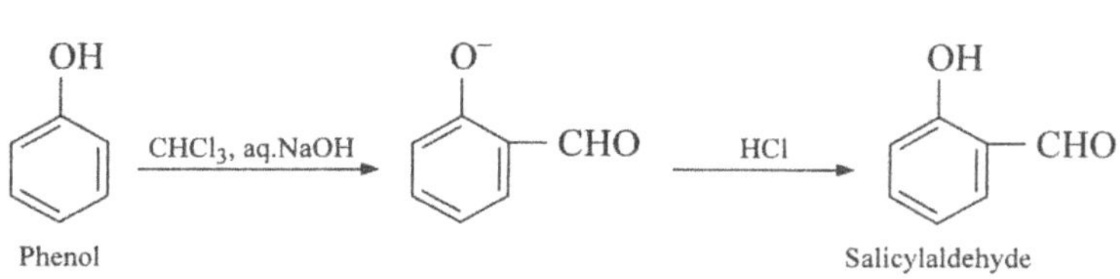

Mechanism This reaction involves electrophilic substitution. Substitution takes place on the highly reactive phenoxide ring. The electrophilic reagent is dichloro carbene ($:CCl_2$) which is generated from $CHCl_3$ by the action of base. Although $:CCl_2$ is neutral, it is strongly electrophilic because the carbon atom is with six electrons.

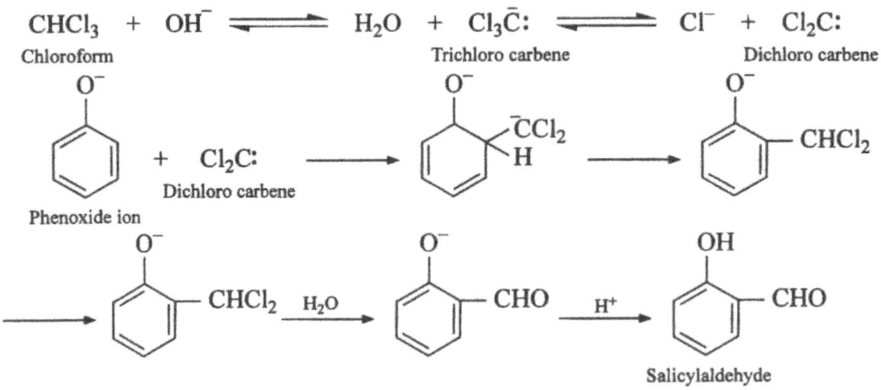

(vii) *Reaction with formaldehyde* Phenols react with formaldehyde to form polymeric substances known as phenol formaldehyde resins. For example, when phenol is reacted with formaldehyde in presence of acid or alkali, a resinous polymer, called bakelite, is obtained.

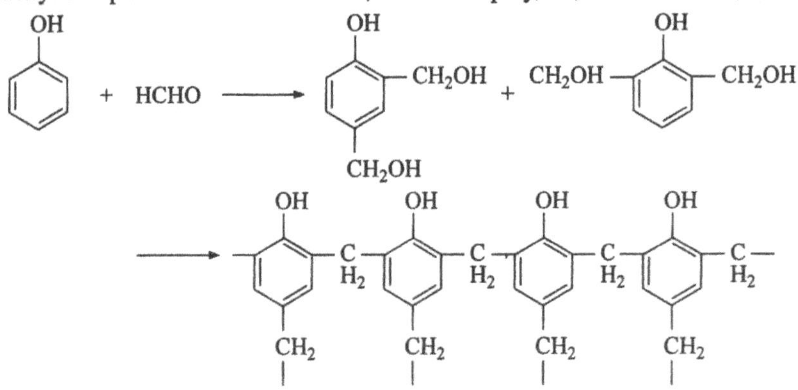

Bakelites (Phenol-formaldehyde resin)

23.5 PHARMACEUTICAL COMPOUNDS

1. *Phenol* Phenol was introduced by Sir Joseph Lister, in 1867, as an antiseptic.

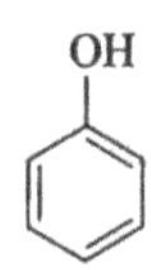

Phenol

Phenol occurs as a colourless to pale pink crystalline solid. It is slightly soluble in water but freely soluble in alcohol, menthol and salol.

Uses

1. Phenol is a good antiseptic and disinfectant against a wide range of microorganisms and viruses.
2. Liquid phenol is used in dentistry and as an analgesic in 5% solution to descensitise the pulp of deciduous teeth.

2. ***Cresol*** It is a mixture of ortho, meta and para isomers of methyl phenol obtained from coal tar. It occurs as colourless or pale brownish yellow colour liquid. It is miscible with water.

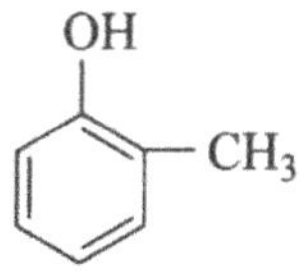

o-Cresol

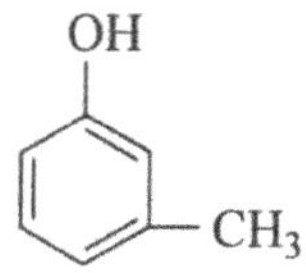

m-Cresol

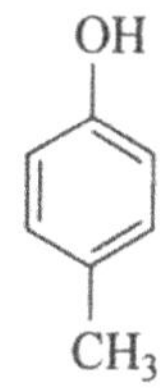

p-Cresol

Uses

1. Cresol exhibits bactericidal activity.
2. Cresol is used to prepare cresol with soap solution (lysol) which is used as a disinfectant in hospitals and homes.

3. ***Thymol*** Thymol is a phenol. It is available from the volatile oils of *Thymus vulgaris* and *Trachspermum ammi*. Chemically, thymol is 2-isopropyl-5-methyl phenol.

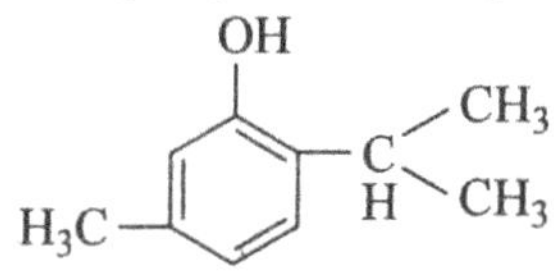

Thymol

Thymol is available as colourless crystalline compound with a pungent odour. It has pungent taste. Thymol is insoluble in water but soluble in organic solvents like alcohol, solvent ether and chloroform.

4. ***Vanillin*** Vanillin is 4-hydroxy-3-methoxy benzaldehyde. It is the active constituent of *Vanilla Planifolia* or other species of *Vanilla*. Vanillin can be synthesised from guaiacol by Reimer-Tiemann reaction.

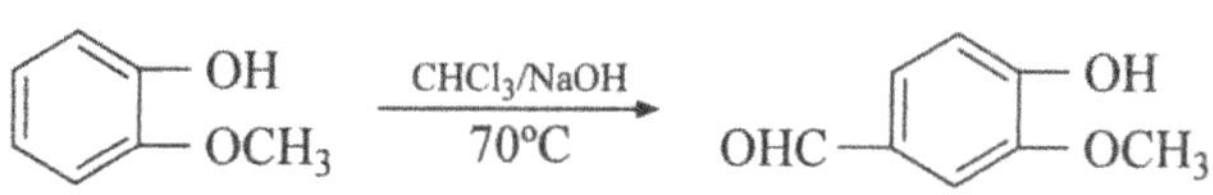

Vanillin is available as colourless or cream-coloured needle-like crystals or powder. It melts at 81°C. The odour and taste of Vanillin are characteristic of Vanilla. It is soluble in 100 parts of water, freely soluble in alcohol, fixed oils and volatile oils.

Use Vanillin is used as a flavouring agent.

5. ***Chlorocresol*** Chlorocresol is a chlorine derivative of phenol. Chemically, chlorocresol is 4-chloro-3-methyl phenol.

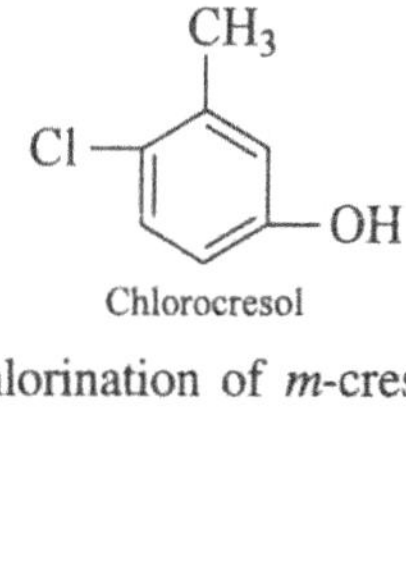

Chlorocresol

Chlorocresol is prepared by chlorination of *m*-cresol.

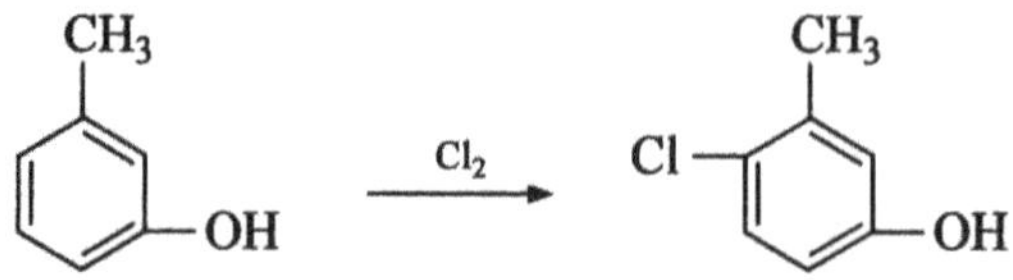

m-Cresol Chlorocresol

Chlorocresol is a colourless crystalline solid and has a characteristic odour. It is slightly soluble in cold water, more soluble in hot water. Chlorocresol is soluble in alcohol, solvent ether, fixed oils and volatile oil.

Uses

1. Chlorocresol is a potent disinfectant against gram positive and gram negative organisms.
2. It is used as preservative for the external preparations.

6. ***Chloroxylenol*** Chloroxylenol is a chlorine derivative of phenol. Chemically, chloroxylenol is 4-chloro-3,5-xylenol.

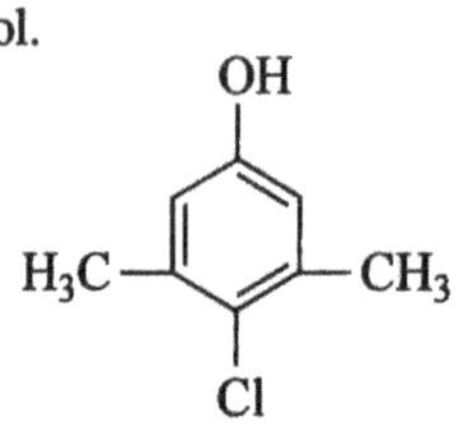

Chloroxylenol

Chloroxylenol is prepared by the reaction of 3,5-xylenol with sulphonyl chloride.

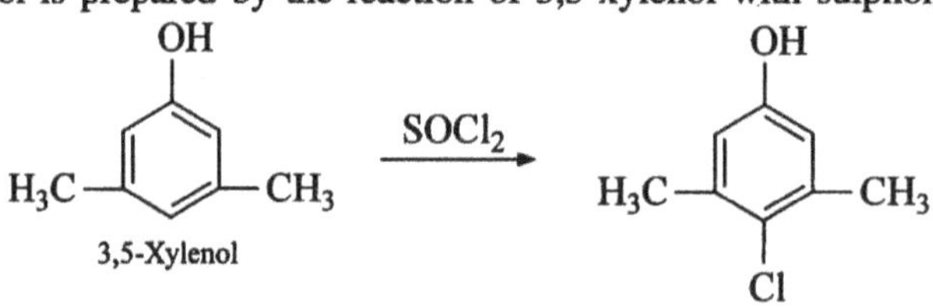

3,5-Xylenol Chloroxylenol

Chloroxylenol is available as colourless or cream coloured crystalline powder. It has a characteristic odour and volatile in steam. Chloroxylenol is insoluble in normal water but more soluble in hot water. It is soluble in alcohol, solvent ether, benzene and fixed oils.

Uses

1. Chloroxylenol is used as an antiseptic agent against gram negative bacteria.
2. Chloroxylenol is used for the treatment of skin wounds and other topical infections.

7. ***Butylated Hydroxyanisole (BHA)*** Butylated hydroxyanisole (BHA) is a derivative of phenol. Chemically, it is 2-*tert*-butyl-4-methoxyphenol.

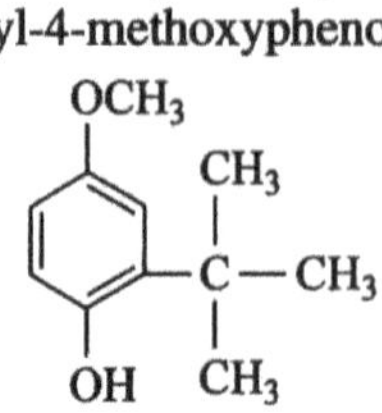

Butylated hydroxyanisole is prepared from hydroquinone by methylation with dimethylsulphate, followed by butylation with 2-methyl propene.

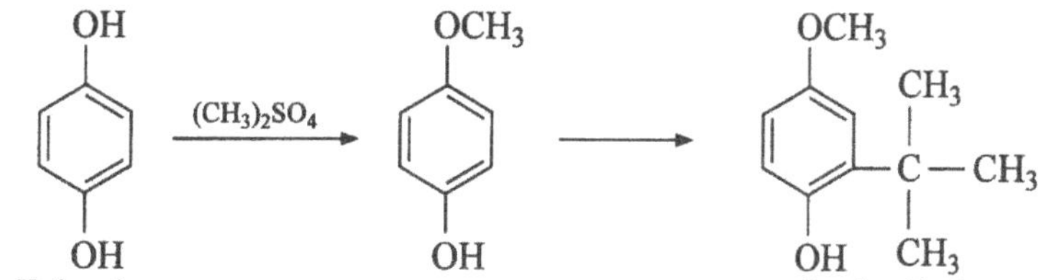

Hydroquinone   Butylated hydroxyanisole

BHA is a colourless, crystalline, water-insoluble powder. It is freely soluble in alcohol, chloroform and ether.

Uses

1. Butylated hydroxyanisole is used as an antioxidant in pharmaceuticals containing fats and oils.
2. BHA is an antioxidant which inhibits oxidation of pharmaceutical products.
3. BHA is also employed in cosmetics and foods.

8. ***Paracetamol (Acetaminophen)*** Paracetamol is a para acetamidophenol derivative. Chemically, paracetamol is 4-hydroxyacetanilide.

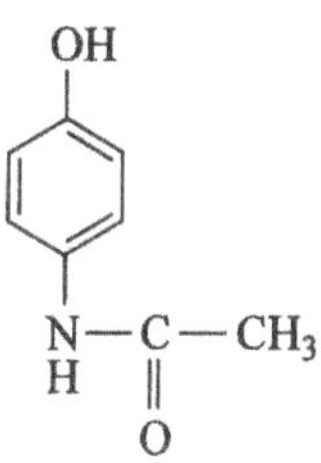

Paracetamol

Preparation of paracetamol involves treating an amine (*p*-aminophenol) with an acid anhydride (acetic anhydride) to form an amide (*p*-acetamidophenol).

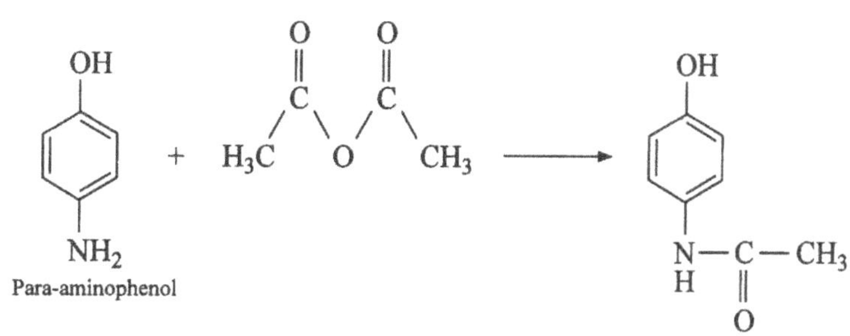

Para-aminophenol   Paracetamol

Paracetamol is colourless, odourless, bitter to taste, crystalline powder. It is insoluble in alkali hydroxides, alcohol and acetone but slightly soluble in water.

Uses

1. Paracetamol is used as antipyretic.
2. Paracetamol has anti-inflammatory activity.
3. It is also used for the treatment of headache, toothache, rheumatism and neuralgia.

9. ***Sodium Amino Salicylate*** Sodium amino salicylate is a sodium salt of 4-amino salicylic acid.

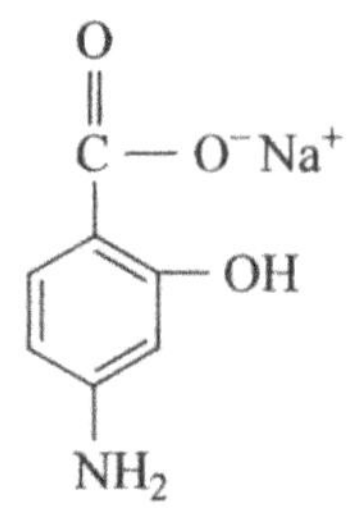

Sodium amino salicylate is available as yellowish-white power or crystalline solid. It is freely soluble in water at *pH* 7.0 (neutral).

Synthesis Sodium amino salicylate is a sodium salt of 4-amino-2-hydroxy benzoic acid. Aminosalicylic acid is prepared from *m*-aminophenol by the following Kolbe-Schmidt reaction:

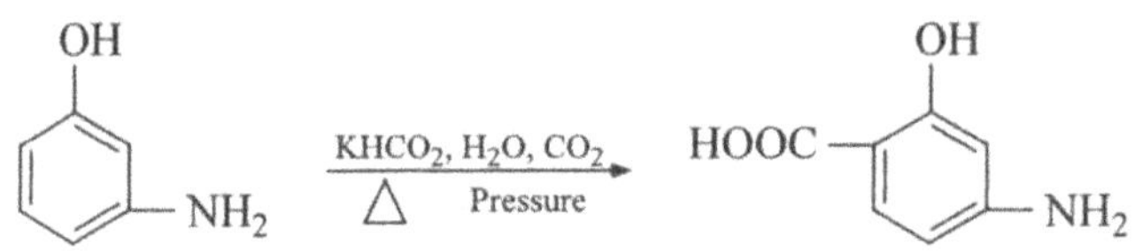

Use Sodium aminosalicylate exhibits good antitubercular action.

PRACTICE QUESTIONS

1. Describe the general methods for the preparation of phenols. Explain why phenol is more acidic than benzyl alcohol. Discuss the chemistry involved in the conversion of phenol into
   (a) salicylaldehyde
   (b) salicylic acid
   (c) anisole
   (d) picric acid
2. Account for the following:
   (a) Why alcohols are weaker acids but stronger nucleophiles than phenols?
   (b) 'Phenols are less acidic than carboxylic acids.'
   (c) Phenol forms 2,4,6-tribromophenol with bromine water, but gives only *o*-bromophenol or *p*-bromophenol with bromine in carbon tetrachloride.
3. (a) Give two methods of preparation of phenols. Account for its acidity.
   (b) Formulate the reactions of phenol with each one of the following reagents.
      (i) Bromine water
      (ii) Dilute nitric acid
      (iii) Benzene diazonium chloride
      (iv) Benzoyl chloride/NaOH

4. How can phenol be made from benzene? Compare and contrast the preparation of phenol and ethanol.
5. Name the reagents and explain the chemistry involved in the following conversions:
   (a) phenol to paracetamol
   (b) Phenol to salicylic acid
6. How is phenol prepared by Dow process? Comment on the reactivity of the above reactions.
7. 'Phenols are more acidic than alcohols and less acidic than carboxylic acids.' Justify the statements.
8. Write short notes on:
   (a) Fries rearrangement
   (b) Kolbe synthesis
9. Give the mechanism of Fries rearrangement and describe its application with respect to any two medicinally useful compounds.

24

CHEMISTRY OF AMINES

24.1 INTRODUCTION

Amines are derivatives of ammonia in which one, two or three of the hydrogen atoms have been replaced by alkyl or aryl groups. Amines are an important class of organic compounds. Many important drugs are amines, the bases present in RNA and DNA are amines, and the fundamental building blocks of proteins are amino acids.

The functional group of an amine is the nitrogen atom connected by three sigma bonds to alkyl groups or aryl groups or hydrogen atoms. The nitrogen atom of an amine can also be included in a ring (heterocycles).

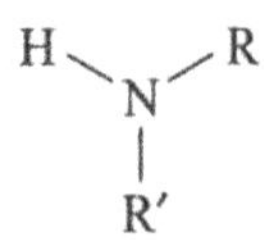

Amine

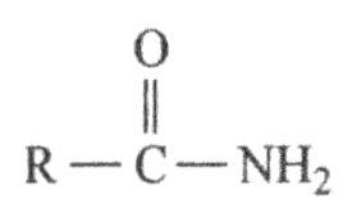

Amide

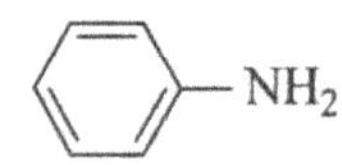

Arylamine

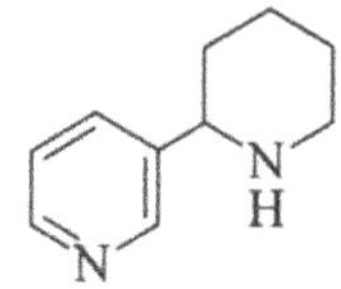

Heterocyclic amine (Nicotine)

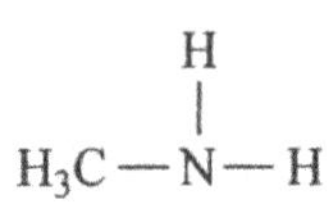

Methyl amine

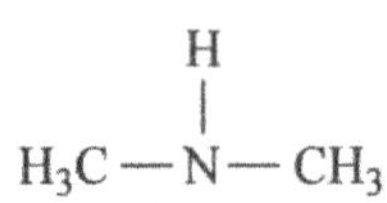

Dimethyl amine

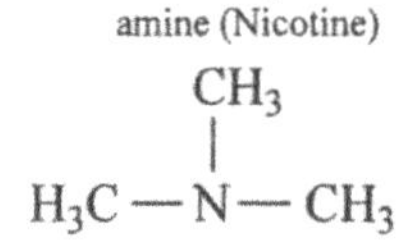

Trimethyl amine

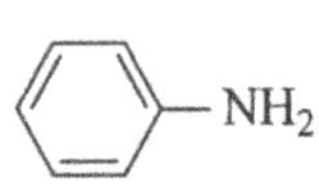

Aniline

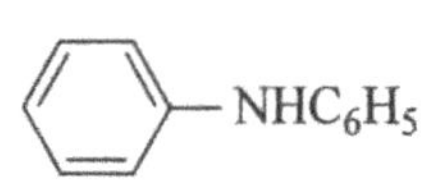

Diphenyl amine

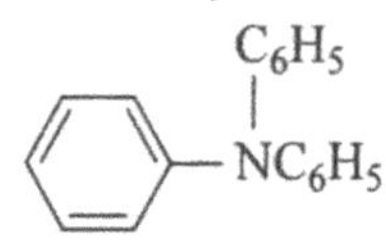

Triphenyl amine

24.2 BONDING IN AMINES

Now, let us look at the bonding around the nitrogen atom of an amine. The nitrogen, in addition to forming three sigma bonds, also carries an unshared electron pair. This means that there are four groups of electrons associated with the nitrogen. Mutual repulsion of these groups leads to a tetrahedral arrangement, much like that of a typical sp^3 carbon

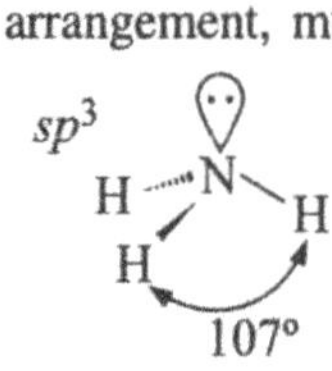

atom. This predicts a bond angle between the N—H bonds of 109.5°, which agrees pretty well with the observed value of 107°, found in ammonia.

Since the bonds connected to the nitrogen are shaped like a flattened pyramid, the arrangement is often called pyramidal. This ignores the unshared electron pair, whose inclusion leads to the tetrahedral description and the corresponding understanding of sp^3 hybridisation in nitrogen. The example used to illustrate this is ammonia, but the nitrogen is also well described as having sp^3 hybridisation in primary, secondary and tertiary amines as well. The N—H bond is more polar than the C—H bond and less polar than the O—H bond. This polarity shows up in a comparison of physical properties of amines and alcohols.

24.3 CLASSIFICATION OF AMINES

The amines are classified as aliphatic and aromatic amines. Each subclass of amines is further subdivided as primary, secondary or tertiary according to the number of carbons bonded directly to the nitrogen atom. Primary amines have one carbon bonded to the nitrogen while secondary amines have two carbons bonded to the nitrogen, and tertiary amines have three carbons bonded to the nitrogen.

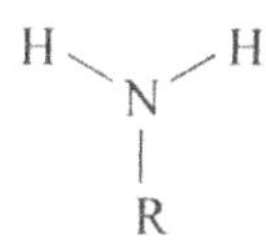
Primary amine

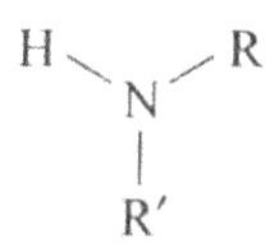
Secondary amine
(General formula)

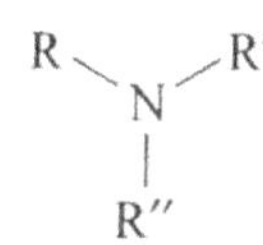
Tertiary amine

24.4 NOMENCLATURE OF AMINES

(a) Amines are commonly named as alkyl amines. Name the alkyl group attached to nitrogen and add the suffix (-amine) as one word. If more than one alkyl group is present, list them in alphabetical order.

(b) If the amine is quaternary, indicate the substituent groups and attach the suffix (-ammonium) and the name of the anion.

$CH_3-CH_2-NH_2$
Ethylamine

$CH_3-CH_2-NH-CH_2-CH_3$
Diethylamine

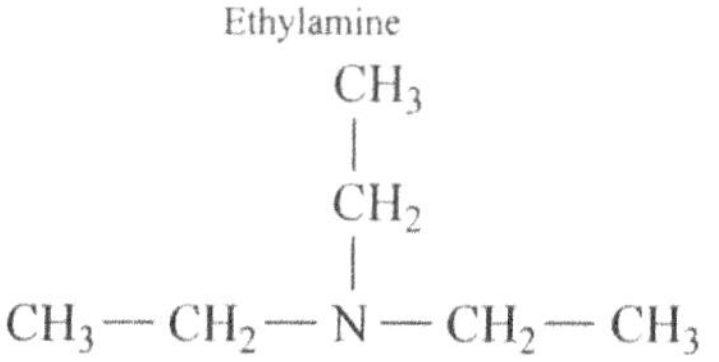
Triethylamine

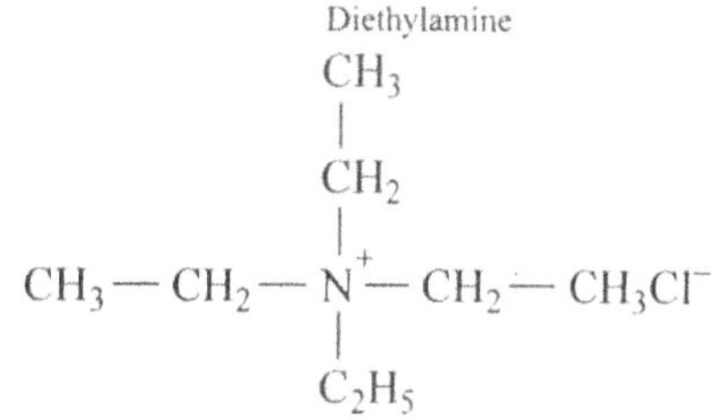
Tetraethyl ammoniumchloride

(c) If the amine group is attached to a group that does not have a simple alkyl name, the amine group as a substituent and indicate it with an amino- prefix and give it a number. If another alkyl group is attached to the amine group designate with an -N prefix.

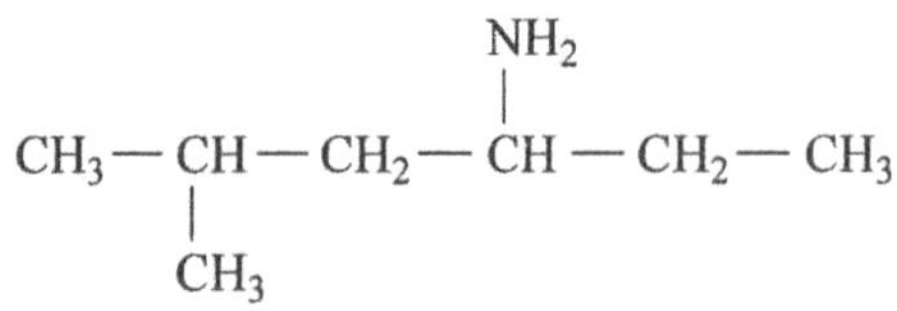

3-Amino-5-methyl hexane

24.4.1 IUPAC Nomenclature of Amines

(i) *Identify the parent hydrocarbon* Find the longest continuous chain of carbon atoms containing the amine group. Change the (-e) ending of the parent alkane to (-amine).

$CH_3-CH_2-CH_2-NH_2$

Propanamine

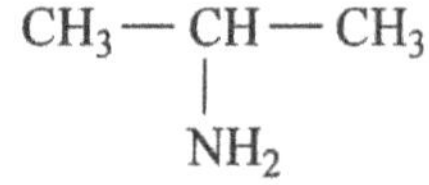

2-Propanamine

(ii) *Number the parent chain and name each substituent* Number the parent chain starting from the end nearest the first branch. Name and number any other substituents and attach them as a prefix to the parent name. Substituents attached to nitrogen are designated by the prefix -N.

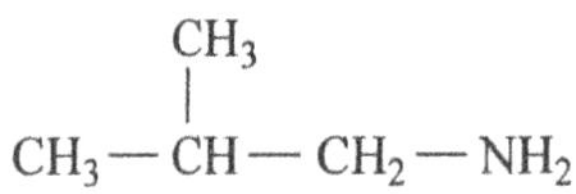

2-Methyl-1-propanamine

$CH_3-CH_2-CH_2-NH-CH_3$

N-Methylpropanamine

(iii) The IUPAC names of simple aromatic amines are based on the parent compound aniline.

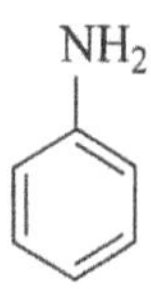

Aniline

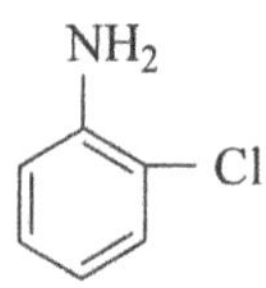

2-Chloroaniline

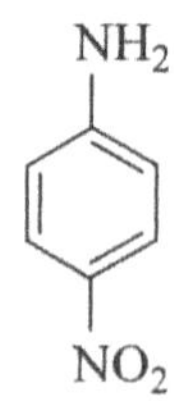

4-Nitroaniline

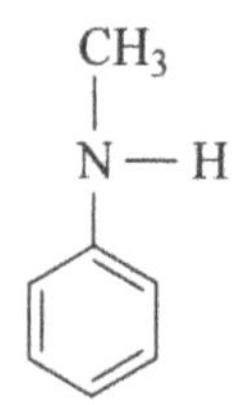

N-Methylaniline

24.5 PREPARATION OF AMINES

The following methods are used to prepare amines.

1. ***From Alkyl Halides*** In this method, an alkyl halide is treated with aqueous or alcoholic solution of ammonia or an amine to yield a primary or secondary or tertiary amine. The reaction is usually carried out either at room temperature or by heating under pressure (Hofmann's method). By this method 1°, 2° or 3° aliphatic amines are prepared.

$$NH_3 \xrightarrow[-HX]{R-X} \underset{\text{Primary amine}}{R-NH_2} \xrightarrow[-HX]{R'-X} \underset{\text{Secondary amine}}{R-NH-R'} \xrightarrow{R''-X} \underset{\text{Tertiary amine}}{R-N(R'')-R'}$$

$$CH_3(CH_2)_6CH_2Br \xrightarrow{NH_3} \underset{(45\%)}{CH_3(CH_2)_6CH_2NH_2} + \underset{(43\%)}{CH_3(CH_2)_6CH_2NHCH_2(CH_2)_6CH_3}$$

2. ***Gabriel's Synthesis*** Potassium phthalimide, on heating with alkyl or aryl halides gives N-substituted phthalimide. This on hydrolysis yields phthalic acid and a primary amine by heating with 20% HCl under pressure.

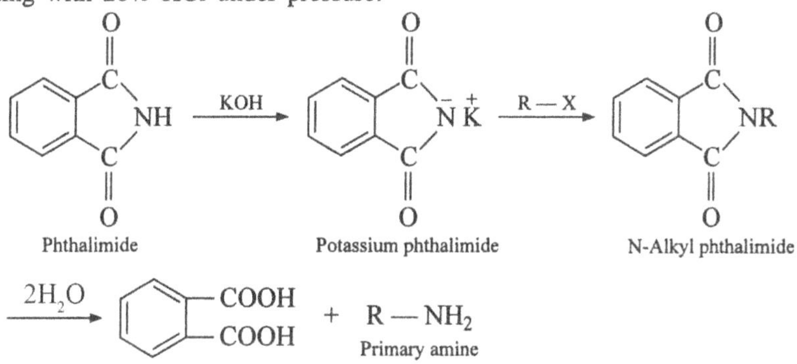

3. ***Reduction of Nitriles*** Aliphatic amines can be obtained conveniently by the reduction of nitriles in presence of catalytic reducing agents or chemical reducing agents.

$$\underset{\text{Alkyl nitrile}}{R-C\equiv N} \xrightarrow{\text{Hydrogen, Ni}} \underset{\text{Primary amine}}{R-CH_2NH_2}$$

$$\underset{n\text{-Propyl nitrile}}{CH_3CH_2CH_2CN} \xrightarrow{\text{Hydrogen, Ni}} \underset{n\text{-Butylamine}}{CH_3CH_2CH_2CH_2NH_2}$$

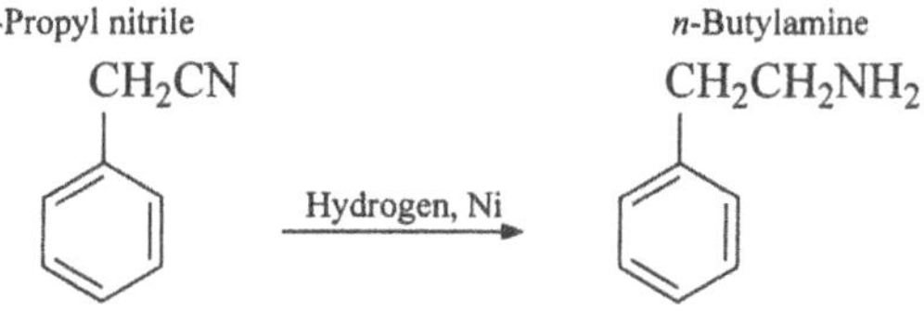

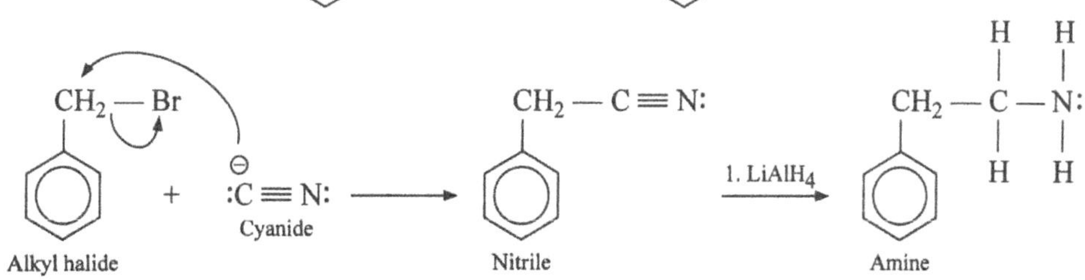

4. ***Reductive Amination (from carbonyl Compounds)*** Aldehydes and ketones by catalytic reduction (H_2, Ni or Pt or Pd) or chemical reduction ($NaBH_3CN$ or $LiBH_3CN$) in presence of ammonia or an amine convert to amines. This process is called reductive amination. Primary, secondary and tertiary amines can be prepared by this process.

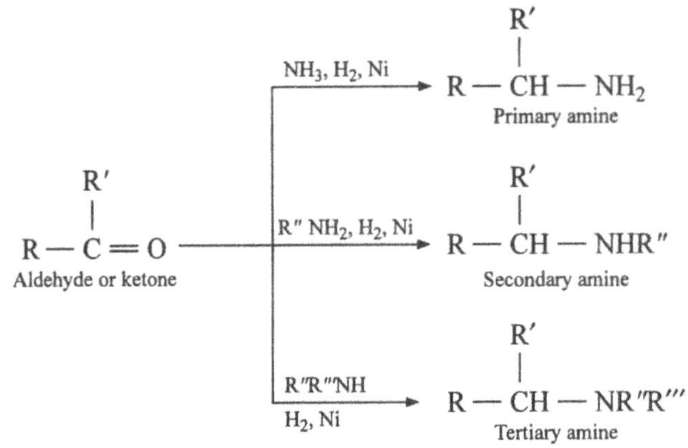

Mechanism

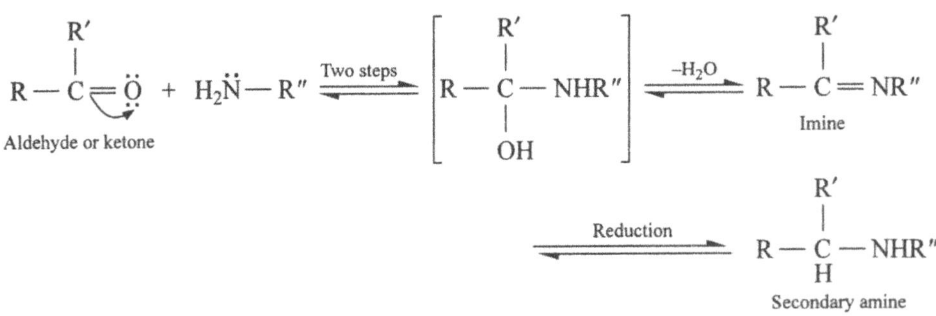

5. ***Reduction of Nitro Compounds*** The nitro group can easily be reduced to an amino group either by catalytic hydrogenation or by chemical reduction. This method is very important to prepare primary aromatic amines.

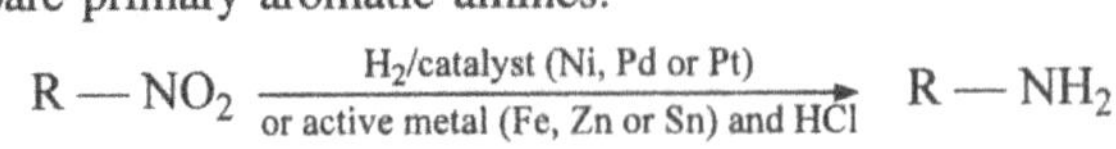

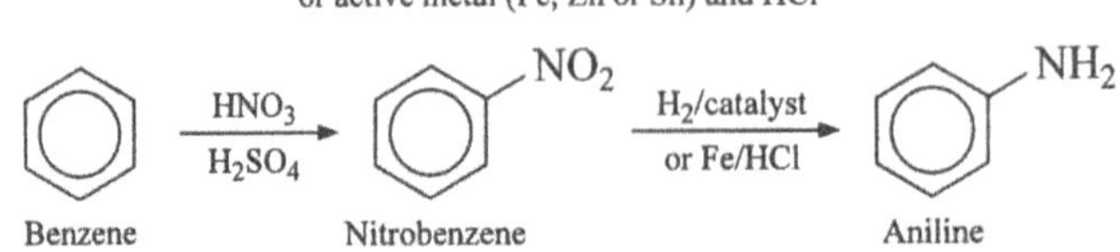

An important application of this reaction is to change the directive effects of the aromatic groups. Reduction changes the meta-directing, deactivating nitro group into the ortho-, para-directing, activating amine group. Thus, changing the sequence of reactions can lead to either *m*-chloroaniline or a mixture of *o*- and *p*-chloroaniline.

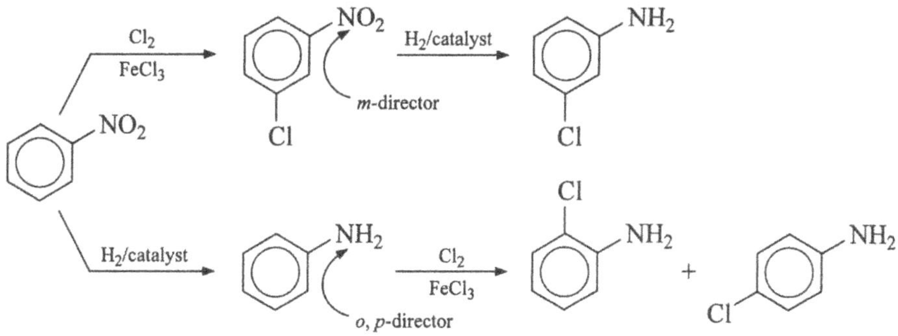

6. ***Reduction of Amides*** Amides can be reduced to amines in presence of lithium aluminium hydride followed by aqueous acid. Amides are prepared by reaction of an amine with an acid chloride or anhydride.

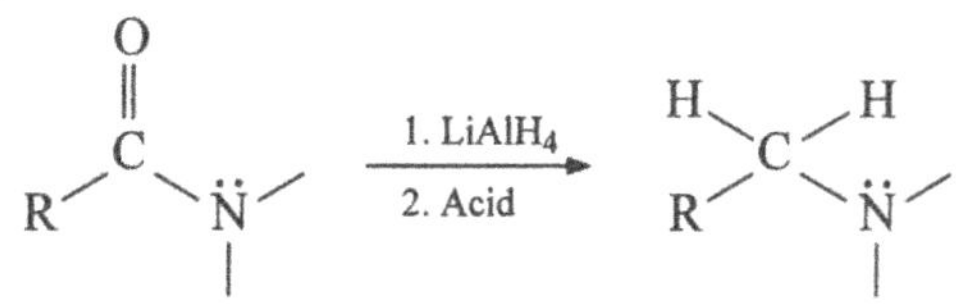

Amide Amine

The following scheme shows the synthesis of benzylamine from benzoyl chloride and ammonia.

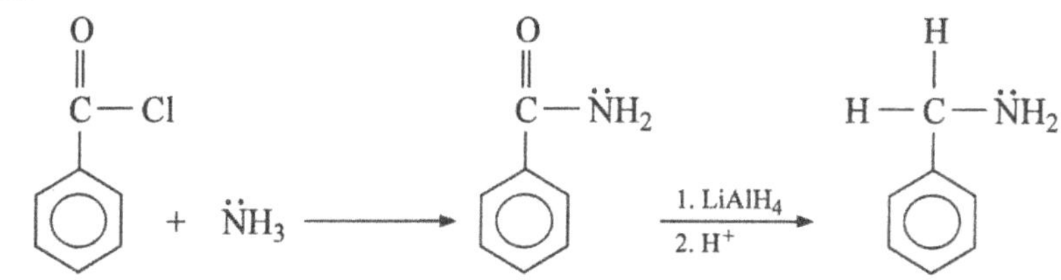

Acid chloride Amide Amine

7. ***Hofmann Degradation of Amides*** Amides, on treatment with bromine or chlorine in presence of alkaline solution, give amines containing one carbon less than the parent amide. This reaction is known as Hofmann degradation of amides.

$$\underset{\text{Amide}}{RCONH_2} + Br_2 + 4KOH \longrightarrow \underset{\text{Amine}}{RNH_2} + 2KBr + K_2CO_3 + 2H_2O$$

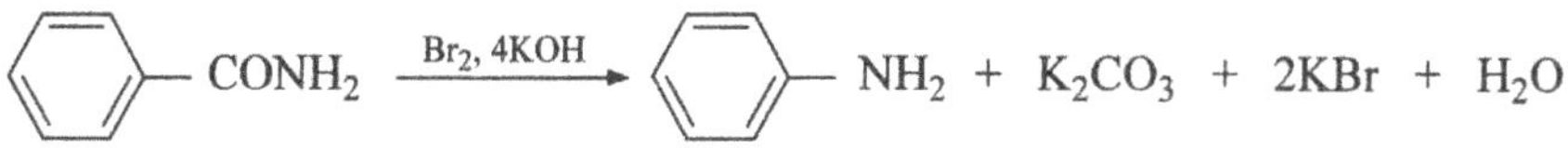

Benzamide Aniline

Mechanism The reaction involves rearrangement of the structure. The hypobromite ion produced by the reaction between bromine and alkali attacks the amide to give amine containing one carbon less than starting amide. The mechanism involves the following steps:

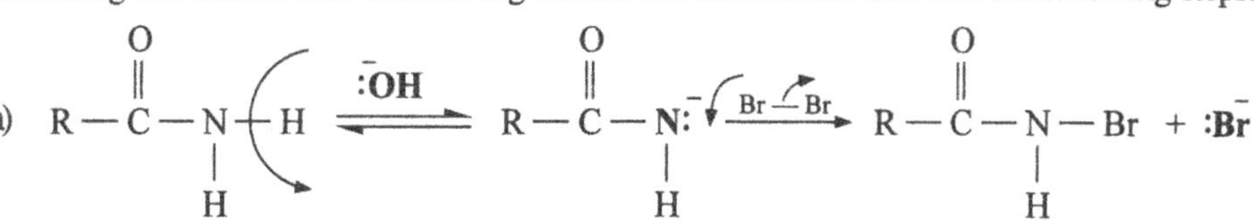

Amide N-Bromo amide

(b) 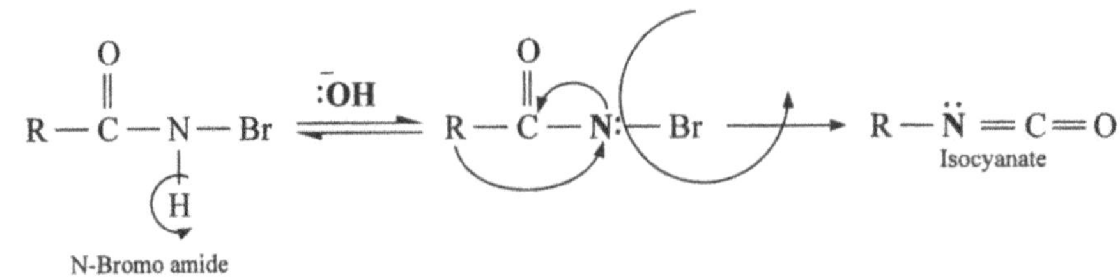

(c) $R-\ddot{N}=C=O + :\bar{O}H \xrightarrow{H_2O} R-NH_2 + CO_3^{--}$

Isocyanate — Amine

24.6 PHYSICAL PROPERTIES OF AMINES

1. Lower amines are gases, higher amines are liquids and the aromatic amines are either liquids or low-melting solids.
2. Amines are basic compounds with strong odours. The odour of amines is often described as 'fishy' since the odour of raw fish comes from the amines contained. Sometimes even 'foul smelling' is an understatement, and two of the amines produced in decaying flesh have suggestive names (cadaverine and putresine).
3. Pure amines are colourless but on exposure to air they get coloured by oxidation with air.
4. Amines form intermolecular hydrogen bonding except tertiary amines hence the lower amines have high boiling points and high solubility in water.

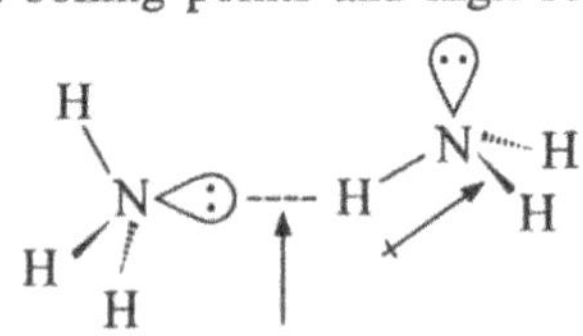

Hydrogen bond

5. The amines are essential to life as constituents of amino acids. They occur in drugs and vitamins, and are essential starting materials for many synthetic processes. The aromatic amine, aniline, is the basis for the synthesis of a whole class of synthetic dyes. Synthetic amines, such as benzedrine, have medical applications.

24.7 CHEMICAL PROPERTIES OF AMINES

1. ***Basicity of Amines*** The distinguishing chemical property of amines is that they are bases like ammonia. This is because of the presence of the unshared electron pair on the nitrogen, which makes them Lewis bases. The basic unshared electron pair is less tightly held by the nitrogen of an amine than the corresponding oxygen of an alcohol, which makes it more available to act as a base. Consequently, amines (and ammonia) are more basic than alcohols (and water), and less basic than alkoxide (RO^-) and hydroxide (OH^-) ions. The basicity of amines is explained by K_b, i.e. the basicity constant. The greater the value of K_b, the greater the basicity of amine. However, pK_a is a generalised method to express the strength of both bases and acids. The high pK_a value represents a strong base.

$$\ddot{N}H_3 + H_2O \rightleftharpoons NH_4^{\oplus} + OH^{\ominus}$$

$$K_b = \frac{[NH_4^{\oplus}][OH^{\ominus}]}{[NH_3]}$$

Basicity of Amines

Amine	*Structure*	K_b
Ammonia	$\ddot{N}H_3$	1.8×10^{-5}
Cyclohexylamine	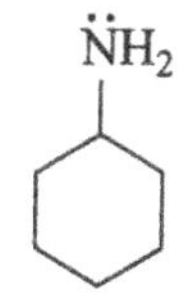	4.7×10^{-4}
Aniline	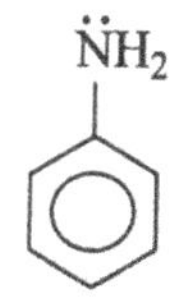	4.0×10^{-10}

(i) *Relative basicity of amines* The relative basicity of amines is determined by the electron density of the amine nitrogen. Groups that increase the electron density, such as alkyl groups, make the nitrogen more basic. Electron-withdrawing groups decrease the electron density and render the nitrogen less basic. As such, any factor that can increase the availability of electron pair on nitrogen, increases the basicity. On the other hand, any factor that has the opposite effect decreases the basicity.

(ii) *Effect of alkyl groups* Cyclohexyl amine is more basic than ammonia because alkyl groups are electron-donating, thereby increasing the electron density of the nitrogen. A secondary amine is more basic than a primary amine because it has two alkyl groups that donate electrons inductively to the nitrogen atom. The tertiary amine is less basic than the other two. The reason is that a tertiary amine has three alkyl groups, which can donate electrons to the nitrogen atom, but this N atom is stearically hindered for protonation due to the presence of three sizeable alkyl groups. Among the primary, secondary and tertiary aliphatic amines the order of basicity is:

Secondary (2°) amine > Primary (1°) amine > Tertiary (3°) amine

Amine	pK_b
Methyl amine	3.36
Trimethyl amine	4.20
Aniline	9.38

(iii) *Effect of aromatic rings* Aromatic amines are weaker bases than ammonia or aliphatic amines. Aniline is strikingly less basic than cyclohexyl amine because the unshared electrons on nitrogen are delocalised into the aromatic ring.

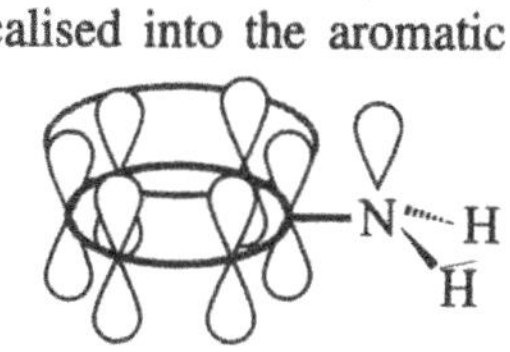

Aniline

Aniline is a resonance hybrid of five contributing structures.

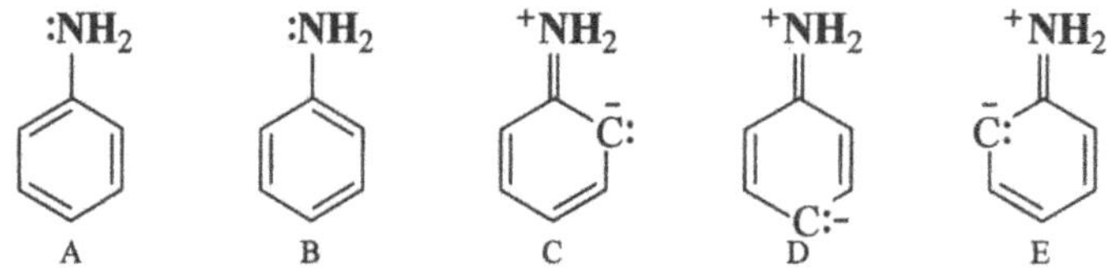

Contributors of aniline

In three of the five contributing structures the electron pair on nitrogen is shared with the aromatic ring. As a result, the electron pair on the nitrogen is less available for sharing with a proton. Aniline is more stabilised by resonance than anilinium ion because anilinium ion has only two contributing structures.

Contributors of Anilinium ion

Thus, aniline is a weaker base than ammonia or aliphatic amine.

Secondary and tertiary aromatic amine are weaker bases than aniline (primary aromatic amine) because the lone pair of electrons on nitrogen of secondary and tertiary amines is delocalised towards benzene rings. Therefore, the order of base strength will be:

Primary aromatic (1°) amine (e.g. aniline) > Secondary aromatic (2°) amine (e.g. diphenylamine) > tertiary aromatic (3°) amine (e.g. triphenylamine)

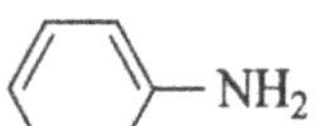

Aniline

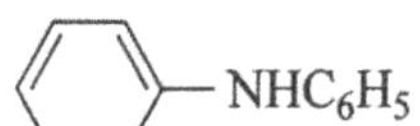

Diphenyl amine

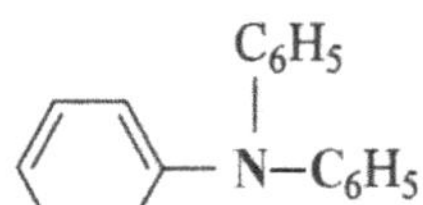

Triphenyl amine

Basicity of aromatic amines is influenced by the substitution in the aromatic nucleus. Electron-releasing groups (e.g —NH_2, —OCH_3, — CH_3) increase basicity by dispersing positive charge of nitrogen and stabilising anilinium ion. The electron-withdrawing groups (e.g. —NO_2, —C = O, —X) decrease basicity as they destabilise the anilinium ion.

2. ***Alkylation*** Primary, secondary and tertiary amines react with alkyl halides to give secondary amines, tertiary amines and quaternary ammonium halides respectively. The starting amine finally changes to a quaternary ammonium halide. These reactions involve nucleophilic attack by the amino group on the positively polarised carbon atom of the alkyl halide.

$$\underset{\text{Primary amine}}{RNH_2} \xrightarrow[-HX]{RX} \underset{\text{Secondary amine}}{R_2NH} \xrightarrow[-HX]{RX} \underset{\text{Tertiary amine}}{R_3N} \xrightarrow[-HX]{RX} \underset{\text{Quaternary ammonium halide}}{[R_4N]^+X^-}$$

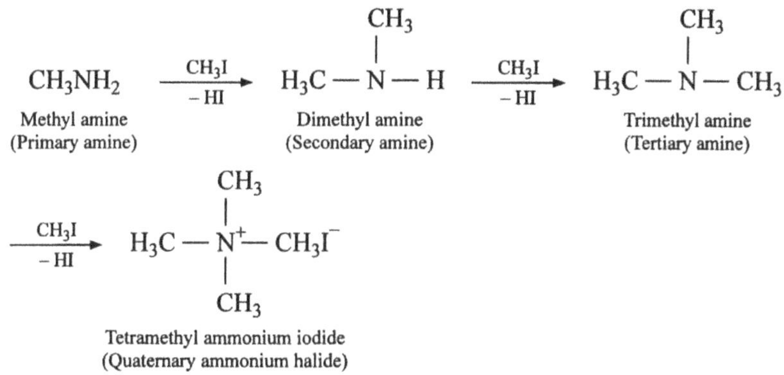

3. ***Acylation*** Primary and secondary amines react with acyl halides or acid anhydrides to form N-substituted amides. Tertiary amines do not react with these acylating agents.

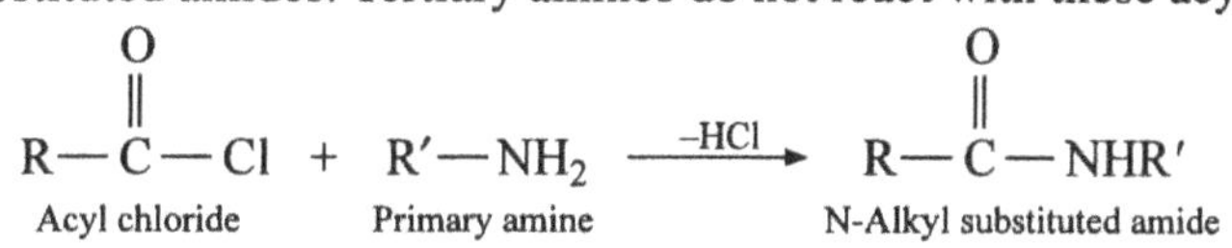

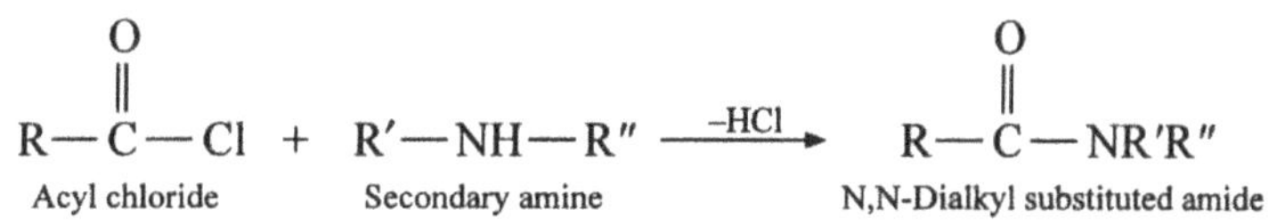

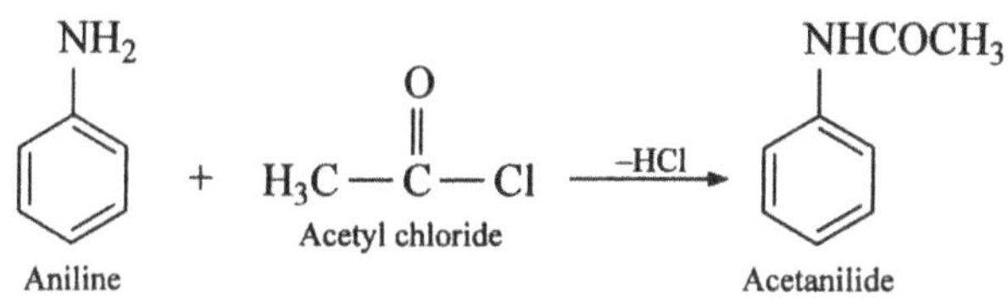

4. ***Reaction of Amines with Nitrous Acid*** The three classes of amines (primary, secondary or tertiary) react differently with nitrous acid. Nitrous acid is a Brønsted acid of moderate strength (pK_a = 3.3). Because it is unstable, it is prepared immediately before use in the following manner:

$$NaNO_2 + H_2SO_4 \xrightarrow{H_2O,\ 0^\circ} H-\ddot{\underset{..}{O}}-\ddot{N}=\ddot{\underset{..}{O}} + NaHSO_4$$

(i) *Primary aromatic amines* react with nitrous acid in the cold to yield diazonium salts. The aromatic diazonium salts are sufficiently stable in cold aqueous solutions to enable them to be used as important intermediates in many synthetic processes.

$$\underset{\text{Aromatic amine}}{ArNH_2} + NaNO_2 + 2HX \longrightarrow \underset{\text{Aromatic diazonium salt}}{ArN_2^+X^-} + NaX + H_2O$$

(ii) *Primary aliphatic amines* also react with cold nitrous acid to yield aliphatic diazonium salts, which are unstable and give a mixture of different products.

$$RNH_2 + NaNO_2 + 2HCl \longrightarrow [R\overset{+}{N}_2]Cl^- \longrightarrow N_2 + \text{Alcohols} + \text{Alkenes} + \text{Alkyl halides}$$

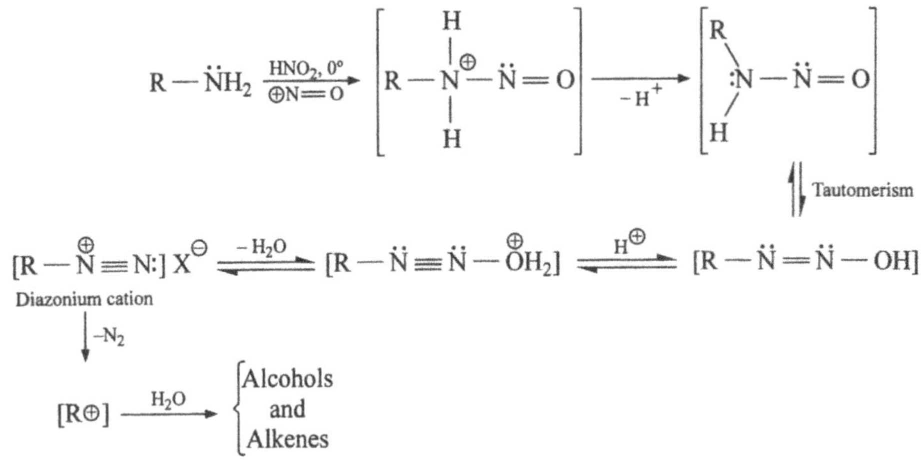

(iii) *Secondary amines (both aliphatic and aromatic)* react with nitrous acid to give N-nitrosamines, which are yellow coloured neutral oily compounds.

$$\underset{\text{Secondary amine}}{R_2NH} + NaNO_2 + HCl \longrightarrow \underset{\text{N-Nitrosamine}}{R_2N-N=O} + NaCl + H_2O$$

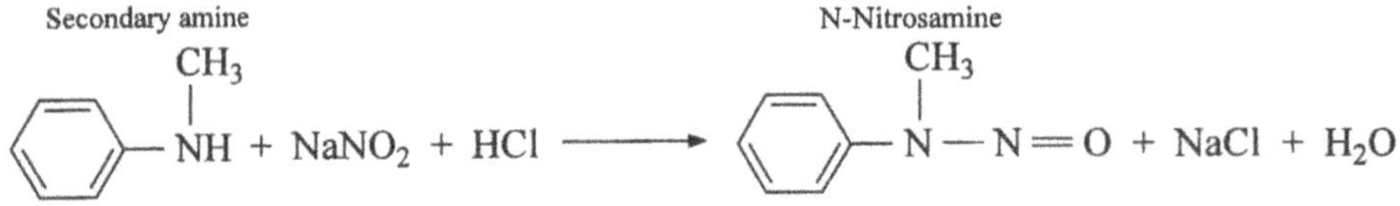

N-Methyl aniline N-Nitroso-N-methyl aniline

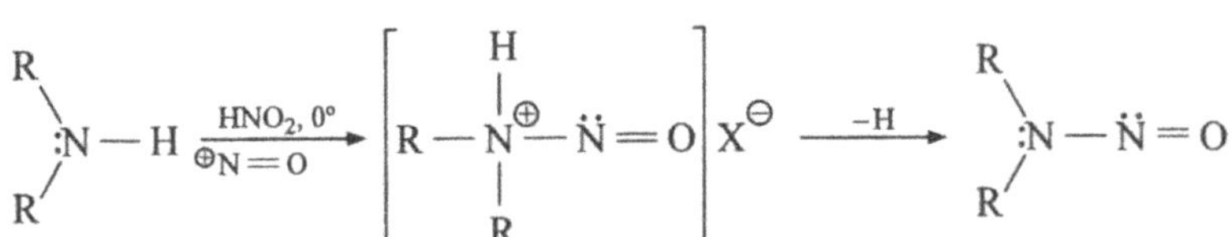

N-Nitrosamine
(A yellow oily liquid)

(iv) *Tertiary aromatic amines* react with nitrous acid to yield ring-substituted product usually the green coloured *p*-nitrosamine.

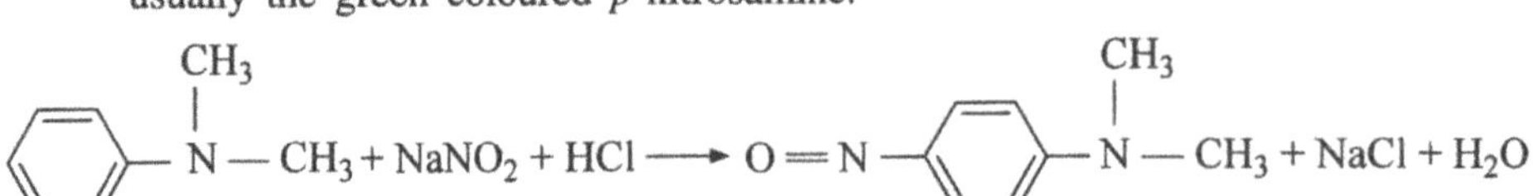

N,N-Dimethyl aniline *p*-Nitroso-N,N-Dimethyl aniline

(v) *Tertiary aliphatic amines* react with nitrous acid only to form water soluble amine salts, trialkyl ammonium nitrites, with no visible change in the appearance of the reacting materials.

$$\underset{\text{Tertiary amine}}{R_3NH} + NaNO_2 + HCl \longrightarrow \underset{\text{Trialkyl ammonium nitrite}}{[R_3NH]^+ NO_2^-} + NaCl$$

5. ***Ring Substitution in Aromatic Amines*** The rings of aromatic amines can undergo electrophilic aromatic substitution reactions, through carbocations as intermediates. In these reactions the —NH_2, —NHR and —NR_2 groups act as strongly activating and ortho, para-directing groups. This is due to presence of the pair of unshared electrons on the nitrogen of

these groups. This donation helps stabilise the intermediate arenium ion. Due to strong activation ring substitution in aromatic amines occurs very rapidly. Often acetylation or benzoylation is carried out to control the rate of electrophilic aromatic substitution of amines.

(i) *Halogenation* Halogenation of aromatic amines proceeds at a very fast rate and all the available ortho and para positions get halogenated even in the absence of a catalyst. To prepare monohalogen derivative, the amino group is deactivated by acetylation. After halogenation, the free amino group is regenerated.

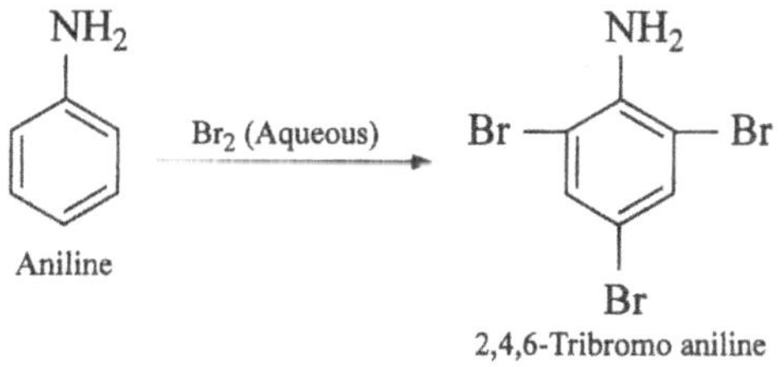

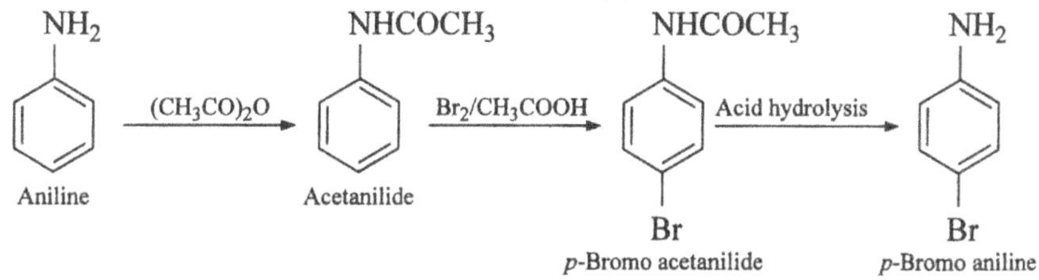

(ii) *Nitration* Direct nitration results in the formation of oxidation products in addition to the desired nitro compounds because nitric acid (of the nitrating mixture) is not only a nitrating agent but also oxidising agent and the highly activated benzene ring can easily get oxidised. In the strongly acidic solution, the amine is converted into the anilinium ion. In the anilinium ion, the nitrogen does not have an unshared pair of electrons but has a positive charge and directs the entering groups to the meta position. Nitration is best carried out using an acetylated amine rather than the free amine.

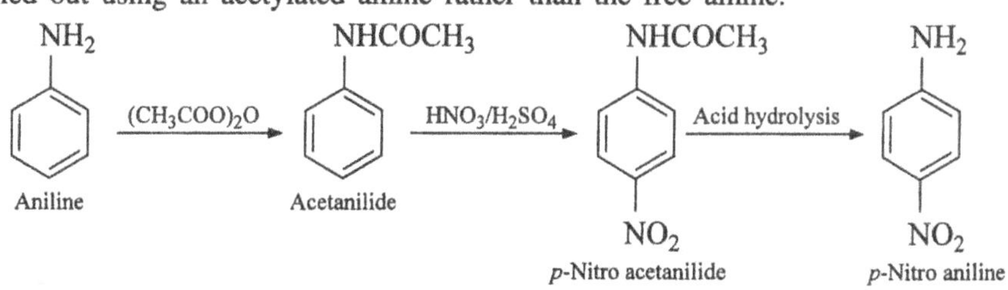

(iii) *Sulphonation* In spite of the strongly activating (amino) group, the sulphonation of aromatic amines takes place under rather drastic conditions. For example, aniline gets sulphonated at 180–90°C with concentrated sulphuric acid.

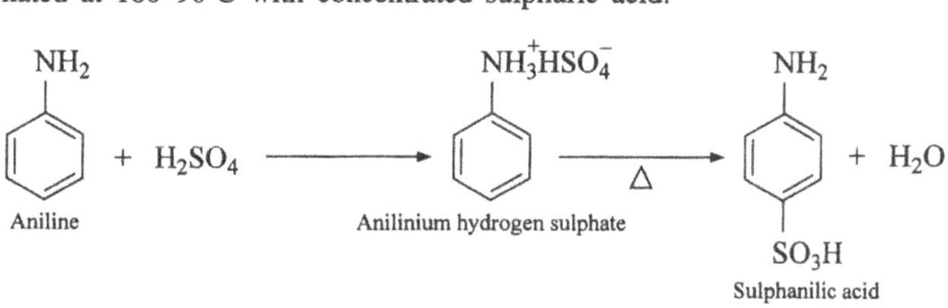

6. ***Reaction with Hinsberg's Reagent (Benzene Sulphonyl Chloride)*** Hinsberg's reagent separates a mixture of primary, secondary and tertiary amines by the following steps:

Step 1 The mixture of amines is treated with benzene sulphonyl chloride and shaken with alkali solution then the three amines behave in different ways.

(i) Primary amine forms alkyl benzene sulphonamide which dissolve in alkali to form sodium or potassium salt of aminoalkyl sulphonamide.

$$\underset{\text{Benzene sulphonyl chloride}}{C_6H_5SO_2Cl} + \underset{\text{Primary amine}}{RNH_2} \longrightarrow \underset{\text{Monoalkyl benzene sulphonamide}}{C_6H_5SO_2NHR} \xrightarrow{KOH} \underset{\text{Potassium salt of benzene sulphonamide}}{C_6H_5SO_2NKR}$$

(ii) Secondary amine forms dialkyl sulphonamide, which does not form salt with alkali and hence remains insoluble in alkali solution.

$$\underset{\text{Benzene sulphonyl chloride}}{C_6H_5SO_2Cl} + \underset{\text{Secondary amine}}{R_2NH} \longrightarrow \underset{\text{Dialkyl benzene sulphonamide}}{C_6H_5SO_2NR_2} \xrightarrow{KOH} \text{No reaction}$$

(iii) Tertiary amine does not react with the Hinsberg reagent.

Step 2 The above alkaline solution is extracted with ether when tertiary amine and dialkyl benzene sulphonamide go to ethereal layer while potassium monoalkyl benzene sulphonamide remains in the aqueous layer. The two layers are then separated. The aqueous layer is acidified with dil. HCl and is followed by heating with conc. hydrochloric acid (HCl) and NaOH to obtain primary amine.

$$C_6H_5SO_2NKR \xrightarrow{\text{Dil. HCl}} C_6H_5SO_2NHR \xrightarrow{H_2O} RNH_2HCl \longrightarrow \underset{\text{Primary amine}}{RNH_2}$$

$$C_6H_5SO_2NR_2 + H_2O \xrightarrow{\text{Con. HCl}} C_6H_5SO_3H + R_2NHHCl \xrightarrow{\text{Distillation}} \underset{\text{Secondary amine}}{R_2NH} + NaCl + H_2O$$

$$\underset{\text{Benzene sulphonyl chloride}}{C_6H_5SO_2Cl} + \underset{\text{Tertiary amine}}{R_3N} \longrightarrow \text{No reaction (Soluble in ether)}$$

To recover the secondary and tertiary amines, the ethereal layer is fractionally distilled. When ether and tertiary amine distills over, it leaves behind the solid dialkyl benzene sulphonamide from which free secondary amine is separated.

7. ***Carbylamine Test*** Warming an alcoholic solution of primary amines (aliphatic or aromatic) with a mixture of alcoholic KOH solution and chloroform to form carbylamines (isocyanides). The carbyl amines have characteristic, unpleasant smell akin to garlic oil by which primary amines can be identified.

$$RNH_2 + CHCl_3 + 3KOH \longrightarrow R{-}NC + 3KCl + H_2O$$

Mechanism

$$CHCl_3 + 3KOH \longrightarrow :CCl_2 + KCl + H_2O$$

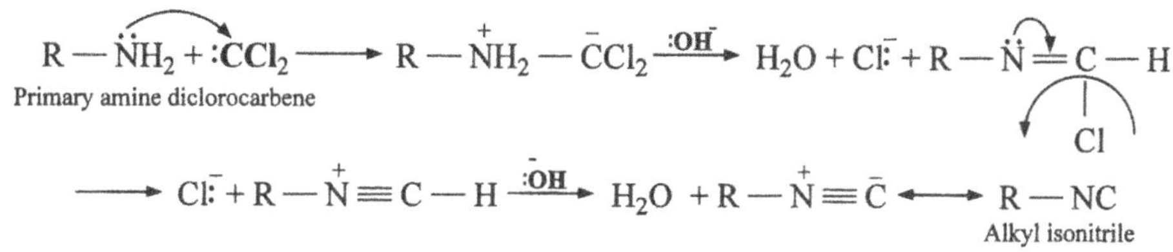

8. ***Mannich Reaction for Amines*** The condensation of an active hydrogen compound (compound capable of forming enol, e.g. acetone) with formaldehyde in presence of a primary or secondary amine is called Mannich reaction in which a hydrogen atom is replaced by an amino alkyl group. The product formed is called Mannich base.

$$C_6H_5.COCH_3 + CH_2O + (CH_3)_2NH:HCl \longrightarrow C_6H_5COCH_2CH_2N(CH_3)_2:HCl$$

The active hydrogen compound may be of an aldehyde, ketone, β-keto ester, nitroalkane or I-alkyne.

Mechanism The Mannich reaction proceeds through the following steps:

In acidic or neutral conditions, the secondary amine first reacts with aldehyde to form an iminium salt, which in the second step is subjected to nucleophilic attack by the active hydrogen compound.

Step 1

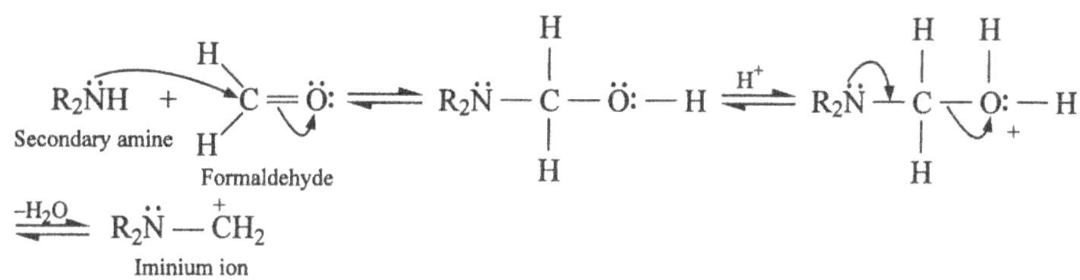

Step 2

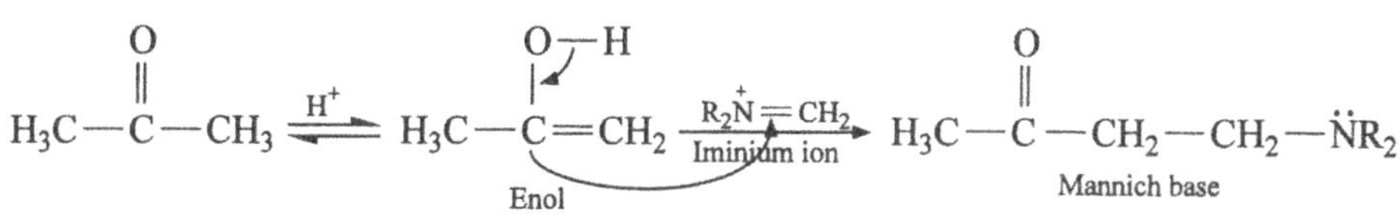

9. ***Reaction with Grignard Reagent*** Primary or secondary aliphatic/aromatic amines react with Grignard reagent and yield alkanes.

$$\underset{\text{Amine}}{RNH_2} + \underset{\text{Grignard reagent}}{R_1MgX} \xrightarrow[\text{THF}]{\text{Ether (or)}} \underset{\text{Alkane}}{R_1H} + RNHMgX$$

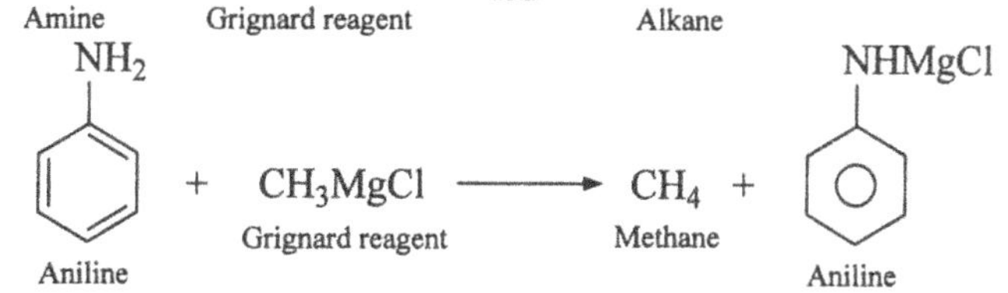

10. ***Reaction with Aldehydes*** Primary aromatic amines react with aldehydes to form Schiff's bases or anils.

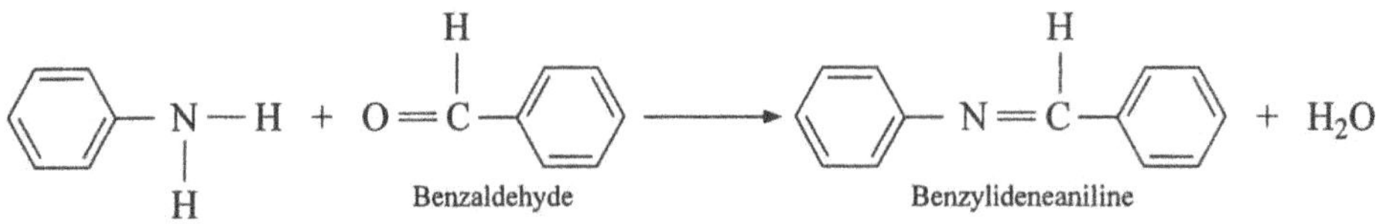

Aniline, Benzaldehyde, Benzylideneaniline

24.8 QUATERNARY AMMONIUM SALTS

Quaternary ammonium salts are tetraalkyl derivatives of ammonium salts. They are obtained by the replacement of all the four hydrogen atoms by alkyl groups. The four alkyl groups may be same or different.

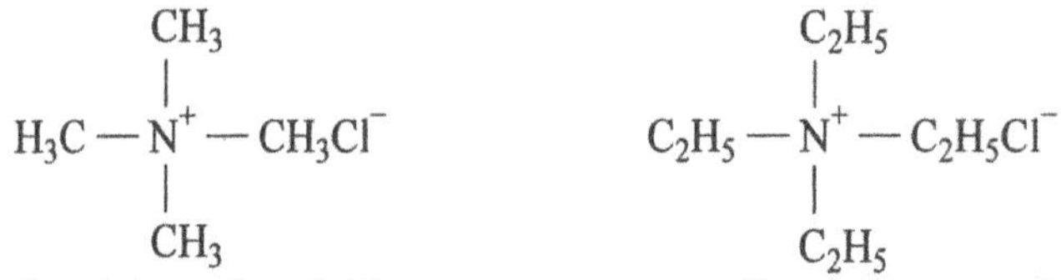

Tetraethylammonium chloride　　　Tetraethylammonium chloride

24.8.1 Preparation

Quaternary ammonium salts are obtained by heating ammonia with excess of alkyl halide in a non-polar solvent like benzene, toluene, xylene, etc.

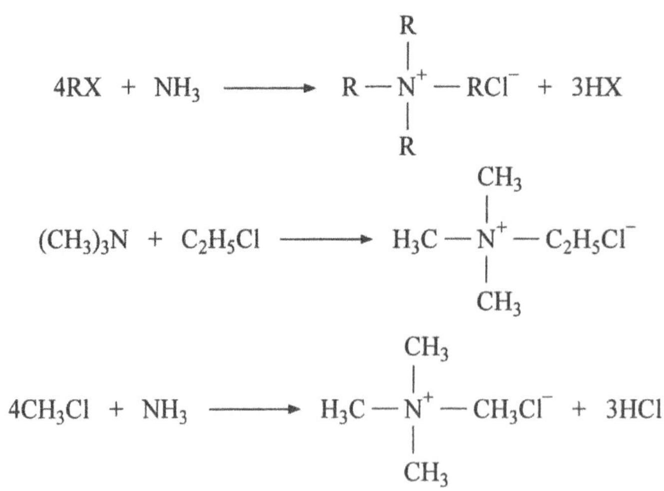

24.8.2 Uses

1. Quaternary ammonium salts have detergent properties, e.g. Cetyl trimethyl ammonium chloride is a detergent.
2. Quaternary ammonium salts have antiseptic and germicidal effects.
3. They stimulate muscles and nerves.

24.9 AROMATIC DIAZONIUM SALTS

24.9.1 Introduction

Aromatic diazonium salts are important aromatic compounds having the general formula $\mathbf{ArN_2^+ X^-}$, where X^- may be an anion such as Cl^-, Br^-, HSO_4^-, NO_3^-, BF_4^-, etc. These compounds contain two nitrogen atoms hence the name diazonium is given. For example,

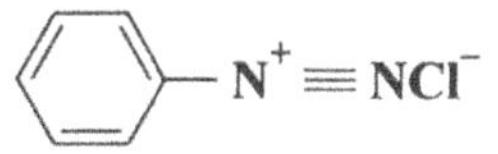

Benzenediazonium chloride

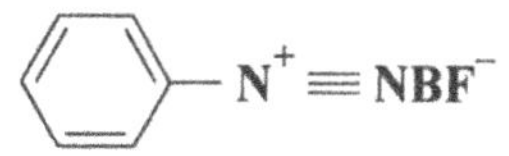

Benzenediazonium fluoroborate

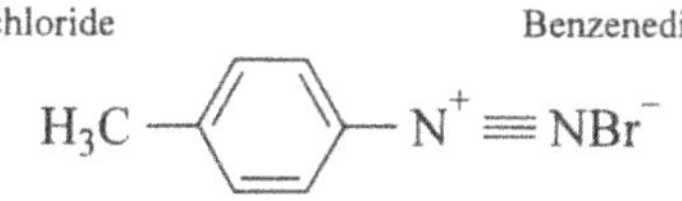

p-Toluenebenzenediazonium bromide

24.9.2 Preparation

Diazonium salts are usually prepared *in situ* by reaction between aromatic primary amine and nitrous acid (obtained *in situ* from $NaNO_2$ + HCl) in cold conditions. This reaction is called diazotisation.

$$ArNH_2 + NaNO_2 + 2HX \longrightarrow Ar\overset{+}{N_2}X^- + NaX + H_2O$$

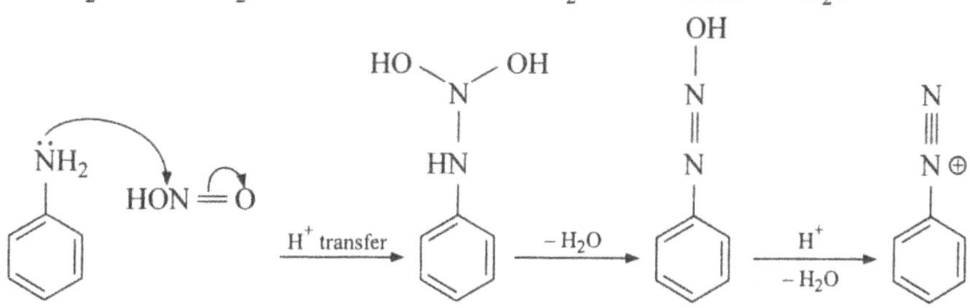

The diazonium salts are prepared by adding well-cooled aqueous solution of sodium nitrite slowly to the cooled solution of aromatic amine in a mineral acid. The addition of sodium nitrite solution is stopped as soon as a few drops of the reaction mixture give blue colour with starch-KI paper. The formation of blue colour indicates the presence of unreacted HNO_2, which is destroyed by adding a small quantity of urea. During the preparation of diazonium salts, the reaction temperature should be maintained between 0°–10°C.

Mechanism of Diazotisation This involves the following steps.

1. *Formation of nitrous acid*

$$NaNO_2 + HCl \rightleftharpoons HO{-}N{=}O + NaCl$$

2. *Protonation of nitrous acid and generation of nitrosonium ion*

$$HO{-}N{=}O \overset{H^+}{\rightleftharpoons} H\overset{H}{\underset{+}{O}}{-}N{=}O \rightleftharpoons O{=}\overset{+}{N}{:} + H_2O$$

3. Nitrosonium ion (electrophile) reacts with nitrogen of amine (due to presence of lone pair of electrons) and leads to formation of N-nitrosamine.

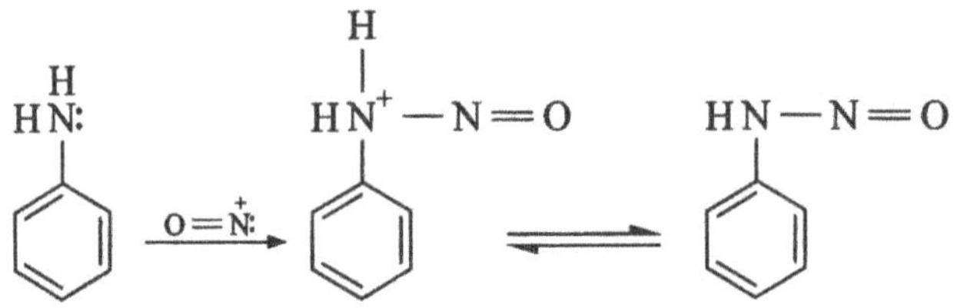

N-Nitrosamine

4. *Formation of diazonium ion from N-nitrosamine*

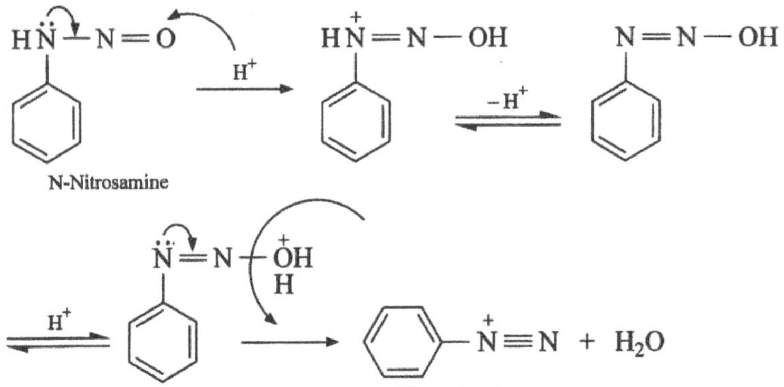

N-Nitrosamine

Diazonium ion

24.9.3 Properties

1. The aromatic diazonium salts such as chloride, bromide, sulphate are water soluble whereas the fluoroborate, naphthalene sulphate, trifluoroacetate are water insoluble. The water-soluble salts ionise and are stable at temperatures below 5°C but decompose above this temperature, losing nitrogen and undergoing reaction with water to form phenols.
2. They also decompose readily in dry state.
3. Diazonium salts are usually colourless, crystalline solids, freely soluble in water. They are highly reactive and are used to prepare many aromatic compounds.
4. The following are chemical reactions of diazonium salts:
   (a) Aryl diazonium salts may be reduced to the corresponding hydrazines by mild reducing agents such as sodium bisulphite, stannous chloride or zinc dust. The bisulphite reduction may proceed by an initial sulphur-nitrogen coupling, as shown in the following equation.

$$Ar-N_2^{(+)}X^{(-)} \xrightarrow{NaHSO_3} Ar-N=N-SO_3H \xrightarrow{NaHSO_3} Ar-NH-NH-SO_3H$$

$$\xrightarrow{H_2O} Ar-NH-NH_2 + H_2SO_4$$

Substitution Reactions Diazonium salts readily undergo substitution of nitrogen with a variety of nucleophilic species. It is a step-wise process and the mechanism of nitrogen loss is either by a purely heterolytic process (producing an *aryl cation*) or a homolytic process (producing an *aryl radical*). The radical pathway is mediated by donation of a single electron from a metal species, for example, Cu (I) or Cu (II). Since the leaving group (N_2) is thermodynamically highly stable, these reactions are favoured.

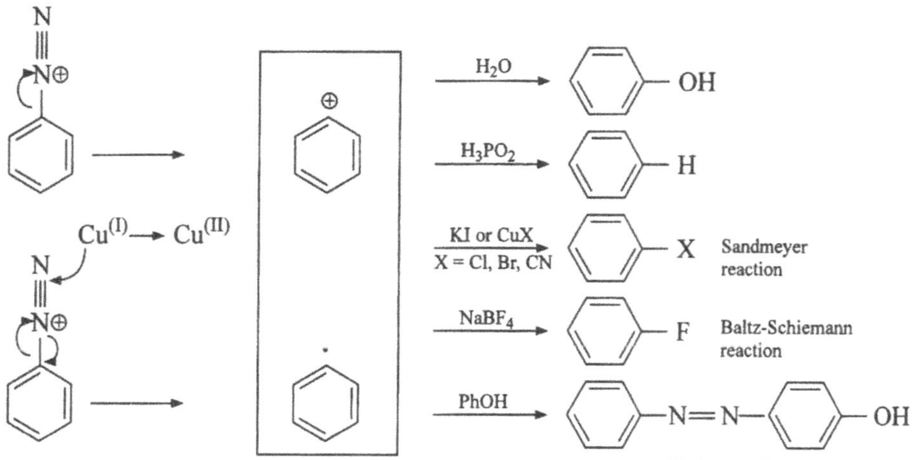

p-Hydroxyazobenzene

(i) *Replacement by hydroxyl group* When a solution of the diazonium salt in dilute H_2SO_4 is boiled, the diazo group is replaced by hydroxyl group and phenol is formed.

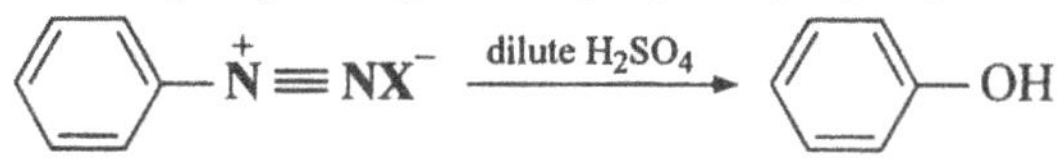

Diazonium salt Phenol

(ii) *Replacement by Cl, Br, I or CN groups* When an aqueous solution of a diazonium salt is treated with potassium halide or potassium cyanide in presence of metallic copper powder, the diazonium group is replaced to yield a halo or cyano derivative. This reaction is known as *Gattermann reaction.*

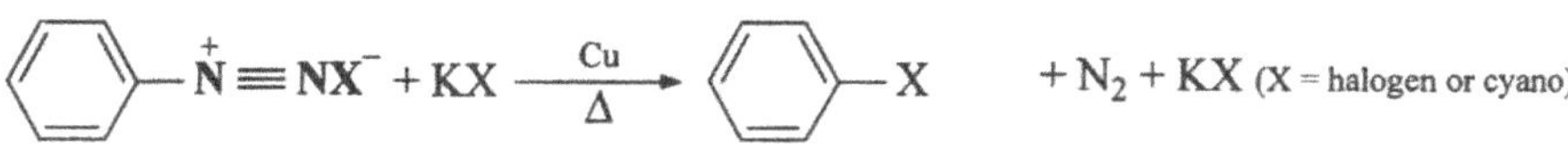

Diazonium salt Halobenzene or Cyanobenzene

Better yields are obtained if the combination of copper powder and potassium halide or potassium cyanide is replaced by cuprous chloride or cuprous bromide or cuprous cyanide in corresponding acid (HCl or HBr or HCN). The substitution reactions that are catalysed by cuprous salts are known as *Sandmeyer reactions.*

(iii) *Replacement by fluorine* When an aqueous solution of diazonium salt is treated with sodium fluoroborate, diazonium fluoroborate is precipitated. Stable diazonium tetrafluoroborate salts may be isolated, which on heating lose nitrogen to give an arylfluoride product. This reaction is known as *Baltz-Schiemann* reaction.

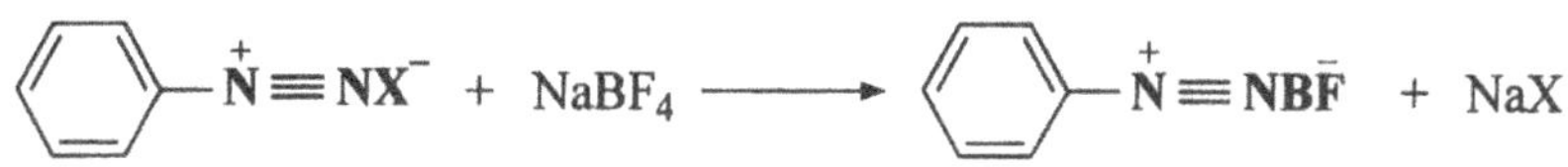

Diazonium salt Diazonium fluoroborate

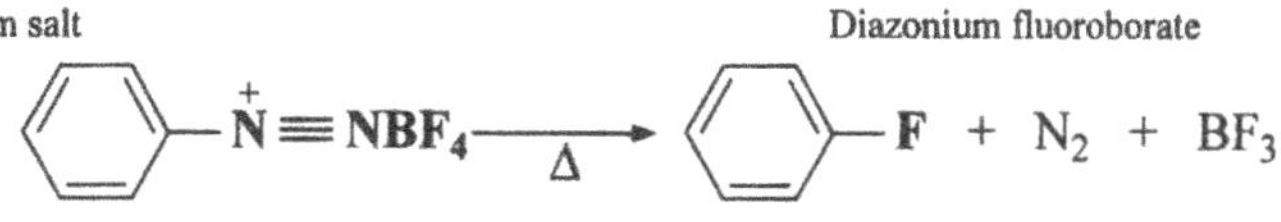

Diazonium fluoroborate Fluorobenzene

(iv) *Replacement by hydrogen* Aryl diazonium salt on treatment with hypophosphorous acid (H_3PO_2) forms the parent aromatic hydrocarbon.

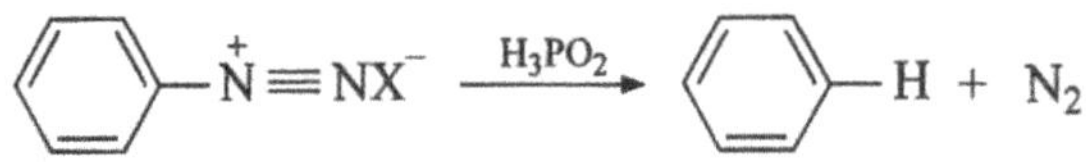

Coupling Reactions In these reactions diazo group is retained. This involves reaction of diazonium ion with aromatic compounds containing powerful electron-releasing substituents (—OH, —NH_2, —NHR, —NR_2) to form compounds called *azo compounds* having the general formula of 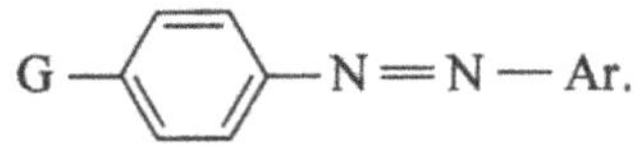

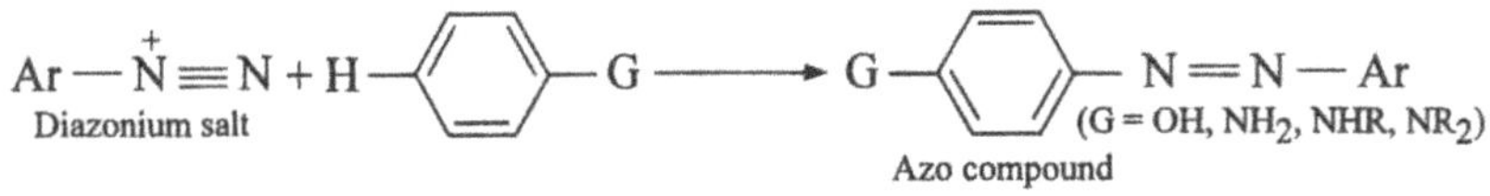

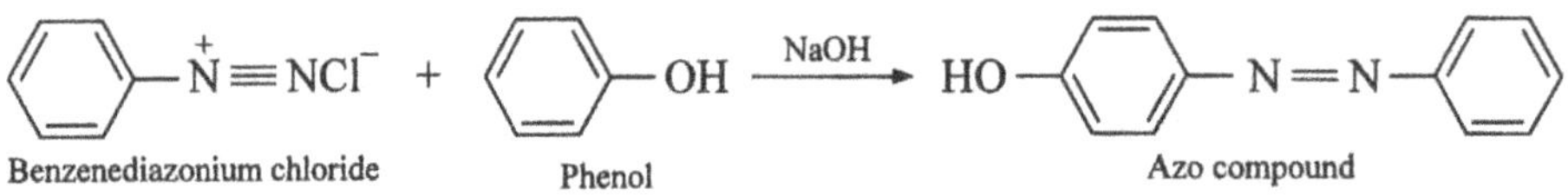

The positive charge of diazonium ions is delocalised over the two nitrogen atoms. It is not possible for nucleophiles to bond to the inner nitrogen, but bonding (or coupling) of negative nucleophiles to the terminal nitrogen gives neutral azo compounds. As shown in the following reaction, this coupling to the terminal nitrogen should be relatively fast and reversible.

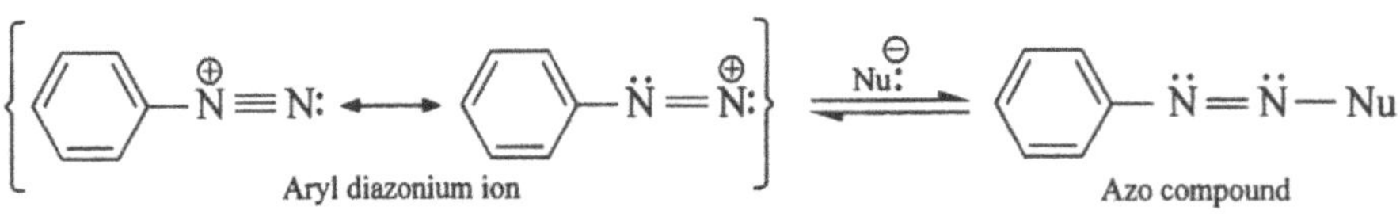

Unless these azo products are trapped or stabilised in some manner, reversal to the diazonium ion and slow nucleophilic substitution at carbon (with irreversible nitrogen loss) will be the ultimate course of reaction. For example, if phenyldiazonium bisulphate is added rapidly to a cold solution of sodium hydroxide – a relatively stable solution of sodium phenyldiazoate (the conjugate base of the initially formed diazoic acid) is obtained.

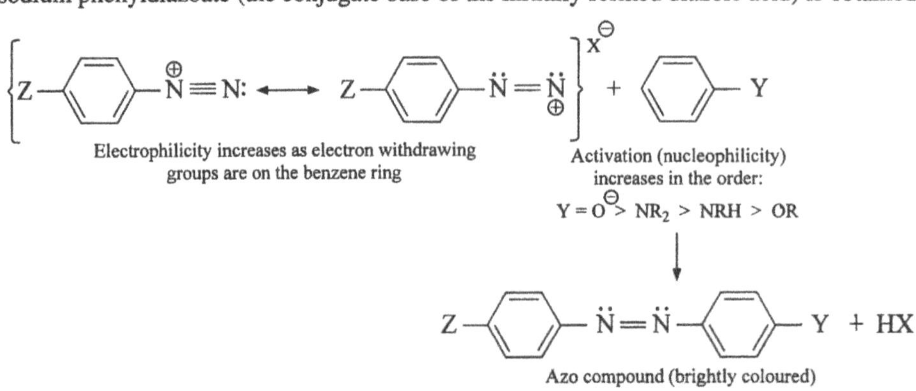

Lowering the *pH* of this solution regenerates phenyldiazoic acid ($pK_a = 7$), which dissociates back to the diazonium ion and, eventually, undergoes substitution to generate phenol. Azo compounds are coloured because of their extended conjugation. They are commercially used as dyes. In these reactions diazonium ion acts as an electrophile.

24.10 PHARMACEUTICAL COMPOUNDS

1. ***Diphenhydramine*** Diphenhydramine is a tertiary amine. It is prepared by treating benzhydryl bromide with 2-dimethylaminoethanol in presence of alcohol.

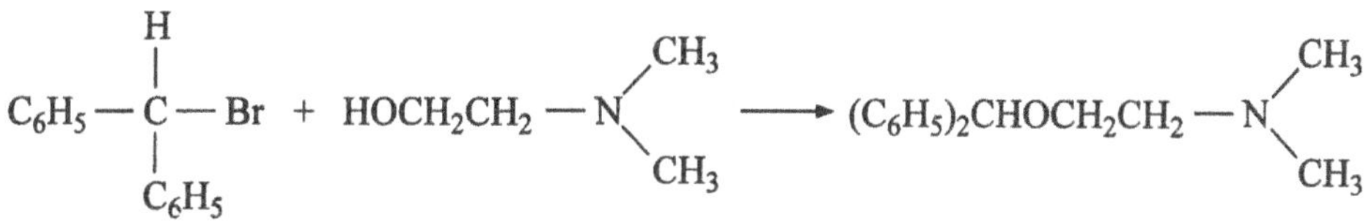

Diphenhydramine is available as diphenhydramine hydrochloride salt. It is available as colourless, odourless, crystalline powder and melts at 166°C. It is soluble in water, alcohol, acetone and chloroform.

2. ***Verapamil*** Verapamil is a tertiary amine. It is available as Verapamil hydrochloride salt. Verapamil hydrochloride is a colourless, water-soluble, crystalline powder. Chemically, it is 5-(N-3,4-dimethoxyphenethyl)-methylamino-2-(3,4-dimethoxyphenyl)-2-isopropyl valesonitrile.

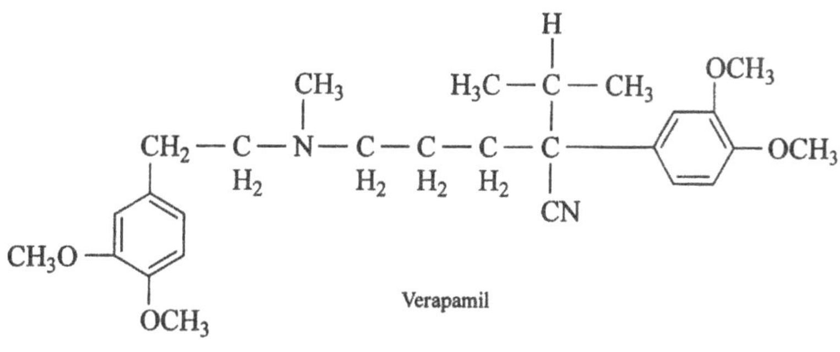

Verapamil

Uses

1. Verapamil hydrochloride is used in the treatment of hypertension.
2. It is also used to control supraventricular tachyarrhythmias and angina pectoris

3. ***Mustine Hydrochloride*** Mustine was the original anti-cancer agent. Mustine hydrochloride is N,N-di(2-chloroethyl) methyl ammonium chloride.

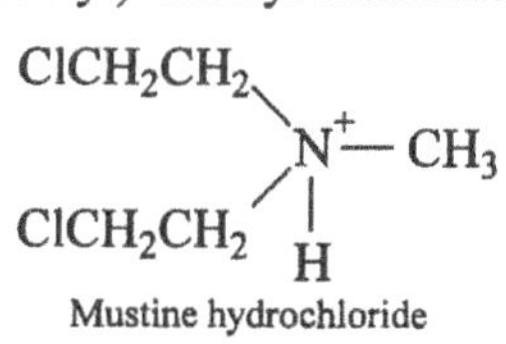

Mustine hydrochloride

Mustine is prepared by mixing di-(2-hydroxy ethyl) methylamine with thionyl chloride.

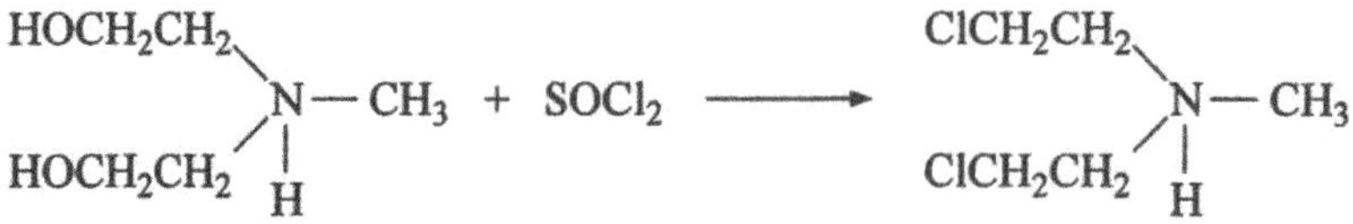

Mustine

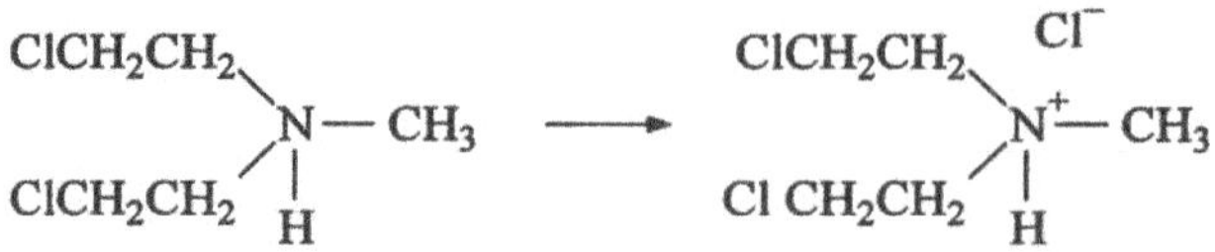

Mustine Mustine hydrochloride

Mustine hydroxychloride is available as colourless crystalline powder. Mustine hydrochloride is used for the treatment of Hodgkin's disease. It is also used to treat other lymphomas and carcinoma of lung.

4. ***Amphetamine*** Amphetamine is a sympathomimetic drug. It is an α-methylphenyl ethylamine.

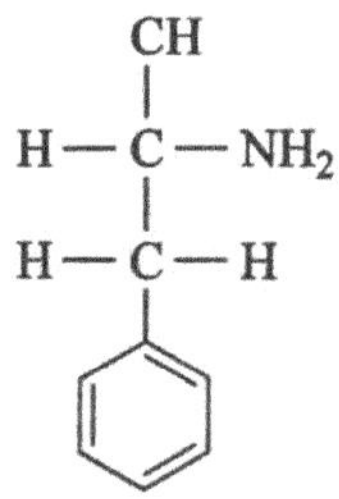

Amphetamine

Amphetamine is prepared from phenylacetone, formic acid and ammonia followed by acidic hydrolysis.

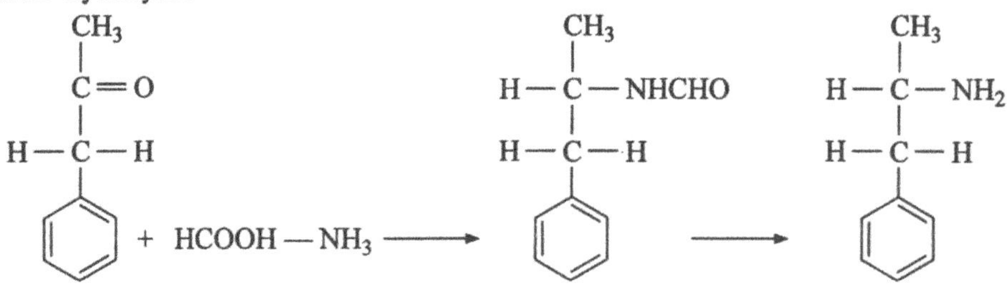

Amphetamine

Amphetamine is available as sulphate. Amphetamine sulphate is available as a white powder. It is freely soluble in water.

Uses

1. Amphetamine has central stimulant effect.
2. It is used in the treatment of narcolepsyal obesity.

5. ***Phenylephrine*** Phenylephrine is 1-(3-hydroxy phenyl)-2-methylamino ethanol.

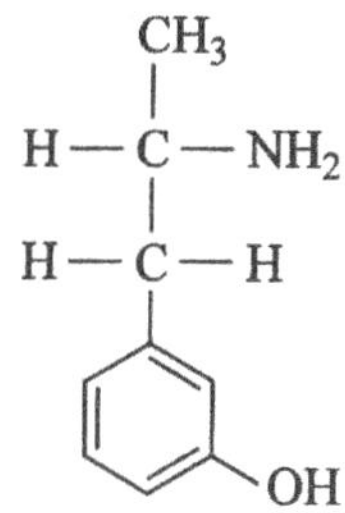

Amphetamine

Phenylephrine is synthesised by a chemical reaction of *m*-chloroacetylphenol with methylamine followed by reduction.

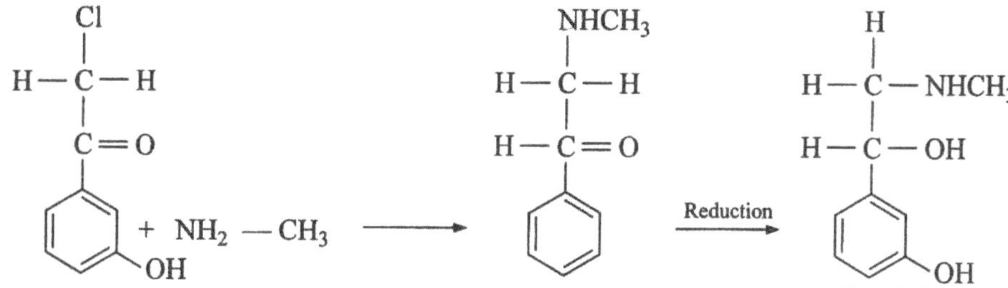

Phenylephrine

Phenylephrine is available as hydrochloride salt. Phenylephrine hydrochloride is a colourless crystalline powder. It is freely soluble in water.

Uses

1. Phenylephrine is used as a nasal decongestant in rhinitis and sinusitis.
2. It is used as a vasoconstrictor along local anaesthetics.
3. It is used as a mydriatic and conjuctival decongestant.

6. ***Thiotepa*** Thiotepa is an aziridine derivative. It is N,N′,N″-triethylenethiophosphoramide.

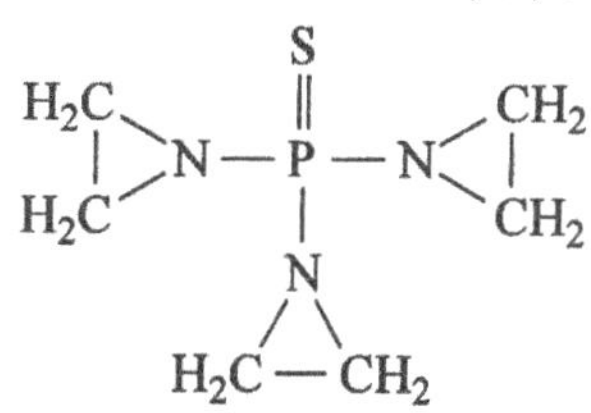

Thiotepa

Thiotepa is prepared by reacting trichlorophosphine sulphide with aziridine.

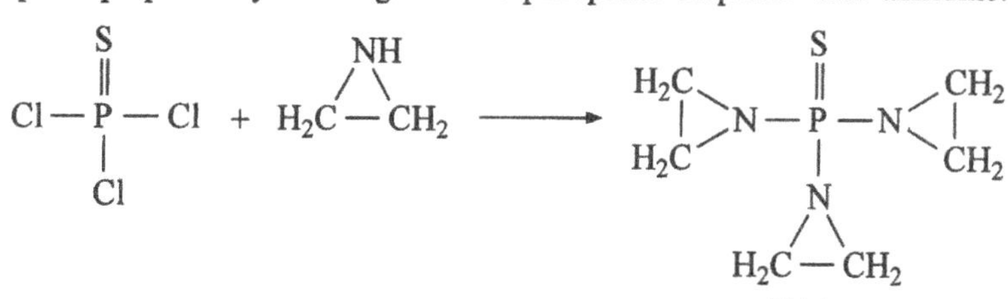

Thiotepa

Thiotepa is available as colourless crystalline flakes. It is freely soluble in water. Thiotepa is used to treat breast and ovary carcinomas.

7. ***Chlorambucil*** Chlorambucil is 4-(di-2-chloroethyl)-aminophenylbutyric acid.

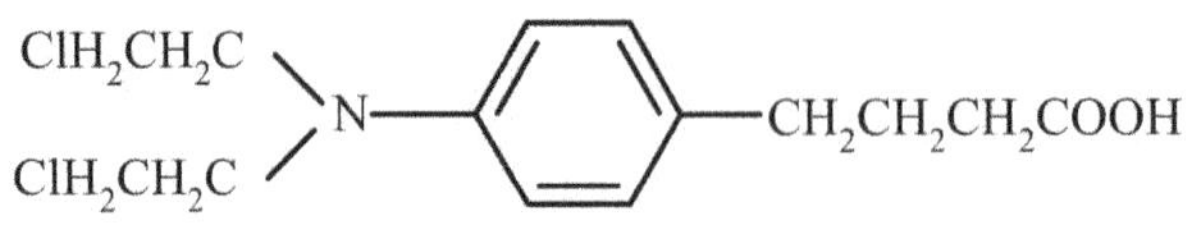

Chlorambucil

Chlorambucil is available as colourless, water-insoluble crystalline powder. It is prepared by adding *p*-aminophenylbutyric acid to ethylene oxide followed by treatment with thionyl chloride.

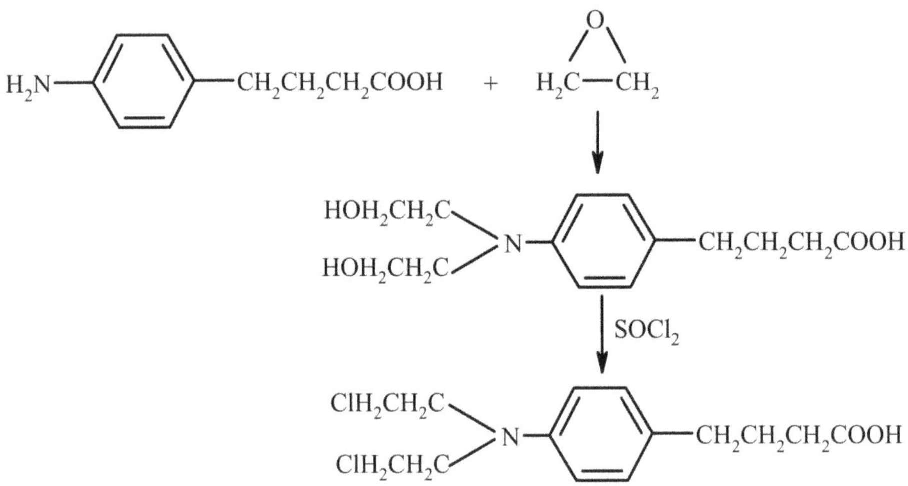

Chlorambucil

Uses

1. Chlorambucil is used to treat cancers like lymphocytic leukaemia and primary macroglobulinemia
2. Chlorambucil is also used to treat lymphosarcoma and Hodgkin's disease.

8. ***Benzocaine*** Chemically, benzocaine is ethyl-4-aminobenzoate. Benzocaine is prepared by reduction of ethyl-4-nitrobenzoate, which is obtained from 4-nitrotoluene by oxidation followed by esterification with ethyl alcohol.

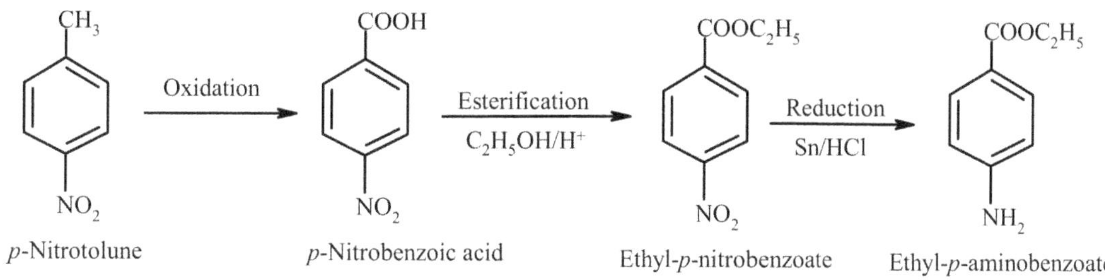

Benzocaine is available as colourless, odourless, water-insoluble crystalline powder. It is soluble in alcohol, ether and chloroform. Benzocaine is used as local anaesthetic.

9. *Ethanol amine* Ethanol amine is also known as 2-amino ethanol or mono ethanolamine. It is an organic compound which is colorless, viscous liquid with an odor reminiscent to that of ammonia. It is widely distributed in biological tissue and is a component of lecithin.

$$H_2N—CH_2—CH_2—OH$$

Uses

1. Ethanolamine is a sclerosing agent
2. It is used as a surfactant and fluorimetric reagent.
3. Used to remove CO_2 and H_2S from natural gas and other gases.

10. *Ethylenediamine* Ethylenediamine is a standardized chemical allergen. It is a clear colorless liquid with an ammonia like odor.

$$H_2N—CH_2—CH_2—NH_2$$

Uses

1. Ethylenediamine is used in corrosion inhibitors and anti-scaling agent.
2. Ethylenediamine is used in ion exchange agents.

PRACTICE QUESTIONS

1. What are amines? How are they prepared in the laboratory? Discuss in detail how the basicity of amines varies with its structure.
2. Starting from aniline suggest schemes and reagents for the preparation of the following:

   (a) Phenol (b) Benzoic acid (c) N,N-dimethyaniline
   (d) P-Nitroaniline (e) Benzanilide (f) Methyl orange
   (g) Benzene sulphanamide (h) Sulphanilic acid (i) Nitrobenzene
   (j) Iodobenzene
3. What are diazonium compounds and how are they prepared? Discuss in detail the various important reactions of diazonium compounds.

4. Describe how an azo dye is prepared. Illustrate your answer with aniline giving the structures and equation.
5. Write structures and uses of:

   (a) Mustine (b) Verapamil (c) Thiotepa
   (d) Phenylephrine (e) Amphetamine

6. How will you convert:

   (a) Methyl amine to ethyl amine
   (b) Secondary amine to tertiary amine
   (c) Aniline to diphenyl amine
   (d) Aniline to phenol
   (e) Aniline to N, N-dimethylaniline

7. How do you differentiate:

   (a) Aniline and N, N-dimethylaniline
   (b) Benzylamine and o-toluidine
   (c) Aniline and N-methylaniline
   (d) N-Methylaniline and N,N-dimethylaniline
   (e) Aniline and methylamine

8. Write notes on:

   (a) Hofmann reaction
   (b) Hofmann's degradation of amides
   (c) Carbylamine reaction
   (d) Hinsberg's reagent
   (e) Gabriel's phthalimide reaction
   (f) Mannich reaction
   (g) Quaternary ammonium salts
   (h) Sandmeyer's reaction
   (i) Diazotisation reaction
   (j) Gattermann's reaction

25

AROMATIC HETEROCYCLIC COMPOUNDS

25.1 INTRODUCTION

Cyclic compounds which contain one or more atoms of other elements along with carbon atoms are called heterocyclic compounds. The non-carbon atoms in the ring are called hetero atoms. The most common hetero atoms are nitrogen, sulphur and oxygen.

25.2 CLASSIFICATION

Depending on the size of the heterocyclic rings, these compounds are classified into three types:

(i) *Five-membered heterocyclic compounds* They contain five atoms in the ring out of which four are carbon atoms and one is hetero atom, for example,

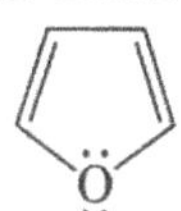

Furan

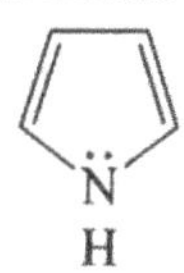

Pyrrole

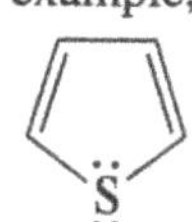

Thiophene

The chemistry of pyrrole, thiophene and furan is dominated by readiness to undergo electrophilic substitution, preferentially at an α-position, but also at a β-position, should the α-positions be blocked. The five-membered heterocycles do not react with electrophiles at the hetero atom.

(ii) *Six-membered heterocyclic compounds* These compounds contain six atoms in the ring, out of which five are carbon atoms and one is a hetero atom.

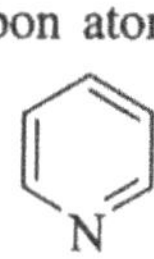

Pyridine

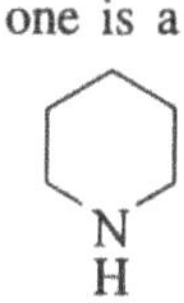

Piperidine

(iii) *Condensed heterocyclic compounds* In these compounds, a benzene ring is fused with a five- or six-membered heterocyclic ring.

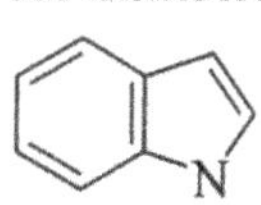

Indole

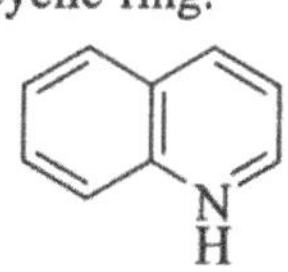

Quinoline

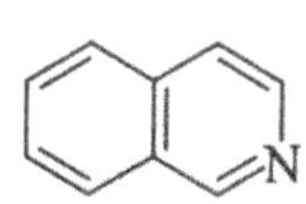

Isoquinoline

25.3 NOMENCLATURE

The following IUPAC rules are followed for naming of heterocyclic compounds.

(i) When a heterocyclic compound contains only one hetero atom the numbering will start from the hetero atom. Exceptions are isoquinoline and isoindole rings.

(ii) If more than one hetero atoms are present in the ring, then numbering will start as preferential series (O, S, N, P, etc.) and such numbering system is selected in which sum of the numbers given to hetero atoms is least.

(iii) The names of monocyclic compounds are derived by a prefix indicating the nature of hetero atom present. For example, *oxa* for oxygen, *thia* for sulphur, *aza* for nitrogen, *sila* for silicon and *phospha* for phosphorus. When two or more hetero atoms of a similar atom are present, then a prefix like *di*, *tri*, *tetra*, etc., are used.

(iv) A suffix indicates ring saturation or unsaturation. For example, the name of five-membered unsaturated ring containing nitrogen ends with ole and a saturated ring ends with -olidine.

(v) There are basic rings having fixed names for IUPAC. Some of the ring structures are given below:

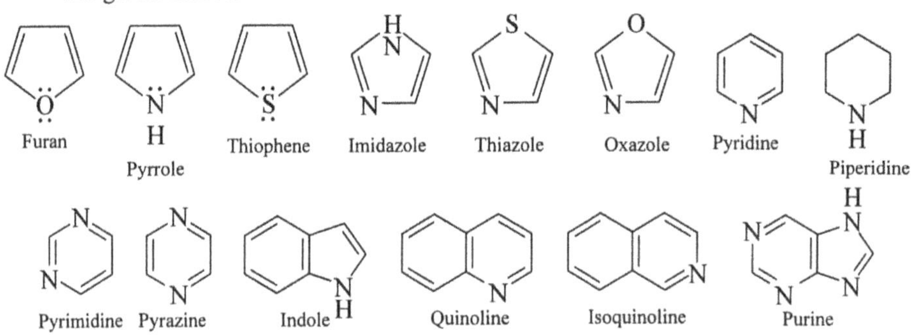

Furan, Pyrrole, Thiophene, Imidazole, Thiazole, Oxazole, Pyridine, Piperidine

Pyrimidine, Pyrazine, Indole, Quinoline, Isoquinoline, Purine

25.4 CHEMISTRY OF FURAN

Furan is a five-membered heterocyclic compound containing oxygen as hetero atom. The molecular formula of furan is C_4H_4O and is a resonance hybrid of the following resonance contributing structures:

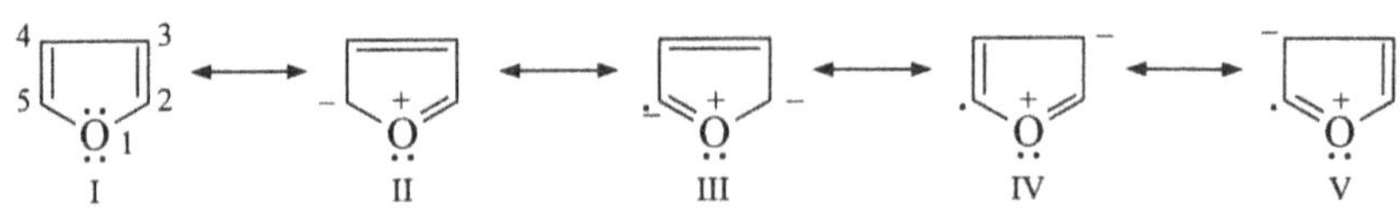

Resonance contributing structures of furan

Among the resonance contributing structures I, II and III are the main contributing structures to the resonance hybrid and hence resonance hybrid has a larger electron density at positions 2 and 5 than at 3 and 4. Furan has four pairs of delocalised π-electrons. Two of the pairs are shown as π bonds and two pairs are shown as non-bonding electrons on the hetero atom. The second pair of non-bonding electrons is not part of the π cloud. These electrons are in a sp^2 hybrid orbital perpendicular to the *p* orbitals. Since furan, is cyclic, planar molecule with three pairs of delocalised π-electrons, fulfils the criteria for aromaticity.

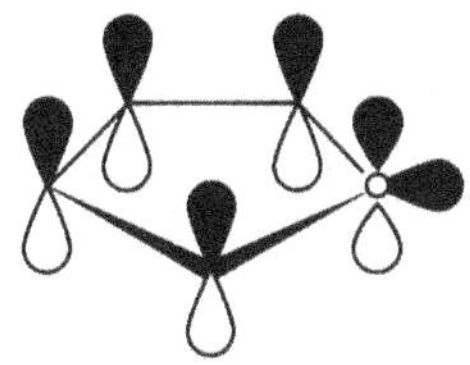

Furan

Furan is slightly soluble in water. Its commercial importance is mainly due to its role as the precursor of the very widely used solvent THF. Furan continues to play an important role in the field of heterocyclic chemistry because their skeletons are present in many naturally occurring molecules.

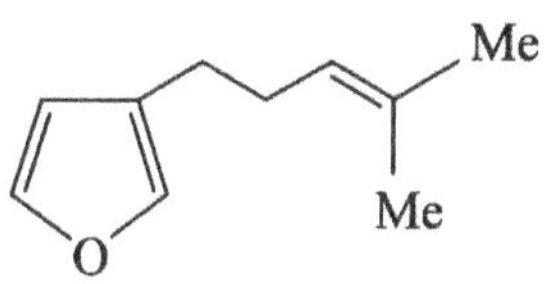

Perillene
(Secondary plant metabolite)

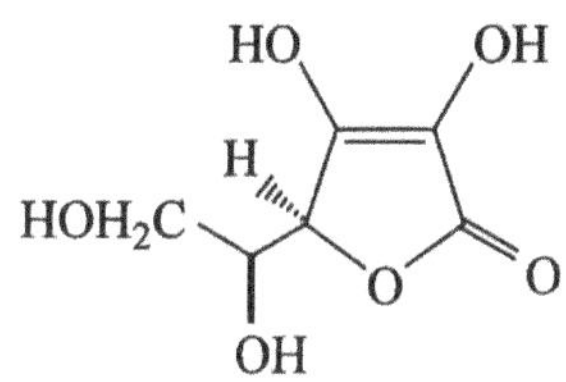

Ascorbic acid
(Antioxidant vitamin C)

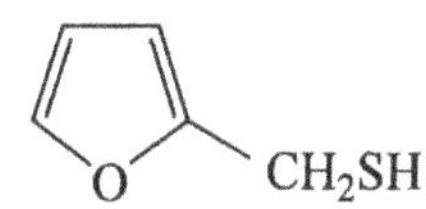

Furfuryl thiol
(Aroma of roasted coffee)

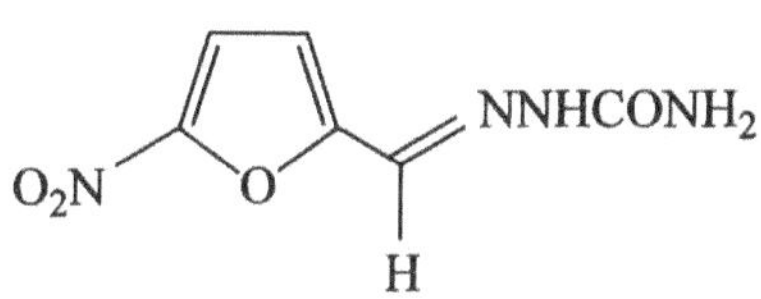

Nitrofurazone
(Bactericide)

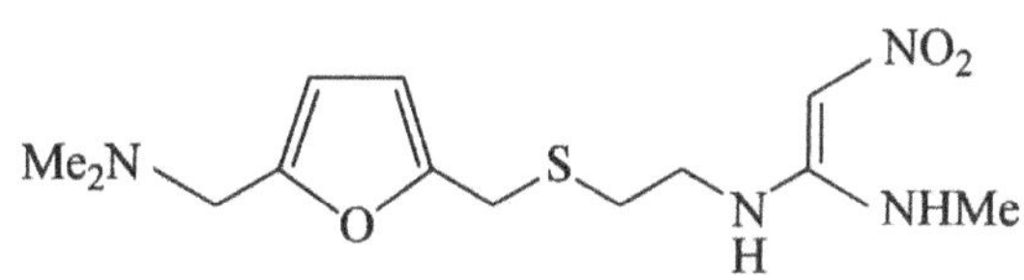

Ranitidine
(Treatment of stomach ulcers)

25.4.1 Preparation

The following methods are used to prepare furan:

(i) Furfural on oxidation gives furoic acid which on heating at 200°C yields furan.

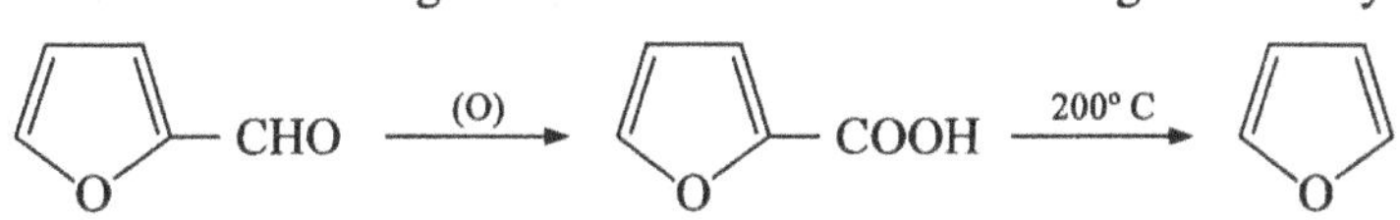

Furfural Furfuroic acid Furan

(ii) Catalytic decomposition of furfural (in steam) gives furan and carbon monoxide.

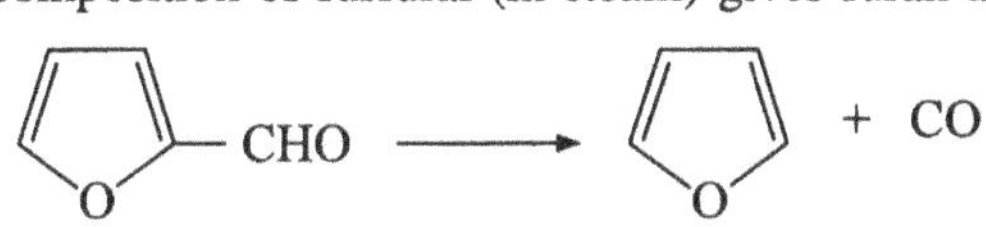

Furfural Furan

(iii) Furfural and furan are available in bulk and represent the starting materials for many syntheses. The aldehyde is manufactured from xylose, obtained in turn from pentosans, which are polysaccharides extracted from any plants, e.g. corncobs and rice husks.

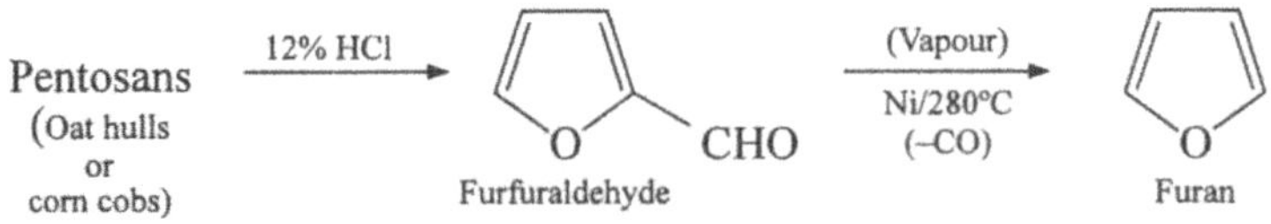

(iv) *The Paal–Knorr synthesis* The most widely used approach to obtain furans is through cyclising dehydration of 1,4-dicarbonyl compounds, which provide all of the carbon atoms and the oxygen necessary for the nucleus.

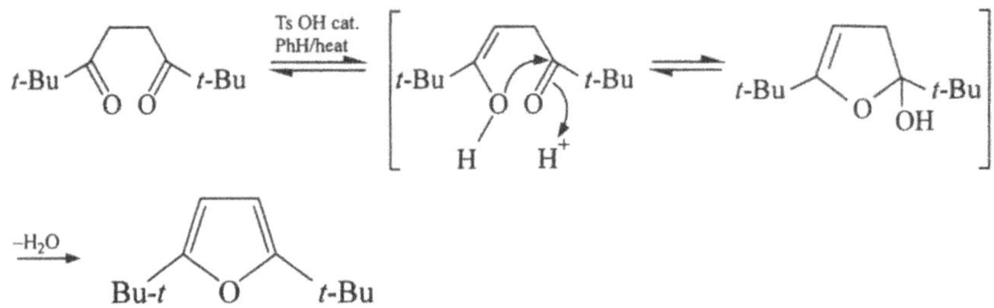

(v) *From γ-hydroxy-α,β-unsaturated carbonyl compounds* γ-Hydroxy-α,β-unsaturated carbonyl compounds can be dehydrated, using mineral or Lewis acids, to form furans.

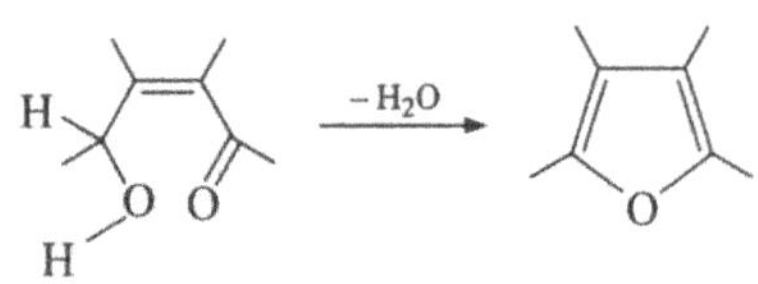

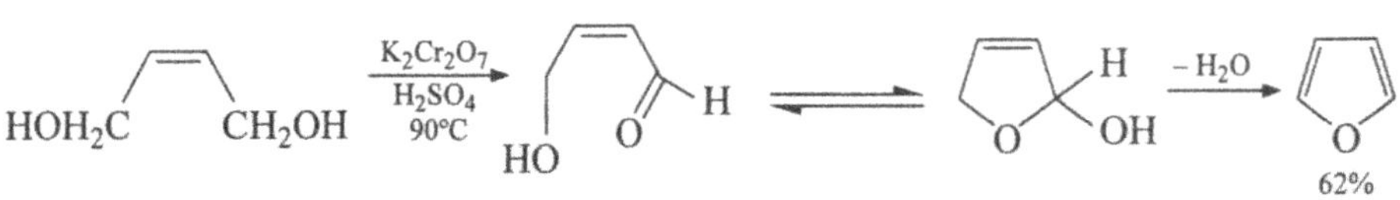

25.4.2 Physical Properties

(i) It is a colourless liquid and having chloroform-like odour.
(ii) It is insoluble in water but easily soluble in common organic solvents.
(iii) Furan boils at 31.4°C.

25.4.3 Chemical Properties

The following are various chemical reactions of furan:

(a) *Reduction* Furan on treatment with hydrogen gas in presence of nickel, platinum or palladium gives tetrahydrofuran.

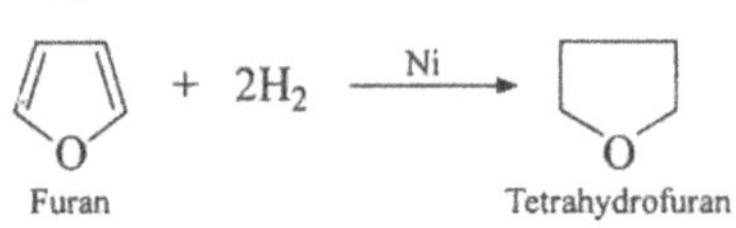

(b) *Reaction with metals* Metallation with alkyllithiums proceeds selectively at an α-position.

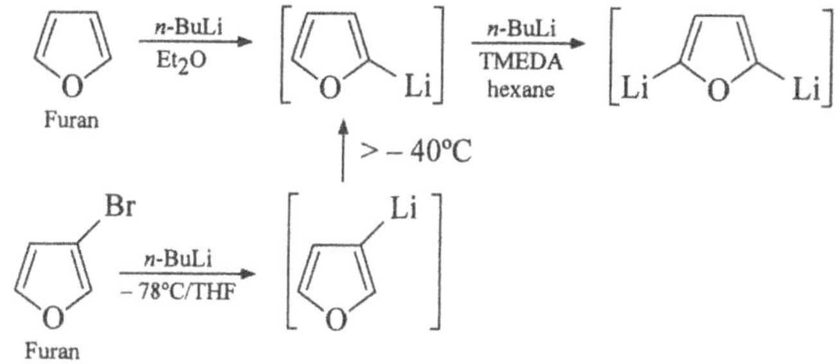

(c) *Mercuration* Mercuration takes place readily with replacement of hydrogen, or carbon dioxide, from an acid.

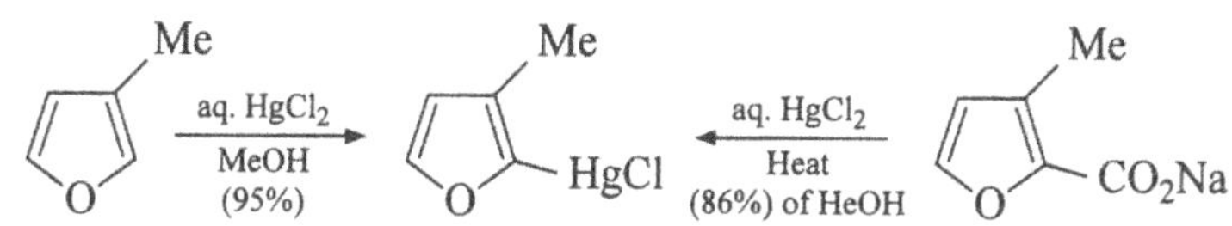

(d) *Condensation with imines and immonium ions*

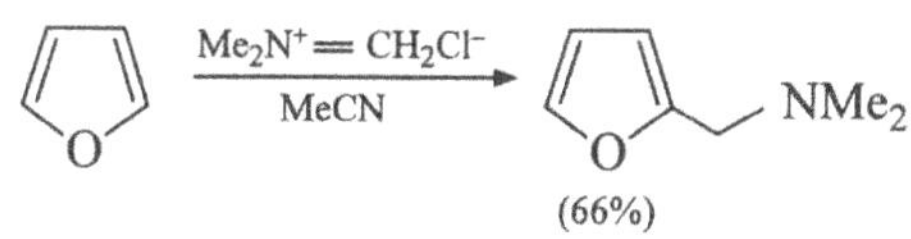

(e) *Gattermann–Koch reaction* Furan on heating with HCN and HCl forms furfural.

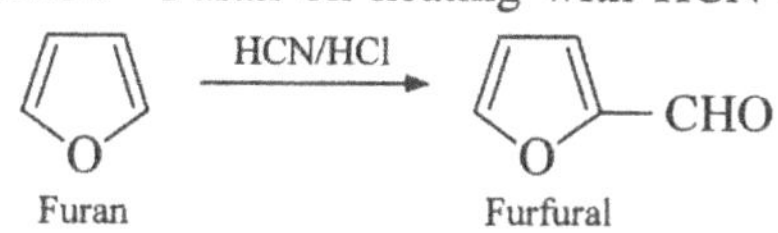

(f) *Diels–Alder reaction* Furan (having diene character) undergoes Diels–Alder reaction with maleic anhydride to form an addition product.

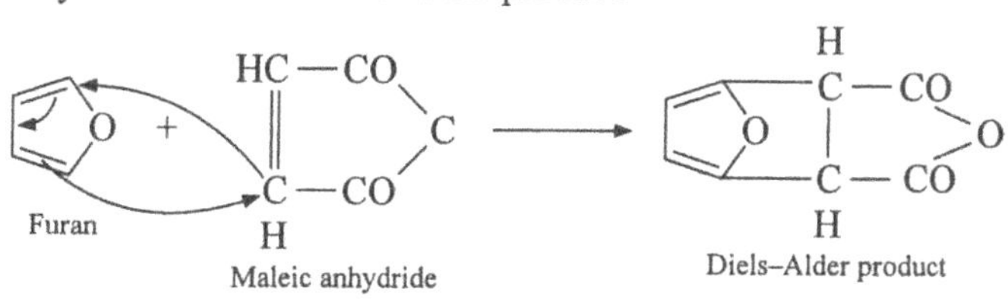

(g) *Ring-opening reaction* Furan gives 1,4-dioxo compounds on treatment with methanol and HCl.

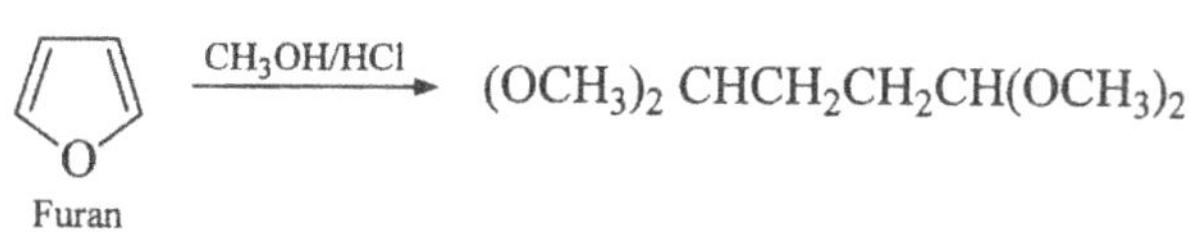

(h) *Protonation* Furan and simple alkyl furans are relatively stable to aqueous mineral acids.

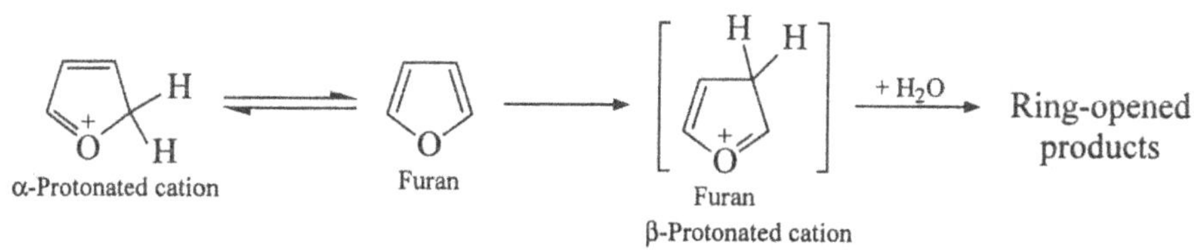

Electrophilic Aromatic Substitution Reactions Furan is an aromatic compound hence undergoes electrophilic aromatic substitution reactions. The substitution occurs preferentially at 2 or 5 positions. In case these positions are blocked, substitution takes place at 3 or 4 position.

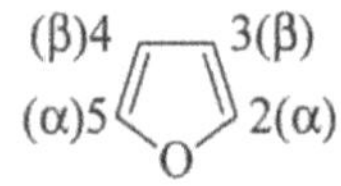

Furan is more reactive than benzene toward substitution reactions because of increased electron density on each carbon. The increased electron density is due to the delocalisation of non-bonding pair of electrons on the ring carbon atoms. The following are some electrophilic aromatic substitution reactions of furan:

(i) *Nitration* Sensitivity precludes the use of concentrated acid nitrating mixtures.

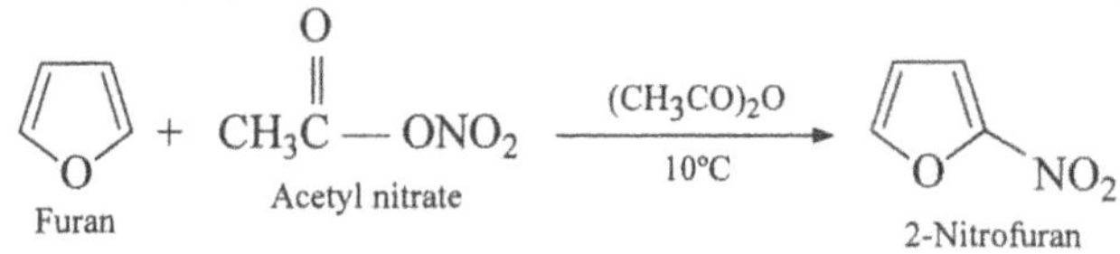

Further nitration of 2-nitrofuran gives 2,5-dinitrofuran as the main product.

(ii) *Sulphonation* Furan and its simple alkyl derivatives are decomposed by the usual strong acid reagents.

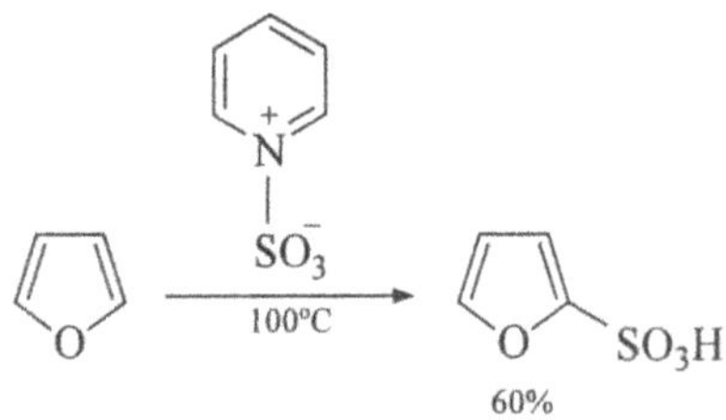

(iii) *Halogenation* Furan reacts vigorously with chlorine and bromine at room temperature to give polyhalogenated products, but does not react at all with iodine.

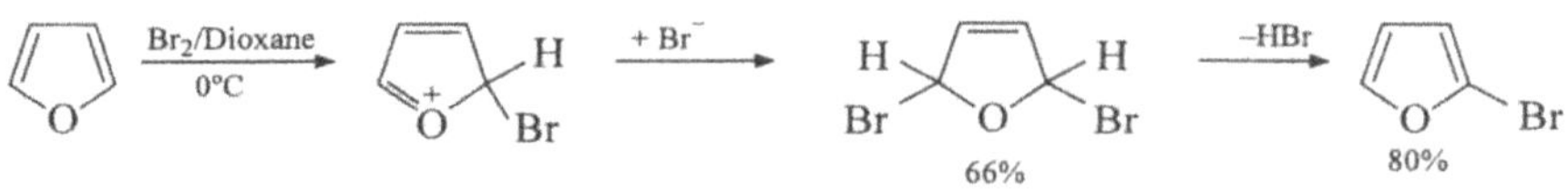

(iv) *Acylation* Carboxylic acid anhydrides or halides normally require the presence of Lewis acid (often boron trifluoride) for Friedel–Crafts acylation of furan, though trifluoroacetic anhydride will react alone.

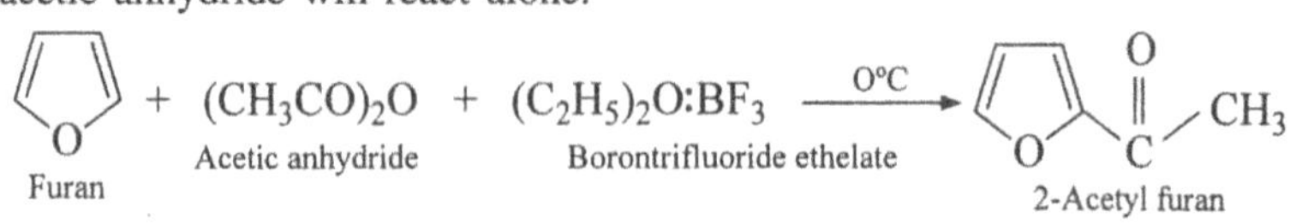

(v) *Alkylation* Traditional Friedel–Crafts alkylation is not generally practicable in the furan series, partly because of catalyst-caused polymerisation and partly because of polyalkylation.

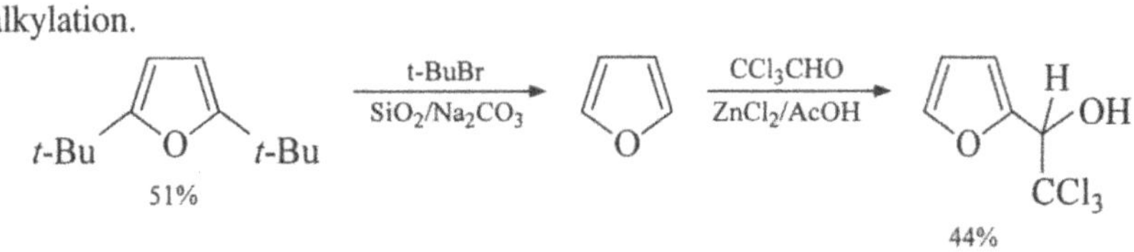

25.5 CHEMISTRY OF PYRROLE

25.5.1 Structure

Pyrrole is another important five-membered heterocyclic compound possessing a nitrogen atom as hetero atom.

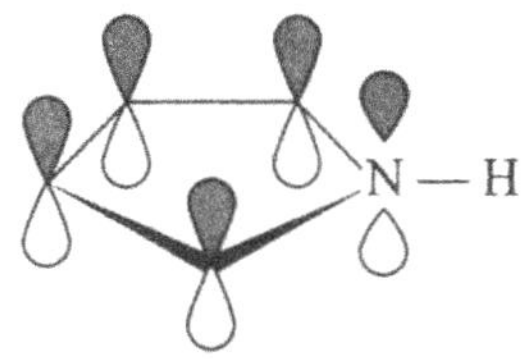

Pyrrole

Pyrrole has three pairs of delocalised π-electrons. Two of the pairs are shown as π bonds and one pair is shown as a pair of non-bonding electrons on the hetero atom. Since pyrrole is cyclic, planar molecule with three pairs of delocalised π-electrons fulfils the criterion for aromaticity.

According to the resonance theory pyrrole is considered as a resonance hybrid of the following contributing structures.

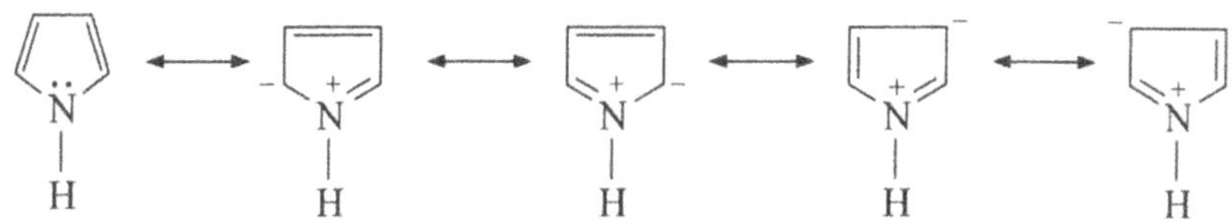

I II III IV V

Resonance contributing structures of Pyrrole

Among the resonance contributing structures (I–V) I, II and III are the main contributing structures to the resonance hybrid and hence resonance hybrid has a larger electron density at positions 2 and 5 than at 3 and 4.

25.5.2 Synthesis of Pyrrole

Pyrrole is obtained commercially by distillation of coal tar. However, it is synthesised in the laboratory by the following methods:

(i) Pyrrole is readily available commercially, and is manufactured by alumina-catalysed gas-phase interaction of furan and ammonia.

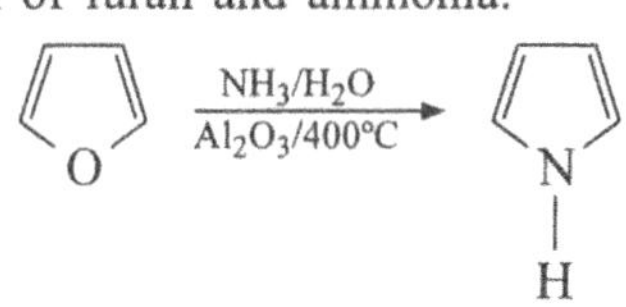

(ii) Pyrrole is also obtained by the distillation of succinimide with zinc dust.

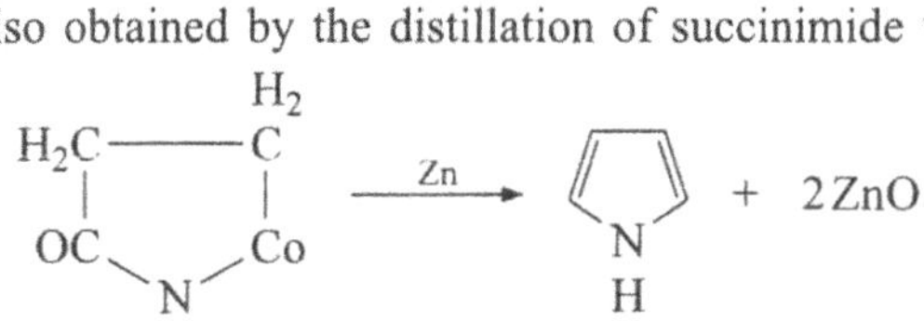

Pyrrole

(iii) Pyrrole can also be prepared by passing acetylene and ammonia through a red-hot tube.

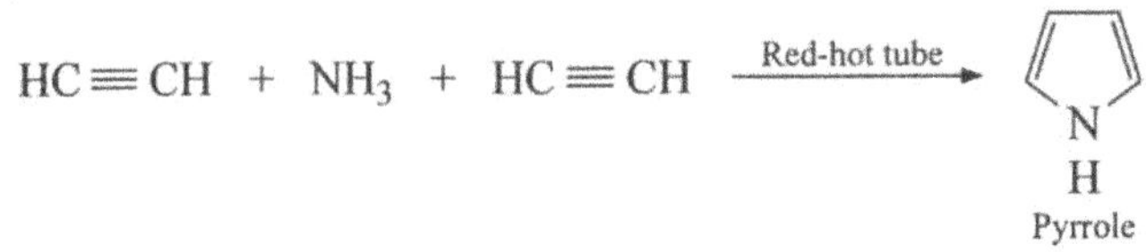

(iv) Pyrrole is synthesised from 1,4-dicarbonyl compounds by cyclising dehydration, through Paal-Knorr synthesis.

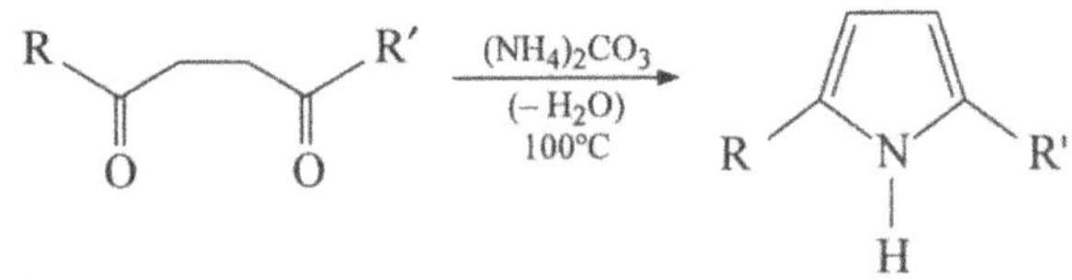

25.5.3 Properties

1. ***Solubility*** Pyrrole is a colourless liquid sparingly soluble in water but easily soluble in organic solvents. It boils at 131°C. The high boiling point and solubility is due to association of hydrogen bonding. Pyrrole behaves both as a weak acid and a weak base and exhibits the following chemical reactions.

2. ***Basicity*** Pyrrole is a weak base because the lone pair of electrons of nitrogen atom contributes to the $(4n + 2)$ π-electron cloud (aromatic sextet). Hence, the availability of these electrons is decreased and consequently pyrrole is a very weak base.

3. ***Reduction*** Pyrrole on reduction with zinc and acetic acid gives 2,5-dihydropyrrole but on reduction with HI and red phosphorus or with hydrogen in presence of nickel catalyst gives pyrrolidine.

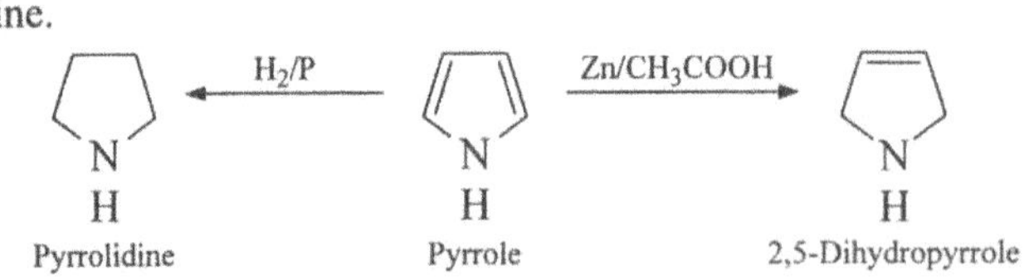

4. ***Oxidation*** Pyrrole is oxidised to maleinimide (imide of maleic acid) with chromium oxide in acetic acid.

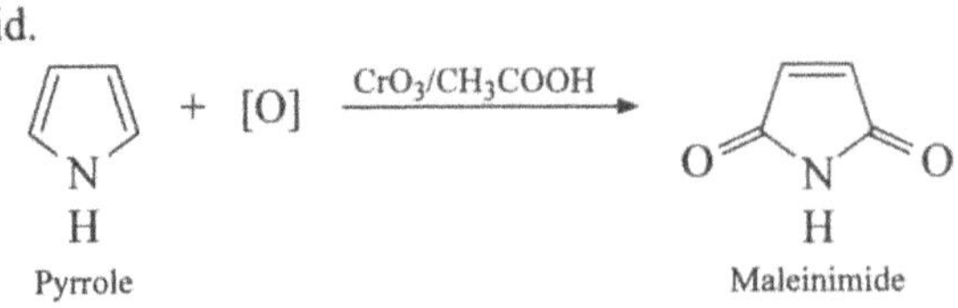

5. ***Ring Expansion Reaction*** Pyrrole ring expands on heating potassiopyrrole chloroform and sodium ethoxide.

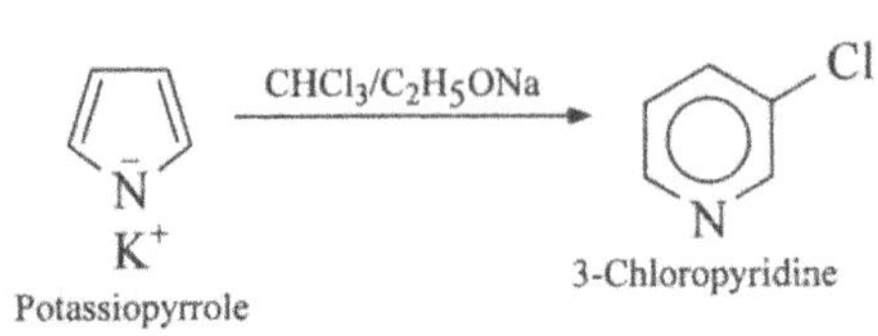

6. ***Ring Opening Reaction*** Pyrrole ring structure opens and forms succinaldehyde dioxime (addition product) on refluxing with ethanolic hydroxylamine.

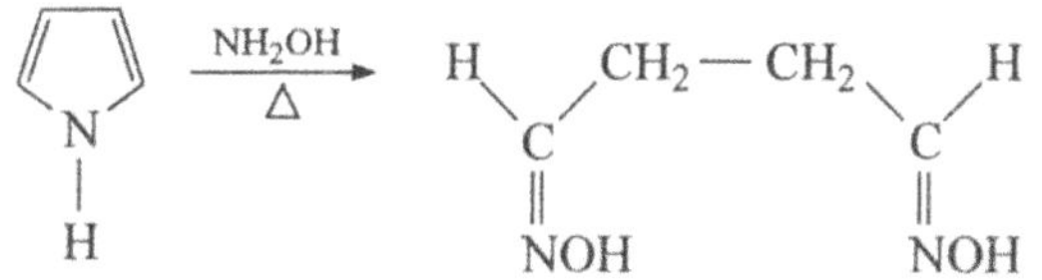

7. ***Diels–Alder Reaction*** Pyrrole undergoes Diels–Alder reaction with maleic anhydride to form an addition product.

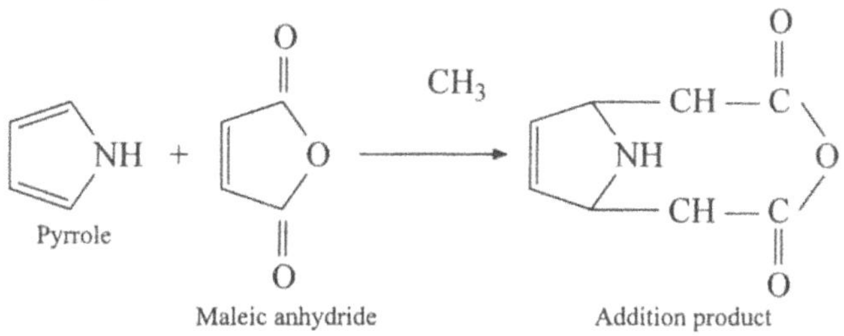

8. ***Electrophilic Aromatic Substitution Reactions*** Pyrrole undergoes electrophilic aromatic substitution more readily at C-2 than the C-3 position. This is because the intermediate carbocation formed by electrophile attack at C-2 is more stable than at C-3 carbon. Among pyrrole, furan and thiophene, pyrrole is by far the most susceptible to electrophilic attack: this susceptibility is linked to the greater electron-releasing ability of neutral trivalent nitrogen, and the concomitant greater stability of a positive charge on tetravalent nitrogen. The following are various electrophilic aromatic substitution reactions of pyrrole.

(i) *Nitration*

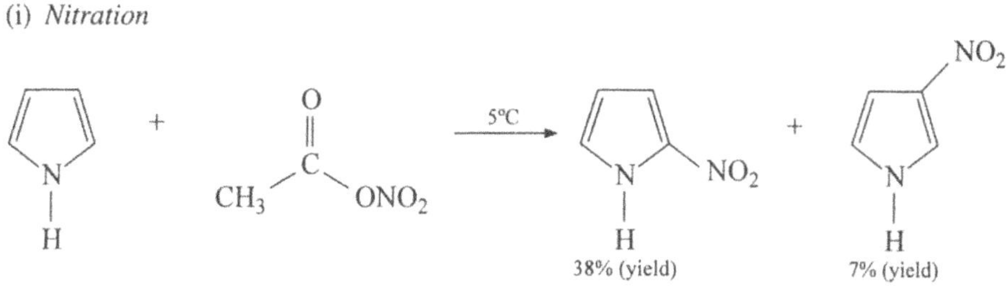

(ii) *Sulphonation*

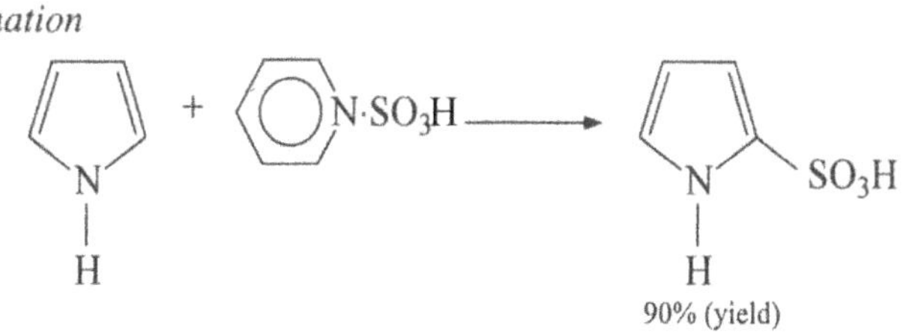

(iii) *Acylation*

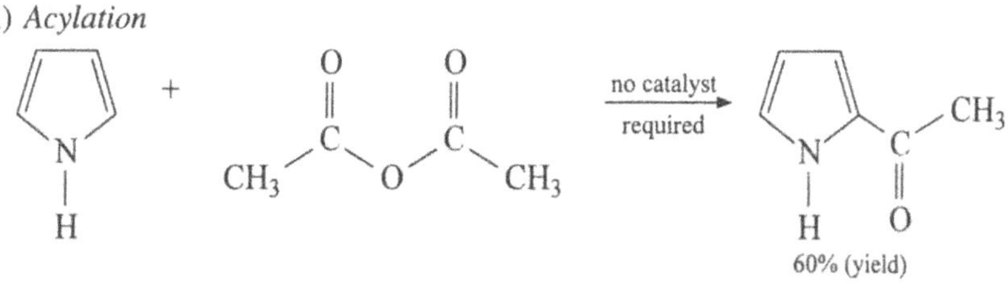

25.6 THIOPHENE

25.6.1 Structure

Thiophene is the 5-membered heterocyclic ring system containing sulphur as the hetero atom. It occurs in coal tar and shale oil along with benzene. Furan has four pairs of delocalised π-electrons. Two of the pairs are shown as π bonds and two pairs are shown as non-bonding electrons on the hetero atom. The second pair of non-bonding electrons is not part of the π cloud. These electrons are in a sp^2 hybrid orbital, which is perpendicular to the *p* orbitals. Since furan is a cyclic, planar molecule with three pairs of delocalised π-electrons, it fulfils the criterion for aromaticity.

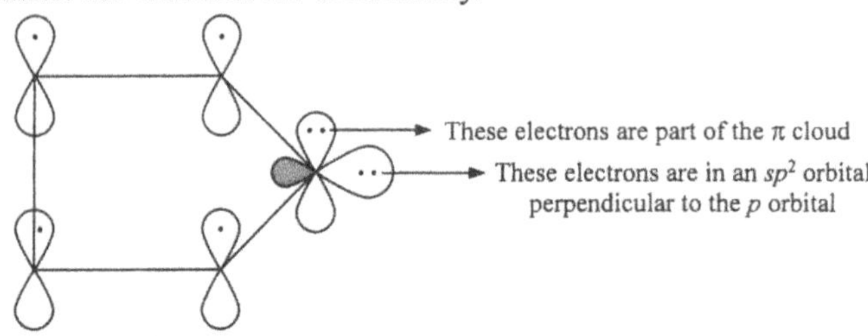

Orbital structure of thiophene

The structure of thiophene is considered as a resonance hybrid of the following resonance contributing structures:

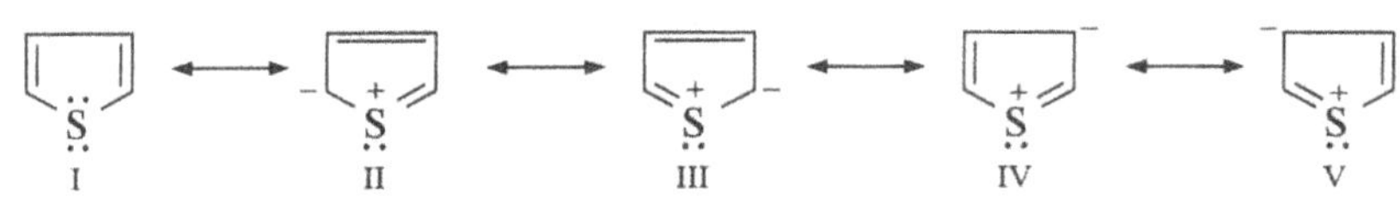

Resonance contributing structures of thiophene

Among the resonance contributing structures (I–V) I, II and III are the main contributing structures to the resonance hybrid and hence resonance hybrid has a larger electron density at positions 2 and 5 than at 3 and 4.

25.6.2 Prepatation

(i) Thiophene is separated from benzene by shaking the mixture with cold concentrated sulphuric acid. Thiophene forms thiophene sulphonic acid as it can be more easily sulphonated than benzene. Finally, thiophene is obtained from thiophene sulphonic acid by heating with steam.

(ii) Thiophene is prepared by the reaction of *n*-butane and sulphur in the vapour phase.

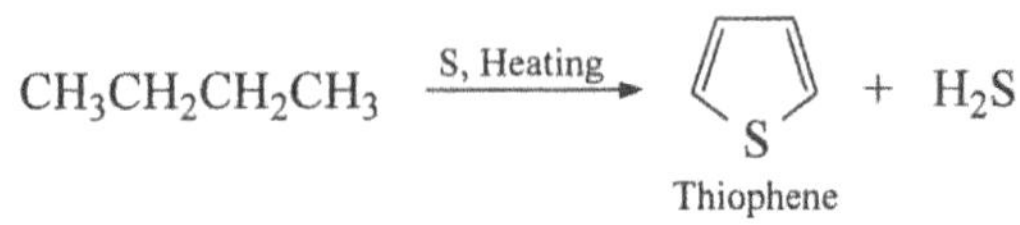

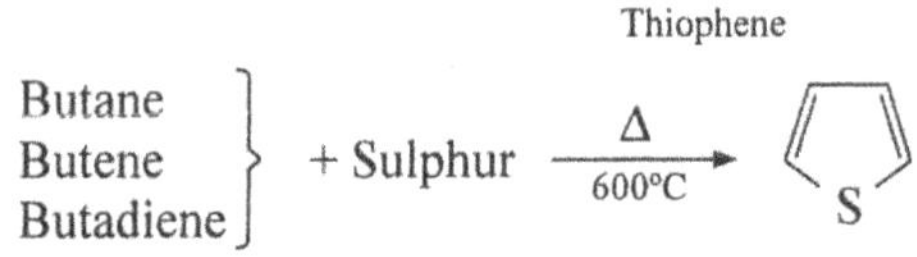

(iii) Thiophene can also be prepared by heating sodium succinate with phosphorous trisulphide (Paal-Knorr Synthesis).

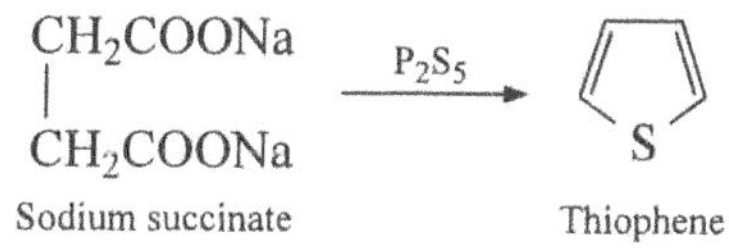

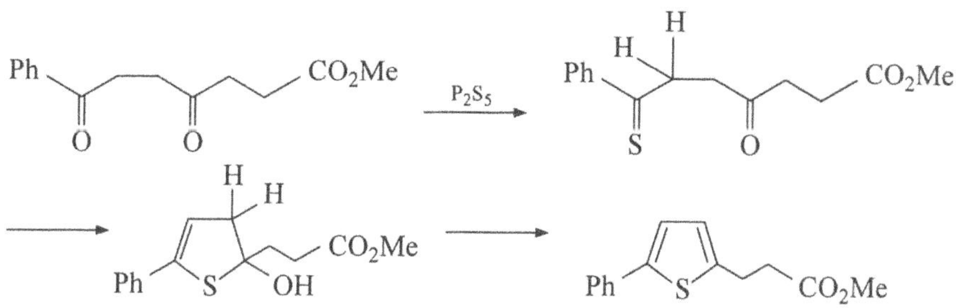

25.6.3 Properties

1. ***Physical Properties*** Thiophene is a colourless liquid having benzene-like odour. It is in soluble in water but soluble in organic solvents and boils at 84°C.

2. ***Reduction*** Thiophene is reduced to tetrahydrothiophene on reaction with hydrogen and large amount of catalyst (palladium) but on reduction with nickel gives *n*-butane by the removal of sulphur.

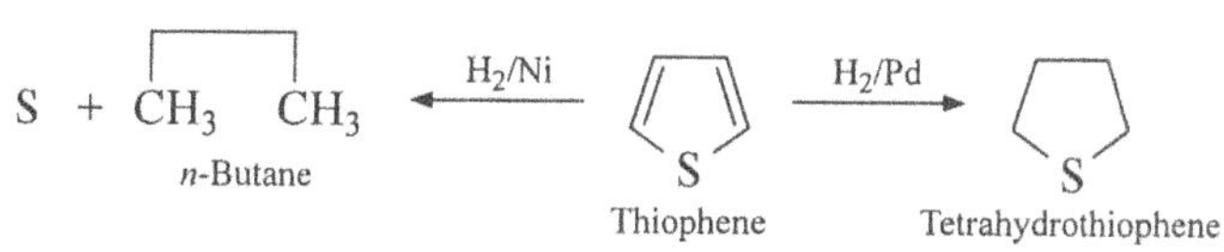

3. ***Oxidation*** Thiophene is not oxidised but tetrahydrothiophene is oxidised to sulphone.

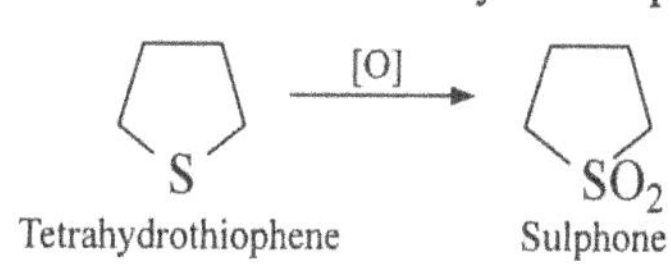

4. ***Electrophilic Aromatic Substitution Reactions*** Thiophene is an aromatic compound hence undergoes electrophilic aromatic substitution reactions at C-2. The following are some electrophilic substitutions reactions of thiophene.

(i) *Nitration*

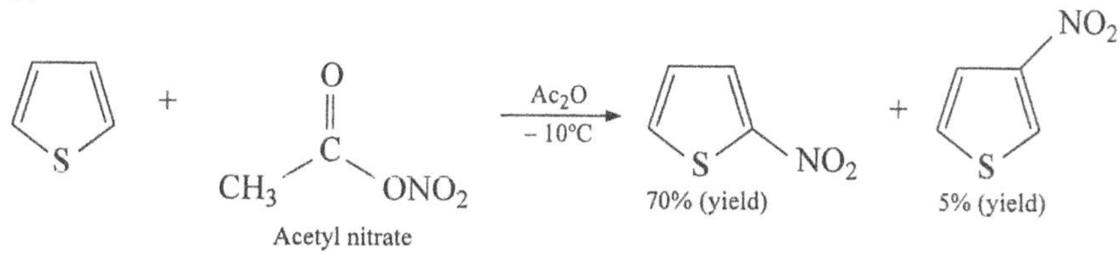

Mechanism

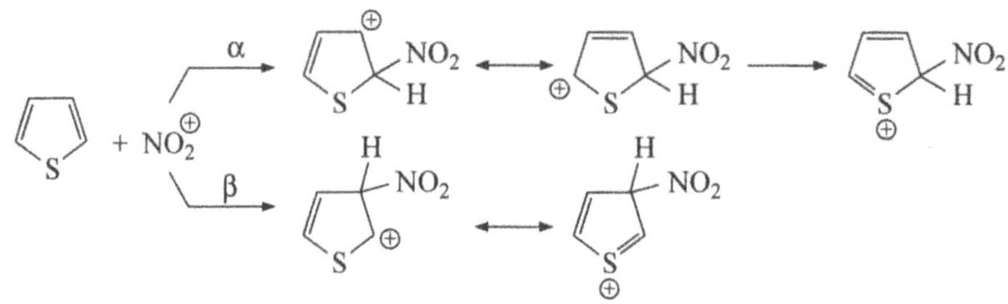

(ii) *Acylation*

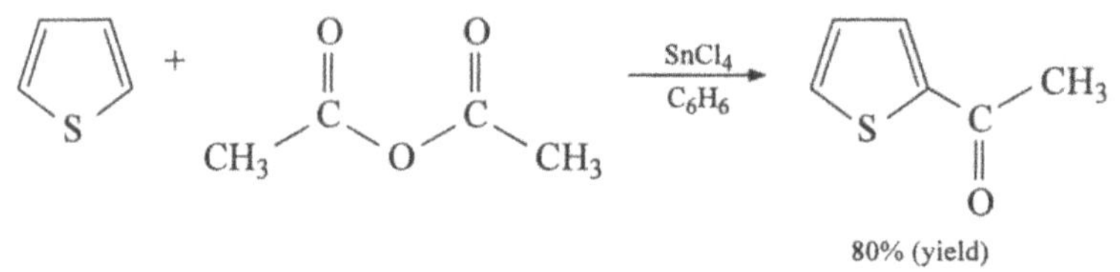

(iii) *Sulphonation*

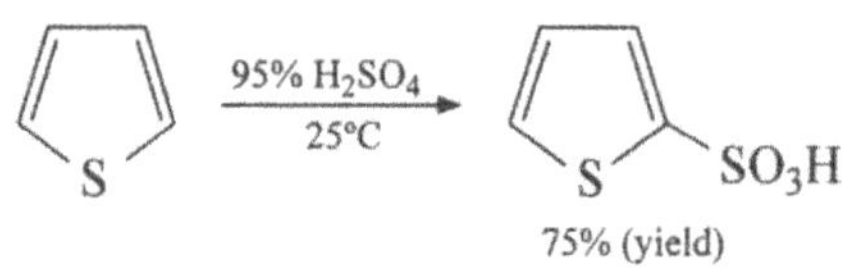

25.7 PYRIDINE

Pyridine is a six-membered heterocyclic ring system containing nitrogen as hetero atom.

25.7.1 Preparation

(i) Pyridine is present in light oil fraction of coal-tar distillation. The light oil fraction is treated with dilute sulphuric acid. This dissolves basic substances including pyridine. The acid layer is isolated, neutralised and fractionated several times to get pure pyridine.

(ii) Pyridine is prepared by passing a mixture of acetylene and HCN through a red-hot tube.

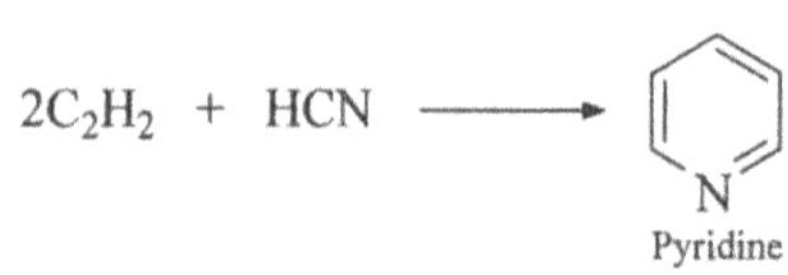

(iii) *Hantzsch synthesis* Hantzsch synthesis involves reaction of 1,3-dicarbonyl compounds with aldehydes and ammonia to give a 1,4-dihydropyridine, which can be aromatised by oxidation with nitric acid or nitric oxide.

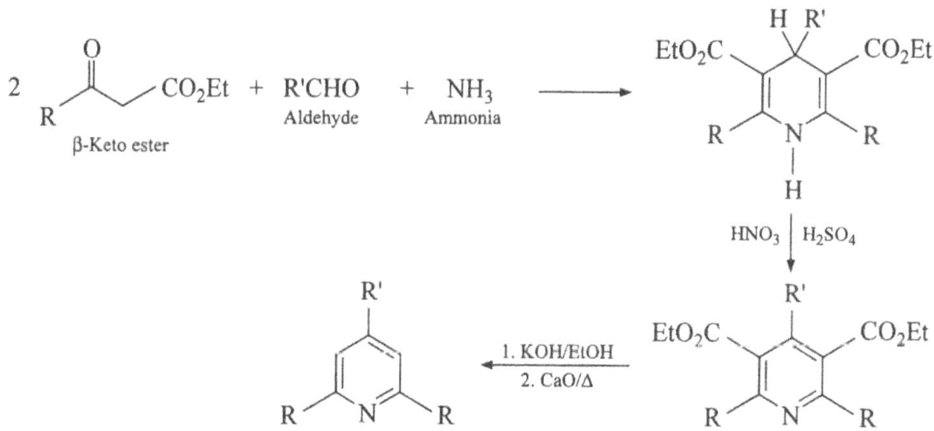

Hantzsch pyridine synthesis

25.7.2 Structure

Pyridine is a cyclic, planar structure. In pyridine, the aromatic sextet is complete without using the nitrogen lone pair of electrons. This unshared electron pair occupies an sp^2 orbital.

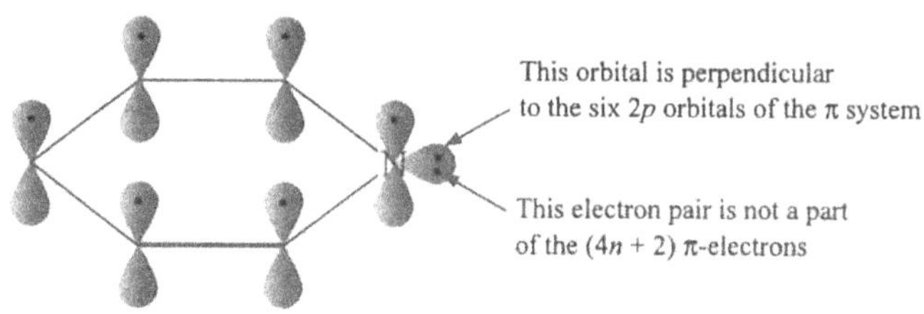

Pyridine

Pyridine is a resonance hybrid of the following contributing structures:

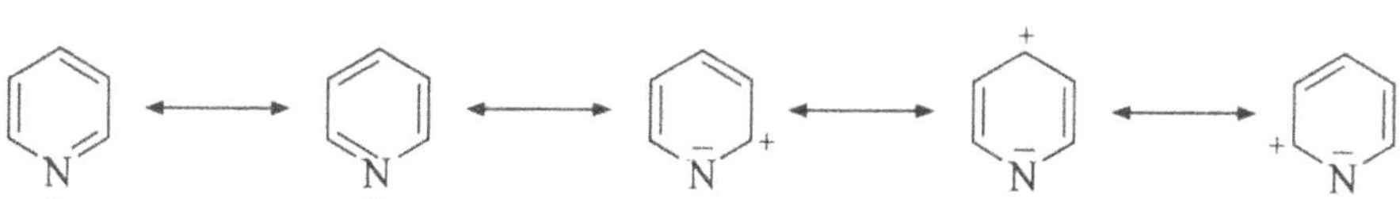

I II III IV V

Resonance contributing structures of pyridine

25.7.3 Properties

1. ***Basicity*** Pyridine like aliphatic amine is a good base (reacts with HCl) due to availability of lone pair of electrons on the nitrogen atom of pyridine structure.

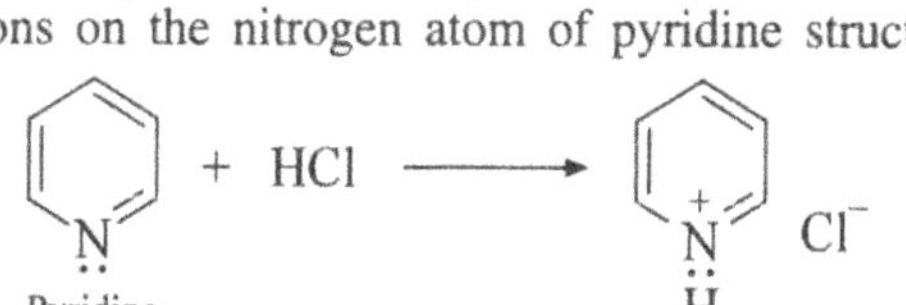

Pyridine

Pyridinium hydrochloride

2. ***Electrophilic Aromatic Substitution Reactions of Pyridine*** Since pyridine is resistant to electrophilic aromatic substitution reactions, drastic conditions are required. This low reactivity of pyridine is due to the presence of non-bonding electrons of nitrogen aligned at right angle to the π-system hence cannot stabilise intermediate carbocation. Further, the hetero atom (N) cannot donate electrons to the carbocation; it, however, withdraws electrons due to electron-withdrawing inductive effect and resonance effect.

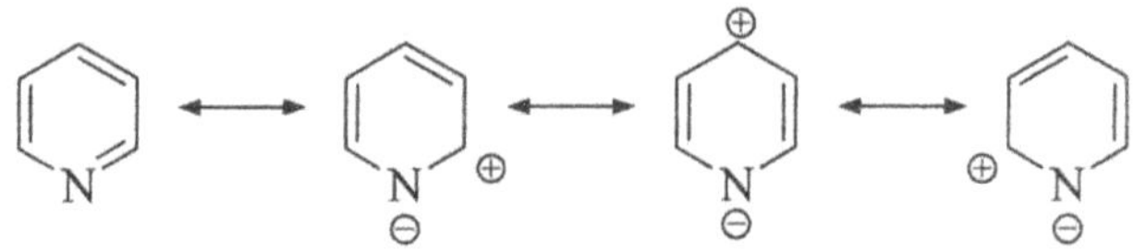

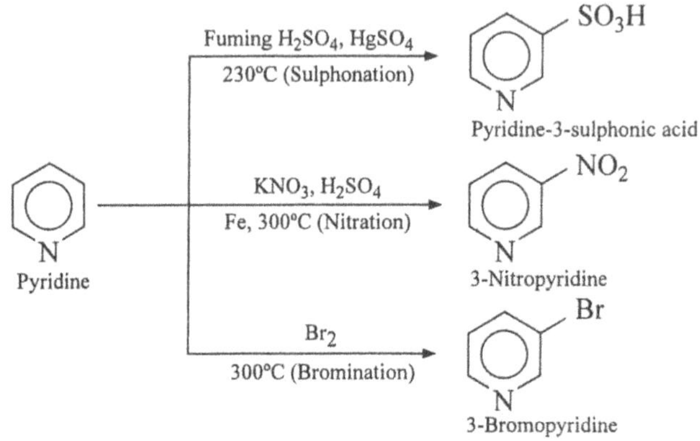

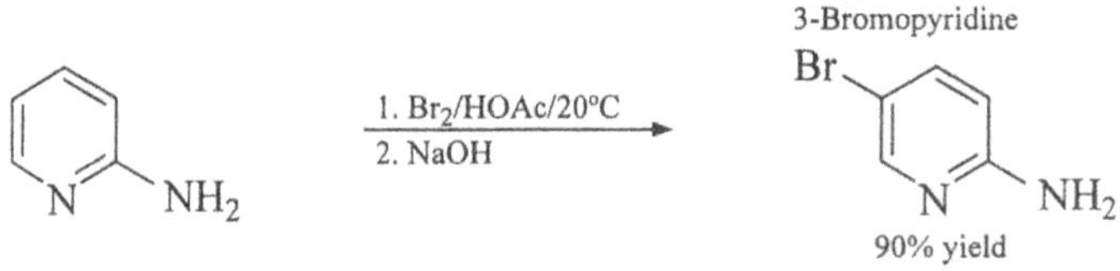

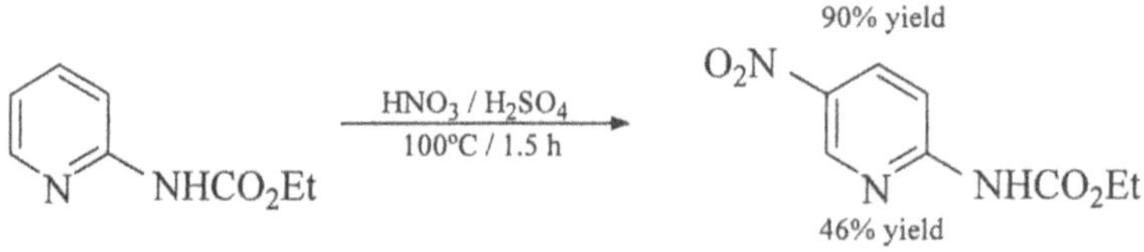

Electron-donating substituents first increase reactivity and then direct attack takes place.

3. ***Nucleophilic Substitution Reactions*** Pyridine undergoes nucleophilic substitution reactions. The electron density at the carbon atoms of pyridine ring is decreased due to electron withdrawal by nitrogen. Substitution usually takes place at the 2 and 4 positions but position 2 is more affected than position 4.

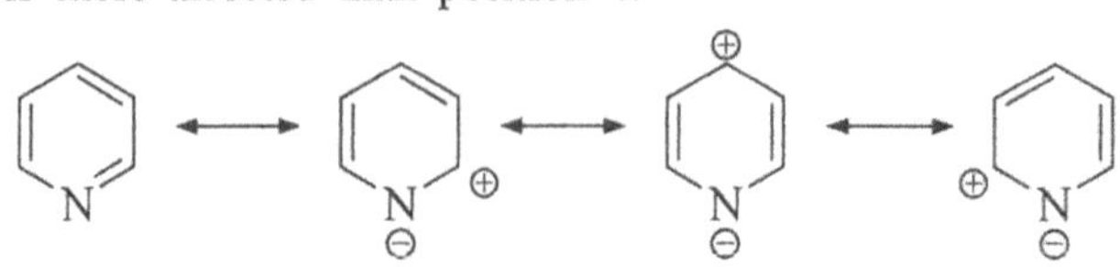

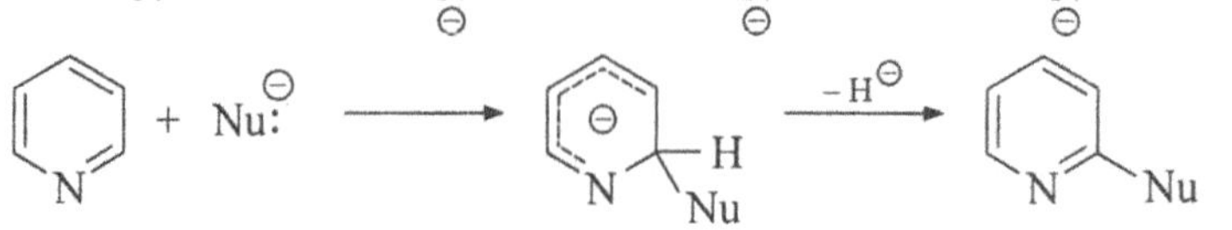

Some of the nucleophilic substitution reactions are given below:

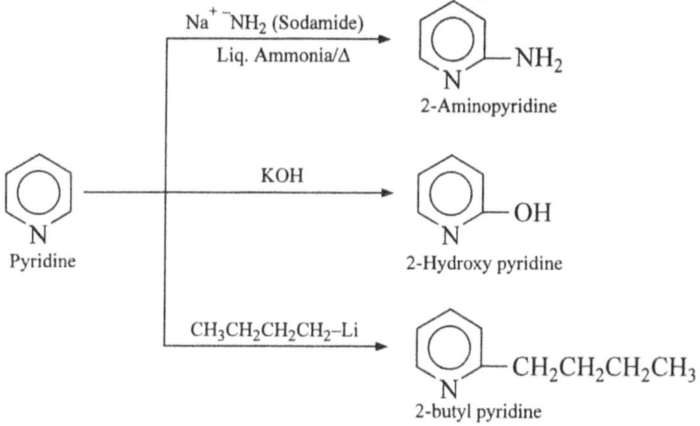

4. *Uses*

Pyridine is used

1. as a solvent
2. as a catalyst in many organic reactions
3. for denaturing alcohol
4. in the preparation of certain drugs

PRACTICE QUESTIONS

1. Describe the classification of heterocyclic compounds with suitable examples.
2. Give the resonating structures of furan and explain why 2-substitution in furan is favoured.
3. 'Furan behaves chemically as an aromatic compound, but in some ways it behaves as a 1 : 3 diene.' Justify this statement by giving all reactions.
4. Write a short note on Paal–Knorr synthesis.
5. Give the different methods of preparation and important reactions of pyrrole.
6. Give the method of preparation and four important reactions of thiazole.
7. Explain the aromatic character of furan, pyrrole and thiophene compounds.
8. What happens when
   (a) *n*-Butane is treated with sulphur at higher temperature.
   (b) Furan is treated with sulphur and sulphur trioxide.
   (c) Pyrrole is treated with H_2, Ni at 250°C.
   (d) Furan is treated with H_2, Ni at 50°C.
9. Write briefly the mechanism of electrophilic substitution reactions of pyridine.
10. Explain why pyridine and $NaNH_2$ give alpha amino pyridine.
11. Account for the following facts:
    (a) Thiophene is more aromatic in nature than furan.
    (b) Electrophilic substititution in naphthalene proceeds faster as 1-position as compared to that at 2 position.
    (c) Pyrrole, furan and thiophene do not contain any benzene ring still they are classed as aromatic compounds.
    (d) Pyridine is more basic than pyrrole.
    (e) The hydrogen in methylene group of diphenyl methane is acidic.
12. Explain the aromaticity of pyridine and give its nucleophilic and electrophilic substitution reactions.

13. Give explanation for the following:
    (a) Why pyridine is more basic
    (b) Why pyridine does not undergo Friedal–Crafts reaction
    (c) Compare the reactivity of pyrrole with pyridine
    (d) Furan acts as dienophile
14. What happens when pyridine is treated with
    (a) Sodamide
    (b) Phenylithium
    (c) Bromine
    (d) Nitric acid
15. Compare the aromaticities of pyrrole, furan, thiophene and pyridine.
16. Discuss the concept of aromaticity in heterocyclic compounds.
17. Discuss the chemistry of thiophene.
18. Give the different methods of preparation and important reactions of furan.
19. Compare the aromaticities of pyrrole, furan, thiophene and pyridine.
20. Give an account of the various reactions of thiophene.
21. Explain what happens when
    (a) Furfural treated with alcoholic potassium cyanide
    (b) Pyrrole is treated with chloroform in the presence of potassium hydroxide
    (c) Pyridine is heated with sodamide
    (d) Furan is heated with maleic anhydride
22. Account for the following statements:
    (a) Pyrrole is more acidic than pyrrolidine
    (b) Outline the preparation of:
        (i) Furan from furfural
        (ii) Thiophene from acetylene
23. What happens when pyridine is treated with
    (a) Bromine at 300°C
    (b) Sulphuric acid at 350°C
    (c) Acetylchloride in the presence of aluminium chloride
    (d) Heating with sodamide
24. Define and classify heterocyclic compounds with examples.
25. Explain how furan is aromatic. Compare any two reactions undergone by furan with that of benzene.
26. Indicate the preferred position of attack on pyridine by electrophilic reagents and give reasons.
27. What happens when
    (a) Furuyl alcohol is treated with methanolic HCl
    (b) Pyrrole is treated with boiling alkali and $CHCl_3$
    (c) Quinoline is treated with benzoylchloride in presence of alkali.
    (d) Pyridine–2,3-dicarboxylic acid heated strongly.
28. Compare the reactivity of benzene, thiophene, furan and pyrrole towards electrophilic substitution.
29. Give the name structure and use of compounds containing the following heterocycles.
    (a) Pyrrole (c) Imiadazole (d) Pyrazole.
30. Write the structure and indicate the numbering of the following heterocyclic systems. Give the structure and uses of two drugs containing each of these ring systems.
    (a) Pyridine (b) Thiophene
31. Discuss the chemistry of pyridine and draw the structural formulae of some pharmaceutically important compounds derived from this.

26

CARBOHYDRATES

26.1 INTRODUCTION

Carbohydrates play a vital role in daily life and are distributed in both plant and animal tissues. They are also known as saccharides (In Greek 'sakcharon' means sugar or sweetness) since many of the carbohydrates are of relatively small molecular weight and have sweet taste. Carbohydrates are the most abundant class of organic compounds found in living organisms. They originate as products of photosynthesis.

Carbohydrates are broadly defined as polyhydroxy aldehydes or ketones and their derivatives or the substances that yield one of these compounds on hydrolysis.

(i) Carbohydrates occur as food reserves in the storage organs of plants and in liver and muscles of animals.
(ii) They are widely distributed molecules in both plants and animals.
(iii) They are indispensable for living organisms, serving as skeletal structures in plants, insects and crustaceans.
(iv) They also serve to lubricate skeletal joints, to provide adhesion between cells and to confer biological specificity on the surface of animal cells.
(v) Ribose and deoxyribose sugars are integral part of ribonucleic acid (RNA) and deoxyribonucleic acid (DNA) respectively. The structural flexibility of these sugars is needed for storage and expression of genetic information.
(vi) Carbohydrates are also linked to many proteins and lipids. These molecules are known as glycoproteins and glycolipids respectively. These molecules perform very important and specific function in biological organisms. For example, human growth hormone is a glycoprotein.
(vii) Carbohydrates play a very important role in cell to cell communication.

26.2 CLASSIFICATION OF CARBOHYDRATES

Carbohydrates are usually classified into three groups:

1. ***Monosaccharides*** The monosaccharides are often called simple sugars. They possess a free aldehyde (— CHO) or keto (— C = O) group and two or more hydroxyl (— OH) groups. Monosaccharides are simple sugars and cannot be hydrolysed into smaller units. Their general formula is $C_n(H_2O)_n$ where *n* is the number of carbonations. The monosaccharides may be further subdivided depending upon the number of carbon atoms as:

(i) *Trioses* These monosaccharides contain three carbon atoms.

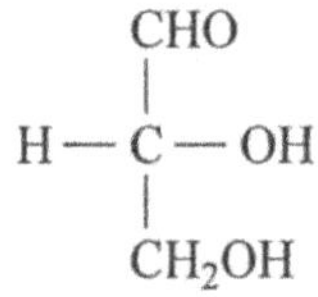

Glyceraldehyde
(Aldose)

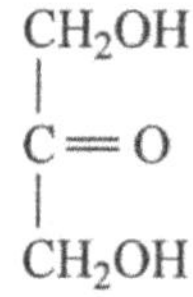

Dihydroxyacetone
(Ketose)

(ii) *Tetroses* Tetroses contain four carbon atoms.

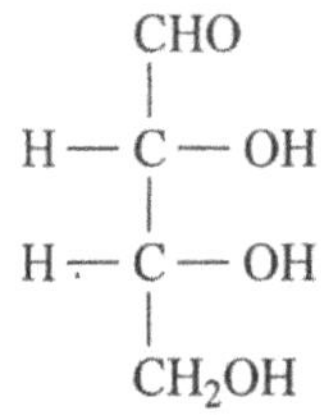

D-Erythrose
(Aldose)

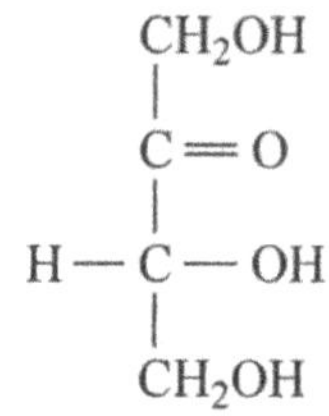

Erythrulose
(Ketose)

(iii) *Pentoses* Pentose monosaccharides contain five carbon atoms.

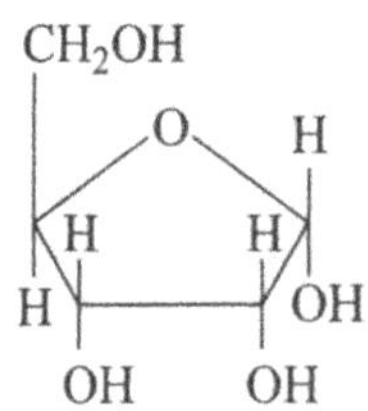

D-Ribose
(Aldose)

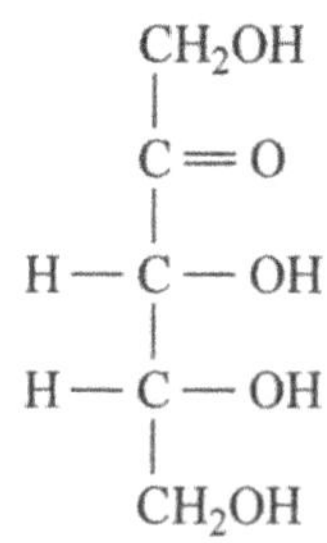

D(–)-Ribulose
(Ketose)

(iv) *Hexoses* Hexose monosaccharides contain six carbon atoms.

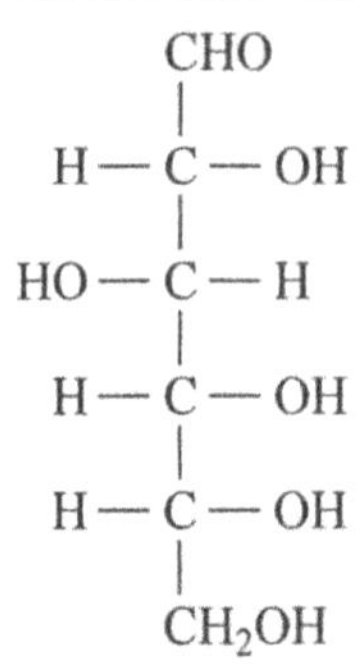

D(+)-Glucose
(Aldose)

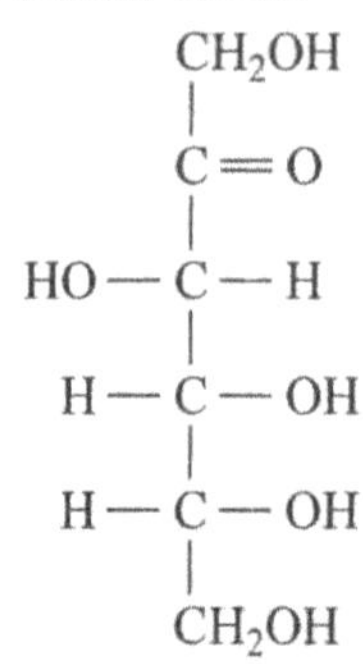

D(–)-Fructose
(Ketose)

2. ***Oligosaccharides*** Oligosaccharides yield 2 to 10 molecules of the same or different monosaccharides on hydrolysis. The general formula of oligosaccharides is $C_n(H_2O)_{n-1}$.

For example

Disaccharides – Sucrose, Maltose, Lactose
Trisaccharides – Rhamninose, Rattinose
Tetrasaccharides – Stachyose, Scorodose
Pentasaccharides – Vertiascose.

3. ***Polysaccharides*** Polysaccharides contain several monosaccharide molecules. They are further subdivided depending on type of monosaccharide molecules obtained by hydrolysis. They are

(i) *Homopolysaccharides* They yield only one type of monosaccharide molecules, e.g. starch, glycogen, cellulose, dextran.
(ii) *Heteropolysaccharides* They are made of more than one type of monosaccharides, e.g. hyaluronic acid, chondroitin.

26.3 GLUCOSE

1. Glucose is an important monosaccharide. It occurs in honey, ripe grapes and most of the sweet fruits.
2. Glucose is a colourless crystalline solid, highly soluble in water, sparingly soluble in alcohol and melts at 146°C.
3. The molecular weight determination shows that the molecular formula of glucose is $C_6H_{12}O_6$. In 1890, Bayer and Fitting proposed the following open-chain structure for glucose.

$$CH_2OH — CHOH — CHOH — CHOH — CHOH — CHO$$

Open chain structure of glucose

4. Baeyer's structure is associated with an aldehydic group and five hydroxyl groups which are attached to five different carbon atoms of carbon chain.
5. Later, Fischer proposed a projection formula for glucose to explain its stereoisomers (16 isomers). All the 16 isomers were identified. D(+)-Glucose is one of the 16 stereoisomers. Fischer designated the following configuration to D(+)-glucose.

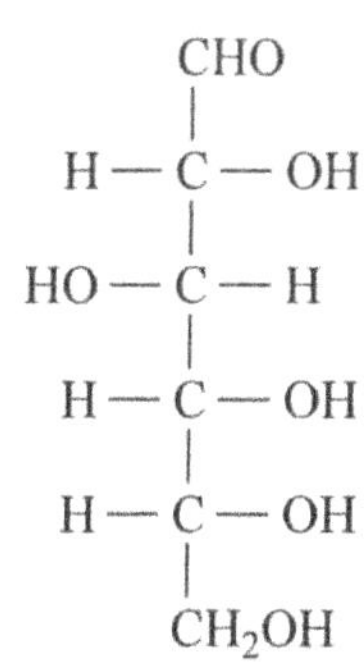

6. However, even Fischer formula failed to describe certain other properties of glucose. Hence, another method of representing the structure was searched for. The aldehyde or ketone group of a sugar can react with alcoholic hydroxyl groups of same molecule forming hemiacetals or hemiketals, respectively.

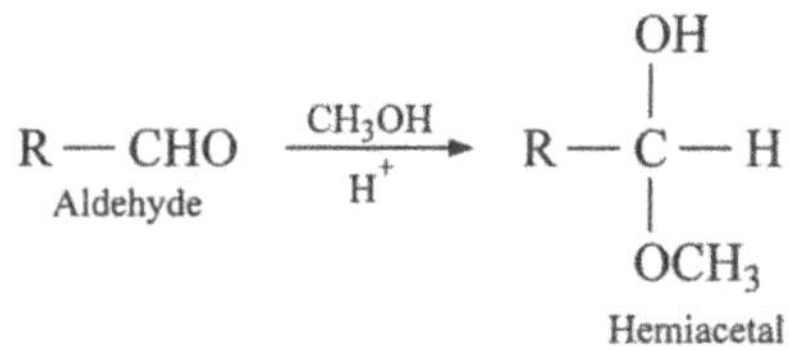

7. Sugar cyclisation normally leads to the formation of 6-membered rings, designated as pyranoses, or 5-membered rings, designated furanoses. The cyclisation creates an asymmetric carbon, the anomeric carbon, with two possible configurations designated alpha and beta.

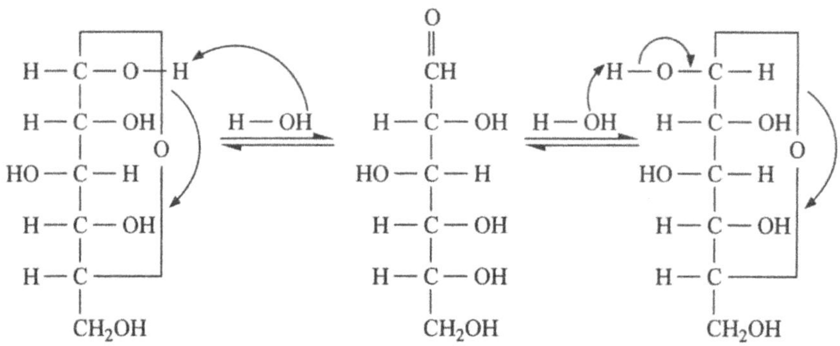

α-D(+)-Glucose D(+)-Glucose β-D(+)-Glucose

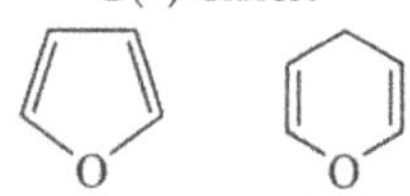

Furan Pyran

8. Two different crystalline forms of glucose were reported in 1895. Each of these gave all the characteristic reactions of glucose, and when dissolved in water equilibrated to the same mixture. This equilibration takes place over a period of minutes, and the change in optical activity that occurs is called mutarotation. These facts are summarised

α-D-Glucose		**equilibrated solution**		**β-D-Glucose**
$C_6H_{12}O_6$	$\xrightarrow[\leftarrow]{H_2O}$		$\xrightarrow[\leftarrow]{H_2O}$	$C_6H_{12}O_6$
M.p. = 146°		[α] = + 52.7°		M.p. = 150°
[α] = + 112°		36% α + 64% β		[α] = + 19°

9. According to Haworth the two glucopyranoses structures for glucose are represented as below:

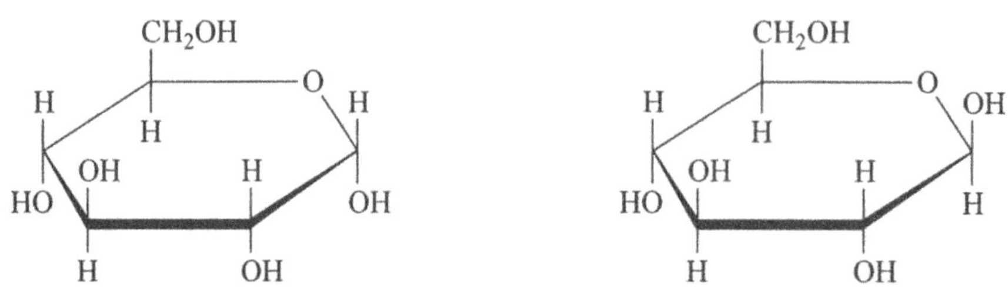

α-D(+)-Glucopyranose β-D(+)-Glucopyranose

26.4 SUCROSE OR SACCHAROSE (TABLE SUGAR, CANE SUGAR)

1. Sucrose is the common sugar of commerce and kitchen (hence, also called household sugar) and is widely distributed in all photosynthetic plants. It is the chief constituent of sugar cane and maple and is also present in pineapple and carrot.
2. Sucrose occurs in varying amounts in different parts of plant such as fruit seeds, flowers and roots. Nectar of flowers is particularly rich in sucrose. It is the raw material for honey. Sucrose is probably the only food constituent used in the crystalline form. It is derived commercially from either sugar cane or beet. In plants, it is formed by elimination of a molecule of water from glycoside hydroxyl groups of α-D-glucose and β-D-fructose.
3. Sucrose is in colourless crystalline form, soluble in water with a melting point 160°C. It is dextrorotatory and has a specific rotation of + 66.5°. It is by far the sweetest of the three common disaccharides (sucrose, lactose, maltose).
4. The molecular formula of sucrose is $C_{12}H_{22}O_{11}$.
5. Sucrose on hydrolysis with dilute acid or enzyme (invertase) yields a mixture of D(+)-glucose and D(–)-fructose in equal amounts. This indicates that sucrose is a disaccharide formed by the condensation of D(+)-glucose and D(–)-fructose.

$$\underset{\text{(+)-Sucrose}}{C_{12}H_{22}O_{11}} + H_2O \xrightarrow[\text{Enzyme hydrolysis (Maltase)}]{\text{Acid hydrolysis (or)}} \underset{\text{D(+)-Glucose}}{C_6H_{12}O_6} + \underset{\text{D(–)-Fructose}}{C_6H_{12}O_6}$$

6. X-ray studies affirms the linkage between two monosaccharide as α-glycosidic linkage and β-glycosidic linkage.
7. Hene sucrose is α-D-glucopyranosyl β-D-fructofuranoside or β-D-fructofuranosyl α-D-glucopyranoside.

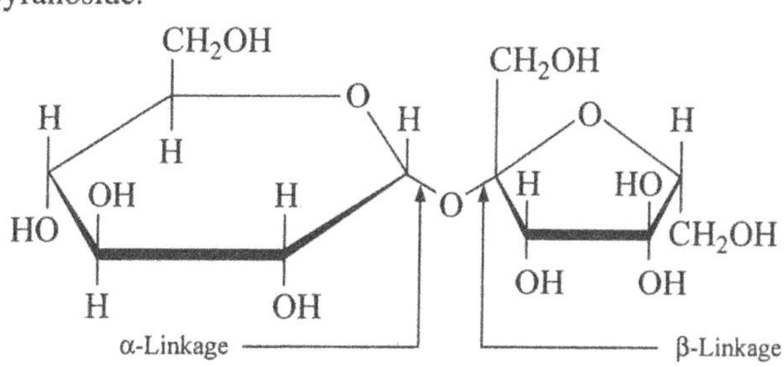

α-D-Glucoyranosyl-β-D-fructofuranoside

26.5 LACTOSE

1. Lactose is solely of animal origin and is found in the milk of mammals. Human milk contain about 6% while cow's milk about 4.5%. A minute quantity of lactose is also present in the milk as neuramin lactose. However, during pregnancy, it may be found in urine.
2. Lactose is also dextrorotatory. The α and β forms have a specific rotation of + 90° and + 35°, respectively. The equilibrium mixture has a specific rotation + 52.5°. It is less soluble in water and much less sweet than sucrose. Upon hydrolysis with the enzyme, lactase, it yields an equimolar mixture of glucose and galactose.

$$\underset{\text{(+)-Lactose}}{C_{12}H_{22}O_{11}} + H_2O \xrightarrow{\text{Dil. Acid of Lactase}} \underset{\text{D-Glucose}}{C_6H_{12}O_6} + \underset{\text{D-Galactose}}{C_6H_{12}O_6}$$

3. Lactose may be formed by elimination of a molecule of water from the glycosidic —OH group of β-D-galactose and the alcoholic —OH group on carbon atom 4 of D-glucose. D-Glucose unit is in hemiacetal form. D-Galactose unit is in full acetal form which develops a linkage through hydroxyl group on C-5.

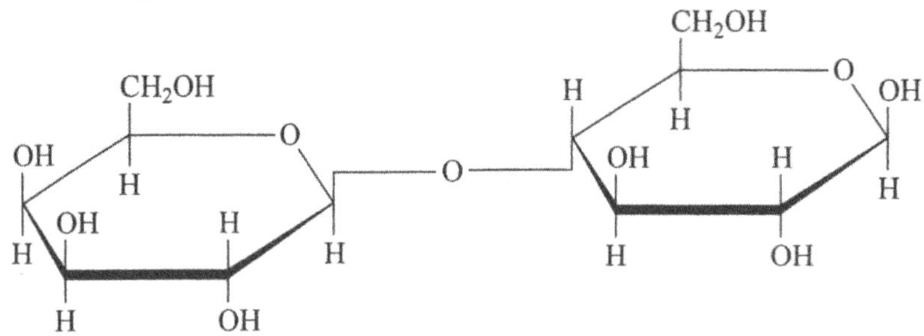

4-O-(β-D-Galactopyranosyl)-D-glucopyranose

26.6 STARCH

1. Starch is the most important reserve food material of the higher plants and is found in cereals, legumes, potatoes, and other vegetables. It is usually present inside the plant cells as compact insoluble grains which may be spherical, lens-shaped or ovoid with a distinctly layered structure.
2. Starch is a white soft amorphous powder and lacks sweetness. It is insoluble in water alcohol and ether at ordinary temperature. The microscopic form of the starch grains is used to characterise the source of starch. Starch is readily hydrolysed by mineral acid with the final production of glucose.
3. Natural starches consist of two components amylose (15–20%), a long unbranched straight chained component and amylopectin (80–85%), a branched chain polysaccharide.
   (i) *Amylose* Amylose has a molecular weight range of 10,000 to 50,000. It may be formed in plant cells by elimination of a molecule of water from glycosidic —OH group of one α-D-glucose molecule and alcoholic —OH group on carbon 4 of the adjacent α-D-glucose molecule. In amylose thus, an α-1,4-glucosidic linkage is seen.

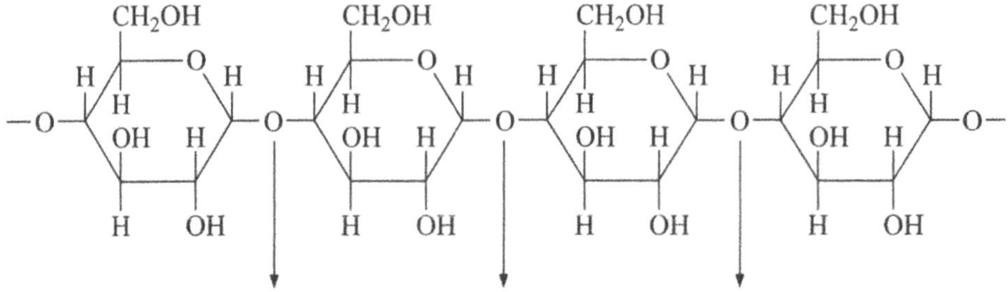

Structure of amylose

(ii) *Amylopectin or isomylose* Amylopectin, upon incomplete hydrolysis, yields the disaccharide isomaltose. It has a high molecular weight range of 50,000 to 1,000,000; thus indicating the presence of 300–5,500 glucose units per molecule. This possesses the same basic chain of α-1,4-glucoside linkage like that of amylose but has, in addition, many side chains attached to the basic chain by α-1,6 glucosides linkages.

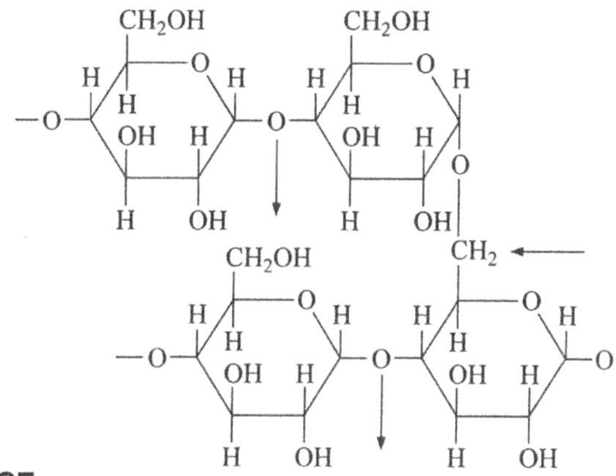

26.7 CELLULOSE

1. Cellulose is not only the abundant extracellular structural polysaccharide of the plant world but is also undoubtedly the most abundant of all biomolecules in the biosphere.
2. It is fibrous, tough, white solid, insoluble in water but soluble in ammonical cupric hydroxide solution (Schweitzer's reagent). It gives no colour with iodine and lacks sweetness.
3. The molecular weight of cellulose ranges between 2,00,000 and 20,00,000; thus corresponding to 1,250–12,500 glucose residues per molecule.
4. Cellulose may be formed by taking out a molecule of water from the glycosidic —OH group on carbon atom 1 of one β-D-glucose molecule and alcoholic —OH group on carbon atom 4 of the adjacent β-D-glucose molecule.
5. Thus, cellulose resembles amylose in structure except that the glucose units are linked together by β-1,4-glucose linkages. Cellulose may, henceforth, be regarded as an anhydride of β-1,4-glucoside linkages.

Cellulose a linear polyglucose joined by β-1-4 bonds

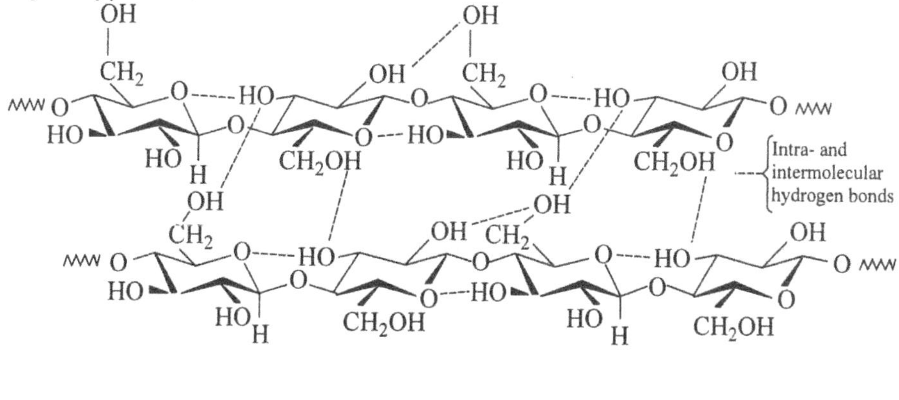

6. Because of the lack of chemical reactivity, the cellulose is of no nutritive value unlike starch. However, the same characteristics have made it useful as fibres for paper and cloth. In man, the cellulose does not get digested since the digestion system of man does not possess an enzyme capable of catalysing the cleavage of β-glucoside bonds. Hence, cellulose serves as an important source of 'bulk' in the diet. However, the ruminants (cattles, sheep, goats, camels, giraffes) and certain wood-eating insects are able to digest it because the microorganisms, present in their digestive tract, do possess such digesting enzymes.

PRACTICE QUESTIONS

1. What are carbohydrates? Classify carbohydrates by giving examples?
2. What is mutarotation? Explain with an example. Give its mechanism.
3. Give a brief account on:
   (a) Glucose
   (b) Sucrose
   (c) Lactose
4. Write the structural features and uses of:
   (a) Starch
   (b) Cellulose

27

PHASE-TRANSFER CATALYSIS

27.1 CATALYSIS

An acceleration of the rate of a process or reaction, brought about by a catalyst, usually present in a small managed quantities and unaffected at the end of the reaction. A catalyst permits reactions or processes to take place more effectively or under milder conditions than would otherwise be possible.

27.2 PHASE-TRANSFER CATALYSIS (PTC)

Phase-transfer catalysis (PTC) is a concept that relates to chemical reactions in which the reactants are in two separate phases, such as in liquid–liquid, solid–liquid, or gas–liquid reactions. In such cases, the rates and yields are very often limited by the slow transport of reactants from one phase to another. It was developed in the mid-1960s. Phase transfer catalysts were found to be instrumental in transporting the reactants, thus increasing considerably yields and rates and facilitating reactions that are otherwise not feasible or very difficult to carry out. PTC is used more and more as a means for facilitating otherwise slow reactions. It is being recognised as a useful tool to improve process efficiency, safety and reduce environmental impact of chemical industry.

For example, alkylhalides are immiscible with water while several nucleophiles they react with are water-soluble. A catalyst, such as a quaternary ammonium salt, can carry the nucleophile from the aqueous to organic phase.

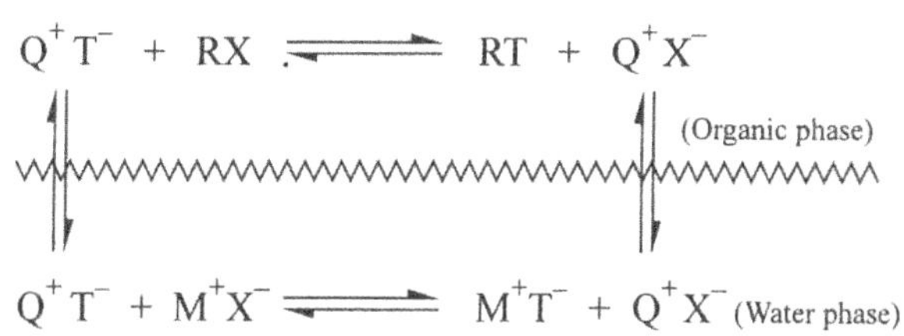

27.3 PHASE-TRANSFER CATALYSTS

Phase-transfer catalysts that participate in PTC process are cations that have finite solubility in both the organic and the aqueous phase. In practice, organic cations are commonly used for this purpose and most typically they are in the form of quaternary ammonium salts (e.g. tetra-*n*-butylammonium bromide and trimethylbenzylammonium hydroxide).

Quaternary ammonium and phosponium salts (with their unique capability to dissolve in both aqueous and organic liquids) are the catalysts of choice for most phase-transfer applications. The ammonium derivatives are the most commonly used (Table 27.1), but the phosphonium-based phase-transfer catalysts (Table 27.2) offer other interesting properties as well, like higher thermal stability. Other phase-transfer catalysts include crown ethers and polyethyleneglycols (PEG), as given in Tables 27.3 and Table 27.4.

Table 27.1 Ammonium Derivatives

1. Tetrabutylammonium bromide
2. Tetrabutylammonium chloride
3. Tetrabutylammonium hydrogen sulfate
4. Tetrabutylammonium iodide
5. Benzyltributylammonium chloride
6. Benzyltriethylammonium chloride
7. Hexadecyltrimethylammonium chloride solution
8. Hexadecyltrimethylammonium hydrogen sulphate
9. Methyltrioctylammonium chloride
10. Tetraethylammonium bromide
11. Tetraethylammonium chloride
12. Tetrahexylammonium hydrogen sulphate
13. Tetramethylammonium bromide

Table 27.2 Phosphonium-based PTC Reagents

1. Tributylhexadecylphosphonium bromide
2. Tetrabutylphosphonium chloride
3. Tetrabutylphosphonium bromide

Table 27.3 Crown Ethers and PEG-based PTC Reagents

1. 12-Crown-4
2. 1-Aza-15-crown-5
3. 15-Crown-5
4. Dibenzo-24-crown-8
5. 18-Crown-6
6. Dicyclohexano-24-crown-8
7. Tris[2-(2-mcthoxycthoxy)ethyl]amine
8. 4,7,13,16,21,24-Hexaoxa-1,10-diazabicyclo [8.8.8]hexacosane
9. Polyethyleneglycol 200

10. Polyethyleneglycol 400
11. Polyethyleneglycol 600
12. Polyethyleneglycol 1000

Table 27.4 PTC-based Reagents on Polymer Support

1. Tributylmethylammonium chloride polymer bound
2. Hexyltributylphosphonium bromide on polymer support
3. Tributylmethylphosphonium chloride polymer bound
4. Hexamethylphosphoramide polymer bound
5. Polyethyleneglycol 600 monobenzyl ether polymer bound
6. Polyethyleneglycol 750 monobenzyl monomethyl ether polymer bound

27.4 METHODOLOGY OF PHASE-TRANSFER CATALYSIS

The PTC methodology involves a substrate (which is soluble in the organic layer) and an anionic reagent (often a nucleophile), which is dissolved in the aqueous layer. The substrate and the anion are then brought together by a catalyst, which transports the anion into the organic phase where reaction can take place with the substrate.

Phase-transfer catalysts can often be used to accelerate the rate of reaction between two chemical species that are initially present in different phases. In the absence of a phase-transfer catalyst such processes often become slow because the two reacting species cannot easily cross the phase boundary in order to react. This can be illustrated by considering the two-phase epoxidation of alpha, beta-unsaturated ketones (Fig. 27.1). This process involves the epoxidation of an enone(1) using hypochlorite ion (ClO^-) in a liquid–liquid two-phase system. In the absence of a phase-transfer catalyst, the reaction is very slow (half-life >7days) because the enone is only soluble in the organic phase and sodium hypochlorite (NaOCl) is only soluble in the aqueous phase.

The driving force for PTC reactions is the potential difference, which is established by a partitioning phase transfer catalyst across the liquid–liquid interface in a two-phase system. This potential difference can also be established by electrochemical instrumentation and PTC reactions can be investigated using electrochemical experiments.

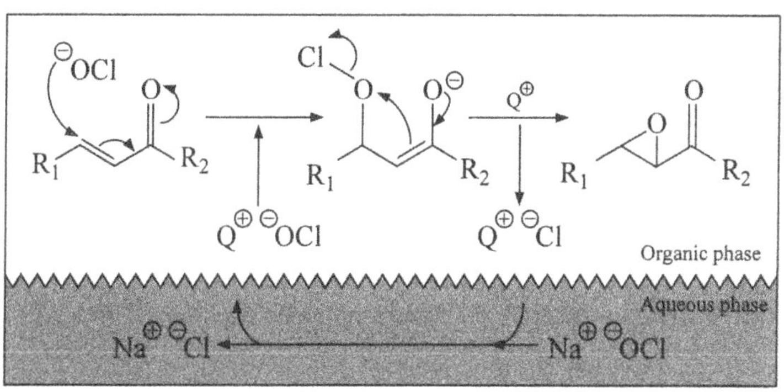

Fig. 27.1 PTC Reactions in a Two-phase System

The catalyst works by moving between the two liquid phases, collecting the hypochlorite ion from the aqueous phase, participating in the epoxidation reaction in the organic phase, and then delivering the by-product chloride ion back to the aqueous phase.

27.5 ADVANTAGES OF PHASE-TRANSFER CATALYSIS

There are several advantages of the phase-transfer catalysis system over single-phase systems, such as

- An increased reaction rate
- A lower reaction temperature
- Avoiding the need for expensive anhydrous or aprotic solvents
- The use of water together with an organic solvent as reaction medium
- Interestingly, some reactions are known to occur in a PTC-system that do not work in a normal system
- The chemical industry strives to increase efficiency, improve process safety and reduce environmental impact; phase-transfer catalysis (PTC) has, therefore, become recognised as a useful a tool for achieving these goals

27.6 FACTORS INFLUENCING PHASE-TRANSFER CATALYSIS

The following variables are required to be considered for phase-transfer catalytic reactions:

- The efficiency of phase-transfer catalysis is influenced by the bulkiness of the groups attached to the phase-transfer catalyst, its lipophilicity as well as that of its counter ion.
- Agitation is a crucial variable in phase-transfer catalytic reactions. Efficient product formation in phase-transfer catalysis needs powerful agitation. The influence of reaction conditions such as agitation parameters, temperature, reaction time, and catalysts can be explored on an automated synthesiser.
- Handling of viscous NaOH solution at low temperature is important for this reaction.

27.7 APPLICATIONS OF PHASE-TRANSFER CATALYSIS

Some examples of well-known phase-transfer catalysed reactions are given here.

1. ***Nucleophilic Substitution Reactions*** Reaction like halogenations and cyanations, e.g. chlorination, bromination: Cl_2/Br_2 addition over a double bond, P—OR → P—Cl, preparation of phosphonic acid dichlorides, R—OH → R—Cl, primary alcohols to alkylchlorides.

2. ***Esterification*** Synthesis of ethers, esters, thioethers, thioesters

3. ***Alkylation and Condensation Reactions*** Alkylation of cyanamide to dialkylcyanamides

4. ***Oxidations and Reductions*** $R\text{-}N_3 \longrightarrow R\text{-}NH_2$, $\text{Aryl-CO-H} \longrightarrow \text{Aryl-CH}_2\text{-OH}$

5. ***Elimination Reactions*** Dehydrohalogenation, dehalogenation, elimination leading to an epoxide.

6. ***Wittig and Wittig–Horner Reactions*** Synthesis of phosphines, synthesis of organo-silicon compounds.

Phase-transfer catalysis can be illustrated by some of the following reactions.

1. ***Diazo Transfer by Means of Phase-Transfer Catalysis*** Preparation of α-diazo carbonyl compounds via phase-transfer catalysis (Scheme 1): The 'diazo transfer reaction' between *p*-toluenesulphonyl azide and active methylene compounds is a useful synthetic method for the preparation of a-diazo carbonyl compounds. However, the reaction of di-*tert*-butyl malonate and *p*-toluenesulphonyl azide to form di-*tert*-butyl diazomalonate proceeded to the extent of only 47% after 4 weeks with the usual procedure. The present procedure, which utilises a two-phase medium and methyltri-*n*-octylammonium chloride (Aliquat 336) as phase-transfer catalyst, effects this same diazo transfer in 2 hours and has the additional advantage of avoiding the use of anhydrous solvents. This procedure has been employed for the preparation of diazoacetoacetates, diazoacetates, and diazomalonates.

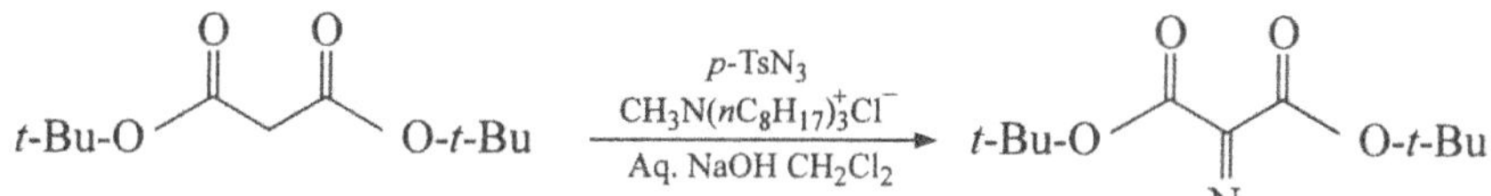

Scheme 1

2. ***Cinchoninium-based Catalysts and Asymmetric Phase-Transfer Catalysis (Scheme 2)*** In 1984, it was reported by researchers at Merck that substituted 2-phenyl-1-indanone systems could be enantioselectively alkylated in the presence of catalytic amounts of substituted N-benzylcinchoninium halides under PTC conditions (50% NaOH/toluene). Further investigations by O'Donnell and co-workers demonstrated that the cinchoninium system was also able to enantioselectively mediate the alkylation of glycine derivatives using PTC conditions (42–66% e.e.). One drawback of this method was that the glycine derivative should have been functionalised as a Schiff-base of benzophenone in order to give good levels of enantioselection, thus necessitating deprotection steps in order to obtain the free enantioenriched α-amino acid. O'Donnell et al. also proposed an ion-paired substrate-catalyst intermediate which determined the enantioselection.

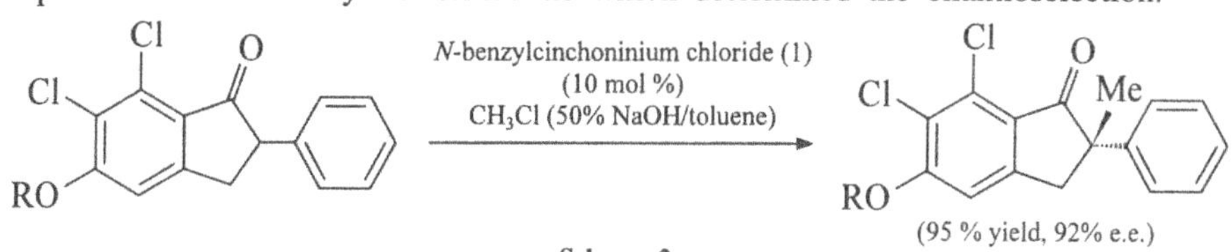

Scheme 2

3. ***Phase-Transfer Catalysis for GC Analysis*** In order to derivitise lipids for GC analysis, phase transfer catalysis procedure has been employed. This procedure involves two immiscible phases of liquid. The top (organic) phase consists of iso-octane containing pentafluorobenzyl bromide at a 20 (pm) picomolar concentration. Pentafluorobenzyl bromide is utilised due to its ability to increase the volatility of the fatty acid and the high electron affinity of fluorine, thus enabling GC/MS analysis.

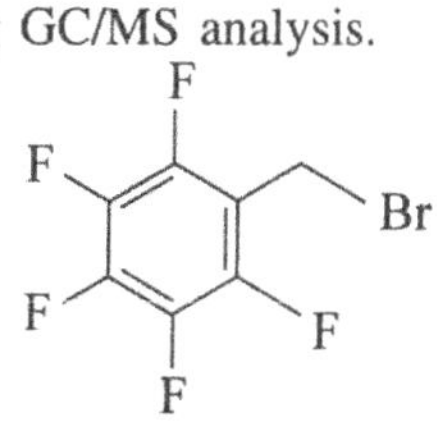

Pentafluorobenzyl bromide ($C_7H_2BrF_5$)
F.W. = 260.99

The bottom phase consists of water at a *pH* of about 8.0 due to the presence of small amount of sodium hydroxide (NaOH). Available fatty acids will settle at the interface of the two liquids such that the negatively charged portion will be located in the aqueous phase. In order to bring the fatty acid into the organic phase, allowing for reaction with the pentafluorobenzyl bromide, a phase transfer catalyst, 18-Crown-6 ether, will be added to the mixture at a 5 picomolar concentration.

4. ***Asymmetric Phase-Transfer Catalysis for the Epoxidation of Chalcone*** A study of asymmetric phase-transfer catalysis using chiral quaternary ammonium salts derived from optically pure amino alcohols is being performed (Scheme 3). The synthesis of these amino alcohols occur through the selective ring opening of (+) limonene epoxide as discovered by other researchers in Professor Singaram's lab.

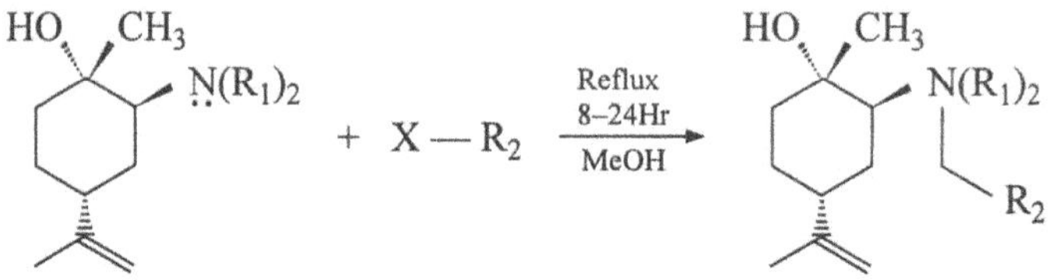

Scheme 3

SUGGESTED READINGS

Agarwal, O.P., *Advanced Practical Organic Chemistry,* Goel Publishing House, Meerut, 1999.

Agami, C., Meynier, F., Puchot, C., Guihem, J. and Pascard, C., *Tetrahedron* 1984, 40, 1031–1038.

Allen, C.F. and Kalm, M.J., *Organic Syntheses*, Wiley, New York, 1963; Collect. Vol. IV, p. 398.

Atkins, P.W., *Physical Chemistry*, Oxford University Press, Oxford, USA, 1998.

Badger, *Chemistry of Heterocyclic Compounds*, Academic Press, New York.

Bentley and Driver's *Textbook of Pharmaceutical Organic Chemistry*, L.M. Atherden, Oxford University Press, Delhi

Brady, James E., *General Chemistry*, Fifth Edition, John Wiley and Sons, New York, 1990.

Boyd, R.N., *Vogel's Textbook of Practical Organic Chemistry*, Revised by Brain S. Furniss, Antony J. Hannaford, Peter W.G. Smith, Austin R. Tatchell (Rev.), ELBS, Singapore, 1994.

Carey, Francis A. and Richard A. Sundberg, *Advanced Organic Chemistry*, Fourth Edition, Kluwer Academic /Plenum Publishers, New York, 2000.

Clayden, J., N. Greeves, S. Warren and P. Wothers, *Organic Chemistry*, Oxford University Press, Delhi, 2001.

Cornils, B., *Angew. Chem.*, 1997, 109, 2147; Int. Ed. Engl. 1997, 36, 2057.

Curran, D.P., *Angew. Chem.*, 1998, 110, 1230; Int. Ed. Engl. 1998, 37, 1174.

Eder, U., G. Sauer and R. Wiechert, *Angew. Chem. Int. Ed.* 1971, 10, 496-497.

Finar, I.L., *Organic Chemistry*, Vol. 1, ELBS, 6th Edition, 1994, Pearson Education Pvt. Ltd., New Delhi, 2003.

Fox, Marye anne James K. Whitesell, *Organic Chemistry*, Second Edition, Jones and Bartlett Publishers, UK, 1997.

Fries, S.L., E.S. Lewis and A.Weissberger, *Investigation of Rates and Mechanisms of Reactions*, Interscience Publishers, New York, 1961.

Foye, William O., *Principles of Medicinal Chemistry*, Third Edition, Varghese Publishers, Delhi, 1989.

Gladysz, J.A., *Science*, 1994, 266, 55.

Gosh, Sachin Kumar, *Advanced General Organic Chemistry*, Books and Allied (P) Ltd., Calcutta, 1998.

Gutsche, C., *The Chemistry of Carbonyl Compounds*, Prentice-Hall, Englewood Cliff, New Jersey.

Hajos, Z.G. and Parrish, D.R. *J. Org. Chem.* 1974, *39*, 1615–1621.

Hanson, James R., *Organic Synthetic Methods*, The Royal Society of Chemistry, Canada, 2002.
Hine, J. *Physical Organic Chemistry*, McGraw-Hill Book., New York.
Horvath, T. and J. Rabai, *Science* 1994, 266, 72.

Juaristi, E., David A. Lightner, Jerome E. Gurst, *Stereochemistry Chemistry of Organic Compounds*, Wiley, New York, 1994.

Kalsi, P.S., *Organic Reactions and Their Mechanisms*, New Age International (P) Ltd. New Delhi, 1998.
Kirmse, W., *Carbene Chemistry*, Second Edition, Academic Press, New York, 1971.
Knochel, P. et al., *Tetrahedron Lett.*, 2000, 41, 4343.
Koldobskii G.I., A.B. Zivich, V.A.Ostrovskii, Review, *J.Obsh.Khim.*, ***62***, No. 1 1992.
Koldobskii G.I., V.A. Ostrovskii, T.F. Osipova, Review, *Khim.Geterotsikl .Soedin.*, #11, 1443–1459 (1983).
Tewari, K.S., et al., *A Textbook of Organic Chemistry*, Vikas Publishing House Pvt. Ltd., New Delhi.

Lerner, R.A. and Barbas III, C.F. *J. Am. Chem. Soc.*, 2000, *122*, 2395–2396.
Lygo, B. and P.G. Wainwright, *Tetrahedron Lett.*, 1997, 38, 8595.
Lygo B. and P.G. Wainwright, *Tetrahedron Lett.*, 1998, 39, 1599.
Lygo, B., J. Crosby and J.A. Peterson, *Tetrahedron Lett.*, 1999, 40, 1385.
Lygo, B., *Tetrahedron Lett.*, 1999, 40, 1389.

Mahan, Bruce H., *University Chemistry*, Third Edition, Narosa Publishing House, New Delhi, 1998.
Mann and Saunders, B.C., *Practical Organic Chemistry*, Fourth Edition, Orient Longman, New Delhi, 1990.
March, Jerry, *Advanced Organic Chemistry*, Fourth Edition, John Wiley and Sons, Inc., USA, 1992.
McElvain, S.M., Kundiger, D., *Organic Syntheses*, Collect. VoI. III, Wiley, New York, 1955, p. 506.
Morrison, R.T. and R.N. Boyd, *Organic Chemistry*, Sixth Edition, Prentice-Hall of India Pvt. Ltd., New Delhi, 1992.

Nadendla, Rama Rao, *Priciples of Pharmaceutical Organic Chemistry (Heterocyclics and Natural Products)*, Vallabh Prakashan, Delhi.
Nogardi. M, *Stereochemistry: Concepts and Applications*, Pergamon Press, New York, 1981.
Nasipuri, D., *Stereochemistry Chemistry of Organic Compounds*, Second Edition, New Age International (P) Ltd, Publishers, New Delhi, 1994.

Osipova, T.F., G.I. Koldobskii and V.A.Ostrovskii, *Zh.Org.Khim.* ***20***, No. 11, 2468-73, 1984.

Paquette, L.A. and Barrett, J.H. *Organic Syntheses*, Wiley, Collect. VoI. V, New York, 1973, p. 467.
Patai Saul, *The Chemistry of Carbon-Carbon Triple Bond*, Edited by Saul Patai, John Wiley, New York, 1978.
Perkins, M. John, *Radical Chemistry: The fundamentals*, Oxford University Press, Oxford, USA, 2001.
Pharmacopoeia of India, Controller of Publications, Delhi, 1985.

Regitz, M., J. Hocker, and A. Liedhegener, *Org. Synth.*, Coll. Vol. 5, 179, 1973.

Remington, *The Science and Practice of Pharmacy*, Mack Publishing Company, twentieth Edition, 2000.

Robinson, Odom Holtzclaw, *General Chemistry*, Tenth Edition, AITBS Publishers and Distributors (Regd.), Delhi, 1998.

Sanyal, S.N., *Reactions, Rearrangements and Reagents*, Bharati Bhawan Publishers and Distributors, Patna.

Schaefer, J.P. and Endres, L., *Organic Syntheses*; Wiley, New York, 1973; Collect. Vol. V, p. 285.

Solomons, T.W.G. and C. Fryhle, *Book's Laws*, Seventh Edition, Wiley, New York, 2000.

Starks, C.M., *J. Am. Chem. Soc.*, 93, 195 (1971).

Studer and D.P. Curran, *Tetrahedron,* 53, 6681, 1997.

Studer, et al., *Science*, 275, 823, 1997.

Solomons, T.W.G., *Organic Chemistry*, John Wiley and Sons Inc., New York, 1996.

Saunders, W.H. and A. F. Cokerill, *Mechanisms of Elimination Reactions,* John Wiley and Sons Inc., New York, 1973.

The Pharmaceutical Codex, The Pharmaceutical Press.

Woodward, R. and T. Katz, *Tetrahedron*, 5, 70, 1959.

Yurkanis, Bruice Paula, *Organic Chemistry*, Prentice-Hall International Inc., Englewood Cliff, New Jewey.

Zard Samir Z., *Radical Reaction in Organic Synthesis*, Oxford University Press, London, 2003.

Index

D

O

S

www.ingramcontent.com/pod-product-compliance
Ingram Content Group UK Ltd.
Pitfield, Milton Keynes, MK11 3LW, UK
UKHW061534190726
13845UKWH00005B/97

9 789386 819628